"CODE RED"

THE DISASTER MANUAL

BY

Surgeon Commander (Dr) K C Sekhar, M.D. (Retd.)

Consultant Anesthesiologist

(Under the Aegis of Visakhapatnam City Branch of Indian Society of Anesthesiologists)

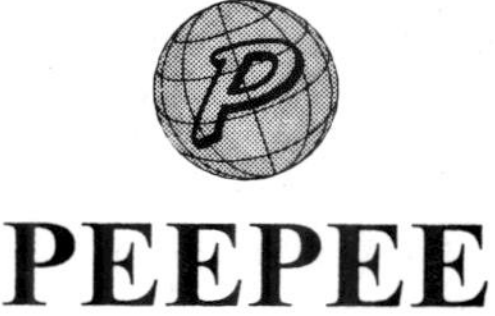

PEEPEE

PUBLISHERS AND DISTRIBUTORS (P) LTD.

"CODE RED" The Disaster Manual

Published by
Pawaninder P. Vij

Peepee Publishers and Distributors (P) Ltd.
Head Office:
160, Shakti Vihar, Pitam Pura
Delhi-110034 (India)

Correspondence Address:
7/31, First Floor, Ansari Road, Daryaganj
Post Box-7243, New Delhi-110002 (India)

Ph: 65195868, 23246245, 9811156083

e-mail: peepee160@yahoo.co.in

e-mail: peepee160@rediffmail.com

e-mail: peepee160@gmail.com

www.peepeepub.com

First Edition: **2011**

ISBN: 81-8445-063-X
978-81-8445-063-7

Printed at
Lordson, C-5/19, Rana Pratap Bagh, Delhi-110 007

FOREWORD

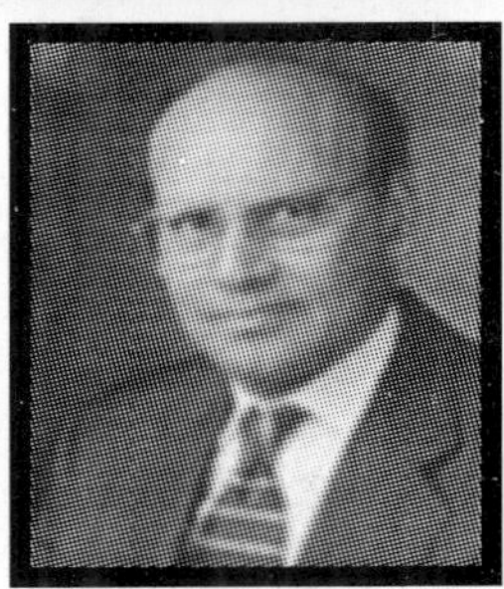

In the aftermath of a disaster, people are left with damaged or destroyed homes, no place to work, no transportation, and destroyed or lost property. Many families must also deal with the greatest tragedy of all – injured, missing or dead loved ones. The first step in disaster assistance is setting up care centers to provide for basic requirements of the victims – food, water, shelter and medical care. When the government declares a major disaster, special aid programs become available and victims can apply online or by phone for basic needs like housing, medical treatement and for rebuilding and repairing damaged property and infrastructure.

The **"CODE RED - The Disaster Manual"** composed by Dr KC Sekhar, Consultant Anesthesiologist at NRI General Hospital, Sangivalasa, Visakhapatnam is a commendable effort, providing a response and knowledge detabase for every known disaster situation imaginable. I am sure that the contents will prove immensely useful to administrators and technocrats alike, in handling and responding appropriately to various polytrauma situations and minimizing mortality and morbidity. Human life is precious and any effort to salvage lives deserves encouragement. I do hope that this book is well received and forms a basis for more effective disaster response in India and abroad.

(Dr. Neerukonda BR Prasad, M.D.)
Chairman Midwest Anesthesia Services
Christ Hospital and Medical Center, Chicago
Chairman and C.E.O., ANITS Engineering College
and NRI General Hospital, Visakhapatnam - 531162

FOREWORD

Disasters have adversely affected humans from the dawn of civilization. The lesson learnt is that nature cannot be ignored and mankind has no choice but to learn to coexist with its unpredictable behaviour.

There has been a dramatic rise in the skills and knowledge required to tackle modern day emergencies. Emergency management is now an important profession and it plays a critical role in protecting the social and economic stability of our communities. Citizens also look to their governments to provide them comprehensive safety and security. On the other side, the compounded effects of natural and man made catastrophes poses escalating threats to humankind and there is an urgent need to find solutions. I am of the opinion that a globally united strategy can provide concrete answers.

For any major disaster, a structured, previously rehearsed, multidisciplinary, proactive approach is a fundamental necessity. Outside help must be sought early and communication lines kept open to request relevant relief resources to save lives and contain collateral damage.

The subject is vast and technology is moving ahead at full throttle to preempt, contain or prevent catastrophes. The Code Red Manual attempts to give a bird's eyeview of the whole problem in a systematic and comprehensive manner. I am sure it will be well received by the entire community at all levels as it contains very useful and practical information.

Dr. T. Ravi Raju, M.D., D.M.
Director for Medical Education
Directorate of Medical Education
Government of Andhra Pradesh
Koti, Hyderabad - 500195

PREFACE

Simply put, any major disaster has calamitous consequences on life and property. Any endeavour to bring a semblance of coherence amidst the chaos needs collective, pre planned response and global support. Any attempt to tackle a devastation of that magnitude in-house, is not sensible. The best part is that you are not alone. All it takes is a timely alert and request for relief to mobilize world wide response. The relief requested must be specific to the situation otherwise you will end up holding redundant stores. Bi annual, planned, dedicated drills/simulations with honest debriefing sessions can afford good hindsight and ensure an appropriate response in real time disaster situations. High tech early warning systems, technology and tools, satellite communications and telemedicine have made a sea change in disaster response. The bottom line in tackling disasters is preparedness and effective mitigation. Nations the world over must concentrate on legislative action to prevent recurrence of events. War and terrorism are great tragedies and political dialogue is essential to prevent them. Political will is also necessary to tackle population explosion, mass education, housing, provision of safe water and sanitation, protection to the vulnerable sections of society and poverty alleviation. Community participation in disaster mitigation is a grass root level essentiality. First response has to be a quick and best response. This can only happen if one is prepared and well rehearsed.

The Disaster Manual attempts to address every possible aspect of Disaster Management and Medicine. Due to the fast paced progress in technology, updates of information is a core issue in today's world. Some chapters may become anachronistic in no time and I hope that newer editions of this manual will keep this manual contemporary and updated.

I have drawn considerably from my own personal experiences while serving on hospital ships in the Indian Navy as well as war like situation in Northern Sri Lanka and the aftermath of the supercyclones in Orissa. An anesthesiologist is trained to be an effective first responder and an efficient, level headed team leader in crisis situations. Improvisation is also an inherent attribute. Hence it should be quite natural that an anesthesiologist has taken the initiative to compile such a manual. I hope it is well received, informative and useful to technical personnel and the laity. Let us stay linked and ensure better responses to future calamities. Error analysis is vital to prevent recurrence and one has to be honest to discuss glitches and circumvent them in the future. Prepare in peacetime to prevail in wartime is a sensible motto. Let us be alert and prepared. Many lives will depend on it.

28 October 2010
Visakhapatnam

K C Sekhar
Author

atha kāle vyatikrānte mahatyati bhayaṅkare|
anāvṛṣṭi anuprāptā rājan dvādaśa vārṣikī|
tasyām dvādaśa-vārṣikyām anāvṛṣṭyām maharṣaya|
vṛtyartham pradravan rājan kṣudhārtā sarvato diśam
na vavarṣa sahasrākṣa pratilomoSbhavat guru|
jagāma dakṣinam mārgam somo vyāvṛtta-lakṣaṇa||
sarāmsi saritāścaiva kupā prasravṇāni ca|
hata-tviṣo na lakṣyante nisargāt daiva-kāritāt||
upa-śuṣka-jala-sthāyā vinivṛtta sabhā prapā|
nivṛtta-yajṇa-svādhyāyā nirvaṣaṭkāra-maṅgalā||
ucchinna-kṛṣi-gorakṣa nivṛtta-vipaṇāpaṇā|
nivṛtta-yūpa-sambhārā vipraṇaṣṭa-mahotsavā||
asthi-saṇcaya-saṅkirṇā mahābhūta-ravākulā|
śūnya-bhūyiṣṭha-nagarā dagdha-grāma-niveśanā||

(śānti .parvan139-141.12-20)

{Translation: After some time, a severe drought occurred for a period of twelve years. In that drought great sages affected by hunger and searching for sustenance, went in all directions. There was no rainfall and Jupiter was retrograde. The Moon went south being eclipsed. Lakes, rivers, wells and springs were without water were not seen due to nature's wrath. Reservoirs dried up, assemblies (of people) dissolved, and scholarly studies, sacrifices and celebrations were withdrawn. Agriculture, dairy, and commerce were given up. Empty cities and burnt down villages filled with the cries of goblins, became the collecting place of bones}

CONTENTS

1 Introduction

> "If you think about disaster you will get it. Brood about death and you hasten your demise. Think positively and masterfully, with confidence and faith, and life becomes more secure, more fraught with action, richer in achievement and experience."
>
> —*Swami Vivekananda*

Since the beginning of time, our fragile planet has suffered, and will continue to suffer from disasters, both natural and man-made. The disasters themselves may not be preventable, but the unnecessary toll of death and injuries can be mitigated. The word disaster **has its origin** (from Middle French désastre, from Old Italian disastro) from the Greek pejorative prefix dis- bad + aster star to signify a divine curse and, traditionally considered as an outcome of divine caprice or judgement. On the average, more than 16 disasters can be expected worldwide each year, with over 65% of natural disasters being either hydrological or meteorological phenomenon. The W.H.O. has recognized the need for international solidarity and co-operation to attenuate the impact of disasters and devoted its 1991 World Health Day theme, to "Should Disaster Strike—Be Prepared". The United Nations General Assembly in its resolution 44/236 dated 22 December 1989 declared the 1990s to be the decade for natural disaster reduction. This was prompted by their observation that the greatest numbers of disasters occurred in countries that were already most affected by poor health and economic conditions. With continued industrialization, population growth and environmental degradation, there is every reason to expect an increase in the frequency of such calamitous events over the coming decades.

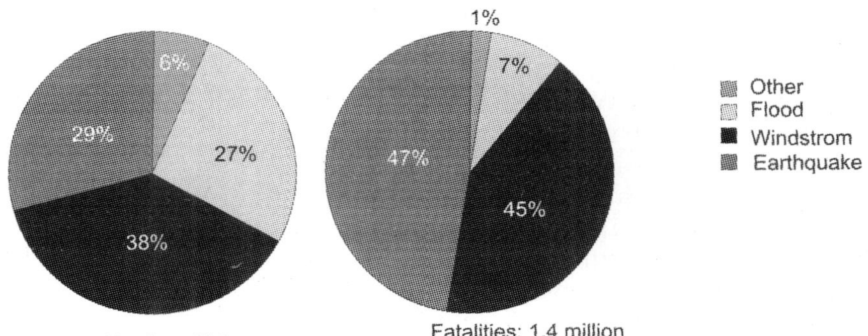

Fig. 1.1: Great natural catastrophes 1950-1999 (*Source:* Munich RE Group)

Deaths from natural disasters do not number amongst the world's top thirty causes of mortality, but represent a rising global trend in sharp contrast to premature mortality from most other causes. In the last half of the 20th century nearly 250 great natural disasters have occurred killing nearly 1.4 million people and **disrupting** the lives of many millions more. 90% of these natural disasters and 96% of deaths they have caused has occurred in the developing world (Fig. 1.1). The approximate number of people affected by disasters annually is at least 130 million and rapidly climbing. The most common disasters have been earthquakes, windstorms and floods. Between 500 to 700 natural catastrophes are recorded every year and associated with extremely large economic losses. During the last decade, the world's human population has increased by another one billion, most of it in the developing world. Millions have moved into cities desperate for work and crowded into substandard buildings in once marginal land. Nearly one billion people live in unplanned shantytowns. Deforestation to maximize farmlands or logging profits and other forms of environmental degradation have increased the vulnerability of human settlements to natural disasters.

Currently, trauma represents a significant portion of the world's morbidity and mortality. It ranks fifth among the leading causes of death after ischemic heart disease, cancer, stroke and respiratory disease. The subject of disaster is in focus at numerous scientific deliberations and various organizations like the World Academy of Emergency and Disaster Medicine (WAEDM), Global Health Disaster Network, Federal Emergency Management Agency (FEMA), Disaster Relief Org, European Centre Disaster Medicine (CEMEC) and Asian Disaster Preparedness Centre (ADPC, Manila). They have attempted to contribute and train professionals from all spheres in the areas of disaster response planning, management of mass casualties, disaster information systems and problems in maxi-catastrophe. Several private organizations also offer training in aspects of disaster management like Disaster Response Technologies Incorporated (USA). A mass of information is available over the internet. Google has nearly 24,600,000 sites on the topic of disaster. Useful sites like ODPEM (Office of Disaster Preparedness and Management), United Nations International Strategy for Disaster Reduction (IDNDR), Disaster Warning Network, Disaster Links, Natural Disaster Early Warning Network, CENAPRED (Centre for National Disaster Prevention), Commonwealth Disaster Management Agency, IRMC (Incident Response Management Concept), FEMA, International Centre for Disaster Mitigation Engineering, National Organization for Victim Assistance, Relief Web, Emergency Preparedness Information Exchange (EPIX), Doctors Without Borders (Medicine Sans Frontiers), Disaster Preparedness and Emergency Response Association (DERA), Life Safety Associates, International Rescue Corps, OXFAM, ResQNet, Survive Alive, Disaster Recovery Institute of Canada, Disaster News Network, Disaster Finder, ClubY2K, iPrepare, Virtual Survival, Secu Safe, World Homes, Angels of Mercy, GEMS (FEMAS Global Emergency Management System) etc. provide vital on-line information on various aspects of disaster management. The 'Stop Disasters' web site even hosts an interactive disaster simulation game. The government's blueprint for disaster response, the Contingency Action Plan for Natural Calamities and the National Fund for Calamity Relief are more reactive than proactive in their approach, with emphasis on provision of relief and not on disaster preparedness and mitigation (Fig. 1.2).

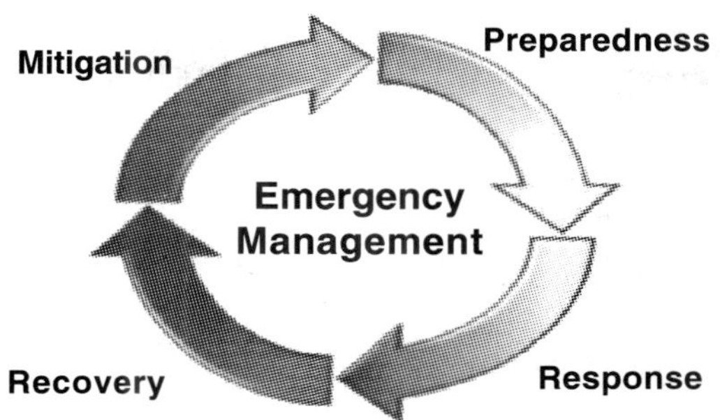

What is Disaster Management?

Preparedness -- activities prior to a disaster.
Examples: preparedness plans; emergency exercises/training; warning systems.

Response -- activities during a disaster.
Examples: public warning systems; emergency operations; search and rescue.

Recovery -- activities following a disaster.
Examples: temporary housing; claims processing and grants; long-term medical care and counseling.

Mitigation - activities that reduce the effects of disasters.
Examples: building codes and zoning; vulnerability analyses; public education.

Fig. 1.2

THE SEVEN CAUSAL FACTORS OF DISASTERS

Common causal factors play a large role in determining the severity and magnitude of a disaster. The following causal factors are general in nature, and not ranked. They may be more or less applicable to any given society and contributes to determining the vulnerability of a society to disasters.

1. **Poverty:** The single most important factor that increases the vulnerability of a people to disaster is poverty. An impoverished people who lack education, usually lack the economic and political

clout to cope with the hazards of their surroundings.

2. **Unregulated population growth:** Unregulated population growth can lead to settlements in hazardous areas susceptibility to disease, competition for scare resources, and civil strife. Disaster losses are significantly reduced when the people of any given society are organized with effective laws and controls to protect the population from potentially hazardous areas, access to public utilities, medical care, education, and economic resources. Vulnerability to disaster increases when a nation's capacity to govern does not consider the impact and trends in population growth in potentially hazardous areas. Even in the most benign climates rapid urbanization can create slowly evolving time bombs which could lead to disaster vulnerability.
3. **Rapid urbanization and migration:** Rapid population growth and migration are related to the major phenomenon of rapid urbanization. It is characterized by the rural poor or civilians in an area of conflict moving to metropolitan areas in search of economic opportunities and security. These massive numbers of urban poor increasingly find fewer options for availability of safe and desirable places to build their houses. Here again, competition for scarce resources, an inevitable consequence of rapid urbanization, can lead to man-made disasters. Many landslides or flooding disasters are closely linked to rapid and unchecked urbanization forcing low-income families to settle on the slopes of steep hillsides or ravines, or along the banks of flood-prone rivers. Many earthquake victims in urban areas have been impoverished families where the physical location vice the structure of their houses were hazardous, as evidenced by landslides onto the house or out from under it.
4. **Transitions in cultural practices.** Many of the inevitable changes that occur in all societies lead to an increase in societies' vulnerability to disasters. Obviously, all societies are in a continual state of transition and change. These transitions are often extremely disruptive and uneven, leaving gaps in social coping mechanisms and technology. These transitions include nomadic populations that become sedentary, rural people who move to urban areas, and both rural and urban people who move from one economic level to another. More broadly, these examples are typical of a shift from non-industrialized to industrializing societies.

   One example of the impact of these transitions is the introduction of new construction materials and building designs in a society that is accustomed to traditional designs and materials. This often results in new materials being used incorrectly. In disaster prone areas, inadequate use of new construction techniques contribute to houses unable to withstand earthquakes or wind storms.

   Compounding the problem is the formation of post disaster communities of survivors who find themselves without social support systems or networks to assist in relief and recovery. Traditional coping mechanisms may not exist in new settlements and the population becomes increasingly dependent on outside intervention for assistance.

   Conflicting cultural practices can also lead to civil conflict and strife. Examples include events leading to violence triggered by religious intolerance.

5. **Environmental degradation:** Many disasters are either caused or exacerbated by environmental degradation. Defores-tation leads to rapid rain runoff, which contributes to flooding. The destruction of mangrove swamps decreases the coastlines ability to resist tropical winds and storm surges. The creation of drought conditions—and the relative severity and length of time the drought lasts—is mainly a natural phenomena. Man-made contributions to drought conditions include: poor cropping patterns, overgrazing, the stripping of topsoil, poor conservation techniques, depletion of both the surface and subsurface water supply, and, to an extent, unchecked urbanization.

6. **Lack of awareness and information:** Disasters can also occur when people who are vulnerable, have not been educated on how to get out of harm's way or take protective measures at the inset of a disaster event. This ignorance may not necessarily be a function of poverty, but a lack of awareness of what measures can be taken to build safe structures on safe building sites. People may be unaware of safe evacuation routes and procedures. Others may be unaware on where to turn for assistance in times of acute distress. Nevertheless, this point should not be taken as a justification for ignoring the coping mechanisms of the majority of people affected by disasters. In most disaster-prone societies, there is a wealth of understanding about disaster threats and responses. This understanding should be incorporated into external assistance initiatives and planning.

7. **War and civil strife:** War and civil strife are regarded as hazards or extreme events that produce disasters. War and civil strife often cause the displacement of the population. The causal factors of war and civil strife include competition for scarce resources, religious or ethnic intolerance, and ideological differences. Many of these are also byproducts of the preceding six causal factors of disasters.

COMPOUND AND COMPLEX DISASTERS

Socio-political forces. Throughout many parts of the world one type of hazard can trigger a domino effect of disasters. For example, a drought may lead to a famine, which in turn leads to civil conflict resulting in a mass displacement of the population. Another example includes flooding which may force people to seek refuge across international borders upsetting the balance of needs and resources and weakening the ability of the government to receive the added population growth. This in turn may lead to civil strife and disorder.

Such compound hazards and disasters need not occur sequentially; they can occur simultaneously. Thus, people may become caught between contending forces in a civil war and also suffer from a major drought with limited means to grow food or to receive outside assistance.

In a growing number of countries, complex disasters are also becoming more evident. Essentially a complex disaster is a form of human-made emergency in which the causes of the emergency as well as the assistance to victims are bound by intense levels of political considerations. The single most prevalent political condition of a complex emergency is civil conflict, resulting in a collapse of political authority.

2 Definitions

> "The disaster that came to my people brought horror, Loving mothers boiled their own children for food Happiness has gone out of our lives; Grief has taken the place of our dance, We are sick at our very hearts And can hardly see through our tears."
>
> —*(From the Book of Lamentations, The Holy Bible, Destruction of Jerusalem, 586 B.C.)*

The International Trauma Foundation defines disaster as a destructive event which, relative to the resources available, causes many casualties, usually occurring within a short period of time, disrupting the structure and function of the community and requiring an extraordinary mobilization of emergency services, and activation and coordination of national and international agencies and resources.

The W.H.O. defines disaster as any occurrence that causes damage, economic disruption, loss of human life and deterioration in health and health services on a scale sufficient to warrant an extraordinary response from outside the community or area. A disaster is a sudden, calamitous event that causes serious disruption of the functioning of a community or a society causing widespread human, material, economic and/or environmental losses which exceed the ability of the affected community or society to cope using its own level of resources.

"Disaster is a situation or event, which overwhelms local capacity, necessitating a request to national or international level for external assistance" (definition considered in EM-DAT or International Emergency Disasters Data Base). Disaster is also described as an unforeseen and often sudden event that causes great damage, destruction and human suffering caused by a combination of hazards, vulnerability and inability to reduce the potential negative consequences of risk.

A disaster is the result of a vast ecological breakdown in the relation between humans and their environment, a serious sudden event (or slow as in the case of drought) on such a scale that the stricken community needs extraordinary efforts to cope with it, often with outside help or international aid. The important element in a disaster is a breakdown in society, which prevents the mounting of a planned response i.e. disorganization of normal functioning to the point of chaos.

Sudden onset disasters strike with no or little warning can be due to:

- Extreme weather events such as severe winds–hurricanes, tropical cyclones, tornadoes and temperate windstorms, heat waves, droughts, floods and storms.

- Geological events like earthquakes, volcanic eruptions.
- Geomorphic events like landslides and debris flows.
- Hydrological events like river and coastal floods and tsunamis.
- Extraterrestrial: Asteroid and comet impacts.

These events can overlap so that a volcanic eruption can trigger a landslide which can then crash into the sea and produce a tsunami that floods the opposite shoreline. Similarly heavy rainfall can cause floods and landslides.

OTHER DISASTER LINKED TERMS DEFINED AND EXPLAINED

Acceptable Risk

The level of loss a society or community considers acceptable given existing social, economic, political, cultural, technical and environmental conditions. In engineering terms, acceptable risk is also used to assess structural and non-structural measures undertaken to reduce possible damage at a level which does not harm people and property, according to codes or "accepted practice" based, among other issues, on a known probability of hazard.

Biological Hazard

Processes of organic origin or those conveyed by biological vectors, including exposure to pathogenic micro-organisms, toxins and bioactive substances, which may cause the loss of life or injury, property damage, social and economic disruption or environmental degradation. Examples of biological hazards: outbreaks of epidemic diseases, plant or animal contagion, insect plagues and extensive infestations.

Building Codes

Ordinances and regulations controlling the design, construction, materials, alteration and occupancy of any structure to insure human safety and welfare. Building codes include both technical and functional standards.

Capacity

A combination of all the strengths and resources available within a community, society or organization that can reduce the level of risk, or the effects of a disaster. Capacity may include physical, institutional, social or economic means as well as skilled personal or collective attributes such as leadership and management. Capacity may also be described as capability.

Capacity Building

Efforts aimed to develop human skills or societal infrastructures within a community or organization needed to reduce the level of risk. In extended understanding, capacity building also includes development of institutional, financial, political and other resources, such as technology at different levels and sectors of the society.

Climate Change

The climate of a place or region is changed if over an extended period (typically decades or longer) there is a statistically significant change in measurements of either the mean state or variability of the climate for that place or region. Changes in climate may be due to natural processes or to persistent anthropogenic changes in atmosphere or in land-use. Note that the definition of climate change used in the United Nations Framework Convention on Climate Change is more restricted, as it includes only those changes which are attributable directly or indirectly to human activity.

Coping Capacity

The means by which people or organizations use available resources and abilities to face adverse consequences that could lead to a disaster. In general, this involves managing resources, both in normal times as well as during crises or adverse conditions. The strengthening of coping capacities usually builds resilience to withstand the effects of natural and human-induced hazards.

Counter Measures

All measures taken to counter and reduce disaster risk. They most commonly refer to engineering (structural) measures but can also include non-structural measures and tools designed and employed to avoid or limit the adverse impact of natural hazards and related environmental and technological disasters.

Disaster Risk Management

The systematic process of using administrative decisions, organization, operational skills and capacities to implement policies, strategies and coping capacities of the society and communities to lessen the impacts of natural hazards and related environmental and technological disasters. This comprises all forms of activities, including structural and non-structural measures to avoid (prevention) or to limit (mitigation and preparedness) adverse effects of hazards.

Disaster Risk Reduction (Disaster Reduction)

The conceptual framework of elements considered with the possibilities to minimize vulnerabilities and disaster risks throughout a society, to avoid (prevention) or to limit (mitigation and preparedness) the adverse impacts of hazards, within the broad context of sustainable development. The disaster risk reduction framework is composed of the following fields of action:

- Risk awareness and assessment including hazard analysis and vulnerability/capacity analysis.
- Knowledge development including education, training, research and information.
- Public commitment and institutional frameworks, including organisational, policy, legislation and community action.
- Application of measures including environmental management, land-use and urban planning, protection of critical facilities, application of science and technology, partnership and networking, and financial instruments.
- Early warning systems including forecasting, dissemination of warnings, preparedness measures and reaction capacities.

Early Warning

The provision of timely and effective information, through identified institutions, that allows individuals exposed to a hazard to take action to avoid or reduce their risk and prepare for effective response. Early warning systems include a chain of concerns, namely: understanding and mapping the hazard; monitoring and forecasting impending events; processing and disseminating understandable warnings to political authorities and the population, and undertaking appropriate and timely actions in response to the warnings.

Ecosystem

A complex set of relationships of living organisms functioning as a unit and interacting with their physical environment. The boundaries of what could be called an ecosystem are somewhat arbitrary, depending on the focus of interest or study. Thus the extent of an ecosystem may range from very small spatial scales to, ultimately, the entire Earth.

EL NIÑO—SOUTHERN OSCILLATION (ENSO)

A complex interaction of the tropical Pacific Ocean and the global atmosphere that results in irregularly occurring episodes of changed ocean and weather patterns in many parts of the world, often with significant impacts, such as altered marine habitats, rainfall changes, floods, droughts, and changes in storm patterns. The El Niño part of ENSO refers to the well-above-average ocean temperatures along the coasts of Ecuador, Peru and northern Chile and across the eastern equatorial Pacific Ocean, while the Southern Oscillation refers to the associated global patterns of changed atmospheric pressure and rainfall. La Niña is approximately the opposite condition to El Niño. Each El Niño or La Niña episode usually lasts for several seasons.

Emergency Management

The organization and management of resources and responsibilities for dealing with all aspects of emergencies, in particularly preparedness, response and rehabilitation. Emergency management involves plans, structures and arrangements established to engage the normal endeavours of government, voluntary and private agencies in a comprehensive and coordinated way to respond to the whole spectrum of emergency needs. This is also known as disaster management.

Disaster management is the discipline of dealing with and avoiding risks and implies the field and hospital management of casualties and their transportation arrangements. It is a discipline that involves preparing, supporting, and rebuilding society when natural or human-made disasters occur. Emergency management is the continuous process by which all individuals, groups, and communities manage hazards in an effort to avoid or ameliorate the impact of disasters resulting from the hazards.

Environmental Impact Assessment (EIA)

Studies undertaken in order to assess the effect on a specified environment of the introduction of any new factor, which may upset the current ecological balance. EIA is a policy making tool that serves to provide evidence and analysis of environmental impacts of activities from conception to decision-making. It is utilised extensively in national programming and for international development assistance projects. An EIA must include a detailed risk assessment and provide alternatives solutions or options.

Environmental Degradation

The reduction of the capacity of the environment to meet social and ecological objectives and needs. Potential effects are varied and may contribute to an increase in vulnerability and the frequency and intensity of natural hazards. Some examples: land degradation, deforestation, desertification, wildland fires, loss of biodiversity, land, water and air pollution, climate change, sea level rise and ozone depletion.

Forecast

Definite statement or statistical estimate of the occurrence of a future event.

Geological Hazard

Natural earth processes or phenomena that may cause the loss of life or injury, property damage, social and economic disruption or environmental degradation. Geological hazard includes internal earth processes or tectonic origin, such as earthquakes, geological fault activity, tsunamis, volcanic activity and emissions as well as external processes such as mass movements: landslides, rockslides, rock falls or avalanches, surfaces collapses, expansive soils and debris or mud flows. Geological hazards can be single, sequential or combined in their origin and effects.

Geographic Information Systems (GIS)

Analysis that combine relational databases with spatial interpretation and outputs often in form of maps. A more elaborate definition is that of computer programmes for capturing, storing, checking, integrating, analysing and displaying data about the earth that is spatially referenced. Geographical information systems are increasingly being utilised for hazard and vulnerability mapping and analysis, as well as for the application of disaster risk management measures.

Greenhouse Gas (GHG)

A gas, such as water vapour, carbon dioxide, methane, chlorofluorocarbons (CFCs) and hydrochlorofluorocarbons (HCFCs), that absorbs and re-emits infrared radiation, warming the earth's surface and contributing to climate change (UNEP, 1998).

Hazard

A potentially damaging physical event, phenomenon or human activity that may cause the loss of life or injury, property damage, social and economic disruption or environmental degradation. Hazards can include latent conditions that may represent future threats and can have different origins: natural (geological, hydrometeorological and biological) or induced by human processes (environmental degradation and technological hazards). Hazards can be single, sequential or combined in their origin and effects. Each hazard is characterised by its location, intensity, frequency and probability.

Hazard Analysis

Identification, studies and monitoring of any hazard to determine its potential, origin, characteristics and behaviour.

Hydrometeorological Hazards

Natural processes or phenomena of atmospheric, hydrological or oceanographic nature, which may cause the loss of life or injury, property damage, social and economic disruption or environmental degradation. Hydrometeorological hazards include: floods, debris and mud floods; tropical cyclones, storm surges, thunder/hailstorms, rain and wind storms, blizzards and other severe storms; drought, desertification, wildland fires, temperature extremes, sand or dust storms; permafrost and snow or ice avalanches. Hydrometeorological hazards can be single, sequential or combined in their origin and effects.

LA NIÑA (SEE EL NIÑO—SOUTHERN OSCILLATION)

Land-use Planning

Branch of physical and socio-economic planning that determines the means and assesses the values or limitations of various options in which land is to be utilized, with the corresponding effects on different segments of the population or interests of a community taken into account in resulting decisions. Land-use planning involves studies and mapping, analysis of environmental and hazard data, formulation of alternative land-use decisions and design of a long-range plan for different geographical and administrative scales. Land-use planning can help to mitigate disasters and reduce risks by discouraging high-density settlements and construction of key installations in hazard-prone areas, control of population density and expansion, and in the siting of service routes for transport, power, water, sewage and other critical facilities.

Mitigation

Structural and non-structural measures undertaken to limit the adverse impact of natural hazards, environmental degradation and technological hazards. Mitigation implies efforts to prevent hazards from developing into disasters altogether, or to reduce the effects of disasters when they occur. The mitigation phase differs from the other phases because it focuses on long-term measures for reducing or eliminating risk. The implementation of mitigation strategies can be considered a part of the recovery process if applied after a disaster occurs. However, even if applied as part of recovery efforts, actions that reduce or eliminate risk over time are still considered mitigation efforts.

Natural Hazards

Natural processes or phenomena occurring in the biosphere that may constitute a damaging event. Natural hazards can be classified by origin namely: geological, hydro-meteorological or biological. Hazardous events can vary in magnitude or intensity, frequency, duration, area of extent, speed of onset, spatial dispersion and temporal spacing.

Preparedness

Activities and measures taken in advance to ensure effective response to the impact of hazards, including the issuance of timely and effective early warnings and the temporary evacuation of people and property from threatened locations or simply a process that entails activities designed to increase control in response to disasters.

Prevention

Activities to provide outright avoidance of the adverse impact of hazards and means to minimize related environmental, technological and biological disasters. Depending on social and technical feasibility and cost/ benefit considerations, investing in preventive measures is justified in areas frequently affected by disasters. In the context of public awareness and education, related to disaster risk reduction changing attitudes and behaviour contribute to promoting a "culture of prevention".

Public Awareness

The processes of informing the general population, increasing levels of consciousness about risks and how people can act to reduce their exposure to hazards. This is particularly important for public officials in fulfilling their responsibilities to save lives and property in the event of a disaster. Public awareness activities foster changes in behaviour leading towards a culture of risk reduction. This involves public information, dissemination, education, radio or television broadcasts, use of printed media, as well as, the establishment of information centres and networks and community and participation actions.

Public Information

Information, facts and knowledge provided or learned as a result of research or study, available to be disseminated to the public.

Recovery

Decisions and actions taken after a disaster with a view to restoring or improving the pre-disaster living conditions of the stricken community, while encouraging and facilitating necessary adjustments to reduce disaster risk. Recovery (rehabilitation and reconstruction) affords an opportunity to develop and apply disaster risk reduction measures.

Relief/Response

The provision of assistance or intervention during or immediately after a disaster to meet the life preservation and basic subsistence needs of those people affected. It can be of an immediate, short-term, or protracted duration.

Resilience/Resilient

The capacity of a system, community or society potentially exposed to hazards to adapt, by resisting or changing in order to reach and maintain an acceptable level of functioning and structure. This is determined by the degree to which the social system is capable of organizing itself to increase its capacity for learning from past disasters for better future protection and to improve risk reduction measures.

Retrofitting (or Upgrading)

Reinforcement of structures to become more resistant and resilient to the forces of natural hazards. Retrofitting involves consideration of changes in the mass, stiffness, damping, load path and ductility of materials, as well as radical changes such as the introduction of energy absorbing dampers and base isolation systems. Examples of retrofitting includes the consideration of wind loading to strengthen and minimize the wind force, or in earthquake prone areas the strengthening of structures.

Risk

The probability of harmful consequences, or expected losses (deaths, injuries, property, livelihoods, economic activity disrupted or environment damaged) resulting from interactions between natural or human-induced hazards and vulnerable conditions. Conventionally risk is expressed by the notation Risk = Hazards × Vulnerability. Some disciplines also include the concept of exposure to refer particularly to the physical aspects of vulnerability. Beyond expressing a possibility of physical harm, it is crucial to recognize that risks are inherent or can be created or exist within social systems. It is important to consider the social contexts in which risks occur and that people therefore do not necessarily share the same perceptions of risk and their underlying causes.

Risk Assessment/Analysis

A methodology to determine the nature and extent of risk by analysing potential hazards and evaluating existing conditions of vulnerability that could pose a potential threat or harm to people, property, livelihoods and the environment on which they depend. The process of conducting a risk assessment is based on a review of both the technical features of hazards such as their location, intensity, frequency and probability; and also the analysis of the physical, social, economic and environmental dimensions of vulnerability and exposure, while taking particular account of the coping capabilities pertinent to the risk scenarios.

Structural/Non-structural Measures

Structural measures refer to any physical construction to reduce or avoid possible impacts of hazards, which include engineering measures and construction of hazard-resistant and protective structures and infrastructure. Non-structural measures refer to policies, awareness, knowledge development, public commitment, and methods and operating practices, including participatory mechanisms and the provision of information, which can reduce risk and related impacts.

Sustainable Development

Development that meets the needs of the present without compromising the ability of future generations to meet their own needs. It contains within it two key concepts: the concept of "needs", in particular the essential needs of the world's poor, to which overriding priority should be given; and the idea of limitations imposed by the state of technology and social organization on the environment's ability to meet present and the future needs. Sustainable development is based on socio-cultural development, political stability and decorum, economic growth and ecosystem protection, which all relate to disaster risk reduction.

Technological Hazards

Danger originating from technological or industrial accidents, dangerous procedures, infrastructure failures or certain human activities, which may cause the loss of life or injury, property damage, social and economic disruption or environmental degradation. Some examples: industrial pollution, nuclear activities and radioactivity, toxic wastes, dam failures, transport, industrial or technological accidents (explosions, fires, spills).

Vulnerability

The conditions determined by physical, social, economic, and environmental factors or processes, which increase the susceptibility of a community to the impact of hazards. For positive factors, which increase the ability of people to cope with hazards, see definition of capacity.

Wildland Fire

Any fire occurring in vegetation areas regardless of ignition sources, damages or benefits.

3 Historical Aspects

> "It is during the periods of apparent disaster, during the sufferings of whole generations, that the greatest improvement in human character has been effected."
>
> —*Sir Archibald Alison*

It is a fact that medical personnel are intimately concerned with disasters. The onset of a disaster presents major problems of response, management and planning in addition to the purely medical problems concerning the treatment of victims. There are very compelling reasons for focusing medical attention upon the period following a disaster, as the prospects of recovery for a victim depends on two key factors— the length of time before the patient receives medical attention (minimum scene time) and the competence of the initial treatment by medical personnel. The statistics on wartime medicine for the past 20 years demonstrates time and again that the survival rate of a victim depends on the time interval without treatment. It is, therefore, quite imperative that early rescue and evacuation of disaster victims with aggressive and expert prehospital care followed by specialized first line treatment at a verified trauma centre is ensured.

Disaster Medicine has been a recognized specialty in France since 1976 and Dr Bernard Nemitz of Amiens, France founded the International Society of Disaster Medicine the same year. In 1981, Dr Pierre Huguenard of Paris initiated a university diploma course in the specialty. In 1985 the European Centre Disaster Medicine (CEMEC) was established in Italy and an annual congress of the World Accident, Emergency and Disaster Medicine (WAEDM) is held to discuss aspects of disaster response planning, information systems, international aid and handling of mass casualty situations. In the U.S.A., the Disaster Relief Organization involving the CNN, IBM Interactive and American Red Cross as well as the Federal Emergency Management Agency (FEMA) provides useful guidelines, updates and on line information during all disaster situations. In France, an anesthesiologist is in charge of ambulances of the Service d'Aide Medicale Urgents (SAMU) while in West Germany, a majority of ambulance and helicopter physicians are anesthesiologists. The International Trauma Anesthesia and Critical Care Society (ITACCS) is a professional society that endeavors to improve trauma management. The Level One Trauma Anesthesia Simulation (LOTAS) project at the University of Maryland uses task analyses, decision trees, algorithms and video analyses of actual trauma patient management to produce a realistic computer simulation for teaching resuscitation and trauma management at all levels. The science aims at improving disaster preparedness by bringing the right technology in a timely, coordinated and effective manner to provide relief, rehabilitation and reconstruction in the wake of disasters worldwide. The syllabus targets aspects of triage, advanced life support, treatment protocols of mass casualties, specific problems of nuclear, chemical and biological disasters, health and psychological aspects of victims and displaced persons. In management aspects, it imparts knowledge about the risks and prevention of disasters (epidemiology), disaster management, evacuation of large populations and aspects of communications, command and coordination and also legislative aspects and media handling. Theoretical and practical exercises are conducted and vital aspects of public health emphasized. Legal issues are included. As an example, the Bavarian Disaster Protection Law conveys special powers to disaster control authorities and hospital administrators to handle mass casualty situations. Owners of installations with a special hazard potential, could be brought to bear the costs of both preventive measures and potential payment of damages in an eventuality, especially relevant in the wake of the Bhopal gas tragedy. Photo-documentation on admission of many sick and injured is encouraged to enable legal decisions on accountability and compensation to be made without delay and prejudice.

4 Classification of Disasters

"Noble souls through dust and heat, rise from disaster and defeat the stronger."

—*Henry Wadsworth Longfellow*

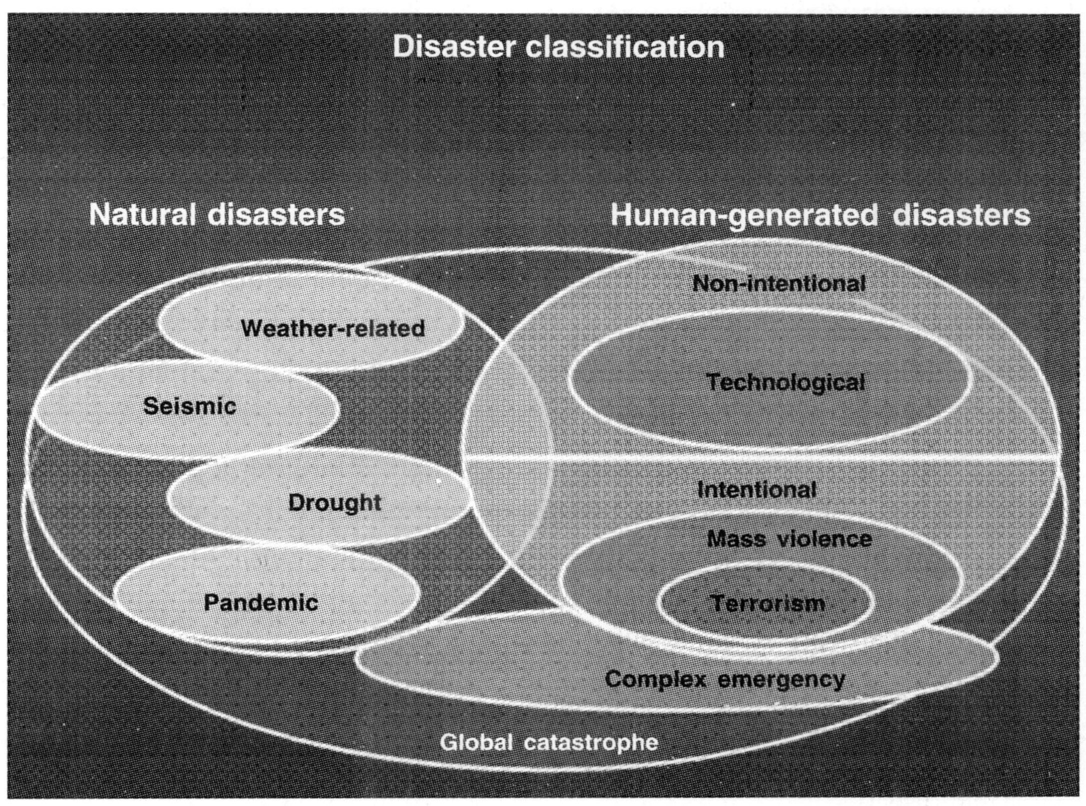

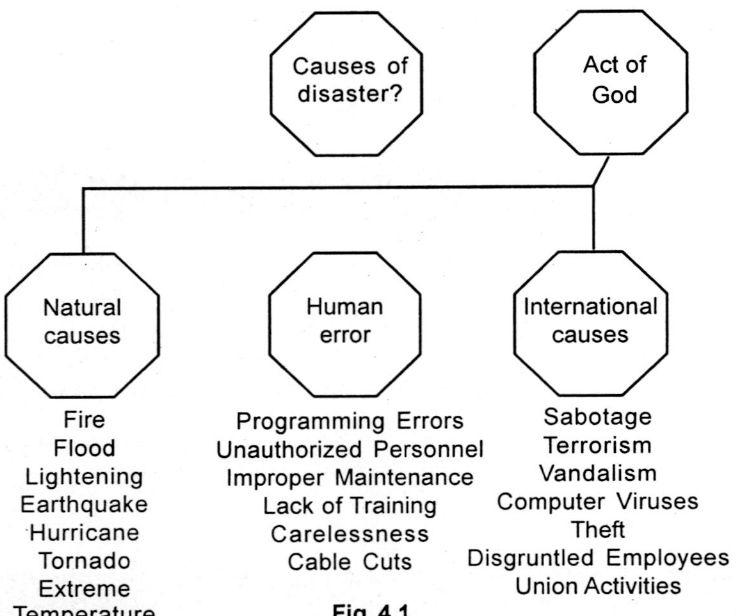

Fig. 4.1

1. *By effect:*
   A. Simple: Where the structure of the community remains intact.
   B. Compound : Where the structure of the community is disrupted.
2. *By cause:*
   A. Natural:
      a. Natural phenomena beneath the earth's surface. Earthquakes, tsunamis and volcanic eruptions.
      b. Natural phenomena of complex physical origin at the earths surface Landslides and avalanches.
      c. Meteorological/Hydrological phenomena—Windstorms (cyclones, typhoons and hurricanes), tornadoes, hailstorms/snowstorms, sea surges, floods, droughts, famines and maritime disasters.
      d. Biological phenomena: Locust swarms and epidemics of communicable diseases.
   B. Artificial or man-made
      a. Caused by warfare:
         i. Conventional warfare, including sieges and blockade.
         ii. Non-conventional warfare–Nuclear, biological, chemical.
      a. Caused by accidents:
         i. Vehicular (planes, trains, ships, automobiles).
         ii. Drowning
         iii. Collapse of buildings or structures.
         iv. Explosions.
         v. Fires.
         vi. Biological.
         vii. Chemical, including poisoning by pesticides and/or pollution.

Another Classification of Natural Disasters

Extreme weather events: Severe winds-hurricanes, tropical cyclones, tornadoes, temperate windstorms.

Geological events: Earthquakes, volcanic eruptions.

Geomorphic events: Landslides, debris flows.

Hydrological events: River and coastal floods, tsunamis.

Extra terrestrial: Asteroid impact.

Extreme weather events: Heat waves, forest fires, famines, droughts and desertification.

Biological: Epidemics/pandemics.

These categories can overlap so that a volcanic eruption can trigger a landslide that can crash into the sea and generate a tsunami and flood the opposite shoreline. Heavy rainfall can cause landslides and floods.

3. *By number of casualties:*
   A. MINOR: 25-99 casualties alive or dead OR 10-49 casualties requiring hospital in-patient treatment.
   B. MODERATE: 100-999 casualties alive or dead OR 50-249 casualties requiring hospital in-patient treatment.
   C. MAJOR: Over 5000 people affected OR over 1000 casualties live or dead OR over 250 casualties requiring hospital in-patient treatment.
4. *By area involved:*
   A. Radius less than 1 km.
   B. Radius 1-100 km.
   C. Radius over 100 km.

Disaster can also be classified by the resultant anticipated necessary response as follows:

- A level I disaster in one in which local emergency response personnel and organizations are able to contain and deal effectively with the disaster and its aftermath.
- A level II disaster requires regional efforts and mutual aid from surrounding communities.
- A level III disaster is of such a magnitude that local and regional assets are overwhelmed, requiring statewide or federal assistance.

PICE

The potential injury creating event (PICE) system is designed to identify common aspects of a disaster and of response capabilities. Such systems are especially valuable tools in planning for disaster mitigation. The PICE system uses 4 modifier to describe a particular disaster. The first modifiers describes the potential for additional casualties. The second identifies the degree to which local resources are disrupted. The third modifier identifies the geographic boundaries of involvement. The final modifier, crisis staging, indicates the likelihood of needing outside assistance to augment or replace local resources. It is important to note that in the PICE methodology, identical disasters may have differing descriptors depending on the location of the event and the availability of resources.

Multiple casualty incidents (MCIs) have, in contrast to disasters, their primary effects (morbidity and mortality) to individuals, while the community infrastructure remain relatively intact. A passenger train accident with 500 injured or dead occupants is considered an MCI. However, if this morbidity and mortality were the result of the release of toxic gas from a hazardous material accident, a much higher potential for additional casualties would exist. Normal operations and activities of daily living disrupted for a longer period, are considered a disaster.

Potential injury-creating event algorithm

A	*B*	*C*	*Stage*
Stable	Static	Local	0
Dynamic	Disruptive	Regional	I
	Paralytic	National	II
		International	III

5. *Color coding of disasters*

   Based on the location and magnitude of the disasters and the local population and their vulnerability, disasters are classified in three classes:

   Green: Very low likelihood of humanitarian disaster.

   Orange: Potential humanitarian disaster

   Red: Very high likelihood of humanitarian disaster.

5

Phases of Disasters

> "The cruelest foe is a masked benefactor. The wars which make history so dreary have served the cause of truth and virtue."
>
> —*Ralph Waldo Emerson*

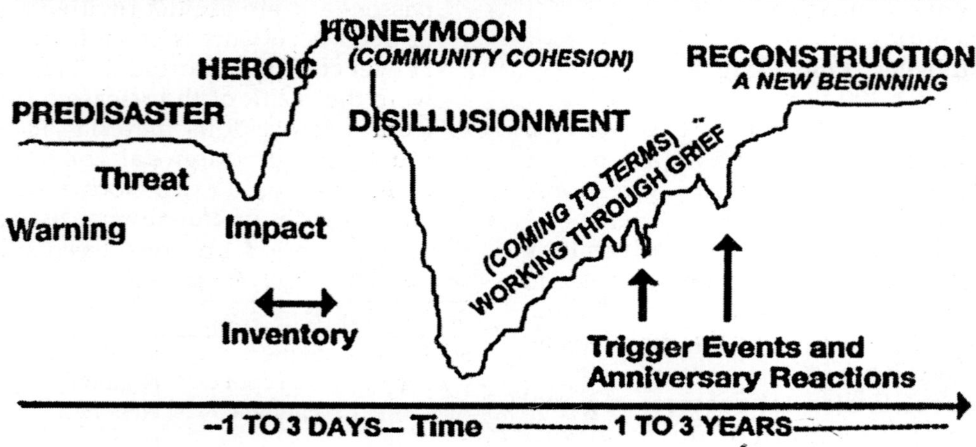

Calvin J Fredrick has proposed that any disaster can be divided into phases, based on the way individuals and the community respond to it. The phases described are:

A. *Warning Period:* Paradoxically, people respond better to a sudden event than when warned in advance. Apparently, people are not able to cope with the anxiety and apprehension. They tend to get alarmed and are unable to respond, overwhelmed by a feeling of helplessness. It becomes vital for community leaders to issue specific tasks to its members during this period for their own safety and emotional stability.

B. *Threat Period:* A time when individuals are required to make critical decisions on the way to respond to the threat. While some people seem to be able to make decisions that are important to their own survival, those, for whom day-to-day decision-making is difficult, respond with an emotional crisis or apathy that may claim their lives.

C. *Impact Period:* As the disaster strikes, people perceive its magnitude. A few respond with panic reactions, while some wander about aimlessly, unable to even follow the directions of others. Some individuals, however, assume leadership and take level-headed decisions for others to emulate and follow.

D. *Inventory Period:* A period of inflection when people try to assess what has happened to them. While some exhibit fear, anger, sorrow, depression and anxiety and soon get over the emotions, some carry emotional scars for the rest of their lives. Some feel isolated and overwhelmed. Some may just stand and stare vacantly, while some women can be seen to hug themselves and display a rocking motion. Children may exhibit a regressive reaction, exhibiting infantile behavior. Most people take grip over their feelings and begin to help the rescue operations or resort to some other purposeful activity.

E. *Rescue Period:* During this post disaster phase, the survivors help each other to cope and re establish shelters and other needs. Some may display a shocked state, apathy and withdrawal.

F. *Remedy Period:* As the victims work together, a spirit of co-operation prevails and the morale of survivors gets upbeat.

G. *Restoration Period:* In this final phase, the victims regain the stability they enjoyed prior to the event. The duration of this period depends upon the type of disaster, the degree of destruction and the amount of help available.

6 Emergency Services

> "The art of losing isn't hard to master; so many things seem filled with the intent to be lost that their loss is no disaster."
>
> —*Elizabeth Bishop*

THE EMERGENCY SERVICES INFRASTRUCTURE

A. *Primary*: Police, Fire, Ambulance services, Hospitals, Medical Administration, and Rescue Services or Teams like Disaster Assistance Rescue Teams (DART) and the Neighborhood Emergency Team (NET).

B. *Secondary:* Armed Forces, General Practitioners, Social and Welfare Services– Governmental or NGOs, News Media. Designated trauma centres have now emerged in strategic locations to provide state-of-the art care in a timely manner to reduce overall mortality. Level I-III organizations give tertiary level care to victims. Level I trauma center possesses capabilities and resources for comprehensive trauma care including research, education, prevention and rehabilitation components. Level II centers possess similar clinical resources without the research and education components. Level III centers possess limited staff and resources for clinical care but capable of handling polytrauma situations and executing precise triage for those who require level I or II center facilities (Table 6.1). Based on clear evidence of serious deficiencies in the management of severely injured patients, the specialty of dedicated trauma care (traumatology) has emerged in several countries to offer focused care to trauma victims.

C. *National and International Agencies Involved in Disaster Planning and Management*: International and National branches of organizations such as Red Cross, United Nations Relief Organization, World Health Organization etc.

D. *Other Services and Organizations.*

Table 6.1: Trauma centre organization

	Level I	*Level II*	*Level III*
Philosophy	Identical commitment to excellent care of severe injuries Trauma quality-assurance process Trauma training programs Trauma public education Teaching program Research 600-1000 cases/year		Best community commitment to stabilization and and transport of severe injuries
Facilities	Lighted heliport	Lighted heliport	
Emergency department	24 h/day with trauma experienced staffing	24 h/day with trauma experienced staffing	24 h/day with trauma experienced staffing
Operating theatre	Staffed and available for trauma 24 h/day	Staffed and available for trauma 24 h/day	Desirable to be staffed and available for trauma 24 h/day
Anaesthesia personnel	Anaesthetist with trauma experience 24 h/day	Nurse anaesthetist or anaesthetist experience with trauma 24 h/day	In-house anaesthesia coverage 24 h/day
Surgery personnel	24 h/day general surgeon and neurosurgeon experienced in trauma; consultants rapidly available	24 h/day general surgeon and neuro-surgeon experienced in trauma; consultants rapidly available	Promptly available general surgeon 24 h/day neurosurgeon availability highly desirable
Surgery case load	At least 50 severely injured patients per trauma general surgeon per year	At least 50 severely injured patients per trauma general surgeon per year	

From Grande CM, Nolan JP, Bernhard WN 1990 Trauma anaesthesia in America: A descrpition of an American trauma centre. Care of the Critically Ill 6:171-175. Used with permission.

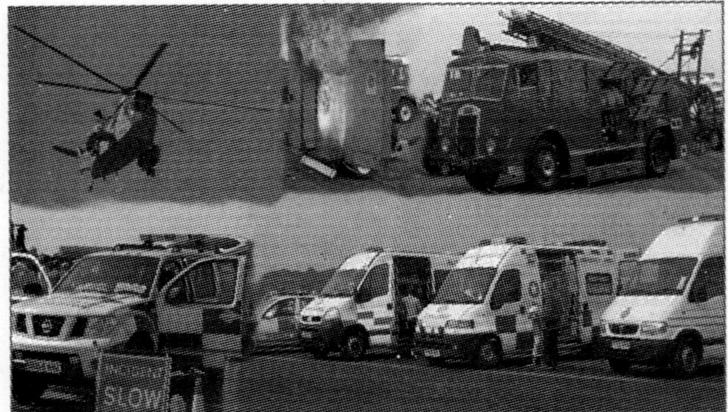

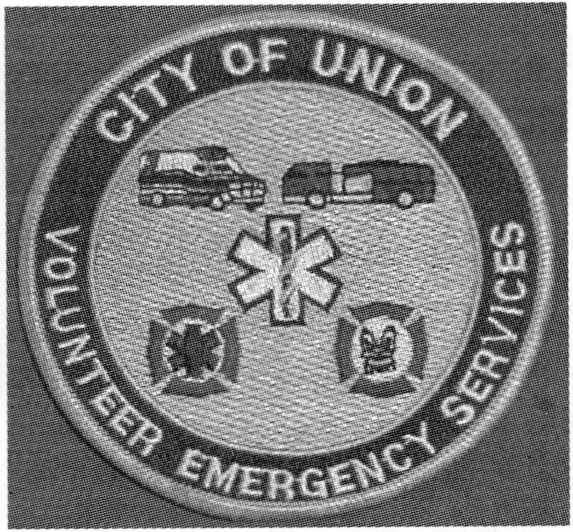

Meteorological services—Satellites, radar, aircraft inputs on location and scale of a calamity; Authorized Co-ordinators and Planners of Disaster Services; Food and Agricultural Authorities; Public Works Departments; National Transportation Safety Board; Education Department; Finance Department; Defence Services; Revenue Commerce Department; Public Health Department; Civil Defence, Home National Guards; Non-Governmental Agencies; Red Cross and Red Crescent Societies, Salvation Army; Philanthropists and Individuals; Press and Media; Individual Helpers/First Responders not connected with Specific Organizations, including physically able victims of the disaster. Relatives of Victims; Amateur Ham Radio Operators Association

7 Public Health Objectives in Disaster Situations

> "I always tried to turn every disaster into an opportunity."
>
> —*John D. Rockefeller*

The major objectives of public health measures instituted during a disaster situation are:

1. To prevent unnecessary morbidity, mortality and economic loss resulting directly from a disaster event.
2. To eliminate morbidity, mortality and economic loss directly attributable to mismanagement of disaster relief efforts.

PUBLIC HEALTH PROGRAMS

Though provision of emergency medical care is an important aspect of disaster relief, true primary preventive services will serve to effectively mitigate the effects of a disaster. These must include:

A. Adequate clothing and shelter.
B. Supply of potable water.
C. Good environmental sanitation.
D. Provision of safe food supplies.
E. Protection of individuals against infectious diseases.

TOP TEN PRIORITIES IN REFUGEE CAMPS

- Initial assessment.
- Measles immunization.
- Water and sanitation.
- Food and nutrition.
- Shelter and site planning.
- Health care and emergency phase.
- Control of communicable diseases and epidemics.
- Public health surveillance.
- Human resources and training.
- Coordination.

Clothing and Shelter

Death from environmental exposure is a distinct possibility after natural disasters as even modest environmental extremes can result in increased energy demand and, thereby, a per capita increase in food requirements.

Shelter provides physical and psychological reassurance and is an important element of well being and health to displaced and dispossessed population. The better the shelter, the better the effect achieved. A sense of ownership provides an anchor in a changing and threatening situation. Local climatic conditions are an important factor for type of shelter provided and a smaller margin for failure as the the climate can be unforgiving of shortfalls in provision.

ADVERSITY IS A MULTIPLICATIVE PROCESS IN DISPLACED PEOPLE AS CLIMATIC, NUTRITIONAL, DISEASE AND

SECURITY DIMENSIONS ALL SEEM TO CONSPIRE AGAINST THE POPULATION. Hence an appropriate level of shelter must be provided. These shelters can be improvised from locally available resources. They should be easily erected and maintained. The act of building a shelter itself represents evidence of self help and return to responsibility and dignity. Shelters help stabilize the situation in camps and helps control population movements.

Children, the aged and the sick are less able to tolerate extremes of temperature and constitute a significant percentage of disaster-affected populations in developing countries. Homeless population will seek out alternative shelters or windbreaks in lee areas to establish personal shelters necessary for survival. They will salvage clothing and waterproofing material such as polythene bits and sheets that have been washed away or buried under debris. It becomes essential, therefore, that displaced persons are housed under conditions that will not lead to the deterioration of public health and the environment. Areas proposed for accommodating displaced persons must be surveyed in order to determine whether basic environmental health services can be provided. Accommodating such population in tent camps should only be considered as a measure of last resort. Existing undamaged structures usually provide the best facilities for temporary shelter. Attempts should be made to rehabilitate victims to houses of their friends and relatives unaffected by the calamity. The sudden creation of areas of high population density such as temporary/transit camps for displaced persons where there has been no prior planning for the sanitary accommodation of large numbers of persons can precipitate numerous public health problems. Once individuals have been located and established on a site, they will usually resist being asked to move again. It is important therefore that relocation sites are well thought out. Most communities have many more buildings than are required for the basic shelter of their population. Existing buildings such as schools, churches, temples, and hotels can be appropriated to serve as dormitories. They are especially useful when they have water supply, kitchen facility and adequate toilets and baths. Many victims will move in with relatives and friends and they should be encouraged to return to their own homes as soon as possible. If adequate resources can be mobilized, they should be provided with materials like thick HDPE sheets, blankets and structural material like aluminium poles for constructing temporary shelters by themselves on their property and home sites. Homeless individuals are often more concerned with maintaining family integrity and guarding personal property than finding an alternative shelter.

Water

Water is the most important and essential item provided to disaster-stricken population. Water supports life as well as constitutes a major medium of disease transmission. Fecal contamination of the water supply is typical after most natural disasters. Contamination of the surface water supply can be presumed in most cases, especially in refugee camps. It can be a significant cause of morbidity among relief workers too. All samples of water that are dark coloured, having an unacceptable odour or manifesting floating material must be considered suspect and prohibited for human consumption. An adequate supply of potable water must be ensured and means of purifying and transporting drinking water must be identified immediately. On the average, a 5 litre supply would be required per person per day and a three day reserve supply for the local population must be catered for.

Potable water: Water which contains no substances posing danger to health when consumed or used for any domestic use.

The absolute minimum physiological quantity of water needed for survival is 3 l/ person/day in a temperate climate. If hygiene needs are added this figure is close to 15 l/ person/day. Requirements for children varies with age and weight. In children over 1 year of age, weight is determined by the formula 2 x (age +4) kg.

For the first 10 kg, fluid requirement per day should be 100 ml/kg body weight. For the second 10 kg, fluid requirement is worked out at 50 ml/kg and for the subsequent kilogram, fluid requirement is 20ml/kg body weight. If child weighs 22 kg:

First 10 kg=1000 ml
2nd 10 kg =500 ml
for the last 2 kg = 40 ml
Total=1540 ml

Fever increases fluid requirements by 12% per degree rise in body temperature (Celsius). If there is vomiting, diarrhea, burns additional fluids will have to be replaced based on estimates.

Tanks available locally from commercial water supply companies, municipality, dairies, breweries, industries, defence establishments and railways can be cleaned and used to transport water. The adaptation of gasoline, chemical and sewage trucks for this purpose must be avoided. Water, however pure, when stored in wooden containers, deteriorates rapidly, and acquires an objectionable taste and odour unless its internal surfaces are burnt or charred. Increasing line pressure to compensate for pressure loss due to leaks can control contamination of partially damaged water distribution systems or breaches in the mains, to prevent reverse flow. Potable water supply must be ensured to hospitals and camps.

Clarification of water is done by sedimentation and/or filtration. It eliminates suspended matter, harmful organisms, cysts, ova, molluscs, cyclops and reduces the chlorine demand of water. Filtration is superior and faster than sedimentation, provided the water is not too turbid. Just standing water in tanks allows coarse suspended matter to settle down in 2 to 6 hours. This process can be hastened by flocculation with pure aluminium sulphate (barber's alum). This causes a precipitate of aluminium hydroxide which engulfs suspended matter and settles down. In a dose of 35 gram of alum per 1000 litres, it rapidly clarifies very turbid water. For exceptionally turbid water, a dose of 70 grams per 1000 litres may be needed. Siphoning the supernatant after 2-6 hours can easily ensure safe potable water. Simple makeshift filters can be improvised by piling 50 cm depth of clean sand topped with 10 cm depth of gravel of grain size 0.5 to 1.0 cm. An improved version using alternate layers of 10cm depth of sand and gravel with a layer of cloth and charcoal sandwiched in between can clarify turbid water considerably. After every 5 hours of use, the layers can be renewed or else recharged by washing out with filtered water (Fig. 7.1).

Sterilization of water means making it fit for drinking by destroying all pathogenic organisms that may be present in it. Boiling is a commonly used method, but fuel may be short in supply in a disaster affected area. If done, 20 minutes of boiling renders water safe for drinking. Where available, distillation by using evaporators and condensers can be utilized. It is expensive and labour intensive. Distilled water is of known purity, clear, odourless and free from deposits and salts responsible for hardness. Other alternatives could be bottled mineral water, aerated drinks

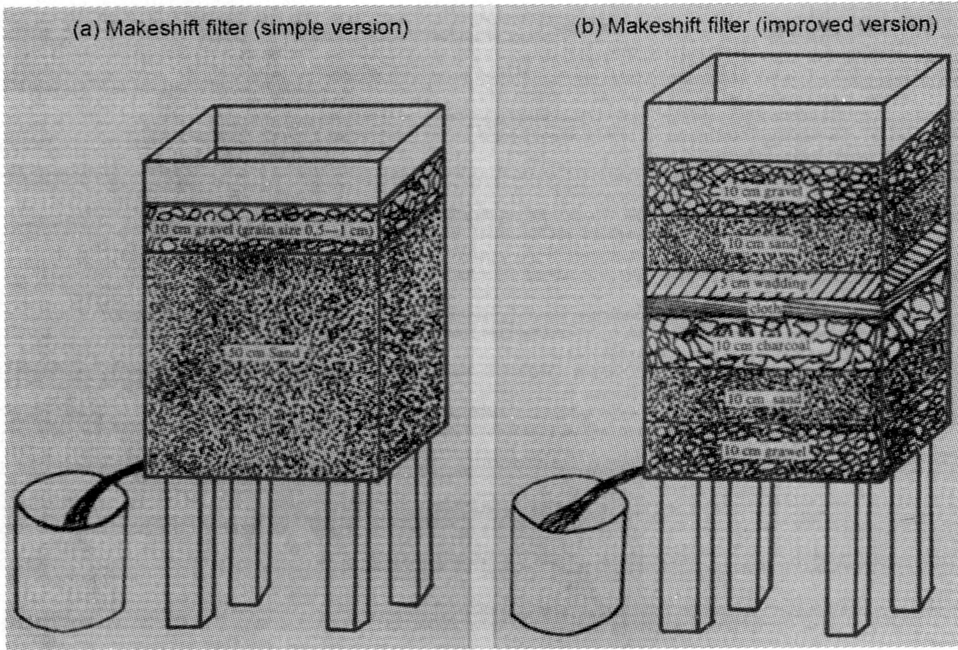

Fig. 7.1

from reliable and certified companies or 5% dextrose from intravenous fluid bottles. Hoses and pumps used for drinking water must not be used for any other purposes. Hoses must have couplings at each end fitted with a cap attached by a short chain to prevent it from being mislaid. The caps exclude entry of dust and dirt when the pipes are not being used. A simpler method of protecting the interior of hoses is to couple the two ends together when not in use. Men handling potable water must be free from infection, adopt good personal hygiene measures and wash their hands frequently with soap and water. If ground water is being used, source it from deep wells or bore wells with sanitary surroundings. Water from streams and ponds should be drawn from the upstream side of dwellings and as far from the banks as possible. Separate areas for drinking water and washing/scrubbing clothes and utensils must be made.

Sterilization of water can be effectively carried out by the use of chlorine. Water must be preferably clarified prior to chlorination. A residual chlorine level of 0.5 ppm (0.4-0.5 mg/l yielding 0.2 mg/l after 30 min contact period) is safe and adequate and it does not give a chlorinous taste to the water. Above 1 ppm, the taste becomes marked and objectionable. In situations where the water quality is doubtful, superchlorination with a residual chlorine of 2 ppm after 30 min contact period may be needed. Chlorination of water by addition of bleach {Ca(ClO)2.CaCl2} or chloride of lime or also known as calcium hypochlorite, is based on its chlorine demand. This is determined by the Horrocks test. Good quality bleach must have 30 to 35% available chlorine, i.e., roughly one third. The powder when exposed to air or moisture, cakes and diminishes in disinfectant potency due to formation of calcium carbonate and liberation of chlorine. These changes are enhanced in the presence of heat and light. Hence bleaching powder must be stored in air tight containers and stored in a cool, dry place. This way, the loss of available chlorine should not exceed 1% per month. When the powder is added to water, it splits into calcium chloride and calcium hypochlorite. The latter is decomposed by the carbonic acid present in water to form hypochlorous acid and insoluble calcium carbonate. Hypochlorous acid is a powerful oxidizing agent and, in the presence of organic material and bacteria , it gives up oxygen and free chlorine.

The chemical reactions involved are represented as following:

$2CaClO,Cl = CaCl_2 + Ca(ClO)_2$

$Ca(ClO)_2 + H_2O + CO_2 = CaCO_3 + 2HClO$

$2HClO = 2HCl + O_2$

$2HClO = H_2O + Cl_2 + O.$

The amount of bleach required depends on the amount of organic and suspended matter, any preliminary treatment such as storage or filtration, and the period of contact. The actual amount of bleach required can be estimated by adding different known quantities of powder and testing the sample chemically. In the Horrock's test, scoops of bleach in increments of 2 grams are added to water samples in measured cups and the sample that turns light blue in colour after an half hour contact with potassium iodide and starch solution is presumed to indicate the chlorine demand of the sample. Bleach is then calculated and added so that the available chlorine in the water sample is 1 part per million (ppm). For all practical purposes, one tablespoon of bleach for 5 litres for drinking purposes and 2 tablespoons for all other purposes must be used, allowing a half hour contact period before consumption or use.

5% bleach:
500 gallon tank=1/2 cup
45 gallon oil drum= 3 tsps
5 gallon bucket=1/2 tsps
2l bottle=6 drops
½ hour contact minimum.

The calculated amount of bleach must be mixed with sterile water (boiled and cooled) or distilled water to make a thin paste and then more sterile water added and stirred. Insoluble calcium carbonate and hydrate settles as a sediment at the bottom and the supernatant is added to the sample to be purified. Another test to detect free chlorine is the orthotolidine test. 0.5 gram of the chemical is dissolved in 50ml 10% hydrochloric acid and one ml of this prepared solution is added to 1ml of the water, mixed and allowed to stand for 5 minutes. Production of a yellow colour indicates the presence of free chlorine. If household bleach (pure sodium hypochlorite solution) is available, 4 drops of 7-10% strength, 8 drops of 4-6% strength or 40 drops of 1% strength per 5 litres water would suffice to make it potable. The bleach must be mixed thoroughly and allowed to stand for 30 min hour before use. Iodine can also be used as an alternative to chlorine when 20 drops of 2% iodine solution per 5 litres of clear water or 40 drops of 2% iodine per 5 litres of turbid water is mixed, stood for 30 minutes and then poured back and forth between two containers to remove the flat taste before being consumed. Water sterilisation tablets are available for purifying small quantities of water. These contain Halozone which is p-sulphondichlo-aminobenzoic acid with a chemical formula $Cl_2NO_2SC_6H_4COOH$. Each tablet contains 4 milligram of the disinfectant made up with dry sodium chloride and dry sodium carbonate, one tablet sufficing for 1 litre of water. A second tablet may be added for extremely contaminated water samples. The tablets must be stored in airtight amber coloured bottles, when they maintain their efficacy at temperatures upto 31°C for 5 months and should be used before one year from the date of manufacture. Addition of calculated amounts of potassium permanganate to give a pink colour persisting for a few minutes, coupled with a weak acid to liberate oxygen can be used. However, its action is feeble when compared to bleach, and costlier. Drinking water must be tested for the presence of Escherichia coli that suggests fecal contamination. E Coli count of 1-10/100 ml water is tolerable, 10-100 indicates need for treatment and >100 is considered unfit for drinking. Water supplies obtained from flooded structures such as wells, rivers, reservoirs, rain collection cisterns must be clarified and then disinfected with bleach to give a 2 ppm residual chlorine level. Chlorine gas or liquid chlorine is also used to sterilize water with the help of a mechanical injector called chloronome. The entire process is automated. Chlorination can also be effectively carried out using osmotic methods across special membranes. Where superchlorination is resorted to, the chlorinous taste can be removed by adding 2.0 grams of sodium thiosulphate to 1000 litres of water. In some instances, ozone, a powerful oxidizing agent can be used to sterilize water. It is rapid in its action but it decomposes fast and has no residual effect, unlike chlorine. Dosage required is 0.2 to 1.5 mg per litre. Ultraviolet ray is an expensive and non-residual germicide and ineffective in the presence of turbidity.

Simple procedures for disinfecting water:

- If the water is cloudy, first use homemade or other filters to eliminate the cloudiness.
- Bring the water to a rolling boil for 20 minutes.
- Or, as an alternative, treat the water with disinfectants such as chlorine (bleach), iodine, silver etc., ensuring appropriate residual concentrations (chlorine 1-2 ppm, silver 100 ppm iodine 1 ppm).

When faced with acute shortage of drinking water fresh fruits, cucumbers, melons, pumpkins and tender coconuts can temporarily provide adequate fluids. Certain types of trees such as birch, linden, sycamore, maple and palm, release ample amounts of palatable liquids. A birch tree can produce nearly 7 litres of fluids per day. The sugary sap can be consumed without boiling and filtering. An empty tin can opened at both ends can be driven into the tree trunk for about 5 cm depth at a height of about 75 cm above ground level, leaving it pointed downwards at an angle. The sap trickles out and can be collected and consumed. Other trees whose peduncle or inflorescence can be tapped for sap are the box elder, black sugar palm, fishtail palm, alam panei, American oil palm and date palm. Green bamboo thickets are an excellent source of fresh water. Water from green bamboo is clear and odorless. To get the water, a green bamboo stalk is bent, tied down, and the top cut off when water will drip freely during the night. Banana and plantain trees can be cut down leaving about a 30-centimeter stump. The centre of the stump can be scooped out to create a bowl-shaped hollow. Water from the roots will immediately start to fill the hollow. The first three fillings of water will be bitter, but succeeding fillings will be palatable and the stump can supply water for four days. Make sure to cover the hollow to keep out insects. Some tropical vines can yield water. A notch is made in the vine as high as reachable and the vine is cut close to the ground. The stream of sap can be collected in a container or drunk straight off. Palms, such as the buri, coconut, sugar, rattan, and nips, contain liquid. A lower frond is bruised and pulled down to "bleed" the tree at the injured site. The 'traveller's tree' has a cuplike sheath at the base of its leaves in which water collects. The leaf bases and roots of the umbrella tree can provide water. The Baobab tree collects water in its bottlelike trunk during the wet season and this can be tapped quite easily.Trees producing milky or coloured sap should not be used. A plastic sheet hung halfway down a trench can also be used to generate water. During the day, the air beneath the sheet becomes saturated with water vapour. This condenses after sunset to form droplets that can be collected at a rate of 0.3 litres per square metre of plastic sheet per hour. Snow and ice can be melted and drunk after treatment. Ice on sea water can be consumed if more than 2 years old, recognized by its bluish hue and rounded corners.

ENVIRONMENTAL SANITATION

Environmental sanitation methods are necessary to prevent contamination of food and water. Latrines must be appropriately constructed and maintained, as needed, in relocation camps, relief worker settlements, and areas of dense population where such facilities have been destroyed. Shallow or deep trench latrines are best suited for camps with an appropriate screen or superstructure to afford privacy and a hand-wash facility. A long trench 30 cm wide and 40 to 60 cm deep is dug and the excavated earth is piled loosely in proximity. Each user has to throw a scoop of the earth over the deposited faeces while the urine falls outside the pit and drains away. A new pit can be dug a metre away from the first pit and used in the same manner. Under warm, dry conditions, the decomposition of faeces takes about eight weeks without attracting fly breeding. Location of such a facility must be well away from dwellings, above flood level in a dry, well drained site and a minimum of 15 metres downstream of any water source Health education on latrine usage and upkeep must be provided to users. Frequent on-site visits by officials and public health workers and professionals will be needed to enforce this. Provision of sanitary garbage disposal including provision of waste receptacles, transportation and incineration or burial must be ensured. Proper waste disposal is critical in preventing communicable disease outbreaks, as fecal contamination of the water supply is a frequent cause of diarrheal disease outbreaks. Domestic flies can transmit conjunctivitis, shigella dysentery, entero virus infection and some parasitic diseases. These will be increased in numbers in warm climates as a result of available breeding places in feces and undisposed garbage. Handling of toxic gases and hazardous substances can be a significant public health problem in certain types of natural and man-made disasters. Volcanic eruption can release a variety of toxic gases as well as poisonous ash that can ravage standing crops and livestock grazing on such contaminated pastures. Thousands of toxic chemicals are being used worldwide and these can be released into the atmosphere during an industrial accident like explosion or fire or during a mishap to a container vehicle during their transportation. Industrial hygienists can estimate the possible levels of exposure to specific gases and provide information regarding the decomposition products of burning material and their monitoring and containment/neutralization. Also military and civil sources of radiation may enter the environment by accident. Chemical and nuclear spills will require rapid assessment in respect of the degree of contamination and immediate implementation of protective measures and evacuation. Industrial hygiene and radiation health personnel should be actively involved in such emergencies. A morgue will be needed in virtually every disaster scenario. An easily accessible central location that is large enough to allow next-of-kin to identify the stored corpses will be necessary. Refrigerated seafood containers may be used as temporary morgues to prevent decomposition and the services of forensic specialists and orthodontists will be required to identify grossly mutilated remnants. The health hazards associated with undisposed bodies are minimal if death has occurred due to trauma and they are not contaminating water supplies. Immediate mass burials or cremation is a relatively low priority. Bodies can be treated with insecticides to prevent vector breeding and mechanical transmission of pathogens. Dead bodies represent a delicate social problem and bodies may be disposed, after identification or detailed photography, by locally traditional methods of burial or cremation. Burial is the simplest and best method if it is physically possible and ritually acceptable. Bodies can also be exhumed for identification later. Cremation requires large amounts of fuel and is not a public health necessity.

Camp Toilet Arrangements

a. If there are no sanitation services, latrines must be built (individual, collective, portable).
b. Before installing a latrine, the soil at the site must be evaluated along with topographical conditions, user access, and the presence of surface and ground water in the surrounding area.
c. If the land is not appropriate for latrine construction (rocky soil or high water table) aboveground latrines with removable tanks must be built. The excreta must be transported to a pit located on appropriate ground, for immediate burial.
d. Estimate the number of latrines to be installed, based on the number of persons in the shelter (1 waterless toilet/25 women and 1 waterless toilet and 1 urinal/35 men).
e. Provide information and instruction to the population on:
   - Throwing used toilet paper into the latrine.
   - Using the sanitation services only for defecating or urinating (do not store tools or other items in the latrine).
   - Washing their hands with soap and water after urinating or defecating.
   - Keeping the floor, walls, and area surrounding the latrine clean.
   - Not defecating or urinating outdoors in the area around the sanitation services or near bodies of water, since this encourages the proliferation of flies and larvae and water contamination through water runoff.

What Not To Do

a. Install excreta disposal systems without first assessing the situation (existence of sanitation services, number of users, and characteristics of the site, among others).
b. Select the location of the sanitation services without taking into account the characteristics of the site (soil type, topography, accessibility, presence of bodies of water, etc.).
c. Try to implement sophisticated excreta disposal technologies.

Solid Waste

Solid waste may be refuse, manure, or animal cadavers. There is a correlation between improper solid waste disposal and the incidence of vector-borne diseases. As a result, arrangements must be made to collect, store, and dispose of refuse and manure.

What To Do

a. Assess the situation, considering the number of people in the shelter, existing services, collection service, topographic conditions, accessibility, and soil type (if the waste must be disposed of on site).

b. Estimate the quantity, type, and capacity of the water storage containers, based on the number of persons and existing services. For a short time, empty food containers, plastic or water-resistant paper bags, and disposable packaging can be used. The capacity of the containers should be 50-100 liters and should not exceed 20-25 kg when full.

c. Provide three or four containers per 100 persons and distribute them so that every family has access to a container (or plastic bag).

d. The containers should not touch the ground, for example they should be on a wooden platform. They must be emptied and washed daily.

e. If there is regular waste collection and final disposal service:
   - Coordinate with the responsible entity to cover refuse collection from the shelter or camp.
   - Check the accessibility of the regular collection service and take the appropriate steps for the shelter or camp.
   - If the regular service does not have access to the shelter or camp, place waste pick-up sites in the surrounding area and locate storage bins or containers away from water sources.

If there is no regular waste collection and final disposal service:

- Organize collection, transport, and final waste disposal service, involving the persons living in the shelter or camp.
- For final disposal, bury the waste by building pits 1.5 meters wide, 1.5 meters long, and 2 meters deep. At the end of each day, cover the refuse with 15 cm of dirt and pack it down. This pit will last 10 days for a population of 200. For larger populations, increase pit size proportionately, up to a maximum of 3 meters x 3 meters. Before the pit is full, cover it with a layer of packed dirt 40 cm thick, so that it is level with the ground. Then dig a new pit.

Recommendations for managing medical waste:

- Separate common, hazardous, and sharp waste, preferably in strong containers with plastic covers.
- Dispose of common waste in the pit described above or other similar ones.
- Hazardous waste will be destroyed in a homemade incinerator that can be built using a fuel drum that must have a ventilation hole on the bottom. Inside there must be a grill to hold the waste. The ashes will be disposed of in the pit for common waste.
- Sharp waste will be disposed of in a hole or pit with 1 m^3 capacity, covered with a heavy concrete slab. A tube 2 inches in diameter will run through the slab and extend roughly 1.5 meters above it. The tube will be used for depositing needles and surgical blades without syringes or venoclysis tubes.

Dead animals and excrement from domestic animals must be buried immediately, since they can be a source of contamination.

Provide information and training to the population on sanitary refuse handling.

What Not To Do

a. Request tools, containers, bins, plastic containers or other devices without first assessing the situation.

b. Mix common waste with medical waste, thus endangering the population.

c. Accept or request sophisticated technology for treating medical waste without having the facilities or trained personnel to operate it.

Food

Food provision is of a fundamental importance to migrant people. Lack of adequate nutrition is a recognized accompaniment to the hardships of mass population movements. Protein calorie deficiency will also render populations susceptible to other afflictions such as infection and disease (particularly measles). Food strategy must meet normal daily nutritional requirements. This a very resource intensive and complex venture. The special requirements of the children as well as pregnant and lactating mothers and the elderly has to be catered for. The weight height ratio and mid arm circumference data can be used to assess nutritional status. Initial nutritional assessment must be followed by a specialized logistic effort and augmented by a medical supervisory role at the beginning of a therapeutic/supplementary feeding programme itself. This must correct nutritional imbalances quickly and effectively in order to allow refugees return to normal feeding and life activities.

Adequate food is usually available to meet the immediate requirement of the local population in most disaster situations. However, destruction of household stocks, disruption of the local transportation and marketing systems can create shortages. Famine can follow in the months after a devastation due to crop damage, loss of land, inundation of cultivable land by sea water and chemical contamination. Floodwaters, insects, rodents and unsanitary handling in mass feeding centres can contaminate existing food stocks. Food degradation and spoilage can occur from long periods of power breaks that may affect the cold/cool chain of storage. Sale of date expired stocks and adulteration by opportunistic traders can occur. Artificial food shortages can also occur due to manipulation of food stocks by unscrupulous traders and political factions to meet their own needs. When mass feeding programs are needed, food should be inspected at distribution points and supervised by an environmental health specialist. Routine microbial analysis of food is not necessary unless a suspected source of a disease outbreak has been identified. To avert health problems the public should be educated about food storage, preparation and safety. When arranging feeding, it must be remembered that even starving populations may not readily accept unfamiliar foods and it would be a better venture to distribute ready-to-eat foods adapted to local tastes, e.g. tamarind rice (puliyohora), poori with dry vegetable preparations, 'khakadas', 'poha'-puffed rice with nuts, dehydrated 'bisi bele baath', bread, 'halwa', long life milk tetrapacks etc. with high nutritive content and good keeping qualities. The Central Food Technological Research Institutes (CFTRI) and the Defence Food Research Laboratories can be contacted for various ready-to-eat and cook-and-serve recipes. Milk powder, boiled sweets and chocolates are the standard contents of many survival ration packs. Food packets may have to be air dropped and their packaging must be distinct for easy location and unlike any explosive and incendiary devices that may be employed in the same run.

Disease Prevention and Control

The range of medical needs in a displaced population will be almost infinite and having no prescriptive answers- one size does not fit all- hence a dynamic approach is required to priorities and task-setting. Suitable vaccination tailored to the threat (endemic diseases) and its incubation period- especially for measles and meningitis. Cold chain to protect vaccines must be ensured. Pediatric, midwifery, geriatric psychological services. Cultural and religious sensitiivites will affect behaviour and coping mechanisms. The transcultural dimension of psychiatric care in refugee camps is particularly demanding. A mix of in patient care and community care approaches may be required. In a disrupted society, the incidence of sexually transmitted diseases can also be expected to be higher. A reservoir of pre existing STD, desperation and destitution may result in part time prostitution in order to eat and/or provide for their families. Education and prophylactic measures will have to be instituted. Religious, social, ethical and historical dimensions will influence the acceptability and ultimate success of specific measures that are largely utilitarian and aiming for the greatest good for the greatest number. The commitment of resources in the acute relief stage must recognize the realities of subsequent development potential–the disaster-development continuum must be worked out based on the bedrock of reality.

With the exception of famines, disasters are generally not followed by major epidemics. However, the potential for the epidemic spread of disease exists, particularly in developing countries. Deterioration of the physical environment, overpopulation, poor sanitation in refugee camps and disruption of the routine disease control programs are the precursors of disease outbreaks. The physical damage done by the disaster can lead to widespread contamination of the water supply and multiplication of disease vector breeding sites. Overcrowding facilitates the outbreak of diarrheal diseases, especially when there has been no commensurate increase in the basic infra structure services. Disease control after disasters should be directed at two areas. Firstly, the hazard of disease must be reduced by appropriate public health interventions like emergency repair of water supply lines and sanitation systems, vector control operations and provision of adequate potable water. The second priority is to establish a surveillance system so that disease outbreak can be promptly identified and controlled. The risk of epidemic disease after a disaster is related to the presence of endemic diseases in the population. Disaster victims are more susceptible to endemic agents because of lack of food and increased environmental exposure. In addition, transmission is intensified due to environmental deterioration, thrusting people into direct contact with pathogens. In general, if a disease did not exist in the population before the disaster, there is little risk of the same occurring, unless a large number of people enter a disaster area and import new disease. The common outbreaks observed following a disaster are diarrheal disease, measles, whooping cough, tuberculosis, malaria and rat-bite fever (leptospirosis). Debris and solid wastes accumulate in empty receptacles along with rain and floodwater allowing insects and rodents to proliferate. This allows for potential disease transmission as well as food contamination and infestation. Vector proliferation and loss of housing can lead to a surge in the incidence of malaria. The washing away of residual pesticides and disruption in control programs compound the problem. The local population must be educated on the need to eliminate breeding sites and adopt personal protection measures. Breakdown in the living conditions and habitat can precipitate outbreaks of plague and louse-borne typhus. Emergency mass immunization is not a good method of disease control but pressures may be brought upon to institute some kind of immunization program. These serve more as a psychic hygiene measure than anything else. However, as donated vaccines are usually available in large quantities and immunization clinics are a highly visible activity, these are construed as a constructive activity by the government and can serve to boost local morale. Routine immunization programs must be continued and camp population may be immunized against measles and whooping cough (pertussis). Tetanus toxoid must be available to trauma victims and relief workers may have to be immunized against cholera and yellow fever in risk areas. The emergency may be utilized to provide immunization to those who would otherwise never seek them. An increase in the incidence of animal bites can be anticipated, especially when stray dogs may move in to gorge on dead carcasses. Human anti rabies vaccine must be available on a case-by case basis and a program to eliminate stray dogs should be considered.

Cholera Vaccine

Oral cholera vaccine is only recommended for populations at *immediate* risk of a cholera epidemic. Vaccination to prevent cholera outbreaks should be undertaken only in concert with other prevention and control measures currently recommended by WHO including; education, safe water and sanitation. Vaccination is not recommended to control ongoing outbreaks.

Parenteral Vaccine

Due to its low efficacy and short duration of protection, this is no longer recommended. Until recently the only cholera vaccine made was from phenol-killed whole cells of V. Cholera, administered in 2 doses, 2 weeks apart. Unfortunately the protective efficacy against severe dehydration was only 50%, the duration of protection hardly exceeded 6 months, and it does not prevent transmission of the infectious agent.

Oral Killed WC/rBS Vaccine

This consists of killed whole-cell V. Cholerae O1, in combination with a recombinant B-subunit of cholera toxin (WC/rBS). It has been marketed since the early 1990s. *Administration:* The vaccine must be diluted with and given with fresh clean water, as per manufacturers instructions. The vaccine should only be given where it can be assured that two doses can be given (10-14 days apart), as only one dose confers very little immunity. Immunity is conferred within one week of the second dose and may be 50%-60% protection for at least three years for all age groups. However, protection in children aged <5 years may decline more rapidly after 6 months. Protection is not conferred against V. cholerae O139. It has also been shown to be safe in pregnancy and breast feeding. *Adverse effects:* occasional mild gastrointestinal disturbances. *Contraindications:* none known, other than hypersensitivity to any of the components. Data are not available on simultaneous immunization of WC/rBS with other vaccines but there is no theoretical risk prohibiting simultaneous administration. A WHO pre-qualified oral killed cholera vaccine is available with SBL Vaccine AB in Sweden.

Oral Live Attenuated CVD 103-HgR Vaccine

A live attenuated oral cholera vaccine containing the genetically manipulated classical V. Cholerae strain CVD 103-HgR has been available since 1994. It is a *single dose* vaccine. Numerous trials have established its safety and immunogenicity, even in immunocompromised individuals, but to date no controlled trial proves its effectiveness in endemic situations. Therefore this vaccine should only be used if there is a high risk of contracting cholera, otherwise the killed WC/rBS vaccine should be used instead. *Administration:* A single dose must be given with clean, fresh water, according to manufacturers instructions. The vaccine provides similar protection levels as the WC/rBS for all age groups after seven days of administration, but this may drop sharply after 6 months. No data exists to confirm whether children <2 years of age are protected, but the vaccine has been well tolerated in children as young as 3 months of age. Protection is not conferred against V. cholerae O139. *Adverse effects:* About 2% vaccines report single episodes of nausea or abdominal cramps. Unfortunately, this vaccine may not be as readily available as the WC/rBS vaccine.

WHO Position on Cholera Vaccine

Oral cholera vaccines should be considered for pre-emptive use in high risk populations before a cholera outbreak has occurred, not reactively as a method of containing an outbreak once it has started. Both WC/rBS and CVD 103-HgR vaccines have proved to be safe and without significant adverse effects. Both vaccines require clean, fresh water for administration. Compared to old parenteral vaccine, they provide better and more long-lasting protection against cholera. However, insufficient protection in children aged less than two years old exclude these vaccines from use in national immunization programme.

Convincing protection in field situations has only been demonstrated only with the WC/rBS vaccine to date. However, the WC/rBS vaccine should be considered in populations at risk of cholera epidemic only if it can be assured that two doses (10-12 days apart, given with clean water) can be administered. If this cannot be assured due to logistical constraints, then the CVD 103-HgR may be considered, but it should be noted that its efficacy has not been demonstrated in controlled trails in endemic areas. The CVD 103 HgR induces protection 7 days after the single dose.

DEAD BODIES IN DISASTERS

The human body is host to many organisms, only some of which are pathogenic. When the body dies, the environment in which pathogens live can no longer sustain them. However, this does not happen immediately, and transmission of infectious agents from a cadaver to a living person may occur. Infectious hazards for individuals who routinely handle cadavers include tuberculosis, group A streptococcal infection, gastroenteritis, transmissible spongiform encephalopathies (such as Creutzfeldt-Jakob disease), hepatitis B, hepatitis C, HIV infection, and possibly meningitis and septicemia (especially meningococcal). Microorganisms involved in the decay process (putrefaction) are not pathogenic. Historically, epidemics resulting in mass casualties have only occurred from a few diseases, including plague, cholera, typhoid, tuberculosis, anthrax, and smallpox. Such infections are no more likely to be present in disaster victims than in the general population. Furthermore, although some of these diseases are highly contagious, their causative agents are unable to survive long in the human body following death. It is therefore unlikely that such epidemics will result from contact with a cadaver. Indeed, survivors present a much more important reservoir for disease. Where dead bodies have contaminated water supplies, gastroenteritis has been the most notable problem, although communities will rarely use a water supply where they know it to be contaminated by dead bodies.

HANDLING THE DEAD

The occupational risks for pathologists and mortuary staff who routinely work with dead bodies are well known, and the risks are unlikely to be different for persons who are dealing with victims of a natural disaster. However, incidents with a large number of fatalities may require a temporary workforce for the collection, transportation, storage, and disposal of the dead. These workers may include military personnel, rescue workers, volunteers, and others who have little or no experience in handling the deceased. Although there is no published literature about the risk of infections for this group, the risk is probably similar to that of public safety workers (e.g., emergency medical personnel, firefighters, and police officers) and funeral workers who are occupationally exposed to infectious agents during the intimate management of cadavers. As noted above, the most likely type of infections are those produced by blood borne viruses, enteric pathogens, and *Mycobacterium tuberculosis*.

Bloodborne Viruses

The risk of infection from blood borne viruses depends on the infection status of the victim (similar to the general population), likelihood and mode of exposure, and, in the case of hepatitis B, the vaccination status of the exposed individual. In many developing countries, especially in sub-Saharan Africa, Southeast Asia, the Middle East, the Pacific, and some countries in Latin America, the prevalence of chronic hepatitis B infection is around 8% to 10%. Hepatitis C virus is estimated to infect about 3% of the world's population, with prevalence being highest in Africa (5.3%), the Eastern Mediterranean (4.6%), the Western Pacific (3.9%), and Southeast Asia (2.2%); the prevalence is lowest in the Americas (1.7%) and Europe (1.0%) (13). The prevalence of HIV infection in those 14-45 years old is as high as 30% to 40% in some African countries; about 0.1% in Asia, Eastern Europe, and Western Europe; and between 0.1% and 6% in Latin America and the Caribbean.

Exposure to blood borne viruses can occur due to direct contact with non intact skin, percutaneous injury from bone fragments and needles, and mucous membrane exposure from splashes of blood or body fluid to the eyes, nose, or mouth. Following one needle-stick injury from an infected individual, the risks of infection have been estimated to be: for hepatitis B, between 6% and 30% in those who have had no prior hepatitis B vaccination, for hepatitis C, 1.8%; and for HIV infection, 0.5%. Infection from non intact skin or mucous membrane exposure is likely to be much lower. Importantly, infectious HIV can survive in cadavers for a considerable amount of time (up to 16 days after death if stored at 2 °C), and viable HIV has also been isolated from bone fragments, spleen, brain, bone marrow, and lymph nodes at autopsy 6 days postmortem.

Gastrointestinal Infections

Because a corpse will commonly leak feces, persons handling dead bodies are more likely to be exposed to gastrointestinal organisms than to bloodborne viruses. Workers may be exposed through direct contact with the victim's body and soiled clothes, and transmission can occur via the fecal-oral route. Contamination of other equipment, such as stretchers and vehicles used for transportation or storage, is also possible. However, common gastrointestinal organisms do not survive long in the environment and present little risk of infection where the body has been decaying for some time, or has been in the water.

Tuberculosis

Around 1% of the world population is infected by tuberculosis each year. Rates are generally much higher in developing countries, especially Africa and Asia, and the increase in HIV infections has led to an increase in the prevalence of tuberculosis. A national study of tuberculosis in the United States of America found that funeral home directors had higher tuberculosis morbidity. This suggests that even when the chest cavity is not opened up, handling intact cadavers presents an increased risk of tuberculosis. Exposure may occur from gurgling at the nose and mouth of the cadaver due to fluid buildup in the chest cavity and putrefaction of tissues and organs. Also, residual air in the deceased's lungs may be exhaled when the body is moved. However, funeral workers have repeated occupational exposures to tuberculosis and so may experience greater risk than is true with the one-time exposure experienced by those handling bodies after a disaster. On the other hand, storage of many cadavers together in temporary mortuaries may present an increased risk of infection; once aerosolized, the tubercle bacilli may remain viable for extended periods of time. The risk of tuberculosis may be reduced by placing a cloth over the deceased's mouth when moving the body and by ensuring suitable ventilation where large numbers of bodies are stored.

Reducing the Risk of Infection

A number of simple measures can be taken to reduce the risk of infection associated with handling dead bodies. Considering that some of the persons doing this work may not have had experience in handling the dead, some basic instruction about the risks and precautions may be required. Universal precautions for blood and body fluids and enteric precautions should be followed. When handling dead bodies, workers should wear gloves, especially if the bodies are badly damaged. Used gloves should be removed and kept in a suitable bag and disposed of appropriately. Where nondisposable gloves are used, they should be cleaned and disinfected. To avoid cross-contamination, personal items should not be handled while wearing soiled gloves, and a new pair is recommended after each body or group of bodies is handled. Other personal protective equipment, such as eyewear, gowns, and masks, are only required where large quantities or splashes of blood are anticipated and are probably not necessary when handling bodies following a natural disaster. Hands should be washed after handling cadavers and before eating, and all equipment, including clothes, stretchers, and vehicles used for transportation, should be washed carefully with a disinfectant. Body bags will further reduce the risk of infection and are useful for the transport of cadavers that have been badly damaged. However, body bags reduce the rate of cooling of the cadaver, thus increasing the rate of decomposition, especially in hot climates. Hepatitis B vaccination will help prevent infection and will be 70% to 80% effective within one week of exposure. Those with prior BCG vaccination may have some protection against tuberculosis, and tuberculin testing may be an appropriate follow-up measure.

DISPOSAL OF DEAD BODIES

There is often considerable concern about the disposal of the dead following a natural disaster. Putrefaction starts soon after death, and suitable storage facilities may not be available for a large number of remains. Concerns about the infectiousness of human remains and the unpleasantness of decaying bodies may lead to rapid unplanned disposal of the dead, sometimes before proper identification of the victim has been made. Concerns about disease may also lead to unnecessary "precautions" such as burying the deceased in common graves and adding chlorinated lime as a "disinfectant".

Cremation

In normal circumstances, human remains are usually buried or cremated. Although cremation will render any remains noninfectious, special equipment and large quantities of fuel are required to achieve high enough temperatures (around 650 °C) for sufficient lengths of time (usually 2.5–3 hours) for complete burning. This makes cremation less practical following mass casualty disasters. Furthermore, cremation should be avoided where victims have not been identified, in which case burial is a more practical option, allowing future disinterment of remains.

Burial

Burial of human remains can be thought of as a particular kind of landfill, similar to that of unlined "dilute and disperse" municipal waste landfill sites. A few studies of cemeteries have detected traceable plumes of indicator bacteria, suggesting that microbiological decay products reach the groundwater. While the pathways and composition of decay products are complex, the principal mechanism of contamination is by rainwater percolating through the soil and coming into contact with buried remains.

The soil in the unsaturated zone (above the water table) is the main line of defense against rainwater leaching from the grave into the groundwater. Pathogens are retained in the unsaturated soil zone, principally due to filtration and adherence to clay particles. Pathogen retention is greater in soils with high clay content but less in soil with a high water content and pH above 7. Pathogens retained in the soil will eventually die off due to lack of nutrients, and die-off increases with reduced soil moisture, increased temperature (die-off rates double with every 10 °C), and soil pH outside the range of 6 to 7.

In a grave site, the disturbed nature of the soil provides an aerated environment that promotes rapid aerobic decomposition. However, it also attracts water, which leads to wetness at grave level, even in otherwise dry areas. Although this favors pathogen survival, decomposition of buried remains produces heat and alkaline soil conditions, possibly increasing pathogen die-off. However, the rate of heat production is highly dependent on burial depth, with significant temperature increases occurring within just a few days after burial at 0.3 m, but taking several weeks at greater depths (1.2 m). While probably similar, it is not clear how the decay and dispersion characteristics may differ where many people are buried simultaneously or where they are buried in communal graves.

Studies of cemetery groundwater have all found evidence of contamination by organic products that are mostly associated with the decay process. No fecal coliforms were found, but pathogenic *Pseudomonas aeruginosa*, streptococci, and clostridia organisms were found in some samples. Groundwater *outside* the cemetery showed that microbiological indicator organisms attenuated rapidly with distance and that the decay plume was better characterized by products associated with the burial process (e.g., coffin materials and embalming substances).

Recommendations for Burial

Although there is some evidence of microbiological contamination in the immediate vicinity of cemeteries, the rapid attenuation of these microorganisms suggests that they pose little risk to the public. However, where it is necessary to choose a new burial site, several issues should be considered. A soil of sand-clay mix of low porosity and a small- to fine-grain texture is likely to maximize pathogen retention in the unsaturated zone. In such soil conditions, the water table should be at least 2.5 m deep in order to allow a "traditional" grave depth of six feet (1.8 m), with a 0.7 m unsaturated zone. This may have to be adjusted for more porous soil conditions, topographic lows, and low points of hydraulic gradients. To protect water supplies, distances of at least 30 m from springs or watercourses and 250 m from any well, borehole, or any source of drinking water have been suggested. However, there are no accepted standards, and distances are best chosen based on local hydrogeological conditions and with the agreement of nearby communities. It may also be likely that following a flood event, soils may be saturated and the water table may be unusually high, making location of a suitable site more difficult.

CONCLUSIONS

There is no evidence that, following a natural disaster, dead bodies pose a risk of epidemics. "Epidemic-causing" acute diseases are unlikely to be more common among disaster victims than among the general population, suggesting that the risk to the general public is negligible. The same is true with casualties of conventional war (as distinct from biological, chemical, or radiological warfare). In both cases it is far more likely that survivors will be a source of disease outbreaks. However, those who handle victims may be exposed to chronic hazards such as blood borne viruses, gastrointestinal infections, and tuberculosis. The risk for this group can be estimated from the disease prevalence in the local population and the likelihood of exposure and transmission.

Simple measures, such as hand-washing and basic hygiene, can reduce the risk of such "occupational" exposures. Those who are likely to be given the task of managing the dead (police, civil defense, military) would benefit from basic instruction as part of disaster preparedness activities. Access to suitable equipment (gloves, body bags, etc.) should also be considered. Following a catastrophic disaster or an event in a remote region, people with no previous instruction may be called upon to assist. Basic messages about suitable precautions would support local authorities and agencies which may themselves be unsure of appropriate methods. Where possible, disposal of the dead should be done according to local custom and practice. Burial is the preferred option in the case of mass casualties and where victims cannot be identified. Burial is unlikely to cause contamination of groundwater if sited correctly. After natural disasters it is important that misinformation about the infectious disease risks of dead bodies do not lead to inappropriate treatment of the victims' bodies.

Epidemiological Surveillance

A system must be established to obtain adequate and timely information on morbidity and mortality in a disaster affected area, especially those with epidemic potential. Reports from medical facilities in respect of admissions, discharges, bed availability, numbers injured and dead at each health center must be garnered. Local press reports, independent reports, rumors in respect of diseases must be taken into cognizance. Both numerator and denominator data must be collected for a more realistic consideration. Morbidity and mortality statistics carry no meaning unless the actual number at risk of disease, injury or death is known. A public health team must be assigned for this function. The return to pre disaster surveillance system should be gradual and planned, as an increased incidence of infectious diseases can be anticipated in an affected area for several months following a catastrophe.

Ideally speaking, attempts to mitigate the results of a disaster would not add to the negative consequences. However, there have been many instances in which inappropriate and/or incomplete management actions taken after a disaster have contributed to unnecessary morbidity, mortality and wastage of resources. Ignorance and/or neglect on the part of individuals and public authorities have led to additional casualties and destruction on several occasions. Many of the same mismanagement problems tend to recur. E.g. Dispatching doctors and paramedics to an area in excess of actual requirements or ignorant of local languages and problems. During the Peruvian earthquake of 1970, volunteers did not speak Spanish and had no disaster relief work experience. Consequently, there was little co-operation or co-ordination between the volunteers and official agencies that were working there. Lack of specific supplies, poor inventory of existing supplies can lead to wasteful indenting, non-positioning of supplies at critical areas and add to casualty figures. During the 1955 hurricanes in Honduras, supplies arrived more than 48 hours after the event.

8 Meta Analysis of Disaster Mismanagement

> "It is not permitted to a man who takes up pen or chisel, to seek originality, for passion is his only business, and he cannot but mould or sing after a new fashion because no disaster is like another."
>
> —*William Butler Yeats*

A retrospective study of disasters has led to an identification of the following gray areas in the management of these phenomena:

- Inadequate appraisal of damages.
- Inadequate problem ranking.
- Inadequate identification of resources.
- Inadequate location of resources.
- Inadequate transportation of resources.
- Inadequate utilization of resources.

Most of the management problems surfaced because relief managers did not know what relief activities were required and/or how they could be accomplished. Existing plans failed to delineate precisely what functions had to be performed, by whom, when, where and in what order to minimize injury, illness, death and damage to property during a disaster.

Failures are largely of the goal or function against standards or agreed criteria, and then failing to identify the lapses in a component or sub system, to end in a catastrophe. High priority must therefore be placed on discussing, locating and minimizing the possibility of such faults in the future by diligent pursuit and improving engineering reliability, instead of just fault finding and scapegoating. Limitation of available data, materials, their functioning under varied stresses and strains may force a designer to adopt some informed guesses in the final assembly or even the goals. This leads to rule of thumb being applied to calculations. Also, there can be no absolute in quality control. Engineering, applied science and design are very much human activities and approximations, and leaps of faith are acknowledged to occur in these fields, especially when novel or path-breaking developments are being pursued. Such procedures are naturally not infallible and this leads to a system having a degree of forgiveness built into it. Ergonomists emphasize the need for studying near-miss phenomenon where little or no damage has occurred and identify the circumstances that could progress to a disaster situation. Other factors such as working conditions, worker selection, absence of safety equipment have also to be analyzed. Hence the need for anticipating disasters and ensuring all round preparedness with rescue and relief plans to tackle it. These emergency plans have to be worked out in earnest, from time to time, as realistic drills followed by a debrief where defects and deficiencies are analyzed and corrected. Focus being kept on probability and the expected and not the unexpected. Acceptable levels of risk must be laid down as guidelines in high-risk areas like the nuclear and chemical industry. Managers must be entrusted with hazard elimination or reduction and also the activation/ implementation of disaster plans to meet all hypothetical emergency situations. Since each disaster is different, one must avoid stereotype responses in such drills, injecting variations to ensure flexibility in responses.

ERROR ANALYSIS: A SIX PRONGED APPROACH

1. THE 5 WHYs STRATEGY

Five iterations of asking why is generally sufficient to get to a root cause. The real key is to encourage the troubleshooter to avoid assumptions and logic traps and, instead, trace the chain of causality in direct increments from the effect through any layers of abstraction to a root cause that still has some connection to the original problem. Very often, the answer to the first "why" will prompt another "why" and the answer to the second "why" will prompt another and so on; hence the name the 5 whys strategy.

History

The technique was originally developed by Sakichi Toyoda and was later used within Toyota Motor Corporation during the evolution of their manufacturing methodologies. It is a critical component of problem solving training delivered as part of the induction into the Toyota Production System. The architect of the Toyota Production System, Taiichi Ohno, described the 5 whys method as "... the basis of Toyota's scientific approach ... by repeating why five times, the nature of the problem as well as its solution becomes clear." The tool has seen widespread use beyond Toyota, and is now used within Kaizen, lean manufacturing and Six Sigma.

Benefits of the 5 Whys

- It helps to quickly determine the root cause of a problem.
- It is easy to learn and apply.

When looking to solve a problem, start at the end result and work backward (toward the root cause), continually asking: "Why?" This will need to be repeated over and over until the root cause of the problem becomes apparent, The 5 Whys technique is a simple technique that can help you quickly get to the root of a problem. But that is all it is, and the more complex things get, the more likely it is to lead you down a false trail. If it doesn't quickly give you an answer that's obviously right, then you may need more sophisticated technique problem solving techniques Because it is so elementary in nature, it can be adapted quickly and applied to most any problem. Bear in mind, however, that if it doesn't prompt an intuitive answer, other problem-solving techniques may need to be applied.

Drawbacks

- Tendency for investigators to stop at symptoms rather than going on to lower level root causes.
- Inability to go beyond the investigator's current knowledge – can't find causes that they don't already know
- Lack of support to help the investigator to ask the right "why" questions.
- Results aren't repeatable – different people using 5 whys come up with different causes for the same problem.

- The tendency to a isolate single root cause, whereas each question could elicit many different root causes.

These can be significant problems when the method is applied through deduction only. On-the-spot verification of the answer to the current "why" question, before proceeding to the next, is recommended as a good practice to avoid these issues.

2. ROOT CAUSE ANALYSIS

Root Cause analysis is a process for identifying the causes that underlie variation in performance, including the occurrence or possible occurrence of a sentinel event. A Sentinel event is a major adverse event that could have been prevented.

- Root Cause analysis helps identify what, how and why something happened, thus preventing recurrence.
- Root causes are underlying, are reasonably identifiable, can be controlled by management and allow for generation of recommendations.
- The process involves data collection, cause charting, rot cause identification and prevention recommendation generation and implementation.

When significant events occur, whether operational failures or injury events, comprehensive methods of approach are key. Beyond accurately determining the root cause of the event, an objective, fact-based method must be developed to ensure that the event will not re-occur. Root cause analysis (RCA) is a process designed for use in investigating and categorizing the root causes of events with safety, health, environmental, quality, reliability and production impacts. The term "event" is used to generically identify occurrences that produce or have the potential to produce these types of consequences. Simply stated, RCA is a tool designed to help identify not only *what* and *how* an event occurred, but also *why* it happened. Only when investigators are able to determine why an event or failure occurred will they be able to specify workable corrective measures that prevent future events of the type observed. Understanding why an event occurred is the key to developing effective recommendations. Imagine an occurrence during which an operator is instructed to close valve A; instead, the operator closes valve B. The typical investigation would probably conclude operator error was the cause.

This is an accurate description of what happened and how it happened. However, if the analysts stop here, they have not probed deeply enough to understand the reasons for the mistake. Therefore, they do not know what to do to prevent it from occurring again. In the case of the operator who turned the wrong valve, we are likely to see recommendations such as retrain the operator on the procedure, remind all operators to be alert when manipulating valves or emphasize to all personnel that careful attention to the job should be maintained at all times. Such recommendations do little to prevent future occurrences. Generally, mistakes do not just happen but can be traced to some well-defined causes. In the case of the valve error, we might ask, "Was the procedure confusing? Were the valves clearly labeled? Was the operator familiar with this particular task?"

The answers to these and other questions will help determine why the error took place and what the organization can do to prevent recurrence. In the case of the valve error, example recommendations might include revising the procedure or performing procedure validation to ensure references to valves match the valve labels found in the field.

Identifying root causes is the key to preventing similar recurrences. An added benefit of an effective RCA is that, over time, the root causes identified across the population of occurrences can be used to target major opportunities for improvement. If, for example, a significant number of analyses point to procurement inadequacies, then resources can be focused on improvement of this management system. Trending of root causes allows development of systematic improvements and assessment of the impact of corrective programs.

Definition

Although there is substantial debate on the definition of root cause, we use the following:

1. Root causes are specific underlying causes.
2. Root causes are those that can reasonably be identified.
3. Root causes are those management has control to fix.
4. Root causes are those for which effective recommendations for preventing recurrences can be generated.

Root causes are underlying causes. The investigator's goal should be to identify specific underlying causes. The more specific the investigator can be about why an event occurred, the easier it will be to arrive at recommendations that will prevent recurrence.

Root causes are those that can reasonably be identified. Occurrence investigations must be cost beneficial. It is not practical to keep valuable manpower occupied indefinitely searching for the root causes of occurrences. Structured RCA helps analysts get the most out of the time they have invested in the investigation.

Root causes are those over which management has control. Analysts should avoid using general cause classifications such as operator error, equipment failure or external factor. Such causes are not specific enough to allow management to make effective changes. Management needs to know exactly why a failure occurred before action can be taken to prevent recurrence.

We must also identify a root cause that management can influence. Identifying "severe weather" as the root cause of parts not being delivered on time to customers is not appropriate. Severe weather is not controlled by the management.

Root causes are those for which effective recommendations can be generated. Recommendations should directly address the root causes identified during the investigation. If the analysts arrive at vague recommendations such as, "Improve adherence to written policies and procedures," then they probably have not found a basic and specific enough cause and need to expend more effort in the analysis process.

Four Major Steps

The RCA is a four-step process involving the following:

1. Data collection.
2. Causal factor charting.
3. Root Cause identification.
4. Recommendation generation and implementation.

Step One—Data Collection

The first step in the analysis is to gather data. Without complete information and an understanding of the event, the causal factors and root causes associated with the event cannot be identified. The majority of time spent analyzing an event is spent in gathering data.

Step Two—Causal Factor Charting

Causal factor charting provides a structure for investigators to organize and analyze the information gathered during the investigation and identify gaps and deficiencies in knowledge as the investigation progresses. The causal factor chart is simply a sequence diagram with logic tests that describes the events leading up to an occurrence, plus the conditions surrounding these events. Preparation of the causal factor chart should begin as soon as investigators start to collect information about the occurrence. They begin with a skeleton chart that is modified as more relevant facts are uncovered. The causal factor chart should drive the data collection process by identifying data needs. Data collection continues until the investigators are satisfied with the thoroughness of the chart (and hence are satisfied with the thoroughness of the investigation). When the entire occurrence has been charted out, the investigators are in a good position to identify the major contributors to the incident, called causal factors. Causal factors are those contributors (human errors and component failures) that, if eliminated, would have either prevented the occurrence or reduced its severity.

In many traditional analyses, the most visible causal factor is given all the attention. Rarely, however, is there just one causal factor; events are usually the result of a combination of contributors.

When only one obvious causal factor is addressed, the list of recommendations will likely not be complete. Consequently, the occurrence may repeat itself because the organization did not learn all that it could from the event.

Step Three—Root Cause Identification

After all the causal factors have been identified, the investigators begin root cause identification. This step involves the use of a decision diagram called the Root Cause Map to identify the underlying reason or reasons for each causal factor. The map structures the reasoning process of the investigators by helping them answer questions about why particular causal factors exist or occurred. The identification of root causes helps the investigator determine the reasons the event occurred so the problems surrounding the occurrence can be addressed.

Step Four—Recommendation Generation and Implementation

The next step is the generation of recommendations. Following identification of the root causes for a particular causal factor, achievable recommendations for preventing its recurrence are then generated.

The root cause analyst is often not responsible for the implementation of recommendations generated by the analysis. However, if the recommendations are not implemented, the effort expended in performing the analysis is wasted. In addition, the events that triggered the analysis should be expected to recur. Organizations need to ensure that recommendations are tracked to completion.

Presentation of Results

Root Cause summary tables can organize the information compiled during data analysis, root cause identification and recommendation generation. Each column represents a major aspect of the RCA process.

- In the first column, a general description of the causal factor is presented along with sufficient background information for the reader to be able to understand the need to address this causal factor.
- The second column shows the Path or Paths through the Route Cause Map associated with the causal factor.
- The third column presents recommendations to address each of the root causes identified.

Use of this three-column format aids the investigator in ensuring root causes and recommendations are developed for each causal factor.

The end result of an RCA investigation is generally an investigation report. The format of the report is usually well defined by the administrative documents governing the particular reporting system, but the completed causal factor chart and causal factor summary tables provide most of the information required by most reporting systems.

THE SIX SIGMA APPROACH

The Six Sigma is a registered service mark and trademark of Motorola, Inc. Six Sigma's implicit goal is to improve all processes to that level of quality or better.

The term "six sigma process" comes from the notion that if one has six standard deviations between the process mean and the nearest specification limit, as shown in the graphic, there will be practically no items that fail to meet specifications. This is based on the calculation method employed in process capability studies. The approach is as follows:-

- *Define* high-level project goals and the current process.
- *Measure* key aspects of the current process and collect relevant data.
- *Analyze* the data to verify cause-and-effect relationships. Determine what the relationships are, and attempt to ensure that all factors have been considered.
- *Improve* or optimize the process based upon data analysis using techniques like Design of experiments.
- *Control* to ensure that any deviations from target are corrected before they result in defects. Set up pilot runs to establish process capability, move on to production, set up control mechanisms and continuously monitor the process.

Six Sigma as a basic version of quality improvement, narrowly designed to fix an existing process and does not help in "coming up with new products or technologies. The Six Sigma model assumes that the process data always conform to the normal distribution "sigma levels". It reflects short-term rather than long-term performance

THE KAIZEN APPROACH

Kaizen is Japanese for "improvement" and referring to a philosophy or practices focusing on continuous improvement in manufacturing activities, all business activities, or even all aspects of life, depending on interpretation and usage. Kaizen is primarily a reactive process where you "check" to see if anything is wrong, then go about fixing it. While this works for lower level processes, it must be advanced to include a creative element where one actively looks for ways of improving - the key being that the worker needs to know what is important to the company to improve. There should also be room for cases where a worker makes a recommendation that doesn't fit the mold of the company's target improvements. Many new companies have started due to workers who saw a means of quantum improvement which their original employer failed to recognize despite being highlighted by the worker.

The cycle of kaizen activity can be defined as:

- Standardize an operation ! measure the standardized operation (find cycle time and amount of in-process inventory) ! gauge measurements against requirements ! innovate to meet requirements and increase productivity ! standardize the new, improved operations ! continue cycle *ad infinitum*.

This is also known as the Shewhart cycle, Deming cycle, or PDCA.

The five foundation elements of kaizen:

- Team work, Personal Discipline, Improved morale, Quality circles and Suggestions for improvement.

Out of this foundation, three key factors arise:

- Elimination of waste (muda) and incorporation of efficiency.
- The Kaizen five - S framework for good housekeeping.
- Seiri – tidiness, Seiton – orderliness, Seiso– cleanliness, Seiketsu – standardized clean-up, Shitsuke – discipline and Standardiza-tion.

T-H-O METHOD OF BEHAVIOUR ANALYSIS

- Trigger + Outcome = Habit.
- Triggers initiate actions/behavior.
- Outcomes control actions/behavior.
- Actions become Habits (*good or bad*).

Consider the model of human behavior that we call THO = Trigger – Habit – Outcome. Research indicates that nearly all accidents happen because of unsafe acts. Some of these acts result from intentional deviations (poor performance or poor behavior), which can and do become bad habits.

There are two things that control the behavior or habit – the trigger and the outcome. This model is based on many observations over decades of study showing that humans can be expected to build habits a certain way depending on the Trigger for an action and depending on the outcome that results from that action.

Habit is someone's usual way of behaving. Trigger is what causes an action or habit. Outcome is the result of an action or habit.

These studies found that outcomes are by far the stronger influence on how we build habits (good or bad). Certain types of outcomes are much more powerful than others. Many safety and reliability programs fail because they focus on the Triggers (such as safety rules, meetings, and procedures). Though these are necessary to get the right habits set, triggers are nearly useless if the right kind of outcome is not present to lock in the right habits.

What is A Trigger?

A trigger causes an action or habit. A trigger can be:

- A one-time happening.
- Or it can be something that has been going on for days, weeks, months or longer.
- A trigger can also be a devastating event – a sudden loss, troubling news – causing you to be distracted or impatient.

Reason People Acquire Poor Behaviors (bad habits).

- Trigger + Outcome = Habit.
- Triggers initiate actions/behavior.
- Outcomes control actions/behavior.
- Actions become Habits (*good or bad*).

Fundamental Theory for Managing Behavior – S-C-P Model:

An action is the way someone acts. An outcome is the result of an action or habit. The most effective outcome in encouraging an improvement in actions or habits is an outcome that is:

- Soon.
- Certain and
- *Positive.*

On the other hand, an outcome that is negative – whether it is soon or certain – is an incentive for a person to work harder at not getting "caught" rather than changing for the better. The stronger outcome (the one that sets the habit most of the time) is the one that is soonest, most certain, and positive. This is a very critical discovery in the understanding of habits and performance.

Here are the three factors determining the power a consequence has on influencing behavior:

- *Timing:* An outcome that follows soon after an action controls the habit more effectively than an outcome that occurs later.
- *Consistency:* An outcome that is certain to follow an action controls the habit more powerfully than an unpredictable or uncertain outcome.
- *Significance:* A positive outcome controls habits more powerfully than a negative outcome.

So, the way to improve Safety Performance (change peoples Habits to the right ones) is to find the optimum outcomes for their actions and then be consistent and certain and soon with the outcomes. The initial soon-certain-positive outcomes in favor of safe behavior build new attitudes toward safety. These new attitudes in turn become the source of both broader and more finely tuned attention to safety, bringing new soon-certain-positive outcomes to bear on the facility's safety performance. In this way the positive and continuous improvement process is established in a facility, becoming a safety mechanism with the goals that are achieved when the new safety-oriented habits are established.

Range of Possible Outcomes

Between the most powerful outcomes (soon-certain-positive) and the weakest ones (late-uncertain-negative) there is a range of outcomes that are mixtures of these three characteristics. Many times, however, each of the outcomes of a particular action is a mixture of strong and weak effects.

Many incentive programs offer rewards that are structured like a savings plan – the workers are expected to spend their energy or their time on a safety effort (similar to saving some money each month) for the sake of an outcome that is positive, but whose power is weak because it is deferred. One thinks of lottery-like safety competitions where winning is beyond the player's control. In the face of these odds, it can be much more pleasant (positive/strong) to spend the money (or spend the time) on some known good (certain/strong) now (soon/strong) than to pay the price (soon) for some safety award or bonus (positive) that they may or may not actually receive (uncertain or late). Similarly, many safety programs are oriented toward penalties and punishments, like the traffic citation for speeding. Such a program is effective thinks of lottery-like safety competitions where winning is beyond the player's control. In the face of these odds, it can be much more pleasant (positive/strong) to spend the money (or spend the time) on some known good (certain/strong) now (soon/strong) than to pay the price (soon) for some safety award or bonus (positive) that they may or may not actually receive (uncertain or late). Similarly, many safety programs are oriented toward penalties and punishments, like the traffic citation for speeding. Such a program is effective in those very rare cases where being caught and cited soon is very certain to follow as an outcome of infringement of the rules. However, even in this case, the management effort is wasteful because resources are spent on delivering *negative outcomes*. Thus, the negative approach (even if it did not have unhelpful side effects) is less effective than a positive approach because, for the same effort, negative outcomes are less powerful in their impact on worker habits than positive outcomes are. In addition, there are always side effects. Most managers know that the punitive approach presents several serious problems. Such a program usually only teaches people not to get caught again, like the speeding example. As a practical matter, in most facilities it is as very expensive to ticket every safety violation as it is for the police to ticket every driver who exceeds the speed limit. Finally, a safety effort that relies solely on the threat of some accumulating physical harm to motivate workers is like a stop-smoking campaign that expects smokers to quit smoking just because they have been educated about associated lung problems.

THO Analysis brings clarity to these matters by insisting on a simple fact:

When a facility's safety effort is not working, it is because the outcomes in favor of safe habits are weaker than the outcomes in favor of unsafe habits.

The Range of Outcomes

Peer Pressure

One of the most powerful Outcomes at work is *peer pressure*, which offers immediate, certain, rewards to the worker who conforms by accepting him or her as *one of the guys*. A supervisor, too, may inadvertently encourage or maintain unsafe habits by praising production performance even though the supervisor saw the workers risking accident or injury while they were hustling. The effect of this praise is further compounded when the worker knows that the supervisor saw him taking risks.

Unnoticed Unsafe Acts – A Positive Outcome

Finally, the most common outcome in favor of unsafe habits is simply that most unsafe acts are not even observed, let alone noted and addressed. In this case, not being observed represents a soon-certain-positive consequence in favor of unsafe acts – the worker knows (certain) that unsafe acts go unnoticed (non-negative=positive) continually (soon).

A Soon/Certain/+ outcome is just twice as powerful as a Late/Uncertain/- outcome, that there is 4 times more chance of the worker not observing safety precautions. However, it turns out that Soon/Certain/+ outcome is 5 to 10 times stronger than a Late/Uncertain/- outcome, so there is *actually a 90% chance that the worker will NOT wear a personal protection when required the first time, after the habit is established, the chances are even higher that he will NOT wear the proper PPE.* So, if increased punishment and enforcement is not the solution, how do we get workers to put on the proper PPE? How do we build safe habits? We must change the Outcomes to be in favor of safety.

CONCLUSION

A safety program that tries to motivate the use of personal protective equipment (PPE) and other routine safety precautions solely by stressing the possibility of possible loss/injury (such as hearing loss) is relying on the weakest kind of consequence-one which occurs slowly or eventually (later), if it happens at all (uncertain), and which is negative. Common sense may indicate that it is illogical to risk something as serious as hearing loss for some very small but immediate convenience or comfort, such as not having to locate and wear protective equipment for hearing.

The fact is that in the give and take of everyday situations most people continually take such risks for precisely these small but immediate, certain, positive outcomes. Whether it is common sense or not, it is human nature to behave this way.

In summary, Soon-Certain-Positive outcomes are the outcomes needed to change behavior. Developing new triggers and outcomes then is necessary to improve safety.

The Safety Task Action Reporting (STAR) system is the main (most successful) process used for improving these work habits.

Management's 2 Key Roles

1. *Improve Human Factors*
   - Provide leadership and resources and follow-through.

- Review each category for "effectiveness," not just compliance.
- Identify what it will take to remedy the weaknesses (especially core issues such as English writing and reading skills),
- Follow-through and continuity ("5–10 year" thinking).

2. *Improve Habits of Workers*
   - Provide leadership and resources; set incentives to activities that will change behaviors.
   - Develop inventory of key behavior issues from incident reports.
   - Implement observation program/tracking program.
   - Set example (do not show them poor habits yourselves).
   - Reward activities (leading indicators) rather than outcomes, to prevent workers from hiding incidents to meet target.
   - Follow-through and continuity.

COGNITIVE RELIABILITY AND ERROR ANALYSIS METHOD (CREAM)

Description

The growing dependence of working environments on complex technology has created many challenges and led to a large number of accidents. Although the quality of organization and management within the work environment plays an important role in these accidents, the significance of individual human action (as a direct cause and as a mitigating factor) is undeniable. This has created a need for new, integrated approaches to accident analysis and risk assessment.

The use of CREAM is, therefore, both timely and useful. It presents an error taxonomy which integrates individual, technological and organizational factors based on cognitive engineering principles. In addition to the necessary theoretical foundation, it provides a step-by-step description of how the taxonomy can be applied to analyse as well as predict performance using a context-dependent cognitive model.

CREAM can be used as a second-generation human reliability analysis (HRA) approach in probabilistic safety assessment (PSA), as a stand-alone method for accident analysis and as part of a larger design method for interactive systems. In particular, the use of CREAM will enable system designers and risk analysts to:

- Identify tasks that require human cognition and therefore depend on cognitive reliability.
- Determine the conditions where cognitive reliability and ensuing risk may be reduced.
- Provide an appraisal of the consequences of human performance on system safety which can be used in PSA.

Audience

For practitioners of human reliability analysis and accident analysis; designers of interactive systems for industrial applications; and researchers in the fields of human error, cognitive engineering and cognitive ergonomics.

9 Relief Measures During Disasters

> "Survival! Living things have been doing just that for a long, long time. Through every kind of disaster and setback and catastrophe. We are survivors."
>
> —*Robert Fulghum*

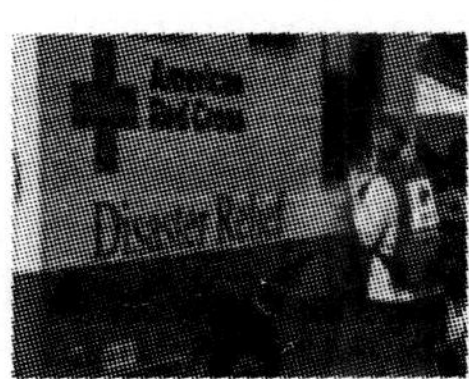

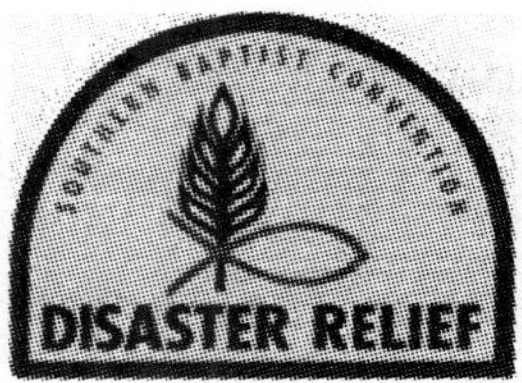

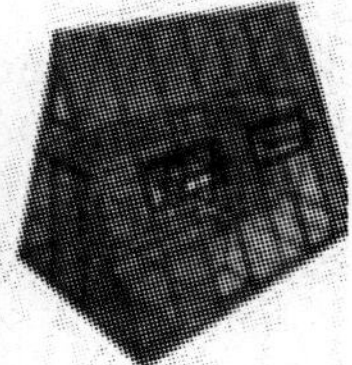

Fig. 9.1

Relief efforts are dependent upon good situation analysis and response. The two activities are very closely inter-related. Inputs like surveillance data etc may be desirable, but what is essential is a single person with sound, practical managerial skills at the helm of any relief operation. The desire to provide immediate relief may lead to hasty decisions that are not based on the actual needs of the affected population. There is a need therefore for surveillance methods to obtain information required for making relief decisions e.g. specific problems in an affected area, the resources available and the relief activities already in progress.

INTERNATIONAL DISASTER RELIEF LAWS, RULES AND PRINCIPLES (IDRL)

(Started 2001 and formally instituted in Nov 2007)

A legal framework contributing to an improvement in the delivery of disaster relief aid is given only after an appeal by the State affected and consent to aid by the affected State. The State must ensure timely appeal after a quick assessment. Aid asked must be specific–types and amounts needed, specified services and expertise.

Goals

1. A decrease in the number of deaths, injuries and impact from disasters.
2. A decrease in the number of deaths, illnesses and impact from diseases and public health emergencies.
3. A increase in local capacity to address the most urgent aspects of vulnerability.
4. Recognize that the principal victims of disasters are families whose lives are turned upside down by a major disaster

and they need immediate, effective support.

Disaster Management Legislations

Provisional rules when a disaster is declared may require modification of existing regulations, plans and procedures.

Be prepared for international aid in a crisis situation.

Domestic laws regarding entry and operation of personnel must be eased– visas, permits must be issued free of cost. Temporary recognition of foreign degrees and qualifications. Temporary registration/ licenses for doctors, paramedics.

Call military in only after first considering civilian alternatives.

Issuer of work permits and licenses to IT and telecommunication personnel with priority access to bandwidth frequencies and satellite sløts for telecommunications and data transfer.

Less administrative and legal barriers to export, transit, import and re-export of medicines and equipments during disasters.

Proper accounting of aid materials to avoid misuse and misappropriation.

Drugs must have 12 months shelf life from day of landing.

All services must be run 24 × 7- no question of fixed working hours.

Air transport to crew.

Provision of buildings for offices and warehouse for storing aid.

Logistics of cargo imported.

Max regional and international support.

Need based aid on priorities.

Provided to all without discrimination.

No political or commercial interests.

Provide respect for human diversity and dignity with zero tolerance for intolerance, discrimination, and social exclusion.

No attempt to gather sensitive information against aid initiatives.

Adequate resources must be provided to all based on International norms.

Permit overflights.

Avoid over regulation, bottlenecks and red tape.

Good liaison with governmental and outside actors at all levels.

Resolution 4

Comprehensive Legal policy and institutional frameworks and planning for disasters preventive, mitigation, preparation, relief and recovery, improved safety and resilience.

To special needs of vulnerable groups– children, displaced, elderly, women, those with disabilities, HIV+. Response must be adequate, consistent with International standards of quality, coordinated by domestic and international actors, sensitive to cultural, religious and social customs and traditions. Involvement of locals and affected persons in design, implementation, monitoring and evaluation. Competent–by adequately trained and qualified personnel.

Actions must strengthen local DRR and decrease future vulnerabilities.

Transparency–share information.

DISASTER RELIEF

Definition

Goods and services provided to meet the immediate needs of disaster affected communities.

Goods

Supplies intended to give relief and help with initial recovery of communities affected by disasters.

Services

Activities (rescue and medical) to assist disaster affected communities.

Ask Why needed?

What is our aim? Clear task statement distinct from purpose.

What are we trying to achieve?

Why are we trying to achieve it?

MISSION STATEMENT

E.g. To provide humanitarian assistance to North West India in order to encourage refugees/displaced to return home.

Decision to Intervene

Can you offer something worthwhile to the situation?

If so, can it be delivered at an affordable cost?

Will the cost be purely financial or are there opportunity costs in addition?

Are there other predictable constraints?

What are the consequences of deployment to the organization?

Hard nosed issues of cost-benefit analysis in a humanitarian operation.

A basic three-step approach closed feedback system would be to:

a. *Collect data:* Both denominator and numerator data are required for realistic determination of the magnitude of a problem e.g. the people at risk of injury as well as the numbers already injured. Without denominator data, one cannot realistically determine the magnitude of a problem, as 10 deaths in a city of 1 million would have a different interpretation from the same number of deaths in a sparsely populated area.

b *Analyze data:* This involves collating and interpreting data. Questions such as the following will have to be asked:
   - What problems are occurring?
   - Why are they occurring?
   - Where all are problems occurring?
   - Who all are affected?
   - What problems are causing the greatest morbidity and mortality?
   - What problems are increasing or decreasing?
   - What problems are self-limiting?
   - What problems will increase if ignored or unattended?
   - What relief resources are available?
   - How can relief resources be used most efficiently?
   - What relief activities are in progress?
   - Are relief activities meeting relief needs?
   - What additional information is needed for decision making?

c. *Respond to data:* Based on the answers to the above lot of questions and the data available, an appropriate response to the situation must be planned after prioritizing the relief activities. An ongoing analysis must be done to measure the results of the relief measures and modifications effected, based on the changing disaster scenario based on the feedback. Like triage, the 3-step approach of data collection, analysis and response has to be subject to a continuous reappraisal of relief needs and their effects.

AFTER A DISASTER, DO

- *Consult with the countries' health disaster coordinators for information about post-disaster health needs.* After a disaster, this coordinator will conduct an assessment, in cooperation with PAHO/WHO and interested NGOs, to determine health needs. Don't start collecting relief items until you have this information.
- *Whenever possible, donate cash or credit directly to the national health authorities, to international agencies, or channel it through well-established private agencies.* Most of the relief items needed can be purchased

locally or in neighboring countries. Cash also can be used to restore the pre-disaster level of health care conditions and to replace national resources that have been diverted from essential programs and used for the emergency.

- *Assist countries during the preparedness, rehabilitation and reconstruction phases.* Unfortunately, disasters are rarely newsworthy once the immediate emergency phase is over. Yet, after a disaster, an affected country will deplete much of its financial and material resources. Later, the affected country will need even more international aid for repairs and reconstruction.
- *Coordinate the efforts* of independent assessment teams or fact-finding missions with those of the affected country and other agencies.

DISCOURAGE SENDING . . .

- *Used clothing, shoes, etc:* In most cases, the local community donates more than enough of these items to meet the demand. It is more economical, convenient and sanitary to purchase items locally than to ship used items. Refer offers of this type of assistance to local charities or voluntary agencies.
- *Household foods:* The same applies for food items. A disaster is not likely to cause a national food shortage in Latin America and the Caribbean, although the international media may highlight local distribution problems.
- *Household medicines or prescriptions:* These items are medically and legally inappropriate. Pharmaceutical products take up needed space and divert the attention of medical personnel from other more pressing tasks to sort, classify, and label them.
- *Blood and blood derivatives:* There is much less need for blood than the public commonly believes. Local blood donors in the affected country will cover the victims' needs. This type of donation is unsuitable because it requires quality and safety controls, such as refrigeration or screening for detection of HIV.
- *Medical or paramedical personnel or teams:* Local health services are able to handle emergency medical care to disaster victims. In fact, most countries have a relatively high physician-to-population ratio.
- *If international aid is needed, neighboring countries are in the best position to assist during the first 24 hours.* Exceptions to this are highly skilled specialists who have been specifically requested by the Ministry of Health. Foreign medical or paramedical personnel who are unfamiliar with local language and conditions should be encouraged to remain at home.
- *Field hospitals, modular medical units:* Considering that this type of equipment is justified only when it meets medium-term needs, it should not be accepted unless it is donated. Equipment specifications, such as weight, volume, freight and installation costs should be provided to the Ministry of Health so that they can decide on its usefulness.

CONSULT FURTHER ABOUT DONATIONS OF

- *Used medical equipment:* Specifications should be provided. If the value of the equipment justifies it, an on-site inspection may be arranged by a technician in the donor country or an international agency such as PAHO/WHO or the Red Cross.
- *New equipment:* When considering these donations, take into account the cost of transportation by air freight, and the

continued availability of spare parts. Most manufacturers are willing to wait several days to allow countries to consult with the proper technical ministry.

- *Tents:* Many countries stock a large quantity of tents that are manufactured locally. The funds that donors are willing to spend to purchase and airlift tents could be put to better use purchasing reconstruction materials locally.
- *Vaccines:* Most often they are neither needed nor approved by the Ministry of Health. Check the presentation, dosage, expiration date, and inform the Ministry of Health, or check with PAHO/WHO.

Logistical and political problems must be resolved to avoid mutual suspicion. Telemedicine networks must be established on priority. A tracking system to record aid that has arrived where it was supposed to and that it had the desired effect to the aid effort.

The Future

Field trained, standing assessment teams will be rapidly injected into a conflict or disaster area at the earliest opportunity. They will be self sufficient in food and shelter etc and will conduct spot assessment using video/still photographs and a pre prepared electronic questionnaire. Once their initial assessment is completed, the team will transmit their data to all interested parties and on the internet. Local infrastructures would be least able to cope with the situation let alone make an assessment. The teams will use high bandwidth to transmit video footages and allow VTC meetings to establish direct links between donors and recipients to ensure a planned response to the affected community's needs based demands.

10 Post Disaster Surveillance

> "We are never ripe till we have been made so by suffering."
>
> —*Henry Ward Beecher*

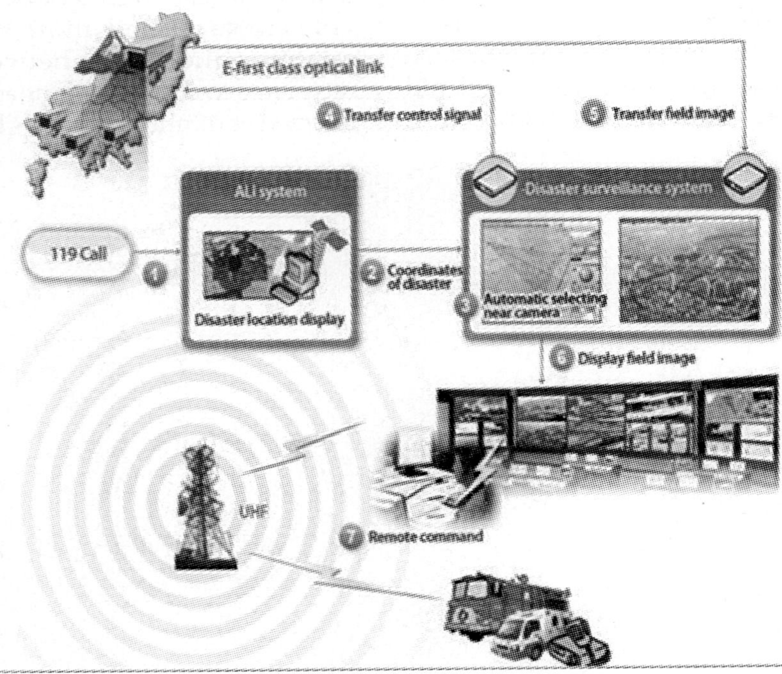

Fig. 10.1

Surveillance following disaster evolves in phases, each one based on the previous one. The first is an immediate assessment, based on the analysis of the available data to determine the forms of relief needed immediately. A short-term assessment is then used to make relief decisions followed by an ongoing assessment procedure to precisely determine maintenance and modifications in relief activities.

IMMEDIATE ASSESSMENT (QUICK AND DIRTY)

The object of this phase of surveillance is to obtain as much general information as possible and as quickly as possible. The most basic information needed at this point in time are:

i. The geographic extent of the disaster-stricken area.
ii. Major problems occurring in the area.
iii. The number of people affected.

An aerial survey would be an effective method to define the geographical extent of the disaster-stricken area and observing major damages and destruction. Census data may be reviewed to arrive at an estimation of population figures affected or at risk. Data regarding the numbers of deaths and injuries may be obtained from all local hospitals and clinics. The most frequent cause of death and major injuries may be determined to predict requirements for further medicare. Forecast of impending problems can sometimes be had from past experience with a particular type of disaster e.g. disruption of water supplies following earthquakes, special problems associated with specific chemical and nuclear disasters etc. As a general picture of a disaster situation is obtained, one must decide if the available data is sufficient to determine immediate relief needs and, if not, what additional information is required to make the decision.

SHORT-TERM ASSESSMENT

This involves a more systematic method of data collection to have a reliable and detailed information about the problems The geographical area affected is divided into smaller areas or blocks to be surveyed simultaneously by different work teams. Their feedback is based on simple, brief and specific reporting forms or questionnaires over a specified time frame. The following composite list of information needed to make relief decisions is suggested, and only those truly needed in a given situation may be requested:

- The number of persons known to be dead, grouped by name, age and sex.
- The number estimated to be seriously injured and/or requiring medicare, grouped as per name, age, sex and type of injury/morbidity.
- The estimated number of homes destroyed, homes uninhabitable and those still capable of affording shelter.
- Conditions of schools, theatres, halls, churches, temples and public buildings.
- Condition and extent of water supply available.
- Condition and extent of food supply.
- Condition and extent of electricity supply.
- The geographical extent of the affected area as defined by streets or other clear boundaries or structures.
- The condition of roads, bridges, communication lines and public utilities.
- Location and condition of health facilities.
- Estimates of medical personnel, equipment and supplies available.
- Descriptions of relief activities already in progress (Search rescue, first aid, food relief, other agencies/NGOs).
- Determine the stricken population's immediate needs and compile a 'needs' list.

Other factors that may affect short-term assessment are the size and terrain at the disaster-affected area, the distances between areas to be surveyed, the types and number of personnel available, the methods of communication, transportation available and usable in the areas to be surveyed. Based on factors like these, short- term assessment can take as little as 4-5 hours or as much as 2 to 3 days. One must make an appreciation of the time factor in a given situation and set a reasonable time frame for return and analysis of data.

Short-term assessment must help one determine relief priorities as soon as possible (ASAP) and estimate resources needed and to be demanded in order to launch a full-scale relief effort. All channels of public information and mass media must be utilized to disseminate the information obtained and relief actions taken e.g. provision of hot meals or a soup kitchen at a school in the affected area etc.

ONGOING SURVEILLANCE

On completion of the short-term assessment and the initiation of relief measures, surveillance becomes an ongoing system. Overall relief operations should be periodically reviewed and altered to correspond to the current situation. House to house and random surveys can be initiated to monitor relief measures and quell rumors and misinformation that can trigger inappropriate and calamitous panic responses. On site personnel must make regular reports to the command and control facility. A reliable overseer or inspector can be sent from time to time to double-check on relief measures or investigate reported problems. Ongoing surveillance can throw light on new problems that may require modified response. Decision-makers must be kept appraised of the ongoing efforts and problems, and the activities of different agencies must be coordinated to prevent duplication of relief efforts.

A relief plan may include all or some of the following activities:

- Rescue of victims and disentanglement.
- Provision of emergency medical care.
- Containment of physical dangers like fires, gas leaks etc.
- Evacuation of population at risk e.g. chemical/nuclear leaks.
- Provision of preventive care like immunization.
- Provision of routine medical care.
- Provision of potable water.
- Provision of survival rations e.g. soup kitchens, distribution of boiled sweets/ chocolates.
- Provision of routine/protective clothing, gas masks, smoke masks.
- Provision of shelter and warmth.
- Field sanitation and excreta disposal.
- Control of vector borne diseases.
- Disposal of the dead by appropriate and sanitary methods after identification.
- Disposal of solid waste.

For the execution of all of the above activities, the relief plan must also address the following support activities:

- Co ordination of volunteer assistance
- Management of facilities.
- Management of the communication systems networks.
- Management of transportation including refrigerated containers for mobile morgue facility where possible and heavy earth moving machinery, cranes, bulldozers etc.
- Management of PRO and front office rumor control services.
- Traffic and crowd control
- Management of video and photographic units.

EVALUATION METHODOLOGY

Evaluation of any endeavour must be an integral part of any relief operation and should consist of comparing what actually happened with what was intended. That is, the actual with the desired, for both the overall disaster management efforts, as well as for each discrete category of the relief efforts.

It is therefore important to set objectives at the very outset, which specify the intended and desirable outcome of the relief. The general objectives would be to eliminate unnecessary mortality, morbidity and economic loss directly attributable to mismanagement of disaster relief efforts. More specific objectives could be the measurement of the levels of mortality, morbidity and economic loss in a given disaster situation against a disaster relief managed with current levels of scientific, technical and operational knowledge elsewhere. Specific and measurable objectives for each of the operational categories of disaster relief, e.g., minimum food requirements for a specified population, for a specified time.

Where these objectives are not met, the evaluation process must be continued to identify the reasons for the discrepancy and give suggestions for remedial actions to prevent such deviations in the future. The role of simulated management can be undertaken to test the various components before actual implementation.

11 Warnings and Alerts During Disasters

> "Many a happiness in life, as many a disaster, can be due to chance, but the peace within us can never be governed by chance."
>
> —*Maurice Maeterlinc*

For many individuals and groups, an encounter with the unfamiliar, unknown situation is likely to generate anxiety. The anxiety is less, of course, if the threat is a recurrent and a familiar one, and the individual response too is attenuated. Another way of looking at a threat is to regard it as a piece of information which must be absorbed and processed appropriately by a psychological or social system so that an individual can respond to it in a considered and analytic manner. If the information input is excessive or distorted, the response is likely to be inadequate. Groups under threat develop collective response based on the inputs of information that affects their anxiety level to a threat. Usually an evaluative and emotional response to the impending danger results in a unified group perception. But in small groups that are dispersed and with inadequate internal solidarity among its members, a major threat is likely to create a dispersive effect. In larger, more cohesive groups, responses may be calm and coping. When the group considers the possibility of danger as remote, they tend to ignore warnings, overcome by a sense of personal invulnerability. When the danger comes a little nearer, the threat is acknowledged as real and personal inconveniences disregarded in order to confront the threat. However, the responses and responsibilities may vary. E.g. some will black out the front windows more fully than the back ones during an air raid threat, as the front of their house was more likely to be seen by official wardens, disregarding the fact that bombers would spot light from either side of the house from the air. Groups may take precautions and feel that they are safe, as they have obeyed instructions rather than take objective personal assessments of the risks indicated. And, by the same token, if they are harmed, they are likely to feel anger and resentment against the authorities for not protecting them adequately, especially if they have complied with the instructions. Individuals affected by disaster often perceive events as if they were directed solely at them – the illusion of centrality. They may feel relief or guilt at being spared while so many others have perished, or else view their suffering and dislocation as their own personal burden, rather than that of the wider group.

The success of a warning depends first upon it reaching those for whom it is intended and secondly upon their reacting to it in an appropriate manner. In turn, the responses of the recipients depends on their present situation, past experiences and the manner in which the warning is interpreted and passed on to them by others. Earlier warnings of disaster events that may not have materialized can lead to public unwillingness and a lack of cooperation to subsequent warnings. Delays and distortions of warnings can also be misleading. Previous faulty warnings will result in subsequent warnings being ignored. Even when a warning is transmitted accurately, the recipients may not completely grasp or fully understand it due to a false sense of security or invulnerability when faced with the danger signs. Pressure of work or distractions can draw their attention away from the emerging signs of danger. They may distrust the source of information and get decoyed into concentrating on their homes and property, placing their implicit trust on the authorities to provide them full safety. Hence a warning must be considered a starting point rather than an end point of a series of stages. A person receiving a warning will tend to verify the message, and if time is available, try to authenticate it before reacting to it. Once satisfied of its genuine nature, he will try to determine the nature, type, severity, location, timing and probability of the danger before determining if the threat is manageable and if his responses to it can be postponed. Alternatively he will want to assess if there are means of escaping the danger and the chances of enduring and surviving the threat.

Because of these complexities, it is clear that warnings must be accurate, unambiguous and reliable. It should be a selective communication and must not be buried in a mass of irrelevant information. It must not be presented at a moment of crisis. The administration must respond to it in a creative, problem-solving manner. Adequate amounts of information must be continuously transmitted to the public and the best available means of coping with the potential hazards presented lucidly and unambiguously. Public address systems and all media must be effectively utilized for this. When the task is daunting or overwhelming, additional help must be sought without any delay. It is difficult to warn people successfully against impending danger when they have not experienced the predicted danger in recent years and when they cannot directly perceive the signs of danger. A warning, when issued, must be a call to action rather than just a sign of imminent danger. When there is a threat of great danger, there exists a need to confirm the message several times over. It is desirable therefore to present a "This is it!" message with a "Yes, this is really it!!" message.

Lead time variations i.e. the time between first signs of a natural hazard developing and when it strikes can vary considerably and affect major population evacuations to prevent large loss of life.

New satellite based technology can give forecast and warning systems to enable evacuation measures and also engineering measures to mitigate and land use planning strategies and assist community preparedness and planning. Seismic resistant construction in areas other than those on the flanks of destructive volcanoes or flood plains. Numerical simulation models and statistics are the main tools for assessing natural hazard risk . But the closer we try to predict the natural world, the less predictable it becomes. Limitations of science is often the basis for shift of blames during disasters to the doors of the scientists. Mankind too harbours an illusion, despite scientific facts to the contrary, that they have a mythical mastery over life and death and control over their environment.

Selected factors influencing response to disaster warnings.

1. Any warning messages broadcasted, especially the early ones, will be accepted at face value only by a minority of the recipients. Most will engage in confirmation efforts for a time.
2. The closer a person is to the target area of a warning, the higher the incidence of face-to-face communication and the

larger the number of sources used in confirmation.

3. Warnings from official sources (police, fire department etc) are more likely to be believed.
4. Message content per se influences belief. The more accurate and consistent the content across several messages, the greater is the belief.
5. The recipient's perception of the senders certainty about the warning is important to credibility.
6. Message credibility is related to what happens in the confirmation process. The response of official sources to questions which call for validation, corroboration, or refutation helps determine believability.
7. A person is more likely to believe a warning of impending danger to the extent that perceived changes in his physical environment support the contents of the message.
8. Past experience may render current warnings less credible if disaster is not part of that experience.
9. As warning messages increase in their accuracy, and/or information about survival choices, and/or consistency with other warnings, and/or clarity about the nature of the threat, the probability of positive response increases.
10. Evacuation tends to be a family phenomenon. The best way to accomplish evacuation appears to be repeated authoritative messages over broadcast media which stimulate discussion within the family and lead to evacuation (if it is going to happen at all).
11. Regardless of the content of a warning message, people tend to define some potential impact in terms of prior experience with that specific disaster agent.

(Ref: UNDRO 1986)

COLOR CODES FOR THREAT LEVELS

Color-coded threat levels are intended to reflect the probability of a threat and its potential gravity and serve to ensure that emergency response personnel are at the desired level of preparedness and ready.

- Severe risk: CODE RED OR CONDITION RED.
- High risk: Code orange or condition orange.
- Elevated/significant risk: Code yellow or condition yellow.
- Guarded /general risk: Code blue or condition blue.
- Low risk: Code green or condition green.

NBC warfare alerts and action.

Level A (Red zone)

Selected when the greatest level of skin, respiratory, and eye protection is required. This is the maximum protection for workers in danger of exposure to unknown chemical hazards or levels above the Immediately Dangerous to Life or Health exposure limit (IDLH) or greater than the AEGL-2 (Acute Exposure Guidelines Levels). AEGLs indicate the concentrations of a chemical in air above which different types of health effects could begin to occur in an unprotected civilian population. AEGLs are to be used by central and state agencies to aid in the development of emergency preparedness plans and to prioritize emergency response actions in the event of a chemical release from an accident or intentional terrorist attack. Required action:

- A NIOSH-certified CBRN full-face-piece SCBA operated in a pressure-demand mode or a pressure-demand supplied air hose respirator with an auxiliary escape bottle.
- A Totally-Encapsulating Chemical Protective (TECP) suit that provides protection against Chemical Biological Radiological Nuclear (CBRN) agents.
- Chemical-resistant gloves (outer).

- Chemical-resistant gloves (inner).
- Chemical-resistant boots with a steel toe and shank.
- Coveralls, long underwear, and a hard hat worn under the TECP suit are optional items.

Level B (Red zone)

Selected when the highest level of respiratory protection is necessary but a lesser level of skin protection is required. This is the minimum protection for workers in danger of exposure to unknown chemical hazards or levels above the IDLH or greater than AEGL-2. It differs from Level A in that it incorporates a non-encapsulating, splash-protective, chemical-resistant splash suit that provides Level A protection against liquids but is not airtight.

- A NIOSH-certified CBRN full-face-piece SCBA operated in a pressure-demand mode or a pressure-demand supplied air hose respirator with an auxiliary escape bottle.
- A hooded chemical-resistant suit that provides protection against CBRN agents.
- Chemical-resistant gloves (outer).
- Chemical-resistant gloves (inner).
- Chemical-resistant boots with a steel toe and shank.
- Coveralls, long underwear, a hard hat worn under the chemical-resistant suit, and chemical-resistant disposable boot-covers worn over the chemical-resistant suit are optional items.

Level C (Yellow zone)

Selected when the contaminant and concentration of the contaminant are known and the respiratory protection criteria factors for using Air Purifying Respirators (APR) or Powered Air Purifying Respirators (PAPR) are met. This level is appropriate when decontaminating patient/victims.

- A NIOSH-certified CBRN tight-fitting APR with a canister-type gas mask or CBRN PAPR for air levels greater than AEGL-2.
- A NIOSH-certified CBRN PAPR with a loose-fitting face-piece, hood, or helmet and a filter or a combination organic vapor, acid gas, and particulate cartridge/ filter combination or a continuous flow respirator for air levels greater than AEGL-1.
- A hooded chemical-resistant suit that provides protection against CBRN agents.
- Chemical-resistant gloves (outer).
- Chemical-resistant gloves (inner).
- Chemical-resistant boots with a steel toe and shank.
- Escape mask, face shield, coveralls, long underwear, a hard hat worn under the chemical-resistant suit, and chemical-resistant disposable boot-covers worn over the chemical-resistant suit are optional items.

Level D (Green zone)

Selected when the contaminant and concentration of the contaminant are known and the concentration is below the appropriate occupational exposure limit or less than AEGL-1 for the stated duration times.

- Limited to coveralls or other work clothes, boots and gloves.

ACUTE EXPOSURE GUIDELINE LEVELS (AEGLS)

These are short-term, one-time, airborne exposure levels with respect to toxic chemicals.

There are 3 levels of health severity and different exposure times and it assists or risk managers to appropriately balance risks and prioritize resources in both emergency planning/prevention and emergency response.

- *AEGL Level 1:* level ***above which*** general population (including susceptible individuals) may have some notable discomfort (non-disabling, transient and reversible).

- *AEGL Level 2:* level ***above which*** general population (including susceptible individuals) may experience serious long-lasting effects or impaired ability to escape.
- *AEGL Level 3:* level ***above which*** general population (including susceptible individuals) could experience life threatening effects or death.

ROLE OF SPACE TECHNOLOGY

Space systems from their vantage position have unambiguously demonstrated their capability in providing vital information and services for disaster management. The earth observation satellites provide comprehensive, synoptic and multi temporal coverage of large areas in real time and at frequent intervals and have become valuable for continuous monitoring of atmospheric as well as surface parameters related to natural disasters. Geo-stationary satellites provide continuous and synoptic observations over large areas on weather including cyclone-monitoring. Polar orbiting satellites have the advantage of providing much higher resolution imageries, even though at low temporal frequency, which could be used for detailed monitoring, damage assessment and long-term relief management. The vast capabilities of communication satellites are available for timely dissemination of early warning and real-time coordination of relief operations. The advent of Very Small Aperture Terminals (VSAT) and Ultra Small Aperture Terminals (USAT) and phased-array antennae have enhanced the capability further by offering low cost, viable technological solutions towards management and mitigation of disasters. Satellite communication capabilities, both fixed and mobile, are vital for effective communication, especially in data collection, distress alerting, position location and co-ordinating relief operations in the field. In addition, search and rescue satellites provide capabilities such as position determination facilities onboard which could be useful in a variety of land, sea and air distress situations.

Applications of space remote sensing in disaster management

Disaster	Prevention	Preparedness (Warning)	Relief
Earthquakes	Mapping geological lineaments land use	Geodynamic measurements of strain accumulation	*Locate stricken areas, map damage*
Volcanic eruptions	**Topographic** and land use maps	**Detection/measurement of gaseous emissions**	Mapping lava flows, *ashfalls* and lahars, *map damage*
Landslides	**Topographic** and land use maps	**Rainfall, slope stability**	*Mapping slide area*
Flash floods	Land use maps	**Local rainfall measurements**	*Map flood damage*
Major floods	Flood plain maps; land use maps	Regional rainfall; evapo-transpiration	Map extent of floods
Storm surge	Land use and land cover maps	Sea state; ocean surface wind velocities	*Map extent of damage*
Hurricanes		**Synoptic weather forecasts**	*Map extent of damage*
Tornadoes		Nowcasts; local weather, Local weather observations	*Map amount, extent of damage*
Drought		**Long range climate models**	Monitoring vegetative biomass

Normal	-Operational or needs very little research
Underlined	-Research and development required
Bold	-Requires improved observation capability
Italics	-Requires improved spatial or temporal resolution

12 The Role of Legislations in Disaster Prone Regions

> "We are often dismayed to find that even disasters cannot cure us of our faults. "
>
> —*Marquis de Vauvenargues*

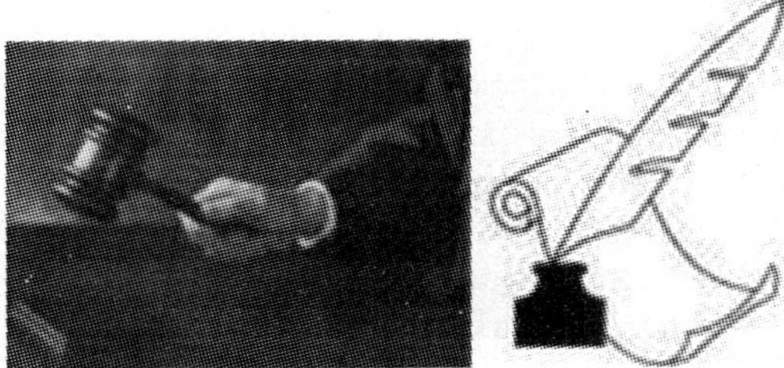

Fig. 12.1

Containment of the adverse effects of disasters using currently available technology and knowledge is an important and often neglected area. Global early warning meteorological systems e.g. Immarsat etc that monitor phenomenon like cyclones, hurricanes and tornado movements using satellite based technology must be accessible to all areas prone to such events. Legislation in respect of constructing residential complexes in flood plains and coastal regions (minimum 5 km distance from coastline in areas prone to ravages by the sea), mandatory seismic housing codes, construction of tornado cellars, mobile home tie-downs, community cyclone shelters, all weather roads, aspects of deforestation, carbon dioxide emissions, toxic waste disposal, transportation of hazardous chemicals, location of industries dealing with potentially lethal chemicals must be developed and implemented. FEMA's BPAT (Building Performance Assessment Team) offers technical know-how on aspects of building safety in disaster-prone areas. The AIT Bangkok has designed low cost timber-frame houses on stilts costing US $20 only that can withstand wind speeds of nearly 180km/h. In India, the National Disaster Management cell with the Ministry of Home Affairs has laid down specifications for all new constructions in seismic zones III, IV and V, recommending reinforced concrete seismic bands at plinth level and level of lintels of doors and windows, and beams at ceiling levels. The cement:sand mixture ratios have also been specified at 1:6 in seismic zones III and IV and 1:4 in zone V.

The long periods of calm between disasters tends to dim the collective memory and develop inaction. Simulated drills and evacuation procedures must be enforced once or twice a year as a civic exercise to effect better co ordination during actual events and also minimize panic /crisis management.

Researchers and investigators must audit each disaster effort to improve the preventive aspects in future situations. Geologists must identify fault areas and flood plains to mitigate the effects of disasters in areas prone to the ravages of earthquakes and floods. Aspects of dam safety based on geological surveys and environmental studies must be taken into consideration before constructing new projects. The Central Water Commission, The National Watershed Development Project for Rainfed Areas, The National Wasteland Board, The Department of Science and Technology, various Urban Planning Development agencies and Meteorological Departments must work in close co-ordination to address issues related to disaster prevention. The National Centre for Disaster Management must create a database, national and international networking and conduct research into all aspects of disasters. Non Governmental Organizations (NGOs), environmental lobbies and volunteer organizations must step up afforestation efforts, closely monitor the air and water in their areas and assist the government implement the legislations and safety recommendations of international watch-dog bodies. Green Peace, Nuclear Regulation Commission, Director General Mine Safety, Explosives Act, Factories Act, Petroleum Act, Gas Cylinder Rules, Dangerous Machines Act, Static and Mobile Pressure Rules, Environment Protection Act, ISI, NIOSH etc have spelt out safety and mitigation protocols in great detail. Improvements in track and signaling, anti-collision technology in the railways, sophisticated instrument landing systems in airports together with phasing out of ageing aircraft, strict implementation of Lloyds Registry safety regulations in shipping will go a long way in preventing major transport disasters. The National Human Rights Commission must look into human rights and gender issues related to disaster situations.

Legal aid must be extended to victims and arbitrary categorization of victims for compensation related issues must be avoided. Archaic and anachronistic laws compounding victims misery must be replaced with ones that alleviate distress. Policy makers and lawmakers must accord high priority to these important issues to minimize recourse to judicial interventions for providing basic necessities. There is need to innovate and improve common information and communication, and also learn from past experiences, always thinking a step ahead to promote community self-help programs. To be truly effective, environmental sanitation needs the understanding, support and active participation of the people. It must be made a subject in primary education as must first-aid and basic life support techniques.

Mere technical improvement of the environment without public education in hygiene and sanitation, based on local customs, traditions, beliefs and mores has proved futile again and again and is self-defeating. Ways must be found to overcome objections and gain popular support and bring people into the programs as partners. Education is vital in overcoming the age-old apathy and the inertia which tends to grip the people. Doing things to the people and for the people is easier, and is vital to get members from all segments of the community to actively participate in the planning and execution of health programs, especially related to excreta disposal and safe water schemes. Public health inspectors and nurses must always remain in touch with the community members to stimulate and educate members in the use and maintenance of privies. Facilities must be simple, economical and ingenious, especially where terrain and attitudes are hostile. Simple designs using local materials are advisable. Part financial contribution from the community is desirable to promote involvement, initiative and self-help. Other governmental, non governmental and corporate financial assistance and sponsorship can also be sought. Pilot schemes and demonstrations in respect of sanitary disposal of excreta must be carried out in health and welfare centers, residences and offices of local health officials, schools, colleges etc. Leaflets and manuals covering the design, construction and operation of these facilities must be prepared and made available to users. Wherever bad construction, poor ventilation and lighting, lack of washing facilities, unsanitary toilets and deficiencies exist, children and youth will absorb wrong ideas and learn harmful habits that may never be eradicated. A simple, well built, well kept lavatory will be safer and have more education value than a porcelain and tile toilet which is allowed to become dirty and a nuisance. Mere classroom teaching of sanitation without actual demonstration will have little effect as people learn better by doing and through example in adopting a sanitary way of life. Campaigns will be useful only if backed by good follow-up, continued health education and inspections. There are innumerable instances of money spent on latrine campaigns where privies have been used as chicken-coops or grain silos in the absence of such follow-up protocols. Public community facilities have their limitations and individual latrines at the rate of one unit per family would be a better long term strategy. Local administration is notoriously poor and ineffective at maintaining such conveniences.

Stocks in warehouses located on high lands, sinking deep tubewells in selected areas must all be carefully planned and implemented in disaster prone areas. Cyclone and tsunami prone areas must adopt energetic afforestation programs and conserve existing mangrove and casuarinas forests along the coastline, as they serve as wind breakers and attenuate the impact of high speed winds, seismic and tidal waves.

FURTHER READING

1. Emergency care in natural disasters – views of the United Nations Disaster Relief Coordinator (UNDRO). WHO Chronicle, Mar198,Vol 34, No.3,p:96-100.
2. Man made disasters. Barry A Turner, Wykeham Publications, London, 1978).

13 Panic Reaction during Disaster

> "Dread of disaster makes everybody act in the very way that increases the disaster. Psychologically the situation is analogous to that of people trampled to death when there is a panic in a theatre caused by a cry of `Fire!'
>
> —*Sir Bertrand Russell*

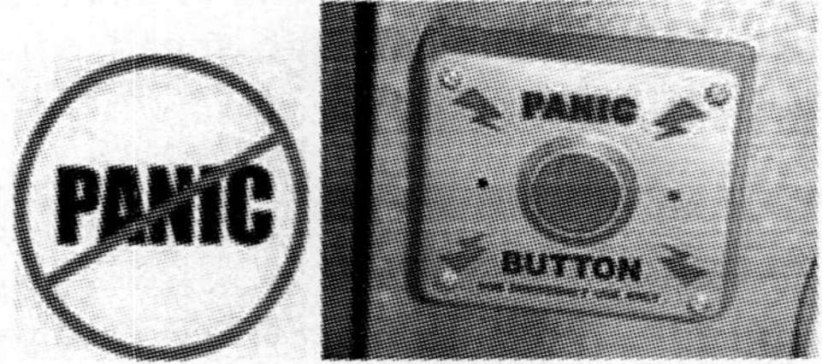

Fig. 13.1

The word panic signifies diffuse, severe (fact-based or hysterical) reactions of individuals or a mass of people to fear and shock. Panic is a primitive reaction to a current real or supposed threat to existence. The determinants in a panic situation are the degree of fear and excitement. These two emotions block the individuals capability of taking level headed decisions, based closeness, causing him or her to become part of the directly suggestive, panicking behavior of a mass of people. During this process, panic transforms individual personalities into a depersonalized, collectively reacting mass, in which the primary characteristics of the participants disappears. Normal inhibitions and feelings of responsibility are eliminated, as is critical ability-leading to abnormal conduct, be it anti social or heroic type. Instinct-based conduct offers an illusion of refuge even when a realistic on sizing up, evaluating and dealing with the given situation. Instead, the individuals actions are determined by the more primitive control mechanisms of self-preservation and herd instinct leading to heedless, ruthless, uncircumspect, unforeseen and incautious flight. It involves the individuals instinctive search for human appraisal would show such conduct to be actually increasing the peril e.g. overloading of life boats when a ship is sinking or the choice of dangerous exits and fatal leaps in a building blaze. The proliferation of infectious fear-laden excitement to the stage of general panic proceeds, via the intensification of an anxiety-ridden uneasiness and a desire to do something. Such a state of mind is not receptive to the calm control of action.

Everyone has a more or less strongly pronounced potentiality for fear and panic. Greek mythology describes the goat-legged God of shepherds, Pan, who amused himself by sounding his conch shell trumpet suddenly and so loudly as to create flight among terrified flocks of goats and cattle. Pans friend, the nymph Echo, had the awful noises created by her master resound from different directions, thereby considerably intensifying the shock and the fear among the grazing animals. Another version describes the legendary commander Pan serving Emperor Dionysus, who devised a phalanx formation of his soldiers in closed ranks during his campaign in India. His foes fought in loosely scattered groups fled in a headlong, unrestrained flight on encountering this terrifying formation. Both versions of the origin of the word panic describe a collective reaction conditioned by terror and fear. Panic reactions tend to occur in many major disasters and in wars. Panic can lead to disasters and disasters can be made worse by panic. Hence the need to understand the phenomenon in greater depth.

The elements of panic are a balance between fear and excitement on one hand and presence of mind on the other. The latter is an accomplishment of reason, involving correct perception of the circumstances, its evaluation and decision making that deliberately distances itself from the situation. Fear and excitement are emotions that promote anxiety and shock-activating protective defense mechanisms. Anxiety is usually accompanied by the conviction that one is at the mercy of the situation, helpless and defenseless, triggering panic or apathy. Primitive control mechanisms then come into play, leading to mindless flights, hectic bodily movement or aggression. These expressions are highly contagious and are a major factor in promoting panic. In some individuals, anxiety results in severe vegetative reactions such as trembling, perspiration, diarrhea, nausea, vomiting, fainting or apathetic whimpering. If the anxiety persists for longer duration, it can cause loss of appetite and libido. Fear is nothing but anxiety with a tangible cause i.e. something specific. Shock, a frequent instigator of panic, is severe, short-lived, unexpectedly-produced state of anxiety that cripples the capability to perceive calmly, to weigh a situation, and to decide. Shock is also accompanied by vegetative symptoms such as trembling, nausea, vomiting, incontinence of urine or stools, fainting and, in extreme cases, stupor state. Vulnerability to shock can be attenuated through familiarity and practice. On the other hand, shocks can also sensitize a person, so that similar situation can lead to a sense of anxious anticipation. Within limits, excitement leads to an increased readiness to react and take action. During panic reaction, the degree of excitement precludes rational behavior resulting in pointless or purposeful violent aggression. Psycho vegetative symptoms include erratic trembling, stuttering, hyperactivity such as running amok.

Panic is a complex interplay of emotions with anxiety, shock, fear and excitement in differently accentuated proportions. Anxiety is based on threat perception, susceptibility and previous conditioning and blocks the capability of reasoning, through emotional contagion, it can be transmitted to others. During an attack of panic, the accompanying anxiety is often overwhelming, and has to be treated thymoleptically and not anxiolytically. Fears can often accelerate into panicky, heedless anxiety. Anxiety intensifies threat, which in turn escalates anxiety setting a vicious cycle in motion. Some individuals exhibit hysterical anxiety with a strong tendency towards dramatic behavior that can whip up emotions and instigate panic in others, lowering the level of reasonable thought and action in others. Most individuals of the same language and ethnic group tend to identify and adjust with the emotions, attitudes, values and demands of the group. This suggestibility that consists of arbitrary adoption of the behavior in one environment is a general human phenomenon, and also links up with the behavior. The socalled herd instinct causes groups of animals to follow a lead animal and also termed as collectivization when the group uncritically accepts that of he leader and behaves in a manner in which it would otherwise not, acting on its own motivation. This group behavior can cause an individual to act in ways alien to his or her own personality. In panic, he can join others in ruthlessly storming towards an exit that seems to lead to rescue, brutally trampling others underfoot in the process. This behavior ranges from brutal killing to heroic behavior seen among martyrs under war conditions. Under suggestibility, a number of individuals become a depersonalized mass, reacting identically. Suggestibility is in inverse proportion of presence of mind and is absent in the mentally unsound.

Under disaster conditions, these disturbances can prompt emotional paralysis or apathy and switch off from his or her environment, failing to take advantage of obvious rescue possibilities and remaining unmindfully exposed to danger.

It is difficult to predict who will panic in a given circumstance, but those with pronounced self-confidence are relatively less prone. Disaster situations can either activate hidden strengths or expose weaknesses and a soft, shy, fearful person can emerge unexpectedly level-headed, brave and be a group leader whilst 'supermen' can emerge as weaklings, becoming confused and frightened.

DEFINITION OF PANIC

It is a heedless, anxiety-filled, excited, collective reaction of a mass of people to a directly experienced threat. Panic extinguishes the composure of the individual so that his actions are based on blind urges for self-preservation and a herd instinct – leading to flight and aggression and a depersonalized reacting group.

A panic situation is triggered by excitement, suppression of composure and real fear.

Circumstances that can touch off panic are:

- Limited space or multiple obstacles that hinder the way of a crowd breaking up fast.
- A lack of algorithms, set protocols/ orders or recognizable authority as seen in sports stadium and hotel fires.
- An absence of internal and external organizational preparation for handling a panic situation.
- Plausible fear of threat including peril of an unspecified extent in a gathering of people.
- The existence of a panic-prone, emotional mass-orientation and heightened excitability that can be intensified by threat or rumors.
- Mutual contagion of a gathering usually by panic-prone individuals.
- Lack of confidence in the competence of law enforcing authorities.

It would be useful, at this juncture, to analyze the patterns of panic under military circumstances in order to better understand those occurring in civil situations. Here, a complex interplay of modifying factors such as training, command structure, logistic facilities and subjection to orders occurs. The following factors can lead to panic in military life are:

- Failure of logistic support e.g. communication, supplies like fuel and ammunitions and medicare.
- Personal conflicts and uncertainties at home.
- Fears about a very risky mission and seemingly impossible assignment.
- Feelings that a mission is pointless.
- Panic-prone commanders who react with uncertainty, ambiguously or irrationally.
- Insufficient confidence in leadership.
- Insufficient confidence in the dependability of subordinates or comrades.

- Shock created by enemy attacks and daunting arsenals.
- Disorientation regarding the current situation with regards to enemy positions and own troop back up.
- Individual panic reactions that can become contagious.

PANIC PROPHYLAXIS

A reserve of presence of mind, based on personal, organizational and material preparations is a pre requisite to cope with a panic situation, which can otherwise blow up into a disaster proportion. The preparations can be in the pre critical phase, long before actual panic breaks out and the other points of time during the critical phase of the situation itself.

PRE CRITICAL PANIC PROPHYLAXIS

Panic avoidance needs thoughtful preparations and build-up of in-house attitudes, alternatives in emergency and action plans that are flexible and easily instituted depending on the situation. Some of these can be as follows:

- Simulation and drills to rehearse for various situations like victim rescue from collapsed or burning buildings, disentanglement procedures in a vehicle smash up or air crash.
- Familiarization drills for passengers with regards to life preservation using life jackets, lifeboats, life buoys, emergency exits etc.
- Orientation to first responder procedures like CPR, first aid in burns, poisoning etc.
- Technical preparations such as inventory of emergency supplies. Transport, evacuation routes, accommodation, medical evacuation chains and communication links, list of places where cranes, earth moving equipment etc can be procured, list of ham operators, e-mail access etc.
- Rapid isolation of panicky persons by decisive and prompt action using sedation with a neuroleptic when required.

PERSONAL PANIC PROPHYLAXIS

This is a more difficult factor, as determination, presence of mind and courage are difficult to teach and assess. It is a matter of internal attitudes based on the knowledge that no one in a disaster situation can be sure that he or she will belong to the lost, the rescuable or the category of a rescuer. It aims at making a person shed his anxiety and remaining calm and level headed according to a situation or a requirement. It counters herd-mentality and moots intense.contemplative preparation for every conceivable disaster situation. A foremost task is to cope with vulnerability to anxiety.

The principles for combating anxiety are the same as that for control of panic state.

- By rechannelizing the anxiety and fears to objective considerations and rational possibilities of doing something about them.
- Diminishing anxiety by counterbalancing it with presence of mind and distancing it by disregarding it and initiating calm responses as during lonely expeditions and long dangerous expeditions.
- Inculcating and exhorting feelings of bravado so that dutiful action replaces irrational fears.

ISLANDS OF REASON

Whenever possible, in the face of impending panic, it is always desirable to create islands of reason. Here authorized personnel, supervisors and volunteers take a determined and serene advocacy of calm and reasonable reaction to a situation. Just as panic and anxiety can be contagious, so can the demonstration of courage, optimistic and rational behavior. The panic-induced mass suggestibility can be effectively countered by the suggestive power of level-headed persons. The herd instinct can be steered by reasonableness. Loud hailers, megaphones or amplifiers lends a tone of authority and be effectively used to augment the instructions and commands.

PRACTICAL STEPS IN PANIC PROPHYLAXIS

Some of the measures recommended are:

- Gatekeepers at entrances must turn away those recognizably drunk.
- No alcoholic spirits should be dispensed on premises of large gatherings.
- Use of electronic surveillance equipment, metal detectors to frisk and identify itinerant trouble-makers.
- Provide for as many doors and exits opening to the outside and capable of being unlocked from a central control point.
- All exits must be signposted clearly and well illuminated.
- Volunteers must wear distinctive apparel and carry megaphones. They must also be well conversant with the layout of the venue.
- The volunteers must be capable of linking up to channelize fleeing throngs rationally towards specific exits and become nuclei of the islands of reason.
- Volunteers must have two way radios to be constantly in touch with a central station or command headquarters to provide real time feedback on status and call for help or back up.
- Adequate medical aid must be available on site for resuscitation and emergency care.
- Crowd control equipments like water jets, tear gas, rubber bullets, foam spray, stun guns and tranquillizers may be stocked in control rooms.

FIGHTING PANIC

Once panic has broken out, the well known principles of disaster control must be set into motion:

1. Panicking streams of people must be split up and led towards the least dangerous, congested directions so that a depersonalized reacting mass is transformed into smaller groups of manageable proportions.
2. Objective decision-making is imperative avoiding all delays and discussions taking a reasonable course of action rather then remaining idle and inconclusive.
3. To absorb panic-fostering drives so that they can be expressed in a less harmful fashion. E.g. by providing timely medical aid, rescue, support etc.
4. To provide dry places to sleep with adequate protection against bad weather and dangers in longer lasting disaster situations. Blankets, provisions and tools can be distributed in order to attenuate anxieties and channelize drives into more constructive purpose, thereby diminishing the sense of panic.

The fundamental prophylaxis is having a reserve of presence of mind so that one is better prepared to prevent a state of helplessness in crisis situations that fosters breaking out of panic and loss of human life and property. Panic is often a rare phenomenon, as an eerie feeling of calm pervades over people during life and death moments, especially with groups who have pre existing knowledge of one another or are well primed with disaster drills in peacetime.

FURTHER READING

1. Panic-Understanding it, Preventing it, Coping with it. HJ Bochnik and W Richtberg. Medical Corps International, 2/1986 p:51-60.
2. Panic anxiety. J Clin Psych,1984, 45, 323-330.
3. Collective behavior. St Milgram, H Toch, Handbook of Social Psychology,2nd Edn,1969, Vol IV, Addison-Wesley(Mass),p:507-610).

14 Psychosocial Management of Disaster Victims

> "There are two big forces at work, external and internal. We have very little control over external forces such as tornadoes, earthquakes, floods, disasters, illness and pain. What really matters is the internal force. How do I respond to those disasters? Over that I have complete control."
>
> —*Leo F. Buscaglia*

Victims of disasters will have a spectrum of psychological and stress related disorders like anxiety, depression, sleep disturbances and insecurity that may require expert help for prompt resolution. Individuals who have experienced core losses, such as the loss of a loved one and/or the loss of a home and all the artifacts of their family existence, will have a prolonged mourning process. It may take more than a few months to truly make peace with the past and turn to the future. The lives of the bereaved may still be strongly affected a year and a half to three years later. Some individuals may experience complicated or pathological bereavement with an intensification, prolongation or even inhibition of normal grief. Adults and children may experience recurrent, deeply disturbing dreams related to their disaster experience. Vivid mental pictures and visions may keep coming back (flashbacks) for several years afterwards and cause great pain and anguish. The aim of mental and social care of victims is to decrease psychological damage, mitigate and prevent development of post traumatic stress disorder and long term mental ill health. Prompt psychological first aid by critical incident stress management, offering educational information and psychological assistance designed to counter the effects of the trauma caused by a disaster experience are essential. This is best tackled by the local social work support groups, supplemented with special support and help measures based on information from different complementary areas of knowledge including ethical considerations, the special needs of different ethnic groups including good interpretation services. All activities must be coordinated with the different public bodies in the disaster organization like the rescue services, police, medical services, social organizations, NGOs, primary health care providers, school health and administrative groups and religious organizations.

A special psychology-psychiatry disaster management group (PDM group) has to be mobilized in the disaster affected area comprising of a specialist in general psychiatry, a specialist in child and adolescent psychiatry, a senior clinical psychologist, a senior social welfare officer and the local priest/pastor/religious leader. Every affected person must have their own support/contact person for a crisis situation and these individuals must be registered in peacetime to enable follow up action. Separation of children from their parents must be avoided as far as possible and those affected must be protected from further traumatic stress. Counseling facilities must be offered round the clock and relatives of deceased must be offered possibilities of traveling to the affected site to assist volunteers in disposing off the bodies of the dead in a comforting and dignified manner. Mental health crisis counseling programs may have to establish hotlines to offer phone counseling to the distressed and give them an opportunity to discuss their thoughts, feelings and come to terms with their emotions, using therapeutic skills such as active listening and cognitive reframing.

Many disaster victims may experience restlessness and fear with the return of the season in which the disaster occurred. Annual storm seasons may trigger anxiety attacks among those who have survived a hurricane in a previous year. Situations, sights and sounds can evoke a stress response. For example, earthquake survivors frequently become jumpy when a truck rumbles by, rattling house windows. Anniversary reactions can occur among those with unresolved grief from significant personal losses and unfinished mourning. Disaster anniversaries also provide an opportunity for emotional healing, as, in many cultures, the first year anniversary of death ends a formal period of mourning and return of psychosocial equilibrium. Some may experience intense feelings of grief, pangs of longing or a resurgence of jumpiness, startle responses and anxiety about personal safety during such commemorations. Some survivors may be so involved and numbed by the paperwork and practicalities of rebuilding after a disaster, that they may not have given themselves time to let down and mourn their losses. Such survivors are bound to experience emotional breakdown and experience waves of grief at anniversary events. Gradual recovery and a phased physical, emotional and spiritual rebuilding process follows. For others, such events may reawaken resentment and anger. The unfairness of fate, things lost, time taken away from their lives, bureaucratic aspects of the recovery process, slowness of rebuilding and healing may manifest as extreme irritation and impatience. Others may indulge in reflection and soul searching and seek mental health counseling. They are more likely to take on a positive stance and recognize the challenges they have overcome and acknowledge the courage, stamina, endurance and resourcefulness within themselves They also turn appreciative of the help given by friends and loved ones through the crisis situation. Others may experience a sense of failure at their real or perceived inability to rebuild their lives or recoup their losses. While most survivors experience relief and welcome the cleansing tears during the fellowship experienced at disaster commemorations, others may ward off anniversary reactions by avoiding reminders and treat the event as just another ordinary day. In conclusion anniversaries help the disaster affected to look back, look within, look around and then look forward to see themselves as survivors, not victims. Psychologists and psychiatrists must educate survivors about common anniversary reactions and help them acknowledge and discuss issues and feelings that are still unresolved. They must view the event as an opportunity and another step towards healing and closure of the disaster experience. Survivors must be allowed to reflect on the profound changes in their lives and encourage them to experience a sense of mastery over an adverse event. Survivors may feel embarrassed or uncomfortable about the intensity of their feelings. Anticipatory guidance and reassurance must be offered by counselors and mental health staff who must also emphasize the importance of survivors reaching out to each other to provide support and share their experiences. Victims must be encouraged to talk about their memories, present thoughts, feelings and concerns and to recognize, articulate and appreciate their own survival strengths and accomplishments so that they are able to look forward to their future with realistic optimism and a proactive attitude.

Critical incident stress debriefing are structured group sessions, backed by a sufficient level of social support for victims following a disaster. The internet is opening up new, unique opportunity for victims to receive social and emotional support. Computer mediated communication helps create virtual communities that help serve as buffers among far flung survivors and greatly improve the ability to debrief each other against the effects of the trauma. E-mail makes it easier to contact strangers as there is less concern about rude intrusions or interpersonal risk and allows self-help discussion groups to form viable and useful groups with significant therapeutic outcome. Disaster mental health teams are now able to facilitate victims of disasters using internet resources to help cope with a tragedy and help persons in a crisis to begin normalize their experiences and maintain a continuous therapeutic contact. The 24 hour availability of the net makes it a great resource for treating flare-ups as they occur. Virtual communities established following disasters can easily provide emotional support, companionship, information and a sense of belonging from the comfort of ones own home.

PSYCHOLOGICAL EFFECTS OF DISASTERS ON CHILDREN

Emotional problems in children triggered by disaster situations are a major challenge to both mental health professionals, as well as to parents and teachers, if long term emotional harm is to be prevented. Children experiencing a catastrophic event exhibit a wide range of reactions. While some may suffer only worries and bad memories that fade with emotional support and time, others may experience deep seated, emotionally painful, distressful or shocking problems that often have lasting mental and physical effects. Psychic trauma is a normal response to an extreme event, and, the more direct the exposure, the higher the risk for emotional harm. Reactions appear immediately after the traumatic event or even days and weeks later. Loss of trust in adults and fear of the event recurring are the commonest features, but emotional reactions vary widely with age.

Children below 5 years of age may cry, whimper, scream, tremble or exhibit immobility, aimless motion, frightened facial expressions, excessive clinging or regressive behaviors like thumb-sucking, bedwetting, fear of darkness and separation from parents. Children of this age group are strongly affected by their parents reactions to the event.

Older children, from ages 6 to 11 years may show extreme withdrawal, disruptive behavior, inattention and regression. They may experience vivid nightmares, sleep problems, irrational fears, irritability, emotional flatness and numbing, outbursts of anger and belligerence. They may also experience psychosomatic and neurotic complaints like tummy pains, especially when it is time to go to school.

Adolescents exhibit responses similar to adults like flashbacks, depression, substance abuse, problems with peers and anti-social behavior. They may be withdrawn, confused or even suicidal and academic performances show a steep decline. They may nurse feelings of extreme guilt over their failure to prevent injury or loss of life and develop revenge fantasies that interfere with their emotional recovery. Those who are victims of child abuse or lacking in family support, or having a history of mental health problems previously, suffer a greater traumatic impact than normal children.

Help and early intervention must begin at the scene of the traumatic event to protect children from further harm and exposure to traumatic stimuli. A safe haven must be created to shelter them from the ongoing event, media and onlookers. A supportive and compassionate verbal or non-verbal exchange like a hug or reassurance helps them feel safe and allays panic responses. Parents and mental health workers would do well to explain the episode in a simple manner to the children in the shelter and encourage them to express their feelings without interference or passing judgment. Children must be told that it is normal to feel upset after a bad event and that it is none of their fault that a disaster has occurred. They must be allowed to cry and be sad and to sleep with lights on for a limited period. The family must attempt to stay together, or else the children may be entrusted to the care of a close relative or friend. The children must be offered art and play therapy and there must be no hurry to rush back to school routines too soon. It is important to identify children with special needs, as they may need more intensive support. Those who avoid eye contact or exhibit avoidance behavior and emotional numbing, nightmares, hyper arousal and disturbing recollections, jumpy and easily startled reactions may need the help of mental health professionals.

Post-traumatic stress disorder (PTSD) is a serious and potentially long lasting problem. It is diagnosed when symptoms like nightmares, flashbacks, increased sleep disturbances, irritability, poor concentration, startle reaction, regressive behavior and a general lack of responsiveness persists for longer than one month after a traumatic event. Incidence rates of PTSD ranges from 2% after a natural disaster to 30% after a man made event like a terrorist attack or a major accident. PTSD may manifest weeks to months after the event and resolve without treatment. Many will require specialized forms of psychotherapy and/or medications.

The child is taught ways to overcome anxiety and depression and modify undesirable behavior. They are specifically instructed on ways to avoid catastrophizing, i.e. that dark clouds do not signify another hurricane. These sessions may run over 6 to 12 weeks with occasional follow up sessions. Support from family and friends plays an important part in recovery. Medications are often prescribed to tackle sleep disturbances, depression and exaggerated startle reflex.

Who is at Risk?

For many children, reactions to disasters are brief and represent normal reactions to abnormal events. A smaller number of children can be at risk for more enduring psychological distress as a function of three major risk factors:

1. Direct exposure to the disaster, such as being evacuated, observing injuries or death of others, or experiencing injury along with fearing ones life is in danger.
2. Loss/grief: This relates to the death or serious injury of family or friends.
3. On-going stress from the secondary effects of disaster, such as temporarily living elsewhere, loss of friends and social networks, loss of personal property, parental unemployment, and costs incurred during recovery to return the family to pre-disaster life and living conditions.

What Creates Vulnerabilities in Children?

In most cases, depending on the risk factors above, distressing responses are temporary. In the absence of severe threat to life, injury, loss of loved ones, or secondary problems such as loss of home, moves, etc., symptoms usually diminish over time. For those that were directly exposed to the disaster, reminders of the disaster such as high winds, smoke, cloudy skies, sirens, or such other events may cause upsetting feelings to return. Having a prior history of some type of traumatic event or severe stress may contribute to these feelings. Children's coping with disaster or emergencies is often tied to the way their parents cope. They can detect adult's fears and sadness. Parents and adults can make disasters less traumatic for children by taking steps to manage their own feelings and plans for coping. Parents are almost always the best source of support for children in disasters. One way to establish a sense of control and to build confidence in children before a disaster is to engage and involve them in preparing a family disaster plan. After a disaster, children can contribute to a family recovery plan.

Age-wise Reactions to Disasters in Children

Below are some common age-wise reactions in children after a disaster or traumatic event:-

Birth through 2 years

When children are pre-verbal and experience a trauma, they do not have the words to describe the event or their feelings. However, they can retain memories of particular sights, sounds, or smells. Infants may react to trauma by being irritable, crying more than usual, or wanting to be held and cuddled. The biggest influence on children of this age is how their parents cope. As children get older, their play may involve acting out elements of the traumatic event that occurred several years in the past and was seemingly forgotten.

Preschool: 3 through 6 years

Preschool children often feel helpless and powerless in the face of an overwhelming event. Because of their age and small size, they lack the ability to protect themselves or others. As a result, they feel intense fear and insecurity about being separated from caregivers. Preschoolers cannot grasp the concept of permanent loss. They can see consequences as being reversible or permanent. In the weeks following a traumatic event, preschoolers play activities may reenact the incident or the disaster over and over again.

School age – 7 through 11 years

The school-age child has the ability to understand the permanence of loss. Some children become intensely preoccupied with the details of a traumatic event and want to talk about it continually. This preoccupation can interfere with the child's concentration at school and academic performance may decline. At school, children may hear inaccurate information from peers. They may display a wide range of reactions sadness, generalized fear, or specific fears of the disaster happening again, guilt over action or inaction during the disaster, anger that the event was not prevented, or fantasies of playing rescuer.

Pre-adolescence to adolescence:11 through 18 years

As children grow older, they develop a more sophisticated understanding of the disaster event. Their responses are more similar to adults. Teenagers may become involved in dangerous, risk-taking behaviors, such as reckless driving, or alcohol or drug use. Others can become fearful of leaving home and avoid previous levels of activities. Much of adolescence is focused on moving out into the world. After a trauma, the view of the world can seem more dangerous and unsafe. A teenager may feel overwhelmed by intense emotions and yet feel unable to discuss them with others.

Meeting the Childs Emotional Needs

Children's reactions are influenced by the behavior, thoughts, and feelings of adults. Adults should encourage children and adolescents to share their thoughts and feelings about the incident. Clarify misunderstandings about risk and danger by listening to children's concerns and answering their queries. Maintain a sense of calm by validating children's concerns and perceptions and discussing concrete plans for safety. Listen to what the child is saying. If a young child is asking questions about the event, answer them simply without the elaboration needed for an older child or adult. Some children are comforted by knowing more or less information than others; decide what level of information a particular child needs. If a child has difficulty expressing feelings, allow the child to draw a picture or tell a story of what happened. Try to understand what is causing anxieties and fears.

Be aware that following a disaster, children are most afraid that:

a. The event will happen again.
b. Someone close to them will be killed or injured.
c. They will be left alone or separated from the family.

Reassuring Children After a Disaster

Suggestions to help reassure children include the following:

- Personal contact is reassuring. Hug and touch your children.
- Calmly provide factual information about the recent disaster and current plans for ensuring their safety along with recovery plans.
- Encourage children to talk about their feelings.
- Spend extra time with children, especially at bedtime.
- Re-establish the daily routine for work, school, play, meals, and rest.
- Involve children by giving them specific chores to help them feel they are helping to restore family and community life.
- Praise and recognize responsible behavior.
- Understand that children will have a range of reactions to disasters.
- Encourage children to help update the family disaster plan.

If the child, despite having tried to create a reassuring environment, continues to exhibit stress, or if the reactions worsen over time, or if they cause interference with daily behavior at school, at home, or with other relationships, it may be appropriate to talk to a professional. One can get professional help from the child's primary care physician, a mental health provider specializing in children's needs, or a member of the clergy/religious group.

Monitor and Limit The Victim's Exposure to the Media

News coverage related to a disaster may elicit fear, confusion and anxiety in children. This is particularly true for large-scale disasters or a terrorist event where significant property damage and loss of life has occurred. Particularly for younger children, repeated images of an event may cause them to believe the event is recurring over and over. If parents allow children to watch television or use the Internet where images or news about the disaster are shown, they must ensure that they are present to encourage communication and provide explanations. This may also include parental monitoring and limiting their own exposure to anxiety-provoking information.

Use Support Networks

Parents help their children when they take steps to understand and manage their own feelings and ways of coping. They can do this by building and using social support systems of family, friends, community organizations and agencies, faith-based institutions, or other resources that work for that family. Parents can build their own unique social support systems so that in an emergency situation or when a disaster strikes, they can be supported and helped to manage their reactions. As a result, parents will be more available to their children and in a better position to support them. Parents are almost always the best source of support for children in difficult times. But to support their children, parents need to attend to their own needs and have a plan for their own support. Preparing for disaster helps everyone in the family accept the fact that disasters do happen, and provides an opportunity to identify and collect the resources needed to meet the basic needs after a disaster. Preparation helps; when people feel prepared, they cope better and so do children.

PSYCHOLOGICAL TRIAGE AFTER DISASTERS

Psychological triage is a technique for determining crisis intervention treatment priorities and needs following a crisis event. Use of this strategy is especially important whenever the number of psychological trauma victims exceeds the number of available crisis interveners. While virtually anyone exposed to a traumatic stressor will be affected to some degree, not everyone will become a psychological trauma victim. Psychological trauma is not simply a consequence of a crisis event; it is also a consequence of how individuals experience the event (personal crisis experiences) and how that experience interacts with a number of individual characteristics (personal vulnerabilities).

Conducting Psychological Triage—Levels of Triage

1. Primary assessment of psychological trauma.
2. Secondary assessment of psychological trauma.
3. Tertiary assessment of psychological trauma.

Preparation

1. Identify mental-health and other community support resources.
2. Develop/Obtain psychological assessment screening tools.
3. Develop crisis intervention referral forms.
4. Understand/Learn about culture specific crisis reactions.

Primary Assessment of Psychological Trauma

- Begins as soon as possible/appropriate and before individual students and/or staff are offered any school crisis intervention.
- Designed to identify those who are considered at risk for becoming psychological trauma victims and to help making initial school crisis intervention treatment decisions.
- Typically includes assessment of the following variables:
  - Crisis exposure (physical and emotional proximity). The physically closer the individual is to the traumatic event, and the longer the exposure, the greater the likelihood of adverse reactions to the

crisis. After exposure to the traumatic event, a relationship with crisis victims is the second most important factor associated with psychological trauma. The stronger the relationships, the greater the likelihood of trauma.

- *Personal vulnerabilities—External Factors like the following:* Family resources, not living with nuclear family, ineffective & uncaring parenting, family dysfunction (e.g., alcoholism, violence, child maltreatment, mental illness), parental PTSD/maladaptive coping with the stressor, poverty/financial stress, social resources, social isolation and lack of perceived social support
- *Personal vulnerabilities—Internal Factors like the following:* Avoidance coping style, pre-existing mental illness, poor self regulation of emotion, low developmental level and poor problem solving, history of prior psychological trauma, self-efficacy and external locus of control, pre-existing mental illness influences the development of acute distress and subsequent psychological trauma, while developmental immaturity may be a protective factor when it comes to initial trauma (i.e., younger children may not comprehend the actual threat of the trauma), once an event is judged threatening, developmentally younger individuals are at greater risk for psychological trauma. A history of prior exposure to trauma increases vulnerability to future trauma and those who dissociate or panic) are at greater risk for psychological trauma.

Secondary Assessment of Psychological Trauma

This begins as soon as school crisis interventions begin to be provided and is designed to identify those who are actually demonstrating warning signs of psychological trauma and to make more informed school crisis intervention treatment decisions. Typically includes assessment of the following risk factors and warning signs:

- Crisis exposure (physical and emotional proximity).
- Personal vulnerabilities.
- Crisis reactions.

Typically involves the following strategies:

- Use of parent, teacher, and self-referral procedures/forms.
- Administering individual and/or group screening measures:
  - Parent, teacher, and self-referral procedures/forms.
- Elements of a referral form:
  - Identifying information.
  - Physical proximity.
  - Emotional proximity.
  - Vulnerabilities.
  - Personal history.
  - Resources.
  - Mental health: Crisis reactions like dissociation, hyperarousal, re-experiencing, avoidance, depression, psychosis, dangerous coping effort (i.e., behaviors that involve any degree of lethality)

Tertiary Assessment of Psychological Trauma

Screening for psychiatric disturbances (e.g., PTSD) typically begins weeks after a crisis event has ended. It is designed to identify that minority of students and/or staff who will require mental health treatment referrals. It typically includes the careful monitoring of crisis reactions/student and staff adjustment as ongoing school crisis intervention assistance is provided.

Personal Crisis Experience

Experiences typically associated with psychological trauma include:

Exposure to the Trauma

The physically closer the individual is to the traumatic event, and the longer the exposure, the greater the likelihood of adverse reactions to the crisis.

Relationships with Victims

After exposure to the traumatic event, a relationship with crisis victims is the second most important factor associated with psychological trauma. The stronger the relationships, the greater the likelihood of trauma.

Severity of Acute Distress

Not only does the immediate response to a traumatic event influence the ability to respond adaptively, but it also appears that those who display more severe reactions (e.g., those who dissociate or panic) are at greater risk for psychological trauma.

Perceived Threat

The individual's subjective impression of the traumatic event can be more important than the event itself. Traumatized individuals will have perceived the event as extremely threatening. Among the factors influencing children's perceptions of the threat are the reactions of caregivers. Crises that are initially not perceived as threatening may become threatening after a child observes the panic reactions of parents or teachers. In addition, children may not view a traumatic event as threatening because they are too young to recognize and understand the potential danger. Conversely, relative cognitive sophistication may make a young child more vulnerable to understanding the magnitude of a traumatic event.

Personal Vulnerabilities

Personal vulnerabilities associated with psychological trauma include both external (familial and social resources) and internal (mental health, developmental level, and previous history of trauma) factors.

External Factors

Family resources like not living with nuclear family, ineffective and uncaring parenting, family dysfunction (e.g. alcoholism, violence, child maltreatment, mental illness), parental PTSD/maladaptive coping with the stressor, poverty/financial stress, social resources like social isolation and lack of perceived social support

- *Familial factors:* Individuals who are no longer able to live with a nuclear family member, come from dysfunctional homes, are exposed to family violence, have a family history of mental illness, and/or live with caregivers who have Acute Stress Disorder or Post-Traumatic Stress Disorder are more likely to become psychological trauma victims.
- *Social factors:* The absence of close peer friendships, access to positive adult models outside of the family, or connections to pro-social organizations or institutions (such as schools) increase vulnerability to psychological trauma. Individuals who must face a trauma without supportive and nurturing friends or relatives suffer more than those who have at lease one source of support.

Internal Factors Like

- Avoidance coping style.
- Pre-existing mental illness.
- Poor self regulation of emotion.
- Low developmental level and poor problem solving.
- History of prior psychological trauma.

- Self-efficacy and external locus of control.
- *Mental health:* A pre-existing mental illness influences the development of acute distress and subsequent psychological trauma.
- *Developmental level:* While developmental immaturity may be a protective factor when it comes to initial trauma (i.e., younger children may not comprehend the actual threat of the trauma), once an event is judged threatening, developmentally younger individuals are at greater risk for psychological trauma.
- *History of trauma:* A history of prior exposure to trauma increases vulnerability to future trauma.

Reactions suggesting the need for an immediate mental health referral.

- Dissociation.
- Hyperarousal.
- Persistent re-experiencing of the crisis event.
- Persistent avoidance of crisis reminders.
- Significant depression.
- Psychotic symptoms.

Post Traumatic Stress Disorder

Exposure to a traumatic event like involved actual or threatened death or serious injury, or threat to physical integrity evokes a response involving fear, helplessness, or horror (disorganized or agitated behavior in children).

Primary Symptoms

- Re-experiencing the trauma (1 or more symptoms).
- Avoidance and numbing (3 or more symptoms).
- Increased arousal (2 or more symptoms).

Duration

More than 4 weeks, acute PTSD, impaired functioning, reactions suggesting the need for an immediate mental health referral.

Maladaptive Coping

- Suicidal and/or homicidal ideation.
- Abuse of others.
- Extreme substance abuse and/or self-medication.
- Extreme rumination and/or avoidance behavior.
- Taking excessive precaution

Developmental Considerations

A. *Preschoolers*
  - Reactions not as clearly connected to the crisis event as observed among older students.
  - Reactions tend to be expressed nonverbally.
  - Given equal levels of distress and impairment, may not display as many PTSD symptoms as older children.
  - Temporary loss of recently achieved developmental milestones.
  - Trauma related play.

B. *School-age children.*
  - Tend to be more directly connected to the crisis event.
  - Event specific fears may be displayed.
  - Reactions are often expressed behaviorally.
  - Feelings associated with the traumatic stress are often expressed via physical symptoms.
  - Trauma related play (becomes more complex and elaborate).
  - Repetitive verbal descriptions of the event.
  - Problems paying attention.

C. *Preadolescents and adolescents.*
  - Reactions become more adult like.
  - Sense of foreshortened future.
  - Oppositional/aggressive behaviors to regain a sense of control.
  - School avoidance.
  - Self-injurious behavior and thinking.
  - Revenge fantasies.

- Substance abuse.
- Learning problem.

Cultural Considerations

Other important determinants of crisis reactions in general, and grief in particular, are family, cultural and religious beliefs. Hence providers of crisis intervention assistance should inform themselves about cultural norms with the assistance of community cultural leaders who best understand local customs.

Traumatized youths do not generally seek professional assistance, and recruiting school personnel to refer trauma-exposed students to school counselors can also leave many of these students unidentified. Hence a more comprehensive assessment of exposure parameters, associated distress, and impairment in functioning is needed to make informed treatment decisions, especially given the possibility of inaccuracies in child and adolescent reports of the degree of exposure and the great variability in responses to similar traumatic events observed among survivors

Summary

A number of factors may play a role in psychological trauma. Although physical proximity to the crisis plays a primary role, and all exposed individuals will be affected to some degree, other variables such as familiarity with victims, reactions to the trauma, perception of the threat, and personal vulnerability are also involved. Knowledge of these factors may be especially helpful when distinguishing those victims who are likely to cope more effectively with a traumatic event, from those who are likely to have ongoing difficulties (e.g., to develop Post-Traumatic Stress Disorder). Not all individuals will be equally affected by a crisis. One size does not fit all. Some will need intensive intervention others will need very little, if any intervention. Recovery from crisis exposure is the norm. Crisis intervention should be offered in response to demonstrated need. Not everyone exposed to trauma either needs or wants professional help.

FURTHER READING

1. Myers, D. (1994)Disaster response and recovery handbook for mental health professionals. Rockville, MD Centre for mental health services.
2. Pollock, GH. Anniversary reactions, trauma and mourning. Psychoanalytic quarterly, 39(3):347-371, 1970.
3. Szekely,L. Anniversaries, unfinished mourning, time and the intervention of the calendar. A psychoanalytic Apercu. Scandinavian psycho-analytic review. Vol 1:115-146, 1978.
4. Storm A King. Using the internet to assist disaster mental health efforts. March, 1996.
5. Osofsky, JD. The effects of exposure to violence on young children. American psychologist.1995; 50(9):782-88.
6. Vogel JM, Vernberg EM. Psychological responses of children to natural and human made disasters. J of Clinical Child Psychology, 1993; 22(4):464-84.
7. Smith EM, Morth, CS, Spitznagel, EL. Post traumatic stress in survivors of three disasters. Journal of Social Behavior and Personality, 1993;8(5):353-68.
8. FEMA guidelines.

15 Breaking Bad News (A Ten Step Approach)

> "The average man is a conformist, accepting miseries and disasters with the stoicism of a cow standing in the rain."
>
> —*Colin Wilson*

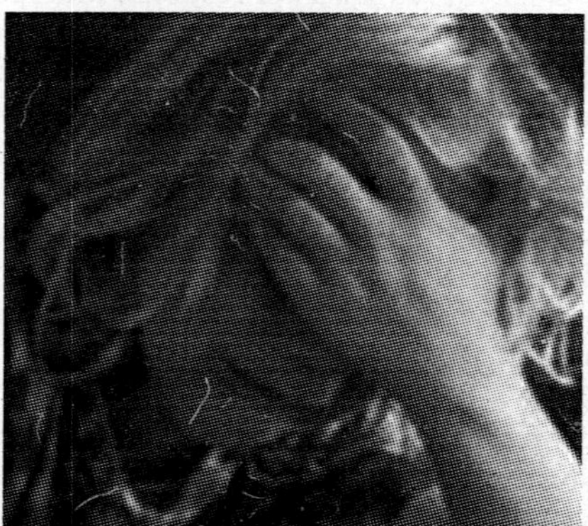

Fig. 15.1

Bad news is any information that drastically alters a persons view of his or her future for the worse. Breaking bad news is similar to breaking an egg a certain amount of skill is needed if one is to avoid making a mess. It is an important skill in disaster situations and it does not have to be time consuming. Many people feel embarrassed, incompetent or awkward while divulging bad news, fearing failure, getting blamed or handling a backlash reaction in the process. Many use the velvet-covered hand grenade approach by dispensing the bad news in a disguised form while others resort to the hit and run approach by giving a curt and frank information to the next-of-kin/relatives. Most would rather not tell and may collude with relatives, giving vague, evasive information and leaving the scene. The ten step approach to breaking bad news is a step-ladder progression to breaking bad news gently and effectively and may prove immensely useful to personnel in a disaster situation.

Step-1: Preparation

It is important to have all the facts correctly and then deciding who should be present. Having a colleague and a few trusted relatives is usual. Timing is important by arranging a meeting which acts like a warning shot, allowing relatives to prepare and brace themselves for the worst. It is important to have everyone seated as it is quite discourteous giving bad news standing up. Also someone can swoon or faint on hearing the news and compound the problem. It is curtsey to introduce oneself and the colleague, preferably of the opposite sex and someone senior in hierarchy to have better credibility. Bad news is best broken in a quiet, private room, devoid of disturbances and interruptions, phone off the hook, bleepers/ pagers and mobile phones switched off and some tissues handy. It would be pertinent to set time limit to the meeting. Avoid giving bad news over the telephone.

Step-2: What is Known?

It is important to find out what the relative already knows with some subtle prompting and probing, addressing their main concerns and expectations.

Step-3: Testing The Waters

Relatives may be frightened to have more information and lost in a conflict between the discomfort of uncertainty, wanting to know more information and the discomfort of fear. Some may prefer to deny and take an ostrich-like stance, not wanting to hear the facts. If they seem to want more information one may proceed to the next step. If they are unsure, it would be advisable to ask them if they want more information or would rather have someone else have the information.

Step-4: Allow Denial

Denial is a way of dealing with fear and should be respected as a coping strategy, especially if they change the topic, making it clear that further information is not wanted at that moment. Giving unsolicited information can cause severe anxiety or reactions of anger. Some may adopt the stance permanently. Only when one has the trust of the relatives can one broach on the note that one has something very serious to convey.

Step-5: The Warning Shot

Here, one puts across that one has something unpleasant to state and talk about the ephemeral state of life. A hierarchy of euphemisms can be employed, pausing after each new piece of new information to allow time for denial, repeating words used by the relatives. The best option is to do this gently, even if full information is demanded, because the relatives can over estimate the amount of details they can handle emotionally.

Step-6: Explain if Requested

Here, the aim is to narrow the information gap and finding the optimal level of information that is needed, without causing excessive fear and anxiety. It is important to be clear, simple, kind, avoiding jargon, being as optimistic as possible and checking the level of understanding by asking if all what is needed has been covered and knowing when to stop. One can know this when the relative changes the topic or looks out of the window or develops fidgety hands. While facts may not be remembered, the way they are given will always be.

Step-7: Elicit Concerns

After explaining the bad news, elicit their painful concerns and prioritize them. This would seem like a positive process during acute grieving and allows verbalization of distress into elements that can be discussed. Premature reassurance and excessive explanations and social chit-chat must be avoided as this can cause dissatisfaction and frustration.

Step-8: Ventilation of Feelings

Convey empathy, trying to understand what the relatives are feeling and also what they are NOT feeling, without getting carried away. Avoid sympathy and stay calm to allow the relatives to think about their own feelings. Probe by discreet queries like, it seems to me that you are feeling? fear? anger etc. So that they acknowledge the same, as this has a therapeutic result. Avoid being too talkative or too brusque.

Step-9: Summary and Plan

Integrate the relatives main concerns and offer all the support and management options available to them, avoiding unrealistic promises and hope. Appointments for further meetings can be made. Keep within the timeframe allotted for the interview, a reminder can be given as to the time left and asking if there are any further points left to be discussed for the moment.

Step-10: Offer Availability

Emotional adjustment to grief takes time, and all details discussed may not be remembered. It is wise to offer further explanation and counseling at a later date/time for which an appointment may be made based on the choice of the relatives. The presence of some other close relatives they may chose to have later can also be finalized at this stage.

In summary, grief reaction or response is characterized by initial disbelief and denial evolving into physical symptoms and social behavior. A sense of loneliness with a blend of feelings of guilt, hostility, anger and emptiness sets in. Eventually death is accepted, and the pain of the loss is integrated into the lives of the next-of-kin permitting normal social interactions and resumption of activities. Sedation in the acute phase must be kept to the minimum and over sedation avoided in order to facilitate normal grieving. The body may be presented for viewing, cleaned and wrapped appropriately and all personal effects presented. Adequate support groups and professional counselors must be offered, especially where pathologic manifestations such as increasing depression, hyperactivity, schizoid symptoms, agitation, antisocial or destructive behavior manifest.

FURTHER READING

Peter Kaye 'Breaking Bad News—A Ten Step Approach', EPL, 1996).

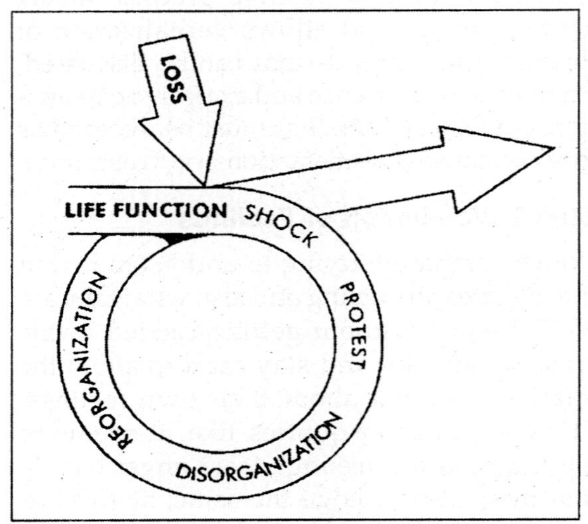

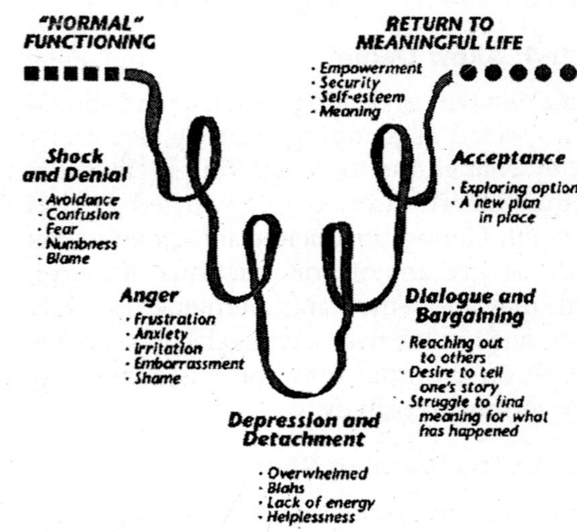

Fig. 15.2

16 Disaster Mitigation and Planning

"An ounce of prevention is worth a pound of cure"

Disasters often cause loss of life, human suffering, loss of income, property loss and damage. These events also disrupt the normal functioning of governments and communities, and adversely affect individuals and families with great severity. Special measures become necessary to assist the efforts of the affected regions in expediting the rendering of aid, assistance, and emergency services, and the reconstruction and rehabilitation of devastated areas.

Natural disasters exert an enormous toll on development. In doing so, they pose a significant threat to prospects for achieving the Millennium Development Goals in particular, the overarching target of halving extreme poverty by 2015. Annual economic losses associated with such disasters averaged US$ 75.5 billion in the 1960s, US$ 138.4 billion in the 1970s, US$ 213.9 billion in the 1980s and US$ 659.9 billion in the 1990s. The majority of these losses are concentrated in the developed world and fail to adequately capture the impact of the disaster on the poor who often bear the greatest cost in terms of lives and livelihoods, and rebuilding their shattered communities and infrastructure. Today, 85 percent of the people exposed to earthquakes, tropical cyclones, floods and droughts live in countries having either medium or low human development.

In many countries the process of development itself has a huge impact—both positive and negative—on disaster risk. It shows how countries that face similar patterns of natural hazards—from floods to droughts—often experience widely differing impacts when disasters occur. The impact depends in large part on the kind of development choices they have made previously. As countries become more prosperous, for example, they are often better able to afford the investments needed to build houses more likely to withstand earthquakes. At the same time, the rush for growth can trigger haphazard urban development that increases risks of large-scale fatalities during such a disaster. The same is true in many other areas. While humanitarian action to mitigate the impact of disasters will always be vitally important, the global community is facing a critical challenge: How to better anticipate—and then manage and reduce—disaster risk by integrating the potential threat into its planning and policies.

To help frame such efforts, a Disaster Risk Index (DRI) can be used to measure the relative vulnerability of countries to three key natural hazards—earthquake, tropical cyclone and flood and then identify development factors that contribute to risk,

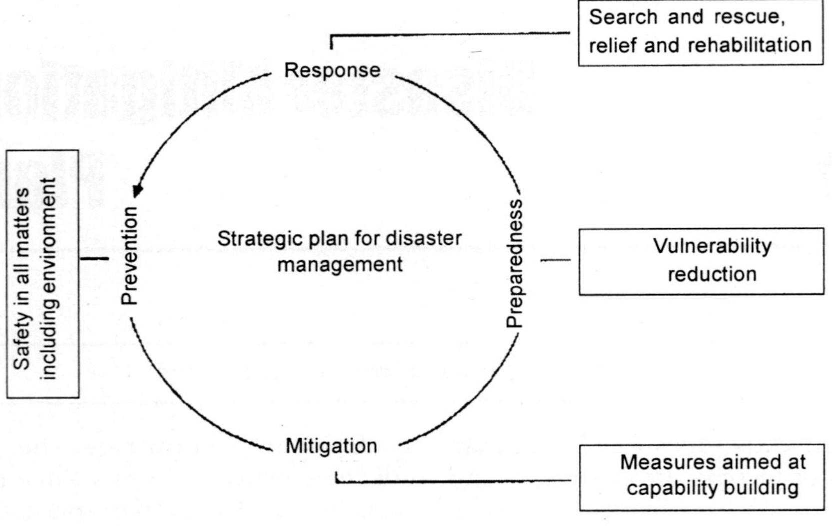

Fig. 16.1

and show in quantitative terms, just how the effects of disasters can be either reduced or exacerbated by policy choices. Disaster mitigation is a critical development issue and it is mandatory that stakeholders are brought together to enable a more careful and coherent planning to mitigate the impact of future disasters (Fig. 16.1).

Mitigation implies a wide variety of measures taken before an event occurs that will prevent illness, injury and death and limit the loss of property. It encompasses any action taken to eliminate or minimize the impact of a disaster on people, property and the environment. Mitigation planning focuses on breaking the cycle of disaster damage, reconstruction, and repeated damage Mitigative measures can be structural or non-structural. Structural measures use technological solutions, like flood levees. Non-structural measures include legislation, land-use planning (e.g. the designation of nonessential land like parks to be used as flood zones), and insurance. Mitigation is the most cost-efficient method for reducing the impact of hazards. However, mitigation is not always suitable and structural mitigation in particular may have adverse effects on the ecosystem.

The mitigation of natural disasters in the 21st century will depend upon the world learning to live with risk and understanding human limits in the face of nature.

Growing human populations in areas exposed to natural hazards are the most important reason why public health impact of disasters will continue to rise inexorably. A wide gap exists between our technical capabilities and their application- accounting for the high human and economic losses in global natural disasters. A major strategy for reducing future losses through mitigation programs is needed. Risk perception is an important limiting factor in taking preventive action. Long term attention to preparedness in disaster-prone areas is required.

A precursor activity to the mitigation is the identification of risks. Physical risk assessment refers to the process of identifying and evaluating hazards. In risk assessment, various hazards (e.g. earthquakes, floods, riots) within a certain area are identified. Each hazard poses a risk to the population within the area assessed. The hazard-specific risk (Rh) combines both the probability and the level of impact of a specific hazard. Catastrophe modeling tools are used to support the calculation. The higher the risk, the more urgent that the hazard specific vulnerabilities are targeted by mitigation and preparedness efforts. However, if there is no vulnerability there will be no risk, e.g. an earthquake occurring in a desert where nobody lives.

The risk reduction strategies include:

- The ability to maintain function of critical services.
- Stringent codes for building design-retrofitting and hardening strategies to physically protect a facility.
- Zoning ordinances-Location/relocation of buildings outside hazard zones.
- Essential building utilities provision.
- Protection methods for building contents.
- Building community shelters.
- Improving drainage and land conditions.
- Insurance.
- Public education.
- Surveillance.
- Warning.
- Evacuation.

Developing a community-wide mitigation plan makes it possible for the community to:

- Save lives and protect property.
- Save money – the costs of mitigation are less than the costs of recovery and rebuilding.
- Strengthen state and city partnerships through the sharing of resources.
- Expedite post—disaster funding by pre-identifying mitigation projects to be implemented when funding becomes available.

Mitigation efforts result in:

- Reduced direct property damage—buildings, bridges, pipelines etc.
- Reduced direct business interruption losses-damage to industrial, commercial, retail facilities.
- Reduced indirect business interruption losses – economic 'ripple effects'.
- Reduced environmental damage—to wetlands, parks, wildlife, historic sites etc.
- Reduced societal losses—casualties, homelessness.
- Reduced need for emergency response-ambulance service, fire protection etc.

Preparedness
The Disaster
Pre-Disaster Risk Reduction Stage
Mitigation
Rescu
Response Stage
Relief
Recovery

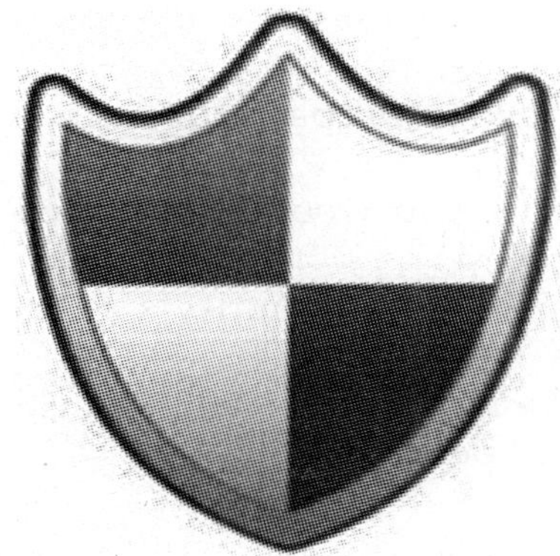

Fig. 16.2

17 Emergency Preparedness Checklist

> "Public calamity is a mighty leveler"
>
> —*Edmund Burke*

The next time disaster strikes, you may not have much time to act. Prepare now for a sudden emergency. Learn how to protect yourself and cope with disaster by planning ahead. This checklist will help you get started. Discuss these ideas with your family, then prepare an emergency plan. Post the plan where everyone will see it - on the refrigerator or bulletin board. For additional information about how to prepare for hazards in your community, contact your local emergency management or civil defense office and your Red Cross chapter.

EMERGENCY CHECKLIST

- Find out what disasters could occur in your area.
- Ask how to prepare for each type of disaster.
- Ask how you would be warned of an emergency.
- Learn your community's evacuation routes.
- Ask about special assistance for elderly or disabled persons.
- Also:
  Ask your workplace about emergency plans.
  Learn about emergency plans for your children's school or day care center.

CREATE AN EMERGENCY PLAN

- Meet with household members. Discuss with children the dangers of fire, severe weather, earthquakes, and other emergencies.
- Discuss how to respond to each disaster that could occur.
- Discuss what to do about power outages and personal injuries.
- Draw a floor plan of your home. Mark two escape routes from each room.
- Learn how to turn off the water, gas, and electricity at main switches.
- Post emergency contact numbers near telephones.
- Teach children how and when to call the police, and fire services.
- Instruct household members how to tune into the radio for emergency information.
- Pick one out-of-state and one local friend or relative for family members to call if separated by disaster (remember it is often easier to call out-of-state than within the affected area during calamities).
- Teach children how to make long distance telephone calls.
- Pick two meeting places in the event of separation.
- Agree to meet at a specific place near your home in case of a fire and also a place

outside your neighborhood in case you cannot return home after a disaster.

- Take a Basic First Aid and CPR instruction.
- Keep family records in a water-and fire-proof container.

PREPARE A DISASTER SUPPLIES KIT

- Assemble supplies you might need in an evacuation. Store them in an easy-to-carry container, such as a backpack or duffel bag.
- Include:
  A supply of water (one gallon/5 litres per day). Store water in sealed, unbreakable containers. Identify the storage date and replace every six months.
  A supply of non-perishable packaged or canned food and a non-electric can opener.
  A change of clothing, rain gear, and sturdy shoes.
  Blankets or sleeping bags.
  A first aid kit and prescription medications.
  An extra pair of spectacle glasses.
- A battery-powered radio, flashlight, and plenty of extra batteries.
- Credit cards and cash.
- An extra set of car keys.
- A list of family physicians and contact numbers.
- A list of important family information; Blood group types, drug allergies, disease information like diabetes, heart ailments, fits etc and the style and serial number of medical devices, such as pacemakers etc.
- Special items for infants, elderly, or disabled family members.

ESCAPE PLAN

In a fire or other emergency, you may need to evacuate your house, apartment, or mobile home on a moment's notice. You should be ready to get out fast.

Develop an escape plan by drawing a floor plan of your residence. Using a black or blue pen, show the location of doors, windows, stairways, and large furniture. Indicate the location of emergency supplies (Disaster Supplies Kit), fire extinguishers, smoke detectors, collapsible ladders, first aid kits, and utility shut off points. Next, use a colored pen to draw a broken line charting at least two escape routes from each room. Finally, mark a place outside of the home where household members should meet in case of fire. Be sure to include important points outside, such as garages, patios, stairways, elevators, driveways, and porches. If your home has more than two floors, use an additional sheet of paper. Practice emergency evacuation drills with all household members at least two times each year.

HOME HAZARD HUNT

- In a disaster, ordinary items in the home can cause injury and damage. Anything that can move, fall, break, or cause a fire is a potential hazard.
- Repair defective electrical wiring and leaky gas connections.
- Fasten shelves securely.
- Place large, heavy objects on lower shelves.
- Hang pictures and mirrors away from beds.
- Brace overhead light fixtures.
- Secure water heater. Strap to wall studs.
- Repair cracks in ceilings or foundations.
- Store weed killers, pesticides, and flammable products away from heat sources.
- Place oily polishing rags or waste in covered metal cans.
- Clean and repair chimneys, flue pipes, vent connectors, and gas vents.

If You need to Evacuate

- Listen to a battery-powered radio for the location of emergency shelters.
- Follow instructions of local officials.

- Wear protective clothing and sturdy shoes.
- Take your Disaster Supplies Kit.
- Lock your home.
- Use travel routes specified by local officials.

If you are sure you have time:

- Shut off water, gas, and electricity mains.
- Let others know when you left and where you are headed.
- Make arrangements for pets as animals are not allowed in public shelters.

PREPARE AN EMERGENCY CAR KIT INCLUDE

- Battery powered radio and extra batteries
- Flashlight and extra batteries.
- Blanket.
- Booster cables.
- Fire extinguisher (5 lb, A-B-C type).
- First aid kit and manual.
- Bottled water and non-perishable high energy foods, such as long life milk tetra packs, chocolate bars, raisins and peanut butter.
- Road maps.
- Shovel.
- Tyre repair kit and pump.
- Flares.

FIRE SAFETY

- Plan two escape routes out of each room.
- Teach family members to stay low to the ground when escaping from a fire.
- Teach family members never to open doors that are hot. In a fire, feel the bottom of the door with the palm of your hand. If it is hot, do not open the door. Find another way out.
- Install smoke detectors. Clean and test smoke detectors once a month. Change batteries at least once a year.
- Keep a whistle in each bedroom to awaken household members in case of fire.
- Check electrical outlets. Do not overload outlets.
- Purchase a fire extinguisher (5 lb., A-B-C type).
- Have a collapsible ladder on each upper floor of your house.
- Consider installing home sprinklers.

BEFORE YOU ENTER YOUR HOME

- Walk carefully around the outside and check for loose power lines, gas leaks, and structural damage. If you have any doubts about safety, have your residence inspected by a qualified building inspector or structural engineer before entering.
- Do not enter:
  If you smell gas.
  Floodwaters remain around the building.
  Your home was damaged by fire and the authorities have not declared it safe.

GOING INSIDE YOUR HOME

When you go inside your home, there are certain things you should and should not do. Enter the home carefully and check for damage. Be aware of loose boards and slippery floors. The following items are other things to check inside your home:

Natural gas: If you smell gas or hear a hissing or blowing sound, open a window and leave immediately. Turn off the main gas valve from the outside, if you can. Call the gas company from a neighbor's residence. If you shut off the gas supply at the main valve, you will need a professional to turn it back on. Do not smoke or use oil, gas lanterns, candles, or torches for lighting inside a damaged home until you are sure there is no leaking gas or other flammable materials present.

Sparks, broken or frayed wires: Check the electrical system. Avoid if you are wet, standing in water, or unsure of your safety. If possible, turn off the electricity at the main fuse box or circuit breaker. If the situation is unsafe, leave the building and call for help.

Do not turn on the lights until you are sure they are safe to use. You may want to have an electrician inspect your wiring.

Roof, foundation and chimney cracks: If it looks like the building may collapse, leave immediately.

Appliances: If appliances are wet, turn off the electricity at the main fuse box or circuit breaker. Then, unplug appliances and let them dry out. Have appliances checked by a professional before using them again. Also, have the electrical system checked by an electrician before turning the power back on.

Water and sewage systems: If pipes are damaged, turn off the main water valve. Check with local authorities before using any water; the water could be contaminated. Pump out wells and have the water tested by authorities before drinking. Do not flush toilets until you know that sewage lines are intact.

Food and other supplies: Throw out all food and other supplies that you suspect may have become contaminated or come in to contact with floodwater.

Your basement: If your basement has flooded, pump it out gradually (about one third of the water per day) to avoid damage. The walls may collapse and the floor may buckle if the basement is pumped out while the surrounding ground is still waterlogged.

Open cabinets: Be alert for objects that may fall.

Clean up household chemical spills: Disinfect items that may have been contaminated by raw sewage, bacteria, or chemicals. Also clean salvageable items.

Call your insurance agent: Take pictures of damages. Keep good records of repair and cleaning costs.

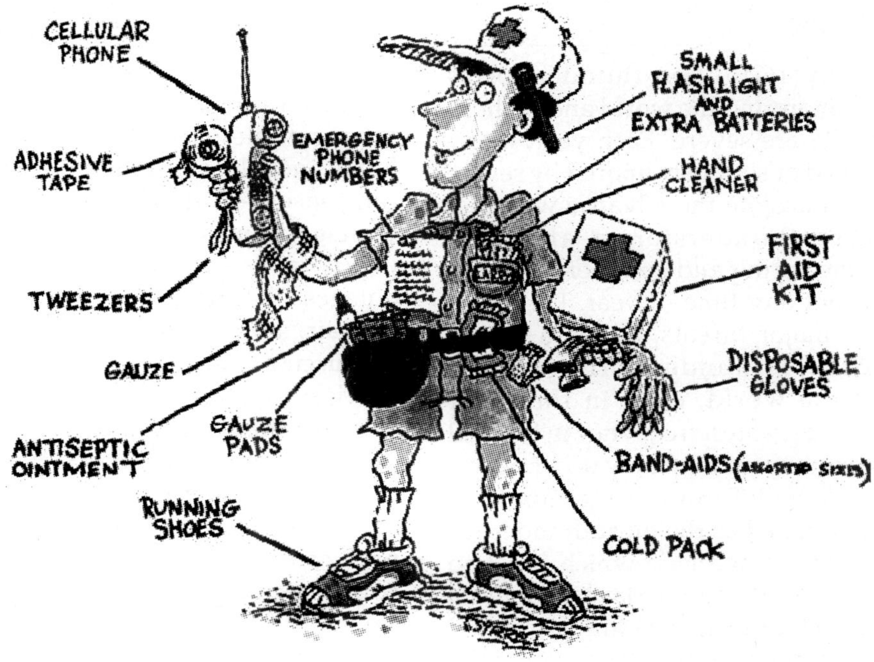

Fig. 17.1

18 Action Plan During Lightning and Thunderstorms

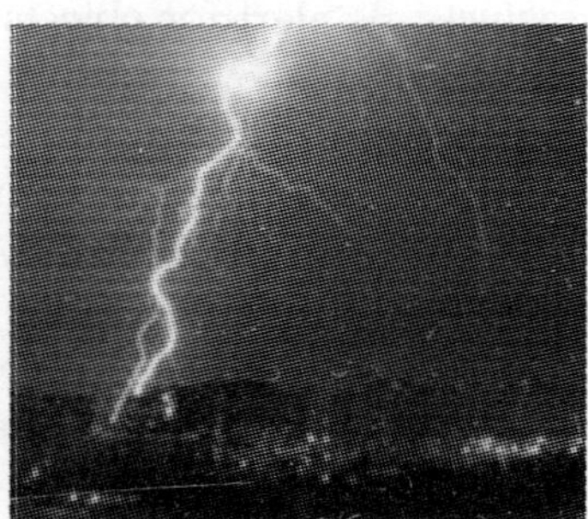

Fig. 18.1

INTRODUCTION

Approximately 16 million thunderstorms occur each year around the world and of those only about 10% are severe. Each year, many people are killed or seriously injured by severe thunderstorms despite the advance warning. While severe thunderstorms are most common in the spring and summer, they can occur just about any time of year. Lightning is one of the major threats during a severe thunderstorm. Thunderstorms occur throughout the world, even in the polar regions, with the greatest frequency in tropical rainforest areas, where they may occur nearly daily. Kampala and Tororo in Uganda have each been mentioned as the most thunderous places on Earth, an accolade which has also been bestowed upon Bogor in Java, Indonesia or Singapore. Thunderstorms are associated with the various monsoon seasons around the globe, and they populate the rainbands of tropical cyclones. In temperate regions, they are most frequent in spring and summer, although they can occur along or ahead of cold fronts at any time of year. They may also occur within a cooler air mass following the passage of a cold front over a relatively warmer body of water. Thunderstorms are rare in polar regions because of cold surface temperatures.

A thunderstorm, also known as an electrical storm, a lightning storm and is usually accompanied by heavy rain and sometimes snow or no precipitation at all. Thunderstorms may line up in series, and strong or severe thunderstorms may rotate. Every thunderstorm produces lightning, which kills more people each year than tornadoes or hurricanes. Heavy rain from thunderstorms can cause flash flooding and high winds can damage homes and blow down trees and utility poles, causing widespread power outages. Warm air has a lower density than cool air, so warm air rises carrying moisture within cooler air and clouds form. As the moist air rises, it cools causing some of the water vapor in the rising packet of air to condense. This releases energy so that the rising packet of air cools less than its surrounding air, so it continues to rise. If enough instability is present in the atmosphere, this process will continue long enough for cumulonimbus clouds to form, which support lightning and thunder. Generally, thunderstorms require three ingredients: (1) moisture, (2) an unstable airmass, and (3) a lifting force.

Mythology

Thunderstorms had a lasting and powerful influence on early civilizations. Romans thought them to be battles waged by Jupiter, who hurled lightning bolts forged by Vulcan. Thunderstorms were associated with the Thunderbirds, held by Native Americans to be a servant of the Great Spirit. Mjolnir, the hammer of the Germanic and Nordic god of thunder, Thor, had the ability to throw lightning bolts.

Definition

A severe thunderstorm is one which produces winds of 58 mph or greater than 1 inch hail or larger or tornadoes. In Canada, a severe thunderstorm is defined as either having tornadoes, wind gusts of 90 km/h or greater, hail of 2 centimeters in diameter or greater, a rainfall rate greater than 50 millimeters in 1 hour, or 75 millimeters in 3 hours.

Stages

All thunderstorms, regardless of type, go through three stages: the cumulus stage, the mature stage, and the dissipation stage. Depending on the conditions present in the atmosphere, these three stages can take anywhere from 20 minutes to several hours to occur.

The first stage of a thunderstorm is the cumulus stage, or developing stage. In this stage, masses of moisture are lifted upwards into the atmosphere. The trigger for this lift can be due to heating of the ground producing thermals, areas where two winds converge forcing air upwards, or where winds blow over terrain of increasing elevation. The moisture rapidly cools into liquid drops of water, which appears as *cumulus* clouds. As the water vapor condenses into liquid, latent heat is released which warms the air, causing it to become less dense than the surrounding dry air. The air tends to rise in an *updraft* through the process of convection. This creates a low pressure zone beneath the forming thunderstorm. In a typical thunderstorm, approximately 5×10^8 kg of water vapor are lifted, and the amount of energy released when this condenses is about equal to the energy used by a city of 100,000 during a month. If the quantity of water that is condensed in and subsequently precipitated from a cloud is known, then the total energy of a thunderstorm can be calculated. In an average thunderstorm, the energy released amounts to about 10,000,000 kilowatt-hours (3.6×10^{13} joule), which is equivalent to a 20-kiloton nuclear warhead. A large, severe thunderstorm might be 10 to 100 times more energetic.

In the mature stage of a thunderstorm, the warmed air continues to rise until it reaches existing air which is warmer, and the air can rise no further. Often this 'cap' is the tropopause. The air is instead forced to spread out, giving the storm a characteristic anvil shape. The resulting cloud is called cumulonimbus incus. The water droplets coalesce into larger and heavier droplets and freeze to become ice particles. As these fall they melt to become rain. If the updraft is strong enough, the droplets are held aloft long enough to be so large that they do not melt completely and fall as hail. While updrafts are still present, the falling rain creates *downdrafts* as well. The simultaneous presence of both an updraft and downdrafts marks the mature stage of the storm, and during this stage considerable internal turbulence can occur in the storm system, which sometimes manifests as strong winds, severe lightning, and even tornadoes.

Typically, if there is little wind shear, the storm will rapidly enter the dissipating stage and 'rain itself out', but if there is sufficient change in wind speed and/or direction the downdraft will be separated from the updraft, and the storm may become a supercell, and the mature stage can sustain itself for several hours.

In certain cases however, even with little wind shear, if there is enough atmospheric support and instability in place for the thunderstorm to feed on, it may even maintain its mature stage a bit longer than most storms.

In the dissipation stage, the thunderstorm is dominated by the downdraft. If atmospheric conditions do not support super cellular development, this stage occurs rather quickly, approximately 20–30 minutes into the life of the thunderstorm. The downdraft will push down out of the thunderstorm, hit the ground and spread out. The cool air carried to the ground by the downdraft cuts off the inflow of the thunderstorm, the updraft disappears and the thunderstorm will dissipate.

The downdraft hitting the ground, may sometimes cause a wind shear, a potential hazardous condition for aircraft flying through it as a substantial change in wind speed occurs, resulting in decrease of lift of the aircraft.

Types of Thunderstorms

There are four main types of thunderstorms: single cell, multicell, squall line (also called multicell line) and supercell. Which type forms depends on the instability and relative wind conditions (shear)at different layers of the atmosphere.

This term technically applies to a single thunderstorm with one main updraft. Within a cluster of thunderstorms, the term "cell" refers to each separate principal updraft.

Thunderstorm cells can and do form in isolation to other cells. Such storms are rarely severe and are a result of local atmospheric instability; hence the term "air mass thunderstorm". These are the typical summer thunderstorm in many temperate locales. They also occur in the cool unstable air which often follows the passage of a cold front from the sea during winter.

While most single cell thunderstorms move, there are some unusual circumstances where they remain stationary. When this happens, catastrophic flooding is possible.

Multicell storms form as clusters of storms but may then evolve into one or more squall lines. They often arise from convective updrafts in or near mountain ranges and linear weather boundaries, usually strong cold fronts or troughs of low pressure.

Multicell line storms, commonly referred to as "squall lines", occur when multi-cellular storms form in a line rather than clusters. They can be hundreds of miles long, move swiftly, and be preceded by a gust front. Heavy rain, hail, lightning, very strong winds and even isolated tornadoes can occur over a large area in a squall line. Bow echoes can form within squall lines, bringing with them even higher winds. An unusually powerful type of squall line called a derecho occurs when an intense squall line travels for several hundred miles, often leaving widespread damage over thousands of square miles.

Occasionally, squall lines also form near the outer rain band of tropical cyclones. The squall line is propelled by its own outflow, which reinforces continuous development of updrafts along the leading edge. This kind of storm is also known as "Wind of the Stony Lake".

Multicell or squall line systems may form within a meteorologically important feature known as Mesocale Convective System (MCS) stretching for hundreds of kilometers. Prior to the discovery of the MCS phenomenon, the individual thunderstorms were thought of as independent entities, each being effectively impossible to predict. The MCS is amenable to forecasting, and a meteorologist can predict with high accuracy the percentage of the MCS that will be affected by thunderstorms.

However, the meteorologist still cannot predict exactly where each thunderstorm will occur within the MCS.

Supercell storms are large, severe quasi-steady-state storms which feature wind speed and direction that vary with height ("wind shear"), separate downdrafts and updrafts (i.e., precipitation is not falling through the updraft) and a strong, rotating updraft (a mesocyclone). These storms normally have such powerful updrafts that the top of the cloud (or anvil) can break through the troposphere and reach into the lower levels of the stratosphere and can be 15 miles (24 km) wide. These storms can produce destructive tornadoes, extremely large hailstones (4 inch or 10 cm diameter), straight-line winds in excess of 80 mph (130 km/h), and flash floods. In fact, most tornadoes occur from this type of thunderstorm.

A back-building thunderstorm is a thunderstorm in which new development takes place on the upwind side such that the storm seems to remain stationary or propagate in a backward direction. Although the storm often appears to be stationary or even moving upwind on radar, this is actually an illusion. The storm in reality is a multi-cell storm with new, more vigorous, cells being formed on the upwind side replacing older cells which continue to drift downstream.

Severity

A severe thunderstorm is a term designating a thunderstorm that has reached a predetermined level of severity. Often, this level is determined by the storm being strong enough to inflict wind or hail damage. In most of the United States, a storm is considered severe if winds reach over 50 knots (58 mph or 93 km/h), hail is ¾ inch (2 cm) diameter or larger, or if funnel clouds and/or tornadoes are reported. Though a funnel cloud or tornado indicates the presence of a severe thunderstorm, a tornado warning would then be issued in place of a severe thunderstorm warning.

Severe thunderstorms can occur from any type of thunderstorm, however multicell and squall lines represent the most common forms. Supercells are often the most powerful type of severe thunderstorm.

Lightning

Lightning is an electrical discharge that occurs in a thunderstorm. It can be seen in the form of a bright streak (or bolt) from the sky. Lightning occurs when an electrical charge is built up within a cloud, due to static electricity generated by supercooled water droplets colliding with ice crystals near the freezing level. When a large enough charge is built up, a large discharge will occur and can be seen as lightning. The temperature of a lightning bolt can be five times hotter than the surface of the sun. Although the lightning is extremely hot, the duration is short and 90% of strike victims survive. Contrary to the popular idea that lightning does not strike twice in the same spot, some people have been struck by lightning over three times, and skyscrapers have been struck numerous times in the same storm. The loud bang that is heard is the super heated air around the lightning bolt expanding at the speed of sound. Because sound travels much more slowly than light the flash is seen before the bang, although both occur at the same moment.

There are several types of lightning:

- In-cloud lightning is the most common. It is lightning within a cloud and is sometimes called intra-cloud or sheet lightning.
- Cloud to ground lightning is when a bolt of lightning from a cloud strikes the ground. This form poses the greatest threat to life and property.
- Ground to cloud lightning is when a

lightning bolt is induced from the ground to the cloud.

- Cloud to cloud lightning is rarely seen and is when a bolt of lightning arcs from one cloud to another.
- Ball lightning is extremely rare and has several hypothesized explanations. It is seen in the form of a 20 to 200 centimeter ball.
- Cloud to air lightning is when lightning from a cloud hits air of a different charge.
- Dry lightning is a misnomer which can refer to a thunderstorm whose precipitation does not reach the ground.
- Heat lightning is a misnomer of a lightning flash that is seen from the horizon that does not have accompanying thunder.

Facts About Lightning

Lightning results from the buildup and discharge of electrical energy between positively and negatively charged areas. The average flash could light a 100-watt light bulb for more than 3 months. Most lightning occurs within the cloud or between the cloud and ground. Your chances of being struck by lightning are estimated to be 1 in 600,000.Lightning's unpredictability increases the risk to individuals and property. Lightning often strikes outside of heavy rain and may occur as far as 10 miles away from any rainfall. "Heat lightning" is actually lightning from a thunderstorm too far away for thunder to be heard. However, the storm may be moving in your direction! Most lightning deaths and injuries occur when people are caught outdoors in the summer months during the afternoon and evening.

Safety Precautions

- *If outside:* move indoors. Most lightning deaths and injuries occur when people are caught outdoors. Once inside avoid doors, windows, and metal objects. Avoid using electrical appliances. Use the telephone only in an emergency. Shutter windows and stay clear away. Do not take bath shower or use plumbing. Stay indoors until 30 min after the last thunderclap.
- *If driving:* Pull over at safety exit and stay inside with emergency flashers on till rain ends. stay indoors until 30 min after the last thunderclap.
- *Stay in your automobile:* An enclosed automobile offers reasonably good protection from lightning.
- *Outdoors:* Stay away from isolated trees. If your hair stands on end or your skin tingles, lightning may be about to strike. Crouch down quickly and make a low target. DO NOT LIE DOWN FLAT. Avoid high ground do not go close to metal fencing. AVOID boating, swimming, golfing, bike riding, riding a lawnmower, loading a truck, playing outdoor games, fishing in a boat, mountain climbing during a thunderstorm.
- If stuck outdoors, avoid high ground do not go close to metal fencing.
- Remember that most lightning casualties occur in the summer months and during the afternoon and early evening.
- The air near a lightning strike is heated to 50,000 degrees Fahrenheit — hotter than the surface of the sun! But lightning strike victims carry no electrical charge and should be attended to immediately.

Lightning Myths and Facts

- **MYTH**:If it is not raining, then there is no danger from lightning
  FACT:Lightning often strikes outside of heavy rain and may occur as far as 10 miles away from any rainfall.
- **MYTH**:The rubber soles of shoes or rubber tires on a car will protect you from being struck by lightning.

FACT:Rubber-soled shoes and rubber tires provide NO protection from lightning. However, the steel frame of a hard-topped vehicle provides increased protection if you are not touching metal. Although you may be injured if lightning strikes your car, you are much safer inside a vehicle than outside.

- MYTH:People struck by lightning carry an electrical charge and should not be touched.

  FACT:Lightning-strike victims carry no electrical charge and should be attended to immediately.
- MYTH:"Heat-lightning" occurs after very hot summer days and poses no threat.

  FACT:What is referred to as "heat-lightning" is actually lightning from a thunderstorm too far away for thunder to be heard. However, the storm may be moving in your direction!

Some thunderstorms can be seen approaching, while others hit without warning. It is important to learn and recognize the danger signs and to plan ahead.

Before

- Learn the thunderstorm danger signs.
- Dark, towering, or threatening clouds.
- Distant lightning and thunder.
- Have disaster supplies on hand.
- Flashlight with extra batteries.
- Portable, battery-operated radio and extra batteries.
- First aid kit and manual.
- Emergency food and water.
- Nonelectric (Manual or battery operated) can opener.
- Essential medicines.
- Cash and credit cards.
- Sturdy shoes.

Check for hazards in the yard. Dead or rotting trees and branches can fall during a severe thunderstorm and cause injury and damage.

Make sure that all family members know how to respond after a thunderstorm.

Teach family members how and when to turn off gas, electricity and water.

Teach children how and when to call the local police, fire department, and which radio station to tune for emergency information.

Severe Thunderstorm Watches and Warnings:

- A severe thunderstorm watch is issued by the National Meteorological Service when the weather conditions are such that a severe thunderstorm (damaging winds 58 miles per hour or more, or hail three-fourths of an inch in diameter or greater) is likely to develop. This is the time to locate a safe place in the home and tell family members to watch the sky and listen to the radio or television for more information.
- A severe thunderstorm warning is issued when a severe thunderstorm has been sighted or indicated by weather radar. At this point, the danger is very serious and everyone should go to a safe place, turn on a battery-operated radio or television, and wait for the all clear by the authorities. Anticipate and prepare for flash floods. When a severe thunderstorm warning is issued, develop an emergency communication plan. In case family members are separated from one another during a thunderstorm (a real possibility during the day when adults are at work and children are at school), have a plan for getting back together.
- Ask an out-of-state relative or friend to serve as the family contact. After a disaster, it's often easier to call long distance. Make sure everyone knows the name, address, and phone number of the contact person.

- Contact you local emergency administrative office or Red Cross chapter for more information on thunderstorms and lightning.

During

If indoors:

- Secure outdoor objects such as lawn furniture that could blow away or cause damage or injury. Take light objects inside.
- Shutter windows securely and brace outside doors.
- Listen to a battery operated radio or television for the latest storm information.
- Do not handle any electrical equipment or telephones because lightning could follow the wire. Television sets are particularly dangerous at this time.
- Avoid bathtubs, water faucets/taps, and sinks because metal pipes can transmit electricity.

If outdoors:

- Attempt to get into a building or car.
- If no structure is available, get to an open space an squat low to the ground as quickly as possible. (If in the woods, find an area protected by low clump of trees—never stand underneath a single large tree in the open.) Be aware of the potential for flooding in low-lying areas.
- Avoid tall structures such as towers, tall trees, fences, telephone lines, or power lines.
- Stay away from natural lightning rods such as golf clubs, tractors, fishing rods, bicycles, or camping equipment.
- Stay away from rivers, lakes, or other bodies of water.
- If you are isolated in a level field and you feel your hair stand on end (which indicates that lightning is about to strike), bend forward, putting your hands on your knees. A position with feet together and crouching while removing all metal objects is recommended. Do not lie flat on the ground.

If in a car:

- Pull safely onto the shoulder of the road away from any trees that could fall on the vehicle.
- Stay in the car and turn on the emergency flashers until the heavy rains subside.
- Avoid flooded roadways.

Estimating the Distance from a Thunderstorm

Because light travels much faster than sound, lightning flashes can be seen long before the resulting thunder is heard. Estimate the number of miles you are from a thunderstorm by counting the number of seconds between a flash of lightning and the next clap of thunder. Divide this number by five.

Important: You are in danger from lightning if you can hear thunder. Knowing how far away a storm is does not mean that you're in danger only when the storm is overhead.

Hail: Hail is produced by many strong thunderstorms. Hail can be smaller than a pea or as large as a tennis ball and can be very destructive to plants and crops. In a hailstorm, take cover immediately. Pets and livestock are particularly vulnerable to hail, so bring animals into a shelter.

After

Check for injuries: A person who has been struck by lightning does not carry an electrical charge that can shock other people. If the victim is burned, provide first aid and call emergency medical assistance immediately. Look for burns where lightning entered and exited the body. If the strike cause the victim's heart and breathing to stop, give cardiopulmonary resuscitation (CPR) until medical professionals arrive and take over.

Remember to help your neighbours who may require special assistance—infants, elderly people, and people with disabilities.

Report downed electric and utility wires.

Drive only if necessary: Debris and washed-out roads may make driving dangerous.

Mitigation

Mitigation includes any activities that prevent an emergency, reduce the chance of an emergency happening, or lessen the damaging effects of unavoidable emergencies. Investing in preventive mitigation steps now, such as installing lightning rods to carry the electrical charge of lightning bolts safely to the ground or purchasing flood/home insurance, will help reduce the impact of severe thunderstorms in the future.

ELECTRIC SHOCK

Introduction

The human body is made up of 60% to 70% water. This makes it a good conductor of electricity. An electric shock occurs upon contact of a human body with any source of voltage high enough to cause sufficient current flows through the body tissues. Death caused by an electric shock is referred to as electrocution and is the second main cause of death at workplace after falls from heights. Incidence is 2.1 deaths per million population or 1:5000 worldwide.

Causes of Electric Shock

Adolescents and adults are prone to high voltage shock caused by mischievous exploration and exposure at work. Most of these deaths are related to on-the-job injuries and death occurs in 3–15 percent of cases, with infection being the most common cause of death in people hospitalized following electrical burns. Electrocution is the second main cause of death at workplace after falls from heights. Incidence is 2.1 deaths per million population or 1:5000 worldwide. Children are not often seriously injured by electricity. They are prone to shock by the low voltage (110-220 volts) found in typical household current. In children aged 12 years and younger, household appliance electrical cords and extension cords caused more than 63% of injuries. Wall outlets were responsible for 15% of injuries. In children older than 12 years, most electrical injuries result from exploring and activities around high-power systems. A bolt of lightning carries as many as 30 million volts.

Skin Resistance

The voltage necessary for electrocution depends on the current through the body and the duration of the current. Using Ohm's law, Voltage = Current × Resistance, we see that the current drawn depends on the resistance of the body. The resistance of our skin varies from person to person and fluctuates between different times of day. In general, dry skin is a poor conductor that may have a resistance of around 100,000 Ù, while broken or wet skin may have a resistance of around 1,000 Ù. The minimum current a human can feel is thought to be about 1 milliampere (mA).

Many variables determine what injuries may occur, if any. These variables include the type of current (AC or DC), the amount of current (determined by the voltage of the source and the resistance of the tissues involved), and the pathway the electricity takes through the body. Low voltage electricity (less than 500 volts) does not normally cause significant injury to humans. Exposure to high voltage electricity (greater than 500 volts) has the potential to result in serious damage.

Electric Shock Values

1. *Electrical sensation:* Tingling sensation occurs at about 0.25 to 0.5 mA for an adult female and between 0.50 and 1 mA for an adult male.

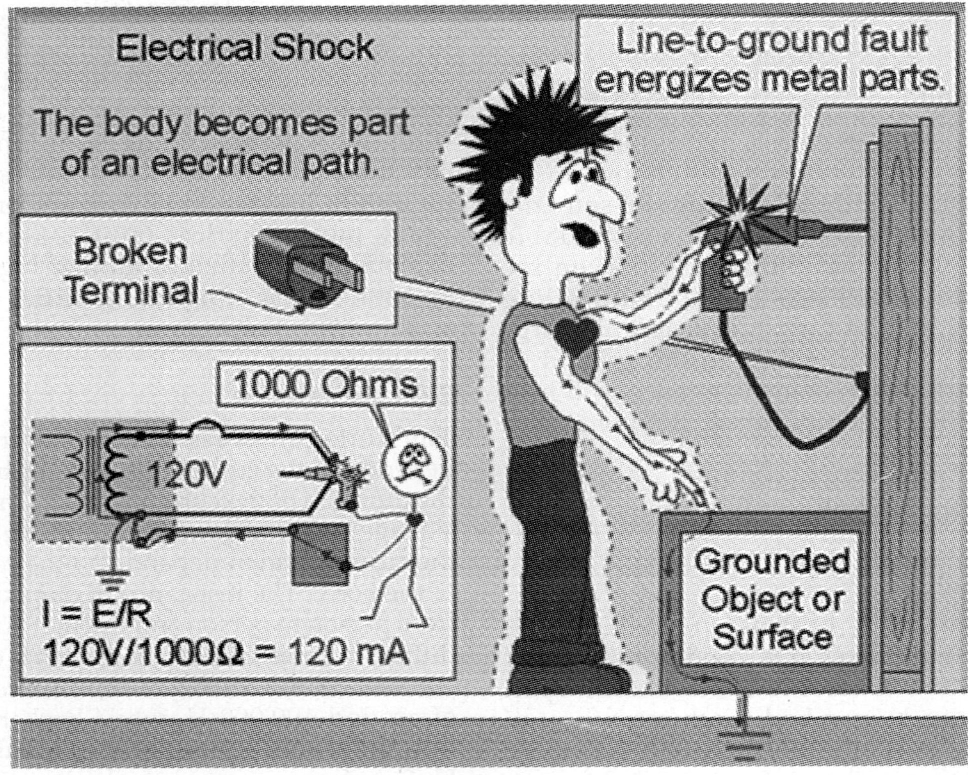

Fig. 18.2

2. *Uncomfortable sensation:* Current over 1-2 mA is very uncomfortable to both sexes.
3. *Maximum Let-Go Level:* The maximum Let Go Threshold level for a female is approximately - 9 mA and for a male it is about - 15 mA.

The "Let Go" Threshold is the current level where we lose control of our muscles and the electricity causes muscles to contract until the current is removed.

The maximum safe shock duration can be determined by the formula:

Seconds = 0.116/(E/R), where R (resistance of person) is assumed to be 1000 ohms.

For a 120V circuit the maximum shock duration = 0.116/(120V/1000) = 1 Second For a 277V circuit the maximum shock duration = 0.116/(277V/1000) = 0.43 Second.

Types of Currents

Comparison between the dangers of alternating current and direct current has been a subject of debate ever since the War of Currents in the 1880s. DC tends to cause continuous muscular contractions that make the victim hold on to a live conductor, thereby increasing the risk of deep tissue burns. On the other hand, mains-magnitude AC tends to interfere more with the heart's electrical pacemaker, leading to an increased risk of fibrillation. AC at higher frequencies holds a different mixture of hazards, such as RF burns and the possibility of tissue damage with no immediate sensation of pain. Generally, higher frequency AC current tends to run along the skin rather than penetrating and touching vital organs such as the heart due to the skin effect. While there will be severe burn damage at higher voltages, it is normally not fatal.

It is sometimes suggested that human lethality is most common with alternating current at 100–250 volts; however, death has occurred below this range, with supplies as low as 32 volts. Danger increase dramatically with voltages over 250 volts. Shocks above 3300 volts are often fatal, with those above 11000 volts being usually fatal.

Electrical discharge from lightning tends to travel over the surface of the body causing burns and may cause respiratory arrest.

Point of entry

- *Macroshock:* Current across intact skin and through the body. Current from arm to arm, or between an arm and a foot, is likely to traverse the heart, therefore it is much more dangerous than current between a leg and the ground. This type of shock by definition must pass into the body through the skin.
- *Microshock:* Direct current path to the heart tissue, the shock is required to be administered from inside the skin, i.e. a malfunctioning pacemaker, or ungrounded catheter etc.

Arc Flash

Up to 80 percent of its electrical injuries involve thermal burns due to arcing faults. The arc flash in an electrical fault produces the same type of light radiation from which electric welders protect themselves using face shields with dark glass, heavy leather gloves, and full-coverage clothing. The heat produced may cause severe burns, especially on unprotected flesh. The blast produced by vaporizing metallic components can break bones and irreparably damage internal organs. The degree of hazard present at a particular location can be determined by a detailed analysis of the electrical system, and appropriate protection worn if the electrical work must be performed with the electricity on.

Effects

1. *Burns:* Heating due to resistance can cause extensive and deep burns. Voltage levels of 500 to 1000 volts tend to cause internal burns due to the large energy (which is proportional to the duration multiplied by the square of the current multiplied by resistance) available from the source. Damage due to current is through tissue heating.
2. *Ventricular fibrillation:* A low-voltage (110 or 230 V), 50 or 60-Hz AC current through the chest for a fraction of a second may induce ventricular fibrillation at currents as low as 60 mA. With DC, 300 to 500 mA is required. If the current has a direct pathway to the heart (e.g., via a cardiac catheter or other kind of electrode), a much lower current of less than 1 mA (AC or DC) can cause fibrillation. If not immediately treated by defibrillation, fibrillations are usually lethal because all the heart muscle cells move independently. current may cause tissue damage or fibrillation if it is sufficiently high. Death caused by an electric shock is referred to as electrocution. Generally, currents approaching 100 mA are lethal if they pass through sensitive portions of the body. Above 200 mA, muscle contractions are so strong that the heart muscles cannot move at all.
3. *Neurological effects:* Current can cause interference with nervous control, especially over the heart and lungs. Repeated or severe electric shock which does not lead to death has been shown to

cause neuropathy. Electrical damage to the brain may result in a permanent seizure disorder, depression, anxiety, or other personality changes. When the current path is through the head, it appears that, with sufficient current, loss of consciousness almost always occurs swiftly. This method is used for execution of criminals in the so called "Electric Chair". In psychiatry treatment electroconvulsive therapy utilizes 0.9 amp current between 200-450 volts, frequency 70 Hertz ,pulse width 1.5 milliseconds and stiumulation duration 2.6 to 5.3 seconds to treat depression.

Management

If you are going to help someone who has sustained a high voltage shock, you need to be very careful that you don't become a second victim of a similar electrical shock. If a high voltage line has fallen to the ground, there may be a circle of current spreading out from the tip of the line. Your best bet may be to call 911. The electric company will be notified so that the power can be shut off. When a severe electric shock injury happens at home, the main power should immediately be shut off. If that cannot be done, and current is still flowing through the child, the alternative is to stand on a dry, nonconducting surface such as a folded newspaper, flattened cardboard carton, or plastic or rubber mat and use a nonconducting object such as a wooden broomstick (never a damp or metallic object) to push the child away from the source of the current. The victim and the source of the current must not be touched while the current is still flowing, for doing so can electrocute the rescuer.

A victim who has fallen from a height or sustained a severe shock causing multiple jerks may have a serious neck injury and should not be moved without first protecting the neck.

A person shocked by high voltage (500 volts or more) should be evaluated in the Emergency Department. It may be prudent to get prehospital care, usually obtained by calling 911. Following a low-voltage shock, go to the Emergency Department for the following concerns:

- Any noticeable burn to the skin (at entry and exit points of current).
- Any period of unconsciousness
- Any numbness, tingling, *paralysis*, vision, hearing, or speech problems.
- Muscle spasms or contractions.
- Sudden immobility or deformity due to fractures.
- Irregular breathing or heartbeats.
- Any electric shock if more than 20 weeks' pregnant.
- A small child who bites or sucks on an electric cord can have a facial injury or distinct burn around the rim of the mouth.

Prevention

- For children younger than 12 years, most electrical injuries are caused by power cords. Inspect your power cords and extension cords. Replace any cords that have broken or cracked external covering and any cord that has exposed wire.
  - Do not allow children to play with any electrical cord.
  - Limit use of extension cords and be sure the cord is rated for the current (measured in amps) that will be drawn by the device being powered.
  - Use outlet covers to protect infants from exploring electrical outlets.
  - Update old, ungrounded electrical outlets to grounded (3-prong) systems. Replace outlets near any water (sink, tub) with fused outlets.
- In children older than 12 years, most electrical injuries result from exploring and

activities around high-power systems. Explain to adolescent children that they should not climb on power towers, play near transformer systems, or explore electrified train rails or other electrical systems.

- Among adults, use of common sense can help reduce electrical injury. People who work with electricity should always check that the power is off before working on electrical systems. Avoid use of any electrical device near water. Be careful of standing in water or when working with electricity.
- Use caution when outdoors during a thunderstorm containing lightning. Protect yourself from lightning strikes by seeking shelter in a sturdy building or crouching low and away from trees and metal objects if caught outdoors.
- To protect against electric shock from dangerous voltages on metal parts of electrical equipment from a ground-fault must be quickly removed by opening the circuit's overcurrent protection device. The time it takes for an overcurrent protection device to open and clear a ground-fault and remove dangerous voltage is inversely proportional to the magnitude of the fault current. This means that the higher the ground-fault current, the less time it will take for the overcurrent device to open and clear the fault.
- An inverse time circuit breaker or fuse most likely will prevent serious electric shock if the ground-fault current is at least six times the rating of the overcurrent protection device. For a 20A circuit, the ground-fault current should be at least 120A. As is apparent, the impedance of the fault current path plays a critical and vital role in removing dangerous voltages from metal parts by facilitating the opening of the branch-circuit overcurrent protection device to prevent electric shock or electrocution.

19 Action Plan During Hurricanes and Cyclones

> "Two thirds of federal disaster aid is weather related and, though we cannot prevent bad weather, we are getting better at predicting it, to help save lives and protect property."
>
> — *William M. Daley*

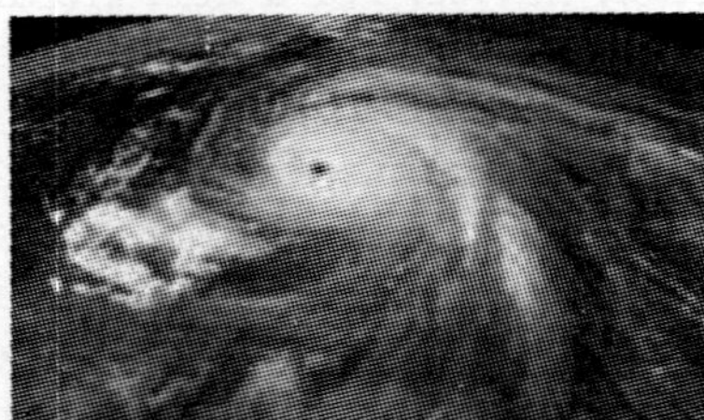

Fig. 19.1

INTRODUCTION

Named after Huracan, the Carib god of evil, the hurricane is an amazing yet destructive natural phenomenon that occurs about 40 to 50 times worldwide each year. Hurricane season takes place in the Atlantic, Caribbean, Gulf of Mexico, and Central Pacific from June 1 to November 30 while in the Eastern Pacific the season is from May 15 to November 30.

HURRICANE FORMATION

Due to the Coriolis effect, the regions between 5° and 20° north and south of the equator are the belts where hurricanes can form (there is not enough rotary motion between 5° north and south.) The term cyclone is used in the Bay of Bengal and Arabian Sea and the term typhoon is used in the Pacific Ocean north of the equator and west of the International Dateline.

The birth of a hurricane starts as a low pressure zone and builds into a tropical wave of low pressure. In addition to a disturbance in the tropical ocean water, the storms that become hurricanes also require warm ocean waters (above 80°F or 27°C down to 150 feet or 50 meters below sea level) and light upper level winds.

GROWTH AND DEVELOPMENT OF TROPICAL STORMS AND HURRICANES

A tropical wave grows in intensity and then develops into an organized area of showers and thunderstorms known as a tropical disturbance. This disturbance becomes an organized area of tropical low pressure that is called a tropical depression based on cyclonic winds (counter-clockwise in the Northern Hemisphere and clockwise in the Southern Hemisphere). A tropical depression's wind speed must be at or below 38 miles per hour (mph) or 62 km/hr when averaged out over one minute. These winds are measured at 33 feet (10 meters) above the surface. Once average winds reach 39 mph or 63 km/hr then the cyclonic system becomes a tropical storm and receives a name while tropical depressions are numbered (i.e., Tropical Depression 4 became Tropical Storm Chantal in the 2001 season.) Tropical storm names are preselected and issued alphabetically for each storm.

There are approximately 80-100 tropical storms annually and about half of these storms become full-fledged hurricanes. It is at 74 mph or 119 km/hr that a tropical storm becomes a hurricane. Hurricanes can be from 60 to almost 1000 miles wide. They vary widely in intensity; their strength is measured on the Safir-Simpson scale from a weak category 1 storm to a catastrophic category 5 storm. Hurricane damage results from three primary causes:

1. *Storm surge:* Approximately 90% of all hurricane deaths can be attributed to the storm surge, the dome of water created by the low pressure center of a hurricane. This storm surge quickly floods low-lying coastal areas with anywhere from 3 feet (one meter) for a category one storm to over 19 feet (6 meters) of storm surge for a category five storm. Hundreds of thousands of deaths in countries such as Bangladesh have been caused by the storm surge of cyclones.
2. *Wind damage:* The strong, at least 74 mph or 119 km/hr, winds of a hurricane can cause widespread destruction far inland of coastal areas, destroying homes, buildings, forests and infrastructure.
3. *Freshwater flooding:* Hurricanes are huge tropical storms and dump many inches of rain over a widespread area in a short period of time. This water can engorge rivers and streams, causing hurricane-induced flooding.

A majority of people living in coastal areas are unprepared for a hurricane disaster. Anyone living along the Atlantic Coast, the Gulf Coast, Indian East coast, Sea of Japan and the Caribbean should be prepared for hurricanes during hurricane season. Fortunately, hurricanes ultimately diminish, reverting to tropical storm strength and then into a tropical depression when they move over cooler ocean water, move over land, or reach a position where the upper level winds are strong. Hurricanes can be dangerous killers. Learning the cyclone/hurricane warning messages and planning ahead can reduce the chances of injury or major property damage.

BEFORE

Plan An Evacuation Route

Contact the local administrative authorities for the community hurricane/cyclone preparedness plan. This plan should include information on the safest evacuation routes and nearby shelters.

Learn Safe Routes Inland

Be ready to travel/drive 2 to 5miles inland to locate a safe place.

Have disaster supplies on hand like flashlight and extra batteries, portable, battery-operated radio and extra batteries, first aid kit and manual, emergency food and water, nonelectric/manual or battery operated can opener, essential medicines, cash and credit cards and sturdy shoes/gum boots and raincoats/caps.

Make arrangements for pets as they may not be allowed into emergency shelters for health and space reasons. Contact your local SPCA for information on local animal shelters.

Make sure that all family members know how to respond after a cyclone/hurricane by teaching family members how and when to turn off gas, electricity, and water and also how and when to call police, or fire department and which radio station to tune to for emergency information.

Protect your windows. Permanent shutters are the best protection. A lower-cost approach is to put up plywood panels. Use 1/2 inch plywood—marine plywood is best—cut to fit each window. Remember to mark which board fits which window. Pre-drill holes every 18 inches for screws. Do this long before the storm.

Trim back dead or weak branches from trees.

Check your home/ flood insurance.

Develop an emergency communication plan. In case family members are separated from one another during a disaster (a real possibility during the day when adults are at work and children are at school), have a plan for getting back together.

Ask an out-of-state relative or friend to serve as the family contact. After a disaster, it's often easier to call long distance. Make sure everyone in the family knows the name, address, and phone number of the contact person.

Hurricane/Cyclone Watches and Warnings

A hurricane/cyclone watch or alert is issued when there is a threat of hurricane conditions within 24-36 hours. A hurricane warning is issued when hurricane conditions (winds of 74 miles per hour or greater, or dangerously high water and rough seas) are expected in 24 hours or less.

DURING A HURRICANE/CYCLONE WATCH /ALERT

- Listen to a battery-operated radio or television for hurricane progress reports.
- Check emergency supplies and fuel car/ transport.
- Bring in outdoor objects such as lawn furniture, toys, and garden tools and anchor objects that cannot be brought inside.
- Secure buildings by closing and boarding up windows. Remove outside antennas.
- Turn refrigerator and freezer to coldest settings. Open only when absolutely necessary and close quickly.
- Store drinking water in clean bathtubs, jugs, bottles, and cooking utensils.
- Review evacuation plan.
- Moor boats securely or move it to a designated safe place. Use rope or chain to secure boat to trailer. Use tie downs to anchor trailer to the ground or house.

DURING A HURRICANE/CYCLONE WARNING

- Listen constantly to a battery-operated radio or television for official instructions.
- If in a mobile home, check tie downs and evacuate immediately.
- Store valuables and personal papers in a waterproof container on the highest level of your home.
- Avoid elevators.

If at home:

- Stay inside, away from windows, skylights, and glass doors.
- Keep a supply of flashlights and extra batteries handy. Avoid open flames, such as candles and kerosene lamps, as a source of light.
- If power is lost, turn off major appliances to reduce power surge when electricity is restored.
- If officials indicate evacuation is necessary: Leave as soon as possible. Avoid flooded roads and watch for washed-out bridges.
- Secure your home by unplugging appliances and turning off electricity and the main water valve.
- Tell someone outside of the storm area where you are going.
- If time permits, and you live in an identified surge zone, elevate furniture to protect it from flooding or better yet, move it to a higher floor.
- Bring pre-assembled emergency supplies and warm protective clothing.

- Take blankets and sleeping bags to shelter.
- Lock up home and leave.

AFTER

- Stay tuned to local radio for information.
- Help injured or trapped persons. Give first aid where appropriate.
- Do not move seriously injured persons unless they are in immediate danger of further injury. Call for help.
- Return home only after authorities advise that it is safe to do so.
- Avoid loose or dangling power lines and report them immediately to the power company, police, or fire department.
- Enter your home with caution. Beware of snakes, insects, and animals driven to higher ground by flood water. Open windows and doors to ventilate and dry your home. Check refrigerated foods for spoilage.
- Take pictures of the damage, both to the house and its contents and for insurance claims.
- Drive only if absolutely necessary and avoid flooded roads and washed-out bridges. Use telephone only for emergency calls.

INSPECTING UTILITIES IN A DAMAGED HOME

- *Check for gas leaks:*If you smell gas or hear blowing or hissing noise, open a window and quickly leave the building. Turn off the gas at the outside main valve if you can and call the gas company from a neighbor's home. If you turn off the gas for any reason, it must be turned back on by a professional.
- *Look for electrical system damage:* If you see sparks or broken or frayed wires, or if you smell hot insulation, turn off the electricity at the main fuse box or circuit breaker. If you have to step in water to get to the fuse box or circuit breaker, call an electrician first for advice.
- *Check for sewage and water lines damage:* If you suspect sewage lines are damaged avoid using the toilets and call a plumber. If water pipes are damaged, contact the water company and avoid the water from the tap. You can obtain safe water by melting ice cubes.

MITIGATION

Mitigation includes any activities that prevent an emergency, reduce the chance of an emergency happening, or lessen the damaging effects of unavoidable emergencies. Investing in preventive mitigation steps now such as strengthening un-reinforced masonry to withstand wind and flooding and installing shutters on every window will help reduce the impact of hurricanes in the future.

20 Action Plan During Tornadoes

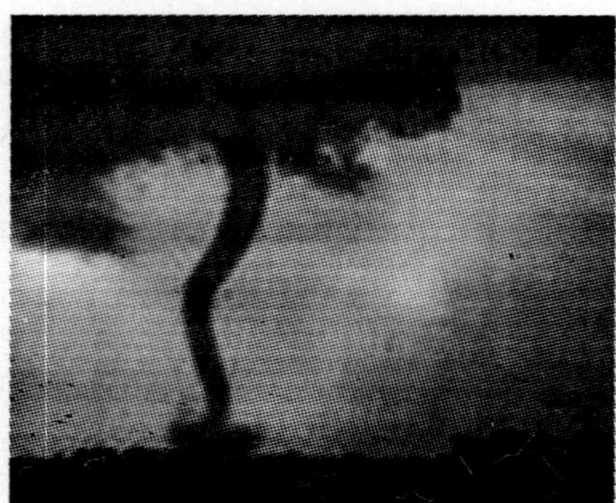

Fig. 20.1

INTRODUCTION

Tornadoes are violently rotating columns of air, pendant from a cumuliform cloud or underneath a cumuliform cloud, and often (but not always) visible as a funnel cloud .Tornadoes form a circular column of low pressure (up to about 100 millibars lower than the surrounding air) which has very fast wind circling around it at speeds of 200 to 500 miles per hour. These 450-1800 foot wide columns can drive straw into wood and wood into metal as they create their path of destruction. In order for a vortex to be classified as a tornado, it must be in contact with the ground *and* the cloud base. Tornadoes, also known as twisters, usually move at about 15 to 30 miles per hour towards the northeast and last from a few minutes to as long as eight hours. Tornadoes are the most destructive of any local atmospheric disturbance and it is the wind, not the low pressure, that causes the most damage. They can make a city look like it was bombed.

Tornadoes occur in all the fifty states of North America, Canada, southern Brazil, South Africa, Australia, Bangladesh, Europe, Japan, and New Zealand.

Formation

Usually when warm moist air meets cold air dry air. Tornadoes can appear from any direction. Most move from southwest to northeast, or west to east. Some tornadoes can change direction or even backtrack. A tornado can double back suddenly, when its bottom is hit by outflow winds. Rain, wind, lightning, and hail vary from storm to storm, from one hour to the next, and even with the direction the storm is moving with respect to the observer. A large hail *can* indicate the presence of an unusually dangerous thunderstorm but neither hail, nor any particular pattern of rain, lightning or calmness, is a reliable predictor of tornado threat.

Tornadoes need a source of instability (heat, moisture, etc.) and a larger-scale property of rotation (*vorticity*) to keep going and last from several seconds to more than an hour. Most tornadoes last less than 10 minutes. A waterspout is a tornado over water and can happen over seas, bays and lakes worldwide. Although waterspouts are always tornadoes by definition; they do not officially count in tornado records unless they hit land. They are smaller and weaker than the most tornadoes over land, but still can be quite dangerous. Waterspouts can overturn boats, damage larger ships, inflict significant damage when hitting land, and kill people. Most tornadoes rotate *cyclonically*, which is counterclockwise in the northern hemisphere and clockwise south of the equator. Multivortex tornadoes contain two or more small, intense *subvortices* orbiting the center of the larger tornado circulation Dr. T. Theodore Fujita developed a damage scale (Fujita 1971, Fujita and Pearson 1973) for winds, including tornadoes, which was supposed to relate the degree of damage to the intensity of the wind. The Enhanced F-scale is a much more precise and robust way to assess tornado damage. It classifies F0 - F5 damage as calibrated by engineers and meteorologists across 28 different types of damage indicators (mainly various kinds of buildings, but also a few other structures as well as trees) and rates the tornado as a whole based on most intense damage within the path. F5 rating implies the most intense possible damage level and a tornado is considered "significant" if it was rated EF2 or greater on the enhanced scale, or at least F2 on the old F-scale. The size or shape of *any particular tornado* does not say anything conclusive about its strength. Some small 'rope' tornadoes can cause violent damage of EF4 or 5 and some very large tornadoes over a quarter-mile wide have produced only weak damage equivalent to EF0 or EF1. The most common tornado sound is a continuous rumble, like a closeby train. Sometimes a tornado produces a loud whooshing sound, like that of a waterfall or of open car windows while driving very fast. Tornadoes which are tearing through densely populated areas may be producing all kinds of loud noises at once, which collectively may make a tremendous roar.

The vertical winds in tornadoes can be strong enough to temporarily levitate even heavy objects if they have a large face to the wind or flat sides (like roofs, walls, trees and cars), and are strong enough to carry lightweight objects tens of thousands of feet high. Though the heaviest objects, such as railroad cars, can only be airborne for short distances, paper can be carried over 100 miles away. The winds from the strongest tornadoes far exceed that from the strongest hurricanes, hurricanes typically cause much more damage individually and over a season, and over far bigger areas. Economically, tornadoes cause about a tenth as much damage per year, on average, as hurricanes. Hurricanes tend to cause much more overall destruction than tornadoes because of their much larger size, longer duration and their greater variety of ways to damage property. The destructive core in hurricanes can be tens of miles across, last many hours and damage structures through storm surge and rainfall-caused flooding, as well as from wind. Tornadoes, in contrast, tend to be a few hundred yards in diameter, last for minutes and primarily cause damage. The highest elevation a tornado has ever occurred is at 10,000 feet above sea level.

Forecasting

Analysis of surface and upper-air data using high-performance computer workstations that intergrate computer model displays, satellite image loops, radar displays, wind profiling, radar wind plots, data from weather stations, upper air data from balloons and planes, lightning strike plots, weather data tables and multiple source overlays. Doppler radar signatures can tell meteorologists a great deal about a thunderstorm's structure and an intense circulation indicates the possibility of a tornado formation.

During a Tornado

Vehicles are notorious as death traps in tornadoes, because they are easily tossed and destroyed. Leave the vehicle for sturdy shelter or drive out of the tornado's path. When the traffic is jammed or the tornado is bearing down on you at close range, your only option may be to park safely off the traffic lanes, get out and find a sturdy building for shelter, if possible. If not, lie flat in a low spot, as far from the road as possible (to avoid flying vehicles). However, in open country, the best option is to escape if the tornado is far away. *If the traffic allows, and the tornado is distant,* you probably have time to drive out of its path. Watch the tornado closely for a few seconds compared to a fixed object in the foreground (such as a tree, pole, or other landmark). If it appears to be moving to your right or left, it is not moving toward you. Still, you should escape at right angles to its track: to your right if it is moving to your left, and vice versa—just to put more distance between you and its path. If the tornado appears to stay in the same place, growing larger or getting closer—but not moving either right or left—it is headed right at you. You must take shelter away from the car or get out of its way fast!

In a basement, the safest place is under a sturdy workbench, mattress or other such protection and out from under heavy furniture or appliances resting on top of the floor above. Safe rooms are reinforced small windowless rooms built in the interior of a home, which are fortified by concrete and/or steel to offer extra protection against tornadoes, hurricanes and other severe windstorms. They can be built in a basement, or if no basement is available, on the ground floor. In existing homes, interior bathrooms or closets are safer. Community tornado shelters are excellent ideas for apartment complexes, schools, mobile home parks, factories, office complexes and other facilities where large groups of people live, work or study.

21 Action Plan During Tsunamis

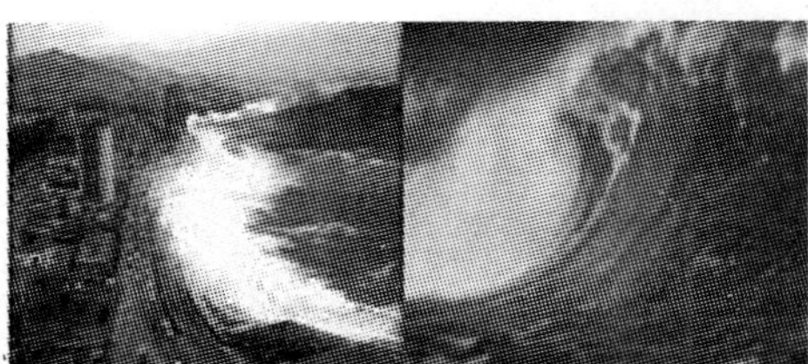

Fig. 21.1

INTRODUCTION

Tsunamis are enormous ocean waves or seismic sea waves, produced by earthquakes or underwater landslides. Tsunami is a Japanese word meaning harbour wave, because of the devastating effects these waves have on low-lying Japanese coastal communities. Tsunamis are not tidal waves, but a series of waves traveling at high speeds averaging 45mph in the open ocean with wavelengths of hundreds of miles and an amplitude of only a few feet, making them imperceptible by ships and unnoticeable from the air. The time between successive wave crests varies from 5 to 90 min. As the waves approach the coast, their speed decreases and their amplitude increases, averaging 15 to 20 feet high and very destructive on impact. Tsunamis are most frequently generated by earthquake-induced movements along the ocean floor. Landslides, eruptions and even meteorite impact can generate tsunamis. If there is a major earthquake, a tsunami can hit the coast in a few minutes even before a warning can be issued. Areas at greatest risk are less than 25 feet above sea level and within one mile of the shoreline (Fig. 21.2). Most deaths due to tsunamis are because of drowning. From an initial source area or epicenter, waves travel outward in all directions and, as they approach the coast, the time between successive wave crests varies from 5 to 9 minutes. The first wave is usually not the largest nor the most significant. A tsunami consists of a series of waves. The danger from a tsunami can last for several hours after the arrival of the first wave. Tsunamis can move faster than a person can run. Sometimes a tsunami causes the water near the shore to recede, exposing the ocean floor. The force of some tsunamis is enormous. Large rocks weighing several tons along with boats and other debris can be moved inland hundreds of feet by tsunami wave activity. Homes and other buildings are destroyed. All this material and water move with great force and can kill or injure people. Tsunamis can occur at any time, day or night. Tsunamis can travel up rivers and streams that lead to the ocean. And one coastal community may experience no damaging waves while another, not that far away, may experience destructive, deadly waves.

WHAT TO DO WHEN A TSUNAMI WARNING IS ISSUED

A tsunami advisory is issued as soon as an earthquake has occurred. A tsunami watch is

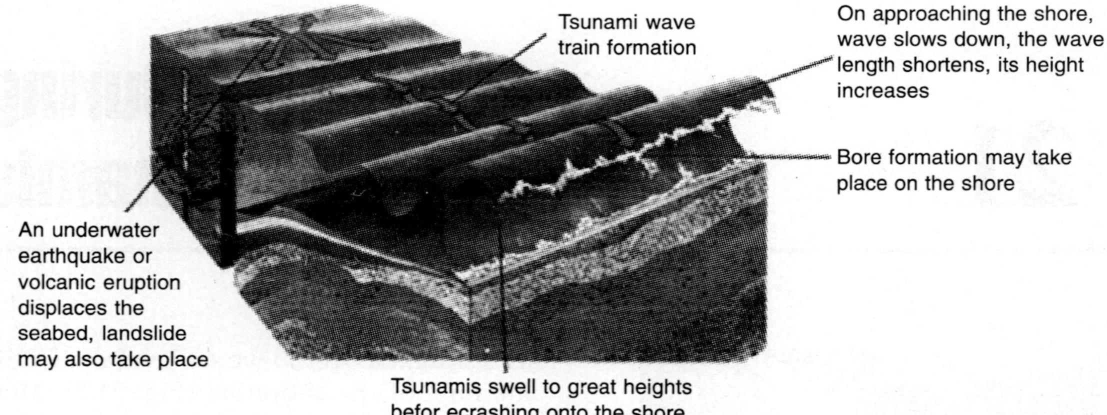

Fig. 21.2: Tsunamis waves

issued when a tsunami has been generated but is at least two hours travel time away from the shoreline. A tsunami warning is issued when a wave has been generated and likely to cause damage, and people in the warned area are strongly advised to evacuate. Listen to the radio and television for more information and instructions from local authorities. A noticeable recession in water away from the shoreline is nature's tsunami warning and should be heeded by moving inland to higher ground immediately. Pick an area that is 10 feet above sea level or a place 2 miles inland, well away from the coastline. Do not be fooled by the modest size of one wave, as the next one may be much bigger. Learn all evacuation routes and determine where and how you would get there if there is a need to evacuate. Check your disaster supplies kit as some supplies may need to be replaced or restocked. Avoid all downed power lines and stay away from buildings and bridges from which heavy objects might fall during an aftershock. If time permits, secure unanchored objects around the house. Return home only after local officials inform you that it is safe. Use your telephone only for emergency calls. Wear sturdy shoes.

WHAT TO DO AFTER A TSUNAMI

Use a battery flashlight when re entering your home, watching every step you take. Examine walls, floors, doors, staircases and windows to make sure that the building is not in danger of collapsing. Inspect foundation for cracks or other damage and look for fire hazards like leaking gas lines, flooded electrical circuits, submerged electrical appliances. Turn off the gas and the mains and call an electrician if there is any doubt. If sewage lines are damaged, do not use the toilets. If the water pipes are damaged avoid using tap water. You can use melted ice cubes from the fridge in the interim. Watch out for snakes and animals that may have entered the building and use a stick to poke through debris. Watch out for loose plaster along the walls and ceilings. Take pictures of the damage for insurance claims. Open all doors and windows to help dry the house and shovel out mud while it is still moist to give walls and floors a chance to dry. Check food supplies and discard all that have come in contact with floodwaters.

LEGISLATIVE REQUIREMENTS IN TSUNAMI PRONE AREAS

Ban on new constructions within several hundred feet of the coastline. If permitted in an odd case allot site that is elevated above 10 feet.

MITIGATION

Under the DART initiative, Tsunami early warning systems (TWS) are geared to provide alerts. Seabed sensors (Bottom pressure recorders) that can detect amplitudes of 1 cm in 6000 metres of water are capable of sending acoustic signal data to modems located in surface buoys. These relay information to ground stations via satellite telecommunications. Alerts are issued on detection of any seismic activity on the ocean floors or any sudden variations in sea level (Fig. 21.3).

IDENTIFICATION OF AREAS AT RISK

Strong coastal ecology program especially with respect to preserving mangroves and coral reefs to safeguard coastal belt.

Shifting of residents near the beach and low lying areas inland to higher ground and safe houses.

If you are on land:
Be aware of tsunami facts. This knowledge could save your life. Share this knowledge with your relatives and friends. It could save their lives.

If you are in school and you hear there is a tsunami warning, you should follow the advice of teachers and other school personnel. If you are at home and hear there is a tsunami

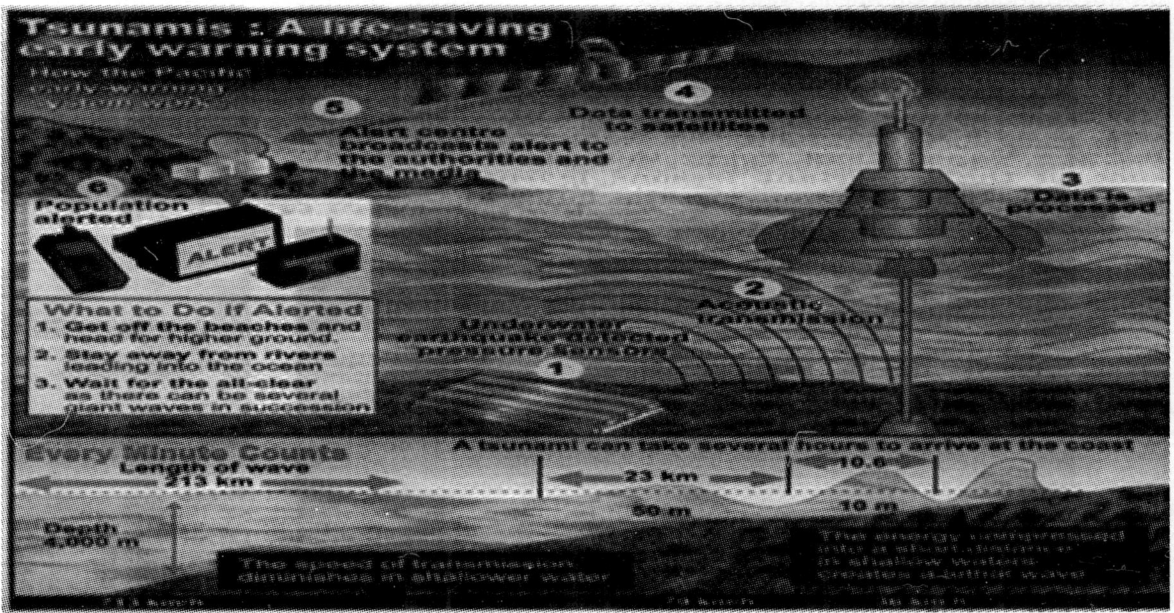

Fig. 21.3: The early warning system that India is now considering to procure. Vishakhapatanam area in the ocean is to be its possible site

warning, you should make sure your entire family is aware of the warning. Your family should evacuate your house if you live in a tsunami evacuation zone. Move in an orderly, calm and safe manner to the evacuation site or to any safe place outside your evacuation zone. Follow the advice of local emergency and law enforcement authorities.

If you are at the beach or near the ocean and you feel the earth shake, move immediately to higher ground, DO NOT wait for a tsunami warning to be announced. Stay away from rivers and streams that lead to the ocean as you would stay away from the beach and ocean if there is a tsunami. A regional tsunami from a local earthquake could strike some areas before a tsunami warning could be announced.

Tsunamis generated in distant locations will generally give people enough time to move to higher ground. For locally-generated tsunamis, where you might feel the ground shake, you may only have a few minutes to move to higher ground.

High, multi-storey, reinforced concrete hotels are located in many low-lying coastal areas. The upper floors of these hotels can provide a safe place to find refuge should there be a tsunami warning and you cannot move quickly inland to higher ground. Local Civil Defense procedures may, however, not allow this type of evacuation in your area. Homes and small buildings located in low-lying coastal areas are not designed to withstand tsunami impacts. Do not stay in these structures should there be a tsunami warning.

Offshore reefs and shallow areas may help break the force of tsunami waves, but large and dangerous wave can still be a threat to coastal residents in these areas. Staying away from all low-lying areas is the safest advice when there is a tsunami warning.

If you are on a boat:
Since tsunami wave activity is imperceptible in the open ocean, do not return to port if you are at sea and a tsunami warning has been issued for your area. Tsunamis can cause rapid changes in water level and unpredictable dangerous currents in harbors and ports.

If there is time to move your boat or ship from port to deep water (after a tsunami warning has been issued), you should weigh the following considerations:

- Most large harbors and ports are under the control of a harbor authority and/or a vessel traffic system. These authorities direct operations during periods of increased readiness (should a tsunami be expected), including the forced movement of vessels if deemed necessary. Keep in contact with the authorities should a forced movement of vessel be directed.
- Smaller ports may not be under the control of a harbor authority. If you are aware there is a tsunami warning and you have time to move your vessel to deep water, then you may want to do so in an orderly manner, in consideration of other vessels. Owners of small boats may find it safest to leave their boat at the pier and physically move to higher ground, particularly in the event of a locally-generated tsunami. Concurrent severe weather conditions (rough seas outside of safe harbor) could present a greater hazardous situation to small boats, so physically moving yourself to higher ground may be the only option.

Damaging wave activity and unpredictable currents can effect harbors for a period of time following the initial tsunami impact on the coast. Contact the harbor authority before returning to port making sure to verify that conditions in the harbor are safe for navigation and berthing.

22 Action Plan During Floods and Flash Floods

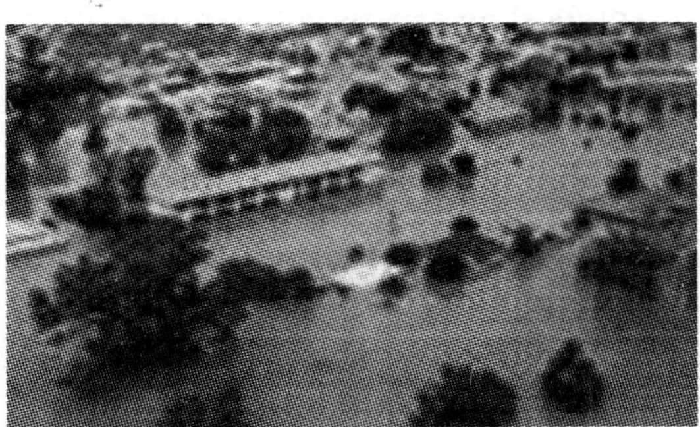

Fig. 22.1

A flood is an overflow or accumulation of an expanse of water that submerges land. The types of floods are:

Riverine Floods

Slow kinds

Runoff from sustained rainfall or rapid snow melt exceeding the capacity of a river's channel. Causes include heavy rains from monsoons, hurricanes and tropical depressions, foreign winds and warm rain affecting snow pack. Unexpected drainage obstructions such as landslides, ice or debris can cause slow flooding upstream of the obstruction.

Fast Kinds

Include flash floods resulting from convective precipitation (intense thunderstorms) or sudden release from an upstream impoundment created behind a dam, landslide or glacier.

Estuarine Floods

Commonly caused by a combination of sea tidal surges caused by storm-force winds. A storm surge, from either a tropical cyclone or an extratropical cyclone, falls within this category.

Coastal Floods

Caused by severe sea storms, or as a result of another hazard (e.g. tsunami or hurricane). A storm surge, from either a tropical cyclone or an extra tropical cyclone, falls within this category.

Catastrophic Floods

Caused by a significant and unexpected event, e.g., dam breakage, or as a result of another hazard (e.g., earthquake or volcanic eruption).

Muddy Floods

A muddy flood is generated by run off on crop land most commonly along hill slopes.

Flash Floods

A flash flood is a rapid flooding of geomorphic low-lying areas – washes, rivers and streams. It is caused by heavy rain associated with a thunderstorm, hurricane, or tropical storm. Flash floods can also occur after the collapse of an ice dam, or a human structure, such as a dam. Flash floods are distinguished from a regular flood by a timescale less than six hours. Flash flooding occurs when the ground becomes saturated with water that has fallen too quickly to be absorbed. The runoff collects in low-lying areas and rapidly flows downhill. Flash floods most often occur in normally dry areas that have recently received precipitation, but may be seen anywhere downstream from the source of the precipitation – even dozens of miles from the source. In areas on or near volcanic mountains, flash floods have also occurred after eruptions, when glaciers have been melted by the intense heat.

In many countries across the world, rivers prone to floods are often carefully managed. Defences such as levees, bunds, reservoirs and weirs are used to prevent rivers from bursting their banks. When these defences fail, emergency measures such as sandbags or portable inflatable tubes are used. Coastal flooding has been addressed with coastal defences such as sea walls, beach nourishment and barrier islands. Global warming and deforestation have been blamed for many of these phenomenon.

Mitigation pays: It includes any activities that prevent an emergency, reduce the chance of an emergency happening, or lessen the damaging effects of unavoidable emergencies. Investing in mitigation steps now such as constructing barriers and purchasing flood insurance will help reduce the amount of structural damage to your home and financial loss from building and crop damage should a flood or flash flood occur. Find out if you live in a flood-prone area from your local emergency management office or Red Cross chapter and also whether your property is above or below the flood stage water level and learn about the history of flooding for your region. Learn flood warning signs and your community alert signals.

Request information on preparing for floods and flash floods.

If you live in a frequently flooded area, stockpile emergency building materials. These include plywood, plastic sheeting, nails, hammer and saw, pry bar, shovels and sandbags.

Have check valves installed in building sewer traps to prevent flood waters from backing up in sewer drains.

As a last resort, use large corks or stoppers to plug showers, tubs, or basins.

Plan and practice an evacuation route.

Contact the local emergency management office or local Red Cross chapter for a copy of the community flood evacuation plan.

This plan should include information on the safest routes to shelters. Individuals living in flash flood areas should have several alternative routes.

- Have disaster supplies on hand.
- Flashlights and extra batteries.
- Portable, battery-operated radio and extra batteries.
- First aid kit and manual.
- Emergency food and water.
- Non electric can opener.
- Essential medicines.
- Cash and credit cards.
- Sturdy shoes/gum boots.
- Develop an emergency communication plan.
- In case family members are separated from one another during floods or flashfloods (a real possibility during the day when adults are at work and children are at school), have a plan for getting back together.
- Ask an out-of-state relative or friend to serve as the family contact. After a disaster, it's often easier to call long distance. Make sure everyone in the family knows the name, address, and phone number of the contact person.
- Make sure that all family members know how to respond after a flood or flash flood. Teach all family members how and when to turn off gas, electricity, and water.

- Teach children how and when to call the police and/or fire department, and which radio station to tune to for emergency information.
- Ask your insurance agent about flood insurance. Home owners policies do not generally cover flood damage.

DURING A FLOOD WATCH

- Listen to a batter operated radio for the latest storm information.
- Fill bathtubs, sinks, and jugs with clean water in case water becomes contaminated.
- Bring outdoor belongings, such as patio furniture, indoors.
- Move valuable household possessions to the upper floors or to safe ground if time permits.
- If you are instructed to do so by local authorities, turn off all utilities at the main switch and close the main gas valve.
- Be prepared to evacuate.

DURING A FLOOD

If Indoors

- Turn on battery-operated radio or television to get the latest emergency information.
- Get your pre-assembled emergency supplies.
- If told to leave, do so immediately.

If Outdoors

- Climb to high ground and stay there.
- Avoid walking through any floodwaters. If it is moving swiftly, even water 6 inches deep can sweep you off your feet.

If In A Car

- If you come to a flooded area, turn around and go another way.
- If your car stalls, abandon it immediately and climb to higher ground. Many deaths have resulted from attempts to move stalled vehicles.

DURING AN EVACUATION

- If advised to evacuate, do so immediately.
- Evacuation is much simpler and safer before flood waters become too deep for ordinary vehicles to drive through.
- Listen to a battery-operated radio for evacuation instructions.
- Follow recommended evacuation routes—shortcuts may be blocked.
- Leave early enough to avoid being marooned by flooded roads.

AFTER A FLOOD

- Flood dangers do not end when the water begins to recede. Listen to a radio or television and don't return home until authorities indicate it is safe to do so.
- Remember to help your neighbors who may require special assistance—infants, elderly people, and people with disabilities.
- Inspect foundations for cracks or other damage.
- Stay out of buildings if flood waters remain around the building.
- When entering buildings, use extreme caution.
- Wear sturdy shoes and use battery-powered lanterns or flashlights when examining buildings.
- Examine walls, floors, doors, and windows to make sure that the building is not in danger of collapsing.
- Watch out for animals, especially poisonous snakes, that may have come into your home with the flood waters. Use a stick to poke through debris.
- Watch for loose plaster and ceilings that could fall.

- Take pictures of the damage—both to the house and its contents for insurance claims.
- Look for fire hazards like broken or leaking gas lines, flooded electrical circuits, submerged furnaces or electrical appliances, flammable or explosive materials coming from upstream.
- Throw away food—including canned goods—that has come in contact with flood waters.
- Pump out flooded basements gradually (about one-third of the water per day) to avoid structural damage.
- Service damaged septic tanks, cesspools, pits, and leaching systems as soon as possible. Damaged sewage systems are health hazards.
- Stay on upper floors/terrace and await relief/ boat patrols or air evacuation. Keep some improvised signaling device ready to attract rescuer attention.

INSPECTING UTILITIES IN A DAMAGED HOME

Check for gas leaks. If you smell gas or hear blowing or hissing noise, open a window and quickly leave the building. Turn off the gas at the outside main valve if you can and call the gas company from a neighbor's home. If you turn off the gas for any reason, it must be turned back on by a professional.

Look for electrical system damage—If you see sparks or broken or frayed wires, or if you smell hot insulation, turn off the electricity at the main fuse box or circuit breaker. If you have to step in water to get to the fuse box or circuit breaker, call an electrician for advice.

Check for sewage and water lines damage—If you suspect sewage lines are damaged avoid using the toilets and call a plumber. If water pipes are damaged, contact the water company and avoid the water from the tap. You can obtain safe water by melting ice cubes.

WATER RESCUE TEAMS AND BOATS DURING FLOODS

Rescue by boats during floods is a vitally important operation to evacuate marooned population and animals and also to salvage property and fight fires. There are a variety of boats and marine crafts for this purpose. The main considerations for these crafts are safety, stability, versatility, durability, low cost, shallow water operational capability and ease of maintenance. Special desirable features are:

1. Wide bottoms that prevent rocking and a non-skid flat floor that provides occupants with extra balance and stability, safe platform in a variety of water conditions.
2. Raised flooring keeps feet dry to prevent slipping.
3. The craft must be diver friendly with ample room to take on and off gear as well as a fold out platform that is connected to the bow of the boat that creates a shelf below the surface of the water. This enables the diver to easily and safely step in and out of the water and for other responders to retrieve gear or other objects from the water surface.
4. Have multi function capability with removable fire pumps that can be assembled in minutes to enable fire fighting.
5. They must be durable in construction. Many inflatable boats are susceptible to tears and punctures. When deployed in locations where elements can damage inflatables, the lives of the responders as well as the victims can be jeopardized. All welded aluminum construction are much more durable enabling the responders to not worry about the conditions and focus on the mission.

Currently, there are 4 levels of classifications of Water Rescue teams:

- Type 1 = consists of 6 people, able to manage search operations, have powered water craft, helicopter transportable, technical rope systems, and haz-mat first responder.
- Type 2 = consists of 4 people, able to make in water contact rescues, assist in search operations, have non-powered water craft, animal rescue certified, and EMT.
- Type 3 = consists of 3 people, low risk/ land based rescue capability. Basically an engine company with throw ropes, throw rings, and pike poles. All teams must have the following:
  1. Must be certified to the Swiftwater Rescue – Technician Level.
  2. Must be certified to the Rope Rescue – Technician Level.
  3. Must be certified in HAZMAT Awareness.
  4. Must have minimum BLS and First Responder certifications.
  5. Must have the minimum safety equipment for each rescuer as needed for the type of team.
  6. Must be capable of supporting 24 hour operations.
  7. Must have UHF, VHF, or Satellite communications capability (minimum of 2 radios per squad).
  8. Must be able to transport team and watercraft (as defined) to designated location safely and all passengers in vehicles must have seatbelts.
  9. Must have the capability to make fuel, food, and water purchases during the deployment and provide documentation of those purchases.

The water rescue team is capable of utilizing state-of-the-art personnel protective and rescue equipment, which includes boats, personal flotation devices and advanced communication equipment, which can be configured to facilitate rescues in any environment or condition. The team is made up of four individual strike teams which consist of five members plus a team leader, assistant team leader, a logistics specialist and a technical support specialist. Most of the members on the water rescue team are also members of technical rescue teams in their own cities. The rescue team must be ready to deploy within one hour of notification unlike the four to six hours required for structural collapse teams. They are trained in ice and swifwater rescue tactics, rescue safety, hydrology,dynamics of moving water and dangers, site survey, boat-based techniques, rigging systems,Hazmat diving and risk and benefit analysis.

The types of rescue boats used during floods are as follows:

A. Conventional Flood Rescue Boats (FRBs)

Most FRBs are less than six metres in length and are propelled by outboard motors. Outboard motors are ideal for smaller boats. They are light and powerful and the modern outboard motors are extremely quiet. Outboard motors provide a completely self-contained propulsion system from engine to transmission to shaft and propeller. They are most often mounted directly on the transom of the boat. However, some boat designs incorporate a motor well or bracket on which the motor is mounted. As the turning propeller pushes the stern, the entire motor swivels about to provide easy steering. Outboard motors come in a large range of sizes, numbers of cylinders and horsepower, and can use different fuel sources. Different types of outboard motors are small electric trolling motors,pre mix (petrol and oil-mixture) two-stroke engines,oil injected two stroke engines, four-stroke engines, diesel-powered outboards and direct-injected two-stroke engines.

Most emergency services use two-stroke and four-stroke outboard motors. Outboard motors work better if used regularly. Avoid long periods of non-use. If stored outside, the motors should be covered. If a boat is left in the water for a long period of time, raise the motor so the water intake is clear of the water to prevent clogging from silt and weed.

There are many different propeller types and shapes. The three main materials used to make them are:

- **Aluminium**—These propellers are best for FRBs, even though they are slightly less efficient than stainless steel propellers (because the blade can flex under load). The big advantages of aluminium propellers are that they are cheap to replace, and if the propeller hits something the aluminium will tear easily and not transfer the shock into the gearbox and damage gears.
- **Stainless steel**—These propellers are very efficient and are much sturdier; however, in the event of a large impact, they are likely to damage the gearbox, leaving crew members and passengers stranded
- **Composite materials (plastic)**—Composite materials are similar to aluminium in performance and offer the same gearbox protection but they are not as cost-effective as aluminium

B. Mercury Hypalon XD Inflatable Boats (Gemini)

Rugged Hypalon XD material that Avon, Achilles, and other inflatable rescue boats have lightweight, but strong aluminum-composite floorboards for more stability in rougher weather and designed to take up to 6-8 people and their gear (750-1000 kg) and accommodate up to a 30hp outboard. Hypalon XD has enhanced resistance to oil, chemicals, weather and damaging UV rays, to give years of trouble-free performance. They have a variety of applications such as swiftwater rescue and ice rescue. They also incorporate standard with internal davit points (Fig. 22.2).

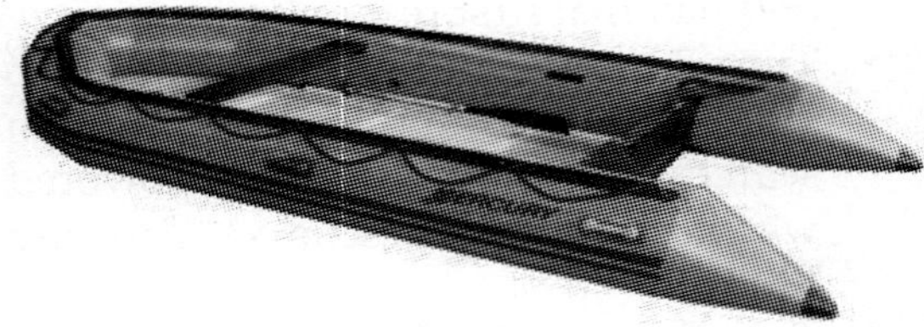

Fig. 22.2

C. *The Universal Flood Rescue Hovercraft*

Manufactured by MAD Hovercraft, these amphibian rescue boats can transport up to 4 persons and used for search and rescue hovercraft operations on land, water, snow and ice, flood rescue and other water rescue where fast response is needed and where standard boats are not able to handle (Fig. 22.3).

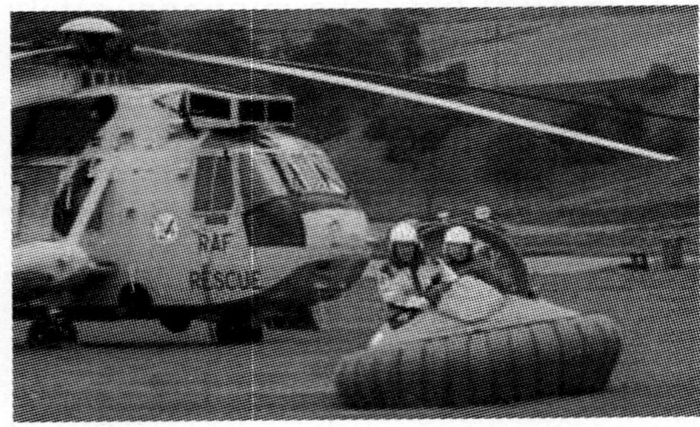

Fig. 22.3

D. Airboats

Airboats are gaining in popularity across the United States of America, and abroad, as highly maneuverable boats that can be deployed for search and rescue, law enforcement, military missions, forestry and other professional uses. Having *no operating*

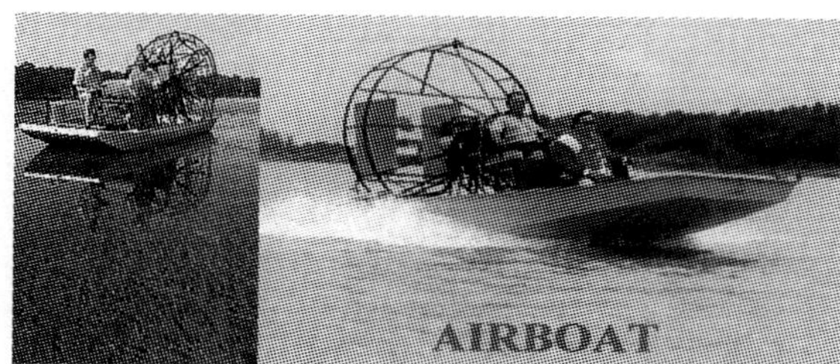

Fig. 22.4

parts below the waterline, the airboat is able to traverse the shallowest of water or no water at all. Additionally, no launching ramps are required and ally speed with maneuverability and safety (Fig. 22.4).

An airboat can be unloaded from its trailer onto dry ground and can even be maneuvered across dry pavement to the water's edge. With a full load capacity, an airboat can maneuver through floodwaters skimming over downed trees submerged fences, automobiles, trash and vegetation. Although airboats do have their limitations, they have been reported to have been operated in up to class 4 whitewater. An aluminum airboat's construction, coupled with a polymer hull covering allows it to withstand the otherwise destructive punishment given it by ice shoves, rocks, logs and tree stumps. An airboat with a polymer-clad aluminum hull can withstand the destructive pounding of jagged ice that would rip the vinyl skirts of a hovercraft to shreds. An airboat's design makes it capable of being launched almost anywhere, regardless of the presence of water or a wet surface. An airboat, equipped with an adequate power plant and a polymer clad bottom, is capable of running on dry ground, even with a full payload.

When being deployed for emergency operations, an airboat can be run directly off its trailer, across dry ground, mud, ice or snow, down an embankment and out onto the body of water or ice with minimal launch time. This capability also makes launching a one-man operation, while being expedient.

Payload

Comparing vessels in length, width and carrying capacity, airboats have a much greater payload than do hovercraft or inflatables, while still maintaining the ability to traverse shallow water or ice. A 16-18 foot aluminum hull airboat, powered by a large block automotive engine, can have a 2,200–2,800 pound load capacity and carry up to 12 people. The same size airboat, specifically designed for search and rescue operation, can accommodate up to four immobilized patients on backboards or in stokes baskets, in addition to the crew and rescue equipment.

Unloaded and under ideal operating conditions, an airboat can travel up to 45-60 mph across water. Carrying a full load, an airboat can be maneuvered over sandbars, dense aquatic vegetation, across mud flats, dry ground and even climb hills.

An airboat is powered by a flow of air, generated by an aircraft style propeller, rotated by either an automotive or aircraft engine. The airflow is directed rearward passing by two vertical rudders that provide steering for the vessel. Like an aircraft, an airboat has only one direction of travel and that is forward. There is no reverse and no brakes on an airboat. However, an experienced airboat operator can turn an airboat on a dime and come to a complete stop within 20 to 30 feet travel at a speed of 30 mph.

Reliability

In years past, airboats have been considered unstable and top heavy vessels with an inherent ability to easily capsize and sink. Those characteristics caused them to be viewed as impractical for deep, open water or swiftwater use. Recent technology has addressed those issues and has resolved those problems, making airboats extremely practical vessels for search and rescue application.

Automotive engines installed on many new airboats make them extremely reliable and easily worked on by anyone with minimal mechanical ability. Automobile engines used on modern airboats range from 60 horsepower engines to the over 600 horsepower, electronic ignition, fuel-injected marine engines. However, the most common and practical automobile engines for a SAR airboat are the Chevrolet 350, 454, 502 or the new 496 cubic inch engines. Matched to the appropriate sized airboat hull, those engines provide both excellent service and reliability.

Automobile engines on airboats require no special parts. Engine parts can be obtained at a local auto parts store. Also, automobile engines require no special fuel. The fuel for an airboat equipped with an automobile engine can be obtained at any gasoline service station. Other than routine maintenance, airboats require no special care. Their uncomplicated design and operational components lend to their easy upkeep.

Every automobile engine installed in an airboat must be equipped with a gear reduction unit to achieve the maximum performance from the engine. This is where modern technology has eliminated the traditional top-heavy characteristic of airboats.

Airboats used for search and rescue operations can now be equipped with what is referred to as a "long-belt gear reduction drive unit". This mechanism allows the automobile engine to be mounted to the interior hull of the boat, eliminating the high center of gravity that previously contributed to the airboat's instability. With the airboat's engine mounted on the bottom deck of the hull, the airboat is capable of operation in extremely rough water conditions, without the risk of capsizing, making it a perfect vessel for search and rescue operations. In addition, the long-belt gear reduction drive unit increases the handling and performance of the airboat. However, let it not be misunderstood that airboats are simple vessels to operate. No different from any other piece of equipment used in emergency services, only formally trained and qualified persons should operate airboats and perform their maintenance.

Innovations and Adaptations

Innovated fire departments have mounted fire pumps with a 500 gallon per minute deckgun mounted on its bow on their airboats to fight fires on islands, to maneuver into shallow marinas to fight boat fires and to extinguish building fires during flooding. When mounted on a trailer, an airboat is nothing more than a big fan on wheels. Fire departments have been known to deploy their airboats during large structure fires and toxic gas leaks for ventilation purposes. The large aircraft like propeller generates a positive pressure airflow unmatched by conventional positive pressure devices. The airflow produced by an airboat propeller provides outstanding performance evacuating smoke from large warehouse fires.

Winter Rescue Operations

Every winter when the lakes, rivers, streams and ponds become covered with ice airboats prove their value. Traditionally, ice rescue operations have been long and laborious events. It has been routinely reported that ice-rescue operations, that would normally require 45 to 60 minutes to execute, have been reduced to 7–12 minutes through the use of an airboat.

23 Action Plan During Landslides and Mudflows

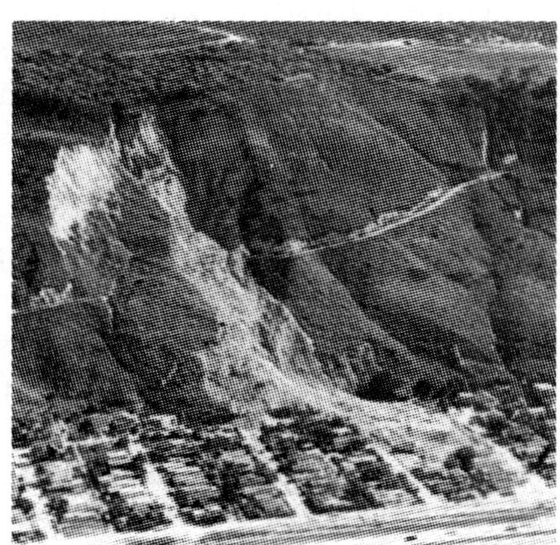

Fig. 23.1

INTRODUCTION

A landslide (or landslip) is a geological phenomenon which includes a wide range of ground movement, such as rock falls, deep failure of slopes and shallow debris flows, which can occur in offshore, coastal and onshore environments. Although the action of gravity is the primary driving force for a landslide to occur, there are other contributing factors affecting the original slope stability. Typically, pre-conditional factors build up specific sub-surface conditions that make the area/slope prone to failure, whereas the actual landslide often requires a trigger before being released. Landslides are caused when the stability of a slope changes from a stable to an unstable condition. A change in the stability of a slope can be caused by a number of factors, acting together or alone.

Natural causes of landslides include:

- Groundwater (porewater) pressure acting to destabilize the slope.
- Loss or absence of vertical vegetative structure, soil nutrients, and soil structure.
- Erosion of the toe of a slope by rivers or ocean waves.
- Weakening of a slope through saturation by snowmelt, glaciers melting, or heavy rains.
- Earthquakes adding loads to barely-stable slopes.
- Earthquake-caused liquefaction destabilizing slopes.
- Volcanic eruptions.

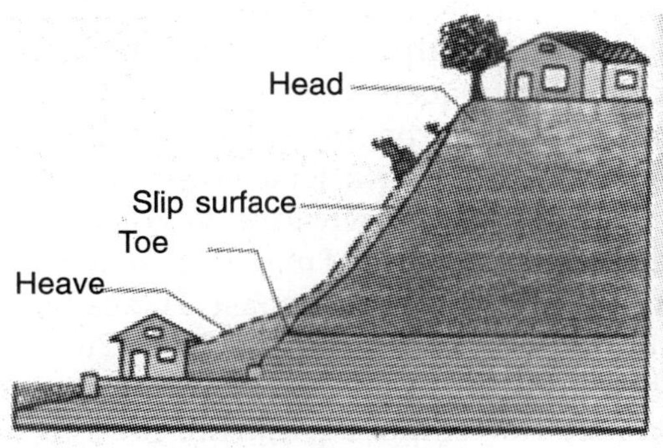

Fig. 23.2: Landslide

Human causes include:

- Vibrations from machinery or traffic.
- Blasting.
- Earthwork which alters the shape of a slope, or which imposes new loads on an existing slope.

- In shallow soils, the removal of deep-rooted vegetation that binds colluvium to bedrock.

Construction, agricultural, or forestry activities(logging) which change the amount of water infiltrates into the soil. Slope material that becomes saturated with water may develop into a debris flow or mud flow. The resulting slurry of rock and mud may pick up trees, houses and cars, thus blocking bridges and tributaries causing flooding along its path.

Muddy-debris flows cause severe damage to structures and infrastructure and often claim human lives. Muddy-debris flows can start as a result of slope-related factors and shallow landslides can dam stream beds, provoking temporary water blockage. The solid-liquid mixture can reach densities of up to 2 tons/m^3 and velocities of up to 14 m/s. These processes normally cause the first severe road interruptions, due not only to deposits accumulated on the road (from several cubic metres to hundreds of cubic metres), but in some cases to the complete removal of bridges or roadways or railways crossing the stream channel. Damage usually derive from a common underestimation of mud-debris flows: in the alpine valleys, for example, bridges are frequently destroyed by the impact force of the flow because their span is usually calculated only for a water discharge.

Earthflows are downslope, viscous flows of saturated, fine-grained materials, which move at any speed from slow to fast. Typically, they can move at speeds from 0.17 to 20 km/h. Though these are a lot like mudflows, overall they are slower moving and are covered with solid material carried along by flow from within. They are different from fluid flows in that they are more rapid. Clay, fine sand and silt, and fine-grained, pyroclastic material are all susceptible to earthflows. The velocity of the earthflow is all dependent on how much water content is in the flow itself: if there is more water content in the flow, the higher the velocity will be.

These flows usually begin when the pore pressures in a fine-grained mass increase until enough of the weight of the material is supported by pore water to significantly decrease the internal shearing strength of the material. This thereby creates a bulging lobe which advances with a slow, rolling motion. As these lobes spread out, drainage of the mass increases and the margins dry out, thereby lowering the overall velocity of the flow. This process causes the flow to thicken. The bulbous variety of earthflows are not that spectacular, but they are much more common than their rapid counterparts. They develop a sag at their heads and are usually derived from the slumping at the source.

Earthflows occur much more during periods of high precipitation, which saturates the ground and adds water to the slope content. Fissures develop during the movement of clay-like material creates the intrusion of water into the earthflows. Water then increases the pore-water pressure and reduces the shearing strength of the material.

A debris avalanche is a type of slide characterized by the chaotic movement of rocks soil and debris mixed with water or ice (or both). They are usually triggered by the saturation of thickly vegetated slopes which results in an incoherent mixture of broken timber, smaller vegetation and other debris. Debris avalanches differ from debris slides because their movement is much more rapid. This is usually a cause of lower cohesion or higher water content and commonly steeper slopes.

Movement

Debris slides generally begin with large blocks that slump at the head of the slide and then break apart as they move towards the toe. This process is much slower than that of a debris avalanche. In a debris avalanche this progressive failure is very rapid and the entire mass seems to somewhat liquefy as it moves down the slope. This is caused by the combination of the excessive saturation of the material, and very steep slopes. As the mass moves down the slope it generally follows stream channels leaving behind a V-shaped scar that spreads out downhill. This differs from the more U-shaped scar of a slump. Debris avalanches can also travel well past the foot of the slope due to their tremendous speed.

A sturzstrom is a rare, poorly understood type of landslide, typically with a long run-out. Often very large, these slides are unusually mobile, flowing very far over a low angle, flat, or even slightly uphill terrain.

Landslides and mudflows usually strike without warning. The force of rocks, soil, or other debris moving down a slope can devastate anything in its path. Take the following steps to be ready.

BEFORE

- Do not build near steep slopes, close to mountain edges, near drainage ways, or natural erosion valleys.
- Get a ground assessment of your property.
- Your county geologist or county planning department may have specific information on areas vulnerable to landsliding. Consult a professional geotechnical expert for opinions and advice on landslide problems and on corrective measures you can take.
- Minimize home hazards. Have flexible pipe fittings installed to avoid gas or water leaks, as flexible fittings are more resistant to breakage (only the gas company or professionals should install gas fittings).

Remember: If you build walls to divert debris flow and the flow lands on a neighbor's property, you may be liable for damages.

Plant ground cover on slopes and build retaining walls.

In mudflow areas, build channels or deflection walls to direct the flow around buildings.

Remember: If you build retaining/deflection walls or channels to divert debris flow and the flow lands on a neighbor's property, you may be liable for damages.

Learn to recognize the following landslide warning signs:

- Doors or windows stick or jam for the first time.
- New cracks appear in plaster, tile, brick, or foundations.
- Outside walls, walks, or stairs begin pulling away from the building.
- Slowly developing, widening cracks appear on the ground or on paved areas such as streets or driveways.
- Underground utility lines break.
- Bulging ground appears at the base of a slope.
- Water breaks through the ground surface in new locations.
- Fences, retaining walls, utility poles, or trees tilt or move.
- Stay alert and awake. Many debris-flow fatalities occur when people are sleeping. Listen to a weather radio bulletin, portable, battery-powered radio or television for warnings of intense rainfall. Be aware that intense, short bursts of rain may be particularly dangerous, especially after longer periods of heavy rainfall and damp weather
- You hear a faint rumbling sound that increases in volume as the landslide nears. The ground slopes downward in one specific direction and may begin shifting in that direction under your feet.

- If you are near a stream or channel, be alert for any sudden increase or decrease in water flow and for a change from clear to muddy water. Such changes may indicate landslide activity upstream, so be prepared to move quickly. Don't delay! Save yourself, not your belongings. Be especially alert when driving. Embankments along roadsides are particularly susceptible to landslides. Watch the road for collapsed pavement, mud, fallen rocks, and other indications of possible debris flows.

Make evacuation plans: Plan at least two evacuation routes since roads may become blocked or closed. Develop an emergency communication plan. In case family members are separated from one another during a landslide or mudflow this is (a real possibility during the day when adults are at work and children are at school), have a plan for getting back together.

Ask an out-of-state relative or friend to serve as the family contact. After a disaster, it's often easier to call long distance. Make sure everyone knows the name, address, and phone number of the contact person.

Home/Flood insurance can be purchased through a local insurance agency.

DURING

- *If inside a building:* Stay inside and take cover under a desk, table, or other piece of sturdy furniture.
- *If outdoors:* Try and get out of the path of the landslide or mudflow. Run to the nearest high ground in a direction away from the path. If rocks and other debris are approaching, run for the nearest shelter such as a group of trees or a building. If escape is not possible, curl into a tight ball and protect your head.

AFTER

- Stay away from the slide area.
- There may be danger of additional slides. Check for injured and trapped persons near the slide area. Give first aid if trained. Remember to help your neighbors who may require special assistance-infants, elderly people, and people with disabilities.
- Listen to a battery-operated radio or television for the latest emergency information.
- Remember that flooding may occur after a mudflow or a landslide. Check for damaged utility lines. Report any damage to the utility company.
- Check the building foundation, chimney, and surrounding land for damage.
- Replant damaged ground as soon as possible since erosion caused by loss of ground cover can lead to flash flooding.
- Seek the advice of geotechnical expert for evaluating landslide hazards or designing corrective techniques to reduce landslide risk.

MITIGATION

Mitigation includes any activities that prevent an emergency, reduce the chance of an emergency happening, or lessen the damaging effects of unavoidable emergencies. Investing in preventive mitigation steps now such as planting ground cover (low growing plants) on slopes, or installing flexible pipe fitting to avoid gas or water leaks, will help reduce the impact of landslides and mudflows in the future. For more information on mitigation, contact your local emergency management office/local administrative authorities.

24 Action Plan During Extreme Heat Wave

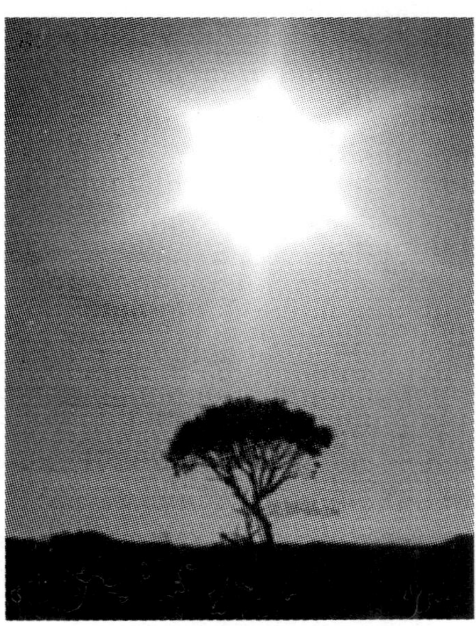

Fig. 24.1

INTRODUCTION

A heat wave is a prolonged period of excessively hot weather, which may be accompanied by high humidity relative to the usual weather in the area. Temperatures that people from a hotter climate consider normal can be termed a heat wave in a cooler area if they are outside the normal climate pattern for that area. The term is applied both to routine weather variations and to extra-ordinary spells of heat which may occur only once a century. Severe heat waves have caused catastrophic crop failures, thousands of deaths from hyperthermia.

Heat waves often occur during the "dog days" of summer. Some regions of the globe are more susceptible to heat waves than others, typically inland desert and semi-desert regions.

Severe heat waves have caused catastrophic crop failures, thousands of deaths from hyperthermia. The loss of human life in hot spells in summer exceeds that caused by all other weather events combined.

DEFINITION

The World Meteorological Organization defines a heat wave when the daily maximum temperature of more than five consecutive days exceeds the average maximum temperature by 5 degrees Celsius (9 degree Fahrenheit)

Doing too much on a hot day, spending too much time in the sun or staying too long in an overheated place can cause heat-related illnesses. Know the symptoms of heat disorders and overexposure to the sun, and be ready to give first aid treatment.

BEFORE

- Contact your local emergency management office or Red Cross chapter for information on extreme heat.
- Install window air conditioners snugly. Insulate spaces around air conditioners for a tighter fit.
- Use a circulating or box fan to spread the cool air.

- Keep heat outside and cool air inside by installing temporary reflectors, such as aluminum foil covered cardboard, to reflect any heat back outside. Keep the cool air inside by weather-stripping doors and windowsills. Consider keeping storm windows up all year. Storm windows can keep the heat of a house in the summer the same way they keep the cold out in the winter.
- Check air-conditioning ducts for proper insulation.

DURING

- Protect windows. Hang shades, draperies, awnings, or louvers on windows that receive morning or afternoon sun. Outdoor awnings or louvers can reduce the heat entering the house by as much as 8 percent. Conserve electricity.
- During periods of extreme heat, people tend to use a lot more power for air conditioning which can lead to a power shortage or outage. Stay indoors as much as possible. If air conditioning is not available, stay on the lowest floor and out of the sunshine. Remember that electric fans do not cool, they just blow hot air around.
- Eat well-balanced, light meals.
- Drink plenty of water regularly. Persons who have epilepsy or heart, kidney, or liver disease and advised fluid-restrictive diets due to fluid retention should consult a doctor before increasing liquid intake.
- Limit intake of alcoholic beverages. Although beer and alcohol beverages appear to satisfy thirst, they actually cause further body dehydration.
- Dress in loose-fitting clothes that cover as much skin as possible. Lightweight, light-colored clothing that reflects heat and sunlight and helps maintain normal body temperature.
- Protect face and head by wearing a wide-brimmed hat or turban.
- Allow your body to get acclimated to hot temperatures for the first 2 or 3 days of a heat wave.
- Avoid too much sunshine. Sunburn slows the skin's ability to cool itself. Use a sunscreen lotion with a high SPF (sun protection factor) rating.
- Avoid extreme temperature changes. A cool shower immediately after coming in from hot temperatures can result in hypothermia, particularly for elderly and very young people.
- Slow down. Reduce, eliminate, or reschedule strenuous activities. High-risk individuals should stay in cool places. Get plenty of rest to allow your natural cooling system to work.
- Take salt tablets only if specified by your physician. Persons on salt-restrictive diets should check with a physician before increasing salt intake.
- Vacuum air conditioner filters weekly during periods of high use.
- Learn the symptoms of heat disorders and know how to give first aid.
- Lower water use. Watering the lawn and washing the car waste water. Whenever possible, re-use water.
- Place a brick or other large, solid object in the flush tank of the toilet to reduce the water used to flush.
- Farmers should opt for drip irrigation techniques to conserve water.

Heat Disorders

Sunburn

Symptoms: Skin redness and pain, possible swelling, blisters, fever, headaches.

First Aid: Take a shower, using soap, to remove oils that may block pores preventing the body from cooling naturally. If blisters occur, apply

HEAT RELATED EMERGENCIES

CONDITION	MUSCLE CRAMPS	BREATHING	PULSE	WEAKNESS	SKIN	PERSPIRATION	LOSS OF CONSCIOUSNESS
HEAT CRAMPS	+	VARIES RAPID	VARIES	+	MOIST-WARM-NO CHANGE	HEAVY	SELDOM
HEAT EXHAUSTION	-	SHALLOW	WEAK	+	COLD CLAMMY	HEAVY	SOMETIMES
HEAT STROKE	-	DEEP THEN SHALLOW	FULL RAPID	+	DRY-HOT	LITTLE OR NONE	OFTEN

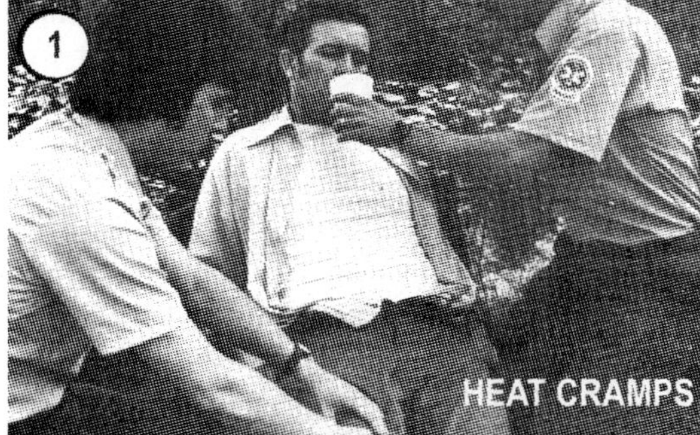

SIGNS AND SYMPTOMS: SEVERE MUSCLE CRAMPS (USUALLY IN THE LEGS AND ABDOMEN) EXHAUSTION,SOMETIMES DIZZINESS OT FAINTNESS

EMERGENCY CARE PROCEDURES:

- MOVE PATIENT TO A NEARBY COOL PLACE
- GIVE PATIENT SALTED WATER TO DRINK, OR COMMERCIAL ELECTROLYTE FLUIDS
- HELPS EASE CRAMPS BY MUSCLE MASSAGE. MASSAGE WITH PRESSURE IS MORE EFFECTIVE THAT LIGHT RUBBING ACTION
- APPLY WARM, MOIST TOWELS TO THE FOREHEAD AND OVER CRAMPED MUSCLES FOR ADDED RELIEF
- IF CRAMPS PERSIST, OR IF MORE SEROUS SIGNS AND SYMPTOMS DEVELOP, READY THE PATIENT AND TRANSPORT

SIGNS AND SYMPTOMS: RAPID SHALLOW BREATHING, WEAK PULSE, COLD CLAMMY SKIN, HEAVY PERSPIRATION, TOTAL BODY WEAKNESS, AND DIZZINESS LEADING TO UNCONSCIOUSNESS

EMERGENCY CARE PROCEDURES:

- MOVE THE PATIENT TO A NEARBY COOL PLACE
- KEEP THE PATIENT AT REST
- REMOVE ENOUGH CLOTHING TO COOL THE PATIENT WITHOUT CHILLING HIM
- GIVE PATIENT SALTED WATER TO DRINK, OR COMMERCIAL ELECTROLYTE FLUIDS. DO NOT ADMINISTER FLUIDS TO UNCONSCIOUS PATIENT
- TREAT FOR SHOCK, BUT DO NOT COVER TO THE POINT OF OVERHEATING PATIENT
- IF UNCONSCIOUS, FAILS TO RECOVER RAPIDLY, HAS INJURIES OR MEDICAL HISTORY, TRANSPORT AS SOON AS POSSIBLE

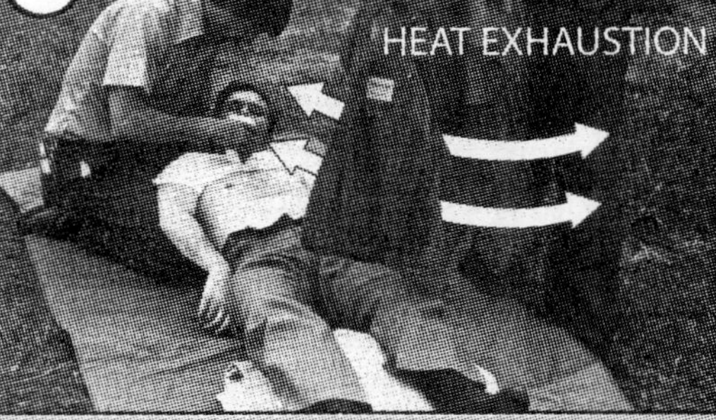

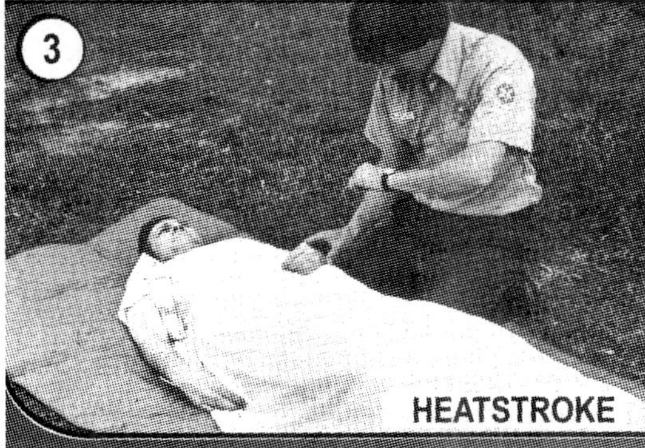

SIGNS AND SYMPTOMS: DEEP BREATHS, THEN SHALLOW BREATHING, RAPID, STRONG PULSE, THEN RAPID WEAK PULSE; DRY HOT SKIN, DILATED PUPILS; LOSS OF CONSCIOUSNESS (POSSIBLE COMA) CONVULSIONS OR MUSCULAR TWITCHING

EMERGENCY CARE PROCEDURES:

- COOL PT. -IN ANY MANNER, RAPIDLY. MOVE PT. OUT OF SUN, OR AWAY FROM HEAT SOURCE. REMOVE CLOTHING-WRAP IN WET TOWELS OR SHEETS. POUR COLD WATER OVER WRAPPINGS, BODY HEAT MUST LOWER RAPIDLY OR BRAIN CELLS DIES!
- WRAP COLD PACKS OR ICE BAGS, IF AVAILABLE & PLACE ONE UNDER EACH ARMPIT, EACH WRIST, EACH ANKLE, AND EACH SIDE OF PATIENT'S NECK
- TRANSPORT AS SOON AS POSSIBLE
- IF TRANSPORT DELAYED, FIND TUB OR CONTAINER-IMMERSE PT. UP TO FACE IN COOLED WATER. MONITOR IN ORDER TO PREVENT DROWNING
- MONITOR VITAL SIGNS THROUGHOUT PROCESS

Fig. 24.2

dry, sterile dressings and get medical attention.

Heat Cramps

Symptoms: Painful spasms usually in leg and abdominal muscles. Heavy sweating.
First Aid: Firm pressure on cramping muscles or gentle massage to relieve spasm. Give sips of water. If nausea occurs, discontinue.

Heat Exhaustion

Symptoms: Heavy sweating, weakness, skin cold, pale and clammy. Weak pulse. Normal temperature possible. Fainting, vomiting.
First Aid: Get victim to lie down in a cool place. Loosen clothing. Apply cool, wet cloths. Fan or move victim to air-conditioned place. Give sips of water. If nausea occurs, discontinue. If vomiting occurs, seek immediate medical attention.

Heat Stroke (Sun Stroke)

Heatstroke is defined typically as hyperthermia exceeding 41°C and anhidrosis associated with an altered sensorium.

It affects people who are unable to control their environment and water intake (eg, infants, elderly persons, individuals who are chronically ill), people with reduced cardiovascular reserve (eg, elderly persons, patients with chronic cardiovascular illnesses), and people with impaired sweating (eg, patients with skin disease, patients ingesting anticholinergic and psychiatric drugs). In addition, infants have an immature thermoregulatory system, and elderly persons have impaired perception of changes in body and ambient temperatures and a decreased capacity to sweat.

Common Symptoms and Signs of Heat Stroke

High body temperature, the absence of sweating, with hot red or flushed dry skin, rapid pulse, CNS symptoms like agitation, disorientation, hallucinations, seizures, cranial nerve abnormalities, cerebellar dysfunction, and opisthotonos, decerebrate posturing or decorticate posturing. Coma may be caused by electrolyte abnormalities, hypoglycemia, hepatic encephalopathy, uremic encephalopathy, and acute structural abnormalities, such as intracerebral hemorrhage due to trauma or coagulation disorders. Cerebral edema and herniation can occur. Examination of the eyes may reveal nystagmus and oculogyric episodes due to cerebellar injury, pupils may be fixed, dilated, pinpoint, or normal. Patients with heatstroke commonly exhibit tachypnea and hyperventilation caused by direct CNS stimulation, acidosis, or hypoxia. Hypoxia and cyanosis may be due to a number of processes, including atelectasis, pulmonary infarction, aspiration pneumonia, and pulmonary edema. Gastrointestinal hemorrhage occurs frequently in patients with heatstroke and patients commonly exhibit evidence of hepatic injury, including jaundice and elevated liver enzymes. Rarely, fulminant hepatic failure occurs, accompanied by encephalopathy, hypoglycemia, and disseminated intravascular coagulation (DIC) and bleeding. Muscle tenderness and cramping are common; rhabdomyolysis is a common complication of exertional heat stroke (EHS) and patient's muscles may be rigid or limp. Acute renal failure (ARF) is a common complication of heatstroke and may be due to hypovolemia, low cardiac output, and myoglobinuria (due to rhabdomyolysis) and patients may exhibit oliguria and a change in the color of urine.

Pathophysiology

The excessive heat denatures proteins, destabilizes phospholipids and lipoproteins, and liquefies membrane lipids, leading to cardiovascular collapse, multiorgan failure, and, ultimately, death. The exact temperature at which cardiovascular collapse occurs varies among individuals because coexisting disease, drugs, and other factors may contribute to or delay organ dysfunction. Full recovery can occur in patients with temperatures as high as 46°C, while death has occurred in patients with much lower temperatures. Temperatures exceeding 106°F or 41.1°C generally are catastrophic and require immediate aggressive therapy.

Morbidity and Mortality

Morbidity and mortality from heatstroke are related to the duration of the temperature elevation. When therapy is delayed, the mortality rate may be as high as 80%; however, with early diagnosis and immediate cooling, the mortality rate can be reduced to 10%. Mortality is highest among the elderly population because of their limited cardiovascular reserves, preexisting illness, and use of many medications that may affect their volume status or sweating ability. Isolated patients with preexisting disease, those confined to a bed are at high risk. Infants and children are at risk for heat illness due to inefficient sweating, a higher metabolic rate, and their inability to care for themselves and control their environment. EHS is the second most common cause of death among high school athletes, surpassed only by spinal cord injury. Lack of acclimatization is a major risk factor for EHS in young adults.

Treatment

Removal of restrictive clothing and spraying water on the body, covering the patient with ice water–soaked sheets, or placing ice packs in the axillae and groin may reduce the patient's temperature significantly. Patients who are unable to protect their airway should be intubated. Patients who are awake and responsive should receive supplemental oxygen. Intravenous lines may be placed in anticipation of fluid resuscitation and for the infusion of dextrose and thiamine if indicated. Hypoglycemia is a common occurrence in patients with EHS and may be a manifestation of liver failure; therefore, infusion of dextrose 50% in water solution (D50W) should be considered in all patients with heatstroke. Intensive care personnel must pay meticulous attention to the airway, reduce the temperature, limit the production of heat, optimize circulation, and monitor for and treat complications. Insert a thermistor probe to monitor temperature continuously. Insert a nasogastric tube to monitor for gastrointestinal bleeding and fluid losses. Place a Foley catheter to monitor urine output. The goal of treatment is to reduce the temperature by at least 0.2°C/min to approximately 39°C. Active external cooling generally is halted at 39°C to prevent overshooting, which can result in iatrogenic hypothermia. Place a flexible indwelling thermistor rectally or an esophageal probe to monitor core body temperature during treatment. Because thermal instability may persist for a few days after the onset of heatstroke, the temperature must be monitored continuously until it is stable. The optimal method of rapidly cooling patients is a matter of debate; each method has its own theoretical advantages and disadvantages.

- Ice-water immersion or an equivalent method is an extremely effective method of rapidly reducing core body temperature and traditionally was the most frequently recommended method. The increased thermal conductivity of ice water can reduce core body temperature to less than 39°C in approximately 20-40 minutes. The practice has been criticized recently. Theoretically, the ice water, which may be extremely uncomfortable to patients who are awake, can cause subcutaneous vasoconstriction, preventing the transfer of heat via conduction. Ice water also increases shivering, which in turn increases internal heat production. Other reasons for the recent criticisms include difficulty monitoring and resuscitating patients.

- Recently, evaporative techniques have been touted to be as effective as immersion techniques without the practical difficulties. However, data on the efficacy of this method are limited. Evaporative body heat loss may be accomplished by removing all of the patient's clothes and intermittently spraying the patient's body with warm water while a powerful fan blows across the body, allowing the heat to evaporate.
- A number of other cooling techniques have been suggested, but none has proven superior to or equal to cold-water immersion or evaporative techniques. These include peritoneal, thoracic, rectal, and gastric lavage with ice water; cold intravenous fluids; cold humidified oxygen; cooling blankets; and wet towels.
- In the most severe cases, cardiopulmonary bypass has been suggested, but this requires highly trained personnel and sophisticated equipment.
- Antipyretics (e.g., acetaminophen, aspirin, other nonsteroidal anti-inflammatory agents) have no role in the treatment of heatstroke because antipyretics interrupt the change in the hypothalamic set point caused by pyrogens. They are not expected to work on a healthy hypothalamus that has been overloaded, as in the case of heatstroke. In this situation, antipyretics actually may be harmful in patients who develop hepatic, hematologic, and renal complications because they may aggravate bleeding tendencies.
- Dantrolene has been studied as a possible pharmacological option in the treatment of hyperthermia and heatstroke, but at present, it has not been proven to be efficacious in clinical trials.

- Along with immediate active cooling, steps to stop excessive production of heat must be taken.
  - Agitation and shivering should be treated immediately with benzodiazepines.
  - Benzodiazepines are the sedatives of choice in patients with sympathomimetic-induced delirium as well as alcohol and sedative drug withdrawals.
  - Neuroleptics, such as chlorpromazine, which were the mainstays of therapy in the past, are best avoided because of their deleterious adverse effects, including lowering of the seizure threshold, interference with thermoregulation, anticholinergic properties, hypotension, hepatotoxicity, and other adverse effects.
- Similarly, convulsions must be controlled.
  - Benzodiazepines and, if necessary, barbiturates are the recommended agents in this setting. Barbiturates may be used despite their theoretical impedance of sweat production.
  - Phenytoin is not effective in controlling convulsions in this situation.
  - Patients whose convulsions are refractory to benzodiazepines and barbiturates should be paralyzed and provided mechanical ventilation. Electroencephalographic monitoring is recommended in all such patients, and anticonvulsant medications should be adjusted accordingly.

- Recommendations on the administration of intravenous fluids for circulatory support differ among patient populations and depend on the presence of hypovolemia, preexisting medical conditions, and preexisting cardiovascular disease.
  - While patients with heatstroke invariably are volume depleted, cooling alone may improve hypotension and cardiac function by allowing blood to redistribute centrally.
  - Aggressive fluid resuscitation generally is not recommended because it may lead to pulmonary edema.
  - Cor pulmonale also is a common finding in patients with heatstroke.
- When pulse rate, blood pressure, and urine output do not provide adequate hemodynamic information, fluid administration should be guided by more invasive hemodynamic parameters, such as central venous pressure (CVP), pulmonary capillary wedge pressure, systemic vascular resistance index (SVRI), and cardiac index (CI) measurements.
  - Patients who exhibit a hyperdynamic state (i.e., high CI, low SVRI) generally respond to cooling and do not require large amounts of intravenous crystalloid infusions.
  - Hypotensive patients who exhibit a hypodynamic response (i.e., high CVP, low CI) traditionally have been treated with low-dose isoproterenol; however, its arrhythmogenicity has raised questions about its continued use. Dobutamine, which is less arrhythmogenic than isoproterenol and more cardioselective, may be the inotrope of choice in these patients.
  - Alpha-adrenergic drugs generally are contraindicated because they cause vasoconstriction and may interfere with heat loss.
- The occurrence of rhabdomyolysis may be heralded by the development of dark, tea-colored urine and tender edematous muscles. This releases large amounts of myoglobin, which can precipitate in the kidneys and result in ARF. Renal failure especially is common in patients who develop hypotension or shock during the course of their disease and may occur in as many as 25-30% of patients with EHS.
  - Treatment of rhabdomyolysis involves infusion of large amounts of intravenous fluids (fluid requirements may be as high as 10 L), alkalinization of the urine, and infusion of mannitol.
  - Fluid administration is guided best by invasive hemodynamic parameters, and urine output should be maintained at 3 cc/kg/h to minimize the risk of renal failure.
  - Alkalinization of the urine (urine pH 7.5-8.0) prevents the precipitation of myoglobin in the renal tubules and may control acidosis and hyperkalemia in acute massive muscle necrosis.
  - Mannitol may improve renal blood flow and glomerular filtration rate, increase urine output, and prevent fluid accumulation in the interstitial compartment (through its osmotic action). Mannitol also is a free radical scavenger and, therefore, may reduce damage caused by free radicals.
  - Once renal failure occurs, dialysis is the only effective therapeutic modality for rhabdomyolysis.
- Metabolic support
  - Muscle necrosis may be so rapid that hyperkalemia, hypocalcemia, and hyperphosphatemia become significant enough to cause cardiac arrhythmias and require immediate therapy.
  - In the presence of renal failure, hemodialysis may be necessary.

- Hypertonic dextrose and sodium bicarbonate may be used to shift potassium into the intracellular environment while more definitive measures (e.g. intestinal potassium binding, dialysis) are prepared.
- Use of insulin may not be necessary in patients who are not diabetic and may be deleterious for patients with EHS and patients with liver failure, who commonly develop hypoglycemia.
- Use of calcium should be judicious because it may precipitate in and cause additional muscle damage. Use of calcium is reserved for patients with ventricular ectopy, impending convulsions, or electrocardiographic evidence of hyperkalemia.
- Various other electrolyte abnormalities have been reported in patients with heatstroke and must be monitored closely and treated carefully. These abnormalities may be related to solute-altering conditions such as vomiting, diarrhea, and use of diuretics. For example, hypokalemia, which is common in the early phases of heatstroke, may develop in response to respiratory alkalosis, diarrhea, and sweating. Similarly, hyponatremia may be due to sodium losses and/or rehydration with salt-poor solutions (e.g. water), and hypernatremia may be due to dehydration.

- Heatstroke commonly leads to severe but reversible hepatic damage.
  - Hepatic injury is represented by elevations in transaminase levels and bilirubin. During this phase, hypoglycemia, abnormal coagulation, cerebral edema, and death can occur, although rarely.
  - Prolonged coagulation times also may signal the development of DIC, which, when present, carries a poor patient prognosis. Clinical manifestations can range from abnormal laboratory values to generalized bleeding occurring approximately 48 hours after the initial insult. DIC also may predispose patients to development of acute respiratory distress syndrome (ARDS), which also increases mortality.
  - Treatment of hepatic failure includes the infusion of dextrose solutions to correct hypoglycemia; the early recognition and treatment of DIC, with replacement of clotting factors, fresh frozen plasma, platelets, and blood; and meticulous respiratory support.
- Pulmonary edema is a common complication of heatstroke and may be due to a number of factors, including fluid overload from aggressive rehydration, fluid over-load from renal failure, congestive heart failure, and ARDS. The latter may develop because of multiple insults, including heat-induced pulmonary damage, aspiration pneumonia, and as a complication of liver failure. ARDS should be treated aggressi-vely, with early mechanical ventilation and positive end-expiratory pressure (PEEP).
- ARF may occur because of direct thermal injury of the kidney, myoglobinuria, hypotension, and/or shock (ATN). Early manifestations of renal failure include oliguria, low-grade proteinuria, and granular casts.
  - ARF initially is treated with intravenous fluids, diuretics, and correction of associated acid-base and electrolyte abnormalities.
  - In the setting of rhabdomyolysis, mannitol may be the diuretic of choice because it does not interfere with the acid-base status of the urine, and it may have antioxidant activity.

- Furosemide may cause tubular acidosis and, therefore, may promote myoglobin deposition within the renal tubules.
- Once renal failure has set in, hemodialysis is the most effective therapy.

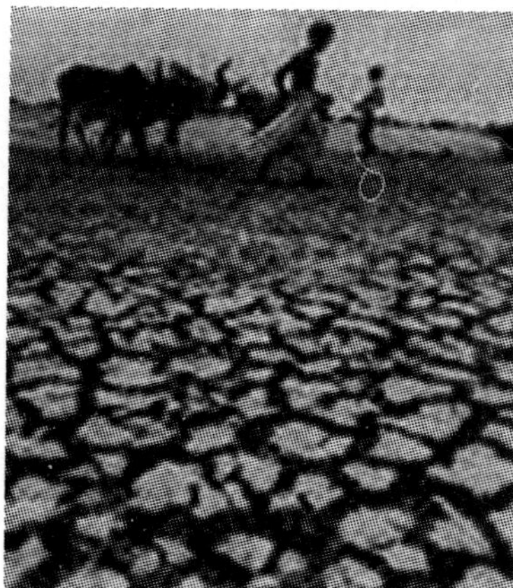

Fig. 24.3

DROUGHT

Definition

Drought is defined as a period in which a region has a deficit in its water supply.

Drought is a normal feature of climate which happens in all climate zones from time to time.

Types

Usually, drought is talked about in one of two perspectives—*meteorological and hydrological*. A drought in terms of meteorology takes into account deficiencies in measured precipitation. Each year's measurements are then compared to what is determined as a "normal" amount of precipitation and drought is determined from there. For hydrologists, droughts are monitored by checking stream flow and lake, reservoir, and aquifer water levels. Precipitation is also considered here as it contributes to the water levels.

In addition, there are *agricultural droughts* that can impact crop production and cause changes to the natural distribution of various species. The farms themselves can cause droughts as soil is depleted and cannot absorb as much water. They can be impacted by natural droughts as well.

Causes of Drought

Because drought is defined as a deficit in water supply, it can be caused by a number of factors. The most important one though relates to the amount of water vapor in the atmosphere as this is what creates precipitation. More rain, sleet, hail, and snow can occur where there are moist, low pressure air systems. If there is an above average presence of dry, high pressure air systems instead, less moisture is available to produce precipitation (because these systems cannot hold as much water vapor). This results in a deficit of water for the areas over which they move.

The same can also happen when winds shift air masses and warm, dry, continental air moves over an area as opposed to cooler, moist, oceanic air masses. El Nino, which affects the ocean's water temperature, also has an impact on precipitation levels because in years when the temperature cycle is present, it can shift the air masses above the ocean, often making wet places dry (drought prone) and dry places wet.

Finally, deforestation for agriculture and/or building combined with the resultant erosion can also cause drought to begin because as soil is moved away from an area it is less able to absorb moisture when it falls.

Stages of Drought

Since many areas, regardless of their climatic region, are prone to drought, different definitions of the stages of drought have developed. They are all somewhat similar however, usually ranging from a drought warning or watch, which is the least severe. This stage is declared when a drought could be approaching. The next stages are mostly called drought emergency, disaster, or critical drought stage. This final stage begins after a drought has occurred for a long period and water sources begin to be depleted. During this stage, public water use is limited and drought disaster plans are put into place.

Regardless of a drought's stage, there are short and long term consequences with any drought because of nature and society's dependence on water. Problems associated with drought can have economic, environmental, and social impacts on both the areas where they occur and areas that have relations with those where the drought happens.

Most of the economic impacts of drought are associated with agriculture and the income generated from crops. In times of drought, the lack of water can often cause a decline in crop yields, and thus a reduction in income for farmers and an increase in the market price of products since there are shortages. In a prolonged drought, unemployment of farmers and even retailers can occur, having a significant impact on the economy of the area and those with economic ties to it.

In terms of environmental problems, drought can result in insect infestations and plant diseases, increased erosion, habitat and landscape degradation, a decrease in air and existing water, as well as an increased risk of fire because of drier vegetation. In short-term droughts, natural environments can often rebound, but when there are long term droughts, plant and animal species can suffer tremendously, and over time desertification can happen with an extreme lack of moisture.

Finally, droughts have social impacts that can cause disputes between users of available water, inequalities in water distribution between wealthy and poor, disparities in areas in need of disaster relief, and a decline in health. In addition, in rural developing countries population migration can begin when one area experiences drought because often people will go to areas where water and its benefits are more prevalent. This then depletes the natural resources of the new area and cause conflicts among neighboring populations besides depleting workers away from the original area. Over time, increased poverty and social unrest is likely to develop.

Drought Mitigation Measures

Because severe drought is often slow in its development, it is relatively easy to tell when one is coming and in areas that are capable, there are several mitigation measures that can be used to reduce the impacts felt by drought.

The most important steps in lessening the effects of drought though are soil and water conservation. By protecting soil, it is better able to absorb precipitation, but it can also help farmers to use less water because it is absorbed and not as much runs off. It also creates less water pollution by the pesticides and fertilizers present in most farm runoff.

In water conservation, public use is often regulated. This mostly includes watering yards, washing cars and outdoor fixtures such as patio tables, and swimming pools. Use of xeriscape landscaping to reduce the need to water outdoor plants in dry environments. In addition, Water conservation devices like low-flow toilets, shower heads, and washing machines can be required for use inside the home.

Finally, desalination of seawater, water recycling, and rainwater harvesting can build on existing water supplies and further reduce the impacts of drought in dry climates. Whatever method is used however, extensive monitoring of precipitation and water usage are the best way to prepare for a drought, inform the public on the problem, and implement conservation strategies.

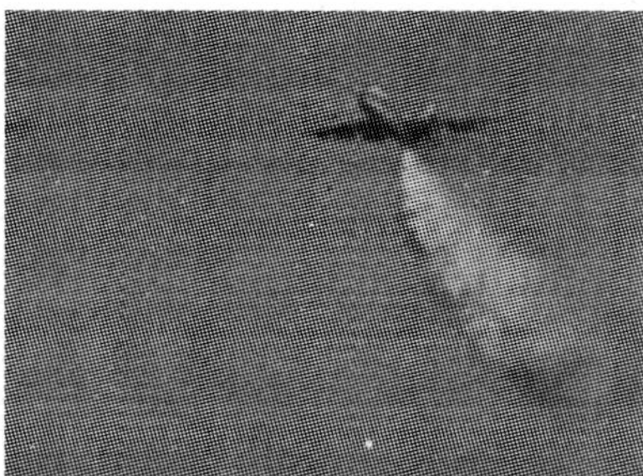

Fig. 24.4

CLOUD SEEDING

"There is no technology that can create rain when there was no potential for it to begin with. Cloud seeding appears to be able to get a little bit more than you would have got otherwise. The conditions are going to have to be just right for cloud seeding to have a measurable impact."
(Keith Seitter, Executive Director of the American Meteorological Society)

Introduction

Annual variations in rainfall are a known phenomenon the world over. There is a huge amount of water vapour in the atmosphere. It is like an ocean and only 10% of the water vapour ever reaches the ground as rainfall or snowfall. A rainstorm happens after moisture collects around naturally occurring particles in the air, causing the air to reach a level of saturation at which point it can no longer hold in that moisture Cloud seeding can be utilized to boost precipitation by at least 25% in specific areas over a whole season depending upon the type of clouds in the affected areas.

Definition

Cloud seeding is a form of *weather modification* attempting to change the amount or type of *precipitation* (rain or snow) that falls from *clouds*. This is done by dispersing substances into the *air* that serve as *cloud condensation* or *ice nuclei*, which alter the microphysical processes within the cloud. Hail and fog suppression over airports is also managed using this technique. About 24 countries currently practice weather modification operationally.

Technique

The first step is to select a cloud mass containing supercooled liquid water—that is, liquid water colder than zero degrees Celsius i.e. whose upper layer temperatures are below freezing. Next hygroscopic chemicals like silver iodide, salt or dry ice (frozen carbon dioxide) is fired into the cloud. Liquid propane into a gas can also been used to produce ice crystals at warmer temperatures than silver iodide This can be done either by dropping flares attached under the wings of an aeroplane or dispersion devices (generators or canisters fired from anti-aircraft guns or rockets) fired from the ground when the fine particles are carried downwind and upwards by air currents after release.

Water droplets attach to the particles forming snowflakes by the process of freezing nucleation. Once these are heavy enough, they fall as first snow then melt into rain at lower altitudes. Essentially, hygroscopic seeding causes the droplet size spectrum in clouds to become more maritime (bigger drops) and less continental, stimulating rainfall through coalescence The trick is getting those seeding materials in the right place at the right time. Dry ice or propane expansion cools the air to such an extent that ice crystals can nucleate spontaneously from the vapor phase. Unlike seeding with silver iodide, this spontaneous nucleation does not require any existing droplets or particles because it produces extremely high vapor supersaturation near the seeding substance. This process is known as "static" seeding.

Seeding of warm-season or tropical cumuliform (convective) clouds using calcium chloride seeks to exploit the latent heat released by freezing. This strategy is called "dynamic" seeding and it assumes that the additional latent heat adds buoyancy, strengthens updrafts, ensures more low-level convergence, and ultimately causes rapid growth of properly selected clouds and translating into more rainfall. Up to 100 times more ice crystals are used in dynamic cloud seeding than in the static method. The process is considered more complex than static clouding seeding because it depends on a sequence of events working properly. Dr. William R. Cotton, a professor of atmospheric science at Colorado State University, and other researchers break down dynamic cloud seeding into 11 separate stages. An unexpected outcome in one stage could ruin the entire process, making the technique less dependable than static cloud seeding.

History

Vincent Schaefer (1906–1993) discovered the principle of cloud seeding in July 1946 through a series of serendipitous events. Following ideas generated between himself and Nobel laureate Irving Langmuir while climbing Mt. Washington in New Hampshire, Schaefer, Langmuir's research associate, created a way of experimenting with supercooled clouds using a deep freeze unit lined with black velveteen. He tried hundreds of potential agents to stimulate ice crystal growth, i.e., salt, talcum powder, soils, dust and various chemical agents with minor effect. Then one hot and humid July day he wanted to try a few experiments at General Electric's Schenectady Research Lab. He was dismayed to find that the deep freezer was not cold enough to produce a cloud using breath air. He decided to move the process along by adding a chunk of dry ice just to lower the temperature. To his astonishment, as soon as he breathed into the chamber, a bluish haze was noted, followed by an eye-popping display of millions of tiny ice crystals, reflecting the strong light rays illuminating a cross-section of the chamber. He instantly realized that he had discovered a way to change supercooled water into ice crystals. The experiment was easily replicated and he explored the temperature gradient to establish the "40°C limit for liquid water. Within the month, Schaefer's colleague, the noted atmospheric scientist Dr. Bernard Vonnegut (brother of novelist Kurt Vonnegut) is credited with discovering another method for "seeding" supercooled cloud water. Vonnegut accomplished his discovery at the desk, looking up information in a basic chemistry text and then tinkering with silver and iodide chemicals to produce silver iodide. Together with Dr. Vonnegut, Professor Henry Chessin, SUNY Albany, a crystallographer, co-authored a publication in Science Magazine and received a patent in 1975. Both methods were adopted for use in cloud seeding during 1946 while working for the General Electric Corporation in the state of New York. Schaefer's altered a cloud's heat budget, Vonnegut's altered formative crystal structure – an ingenious property related to a good match in lattice constant between the two types of crystal. The first attempt to modify natural clouds in the field through "cloud seeding" began during a flight that began in upstate New York on 13 November 1946. Schaefer was able to cause snow to fall near Mount Greylock in western Massachusetts, after he dumped six pounds of dry ice into the target cloud from a plane after a 60 mile easterly chase from the Schenectady County Airport.

From March 1967 until July 1972, the U.S. military's Operation Popeye cloud-seeded silver iodide to extend the monsoon season over North Vietnam, specifically the Ho Chi Minh Trail. The operation resulted in the targeted areas seeing an extension of the monsoon period an average of 30 to 45 days. The 54th Weather Reconnaissance Squadron carried out the operation to "make mud, not war".

In 1969 at the Woodstock Festival, various people claimed to have witnessed clouds being seeded by the U.S. military. This was said to be the cause of the rain which lasted throughout most of the festival.

An attempt by the United States military to modify hurricanes in the Atlantic basin using cloud seeding in the 1960s was called Project Stormfury.

The United States Bureau of Reclamation (Reclamation; Department of the Interior) and the National Oceanic and Atmospheric Administration (NOAA; Department of Commerce). Reclamation sponsored several cloud seeding research projects under the umbrella of Project Skywater from 1964 to 1988, and NOAA conducted the Atmospheric Modification Program from 1979 to 1993.and the Weather Damage Modification Program, from 2002–2006. In the United States, cloud seeding is used to increase precipitation in areas experiencing drought, to reduce the size of hailstones that form in thunderstorms, and to reduce the amount of fog in and around airports. Cloud seeding is also occasionally used by major ski resorts to induce snowfall A number of commercial companies, such as Aero Systems Incorporated , Atmospherics Incorporated, North American Weather Consultants, Weather Modification Incorporated, Weather Enhancement Technologies International, Seeding Operations and Atmospheric Research (SOAR) , offer weather modification services centered on cloud seeding. The USAF proposed its use on the battlefield in 1996, although the U.S. signed an international treaty in 1978 banning the use of weather modification for hostile purposes.

In Australia, CSIRO conducted major trials between 1947 and the early 1960s.The Hydro-Electricity Commission catchment area on the Central Plateau achieved rainfall increases as high as 30% in autumn. The Tasmanian experiments were so successful that the Commission has regularly undertaken seeding ever since in mountainous parts of the State.

In Austrian silver iodine seeding for hail prevention began in 1981–2000, and the technique is still actively deployed there.

The largest cloud seeding system in the world is that of the People's Republic of China Northern China, where Beijing is located, doesn't receive much rain—its rainfall levels are 35 percent below the world average, and some of its water supplies are significantly polluted. The area relies heavily on cloud seeding. Zhiang Qiang, who runs the Beijing Weather Modification Office, told the Asia Times that water levels in Beijing's water basins have increased up to 13 percent due to cloud seeding. Cloud seeding also has been used to cool Beijing on hot days. There is even political strife caused by neighboring regions which accuse each other of "stealing rain" using cloud seeding. In February 2009, China also blasted iodide sticks over Beijing to artificially induce snowfall after four months of drought, and blasted iodide sticks over other areas of northern China to increase snowfall. The snowfall in Beijing, which rarely experiences snow, lasted for approximately three days and led to the closure of 12 main roads around Beijing.

Russian military pilots seeded clouds over Belarus after the Chernobyl disaster to remove radioactive particles from clouds heading toward Moscow. In Moscow. The Russian Air Force tried seeding clouds with bags of cement on Jun 17, 2008. One of the bags did not pulverize and went through the roof of a house!

In Southeast Asia, open burning produces haze that pollutes the regional environment. Cloud-seeding has been used to improve the air quality by encouraging rainfall.

In India, pioneering attempts in the field of rainmaking were made by a Tata firm in 1951 over Western Ghats using ground based silver iodide generators. Dr. Banerji in the year 1952 attempted cloud seeding with salt and silver iodide by means of hydrogen filled balloons released from the ground. Cloud seeding operations were conducted during the years 2003 and 2004 through U.S. based Weather Modification Inc. in state of Maharashtra . In 2008, 12 districts of state of Andhra Pradesh were shortlisted for cloud seeding.

Adverse Effects

Several detailed ecological studies that showed negligible environmental and health impacts and the present scale of cloud seeding is considered to be 100 times less than industry emissions into the atmosphere in many parts of the world, or individual exposure from tooth fillings. Cloud seeding could provoke legal disputes between nations, if rain was increased in one area but reduced in another. Cloud seeding may also suppress precipitation.

Part of the problem is that it is difficult to discern how much precipitation would have occurred had the cloud not been seeded. The process is also dependent on specificity of clouds, wind speed and direction, terrain and other factors.

There are reports that cloud seeding has affected the pygmy possum amongst other species as well as causing recent high level algal blooms in once pristine glacial lakes.

25 Action Plan During a Wildfire

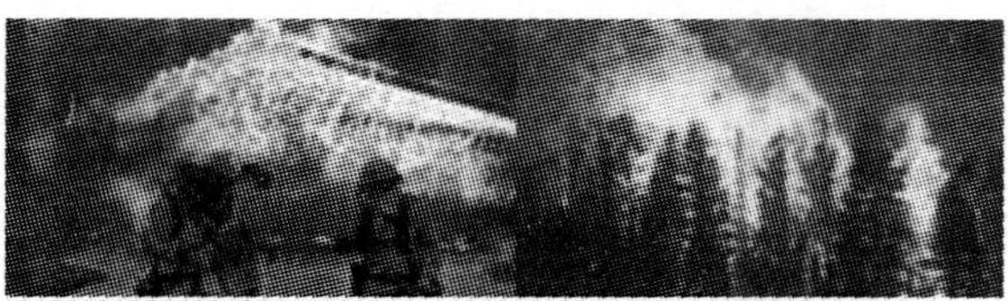

Fig. 25.1

INTRODUCTION

A wildfire is any uncontrolled fire that occurs in the countryside or wilderness. Other names such as brushfire, bushfire, forest fire, grass fire, hill fire, peat fire, vegetation fire and wildland fire may be used to describe the same phenomenon. A wildfire differs from other fires by its extensive size; the speed at which it can spread out from its original source; its ability to change direction unexpectedly; and to jump gaps, such as roads, rivers and fire breaks. Wildfires are characterized in terms of their physical properties such as speed of propagation; the combustible material present; the effect of weather on the fire; and the cause of ignition.

Fossil records and human history contain accounts of wildfires, and wildfires occur on every continent except Antartica and can be cyclical events. Wildfires can cause extensive damage, both to property and human life. Along with the damage caused, they also have various beneficial effects on wilderness areas, such as plant species that are dependent on the effects of fire for growth and reproduction. However, large wildfires may have negative ecological effects.

The strategies of prevention, detection, and suppression have varied over the years, but improved technology and research has resulted in newer and more effective weapons against wildfires around the world. Current techniques may permit and even encourage smaller fires in some regions as a means of minimizing or removing sources of fuel from any wildfire that might develop. While some wildfires burn in remote forested regions they can cause extensive destruction of homes and other property located in the *wildland-urban interface*: a zone of transition between developed areas and undeveloped wilderness. The name wildfire was once a synonym for Greek fire as well as a word for any furious or destructive conflagration. Wildfires differ from other fires in that they take place outdoors in areas of grassland, woodlands, bushland, scrubland, peatland, and other woody materials that act as a source of fuel or combustible material. Buildings are not usually involved, unless the fire spreads to adjacent communities and threatens these structures.

Some of the features of wildfires include the *forward rate of spread* (FROS), especially in "continuous fuels, thick vegetation and continuous overhead tree canopies", which can be as fast as 10.8 kilometers per hour (6.7 mph) in forests and 22 kilometers per hour (14 mph) in grasslands; and the ability of the burning front to unexpectedly change direction and to jump across fire breaks. The intense heat and smoke can lead to disorientation and loss of appreciation of the direction of the fire. These factors make fires particularly dangerous.

While wildfires may be categorized as large, uncontrolled disasters that burn through 0.4 to 400 square kilometres (100 to 100,000 acres) and higher, wildfires can be as small as 0.25 acres (0.0010 km^2) or less. However, even though smaller events may be included in fire behavior analysis. Catastrophic wildfires influence fire policies more so than small fires.

Wildfires start when an ignition source is brought into contact with a combustible vegetation that is subjected to sufficient heat and has an adequate supply of oxygen from the ambient air. A high moisture content usually prevents ignition and slows down propagation because higher temperatures are required to evaporate any water within the material and heat the material to its fore point. Dense forests usually provide more shade, resulting in lower ambient temperatures and greater humidity. Less dense material such as grasses and leaves are easier to ignite because they contain less water than denser material such as branches and trunks. Plants continuously lose water by evaporation, but water loss is usually balanced by water absorbed from the soil, humidity or rain. When this balance is not maintained, plants dry out and are therefore more flammable, often a consequence of a long, hot, dry periods.

A wildfire *front* is the portion sustaining continuous flaming combustion, where unburned material meets active flames, or the smoldering transition between unburned and burned material. As the front approaches, the fire heats both the surrounding air and woody material through convection and thermal radiation. First, wood is dried as water is vaporized at a temperature of 100 °C (212 °F). Next, the pyrolysis of wood at 230 °C (450 °F) releases flammable gases. Finally, wood can smolder at 380 °C (720 °F) or, when heated sufficiently, ignite at 590 °C (1,100 °F). Even before the flames of a wildfire arrive at a particular location, heat transfer from the wildfire front can precede the flames, warming the air to 800 °C (1,470 °F) and drying and pre-heating flammable materials. Also, high-temperature and long-duration surface wildfires may encourage flashover or *torching*: the drying of tree canopies and their subsequent ignition from below.

Wildfires in forested areas can move at speeds of 10.8 kilometers per hour (6.7 mph), while grass fires have been recorded at up to 22 kilometers per hour (14 mph). Wildfires can advance tangential to the main front to form a *flanking* front, or burn opposite the direction of the main front by *backing*. Wildfires may also spread by *jumping* or *spotting*, as winds and vertical convection columns carry hot wood embers and other burning materials through the air over roads, rivers, and other natural barriers or firebreaks. Torching and crown fires are prone to spotting, and dry ground fuels that surround a wildfire are especially vulnerable to ignition from firebrands.

Air rises as it is heated, and large wildfires create powerful updrafts that will draw in new air from surrounding areas (thermal column/ stack effect) Great vertical differences in temperature and humidity encourage pyro-cumulus clouds and tornado-force fire whirls and winds of speeds of more than 80 kilometers per hour (50 mph) Extreme fire behavior includes wide rates of spread, prolific crowning and/or spotting, the presence of fire whirls, and a strong convection column.

Wildfires and their spread vary based on the flammable material present and its vertical arrangement. Fuel density is governed by topography, as land shape determines factors such as available sunlight and water for plant growth. For example, fuels uphill from a fire are more readily dried and warmed by the fire than those downhill, yet burning logs can roll downhill.

Overall, *fire types* can be generally characterized by their fuel as follows:

- ***Ground:*** Subterranean roots, duff and other buried organic matter. This fuel type is especially susceptible to ignition due to spotting. Ground fires typically burn by smoldering and can burn slowly for days to months, e.g. peat fires.
- ***Crawling*** or ***surface:*** Low-lying vegetation such as leaf and timber litter, debris, grass, and low-lying shrubbery. Ground-clearing fires lit by humans near the rain forests creates knee-high surface fires that cause significant damage in an ecosystem not well adapted to fire.
- ***Ladder:*** Material between low-level vegetation and tree canopies, such as small trees, downed logs, vines and invasive plants.
- ***Crown, canopy,*** or ***aerial:*** Suspended material at the canopy level, such as tall trees, vines, and mosses. The ignition of a crown fire is dependent on the density of the suspended material, canopy height, canopy continuity, and sufficient surface and ladder fires in order to reach the tree crowns.

Heat waves, drought conditions, global warming and cyclical climate changes like El Nino and other weather patterns can also dramatically increase the risk and alter the behavior of wildfires. Years of precipitation followed by warm periods have encouraged more widespread fires and longer fire seasons. The intensity also increases during daytime hours. Burn rates of smoldering logs are up to five times greater during the day due to lower humidity, increased temperatures, and increased wind speeds. Sunlight warms the ground during the day and causes air currents to travel uphill, and downhill during the night as the land cools. Wildfires are fanned by these winds and often follow the air currents over hills and through valleys.

The four *major natural causes* of wildfire ignitions are lightning, volcanic eruption, sparks from rockfalls, and spontaneous combustion. Smoldering underground coal fires can also flare up and ignite nearby flammable material. However, many wildfires are attributed to *human sources* such as arson, discarded cigarettes, sparks from equipment, and power line arcs. Slash and burn farming is often considered the least expensive way to clear and prepare land for future use Forested areas cleared by logging encourages the dominance of flammable grasses, and abandoned logging roads overgrown by vegetation may act as fire corridors.

If you see a wildfire, inform the police and fire department. Don't assume that someone else has already called. Describe the location of the fire, speak slowly and clearly, and answer any questions asked by the dispatcher.

Before the Fire Approaches Your House

- *Evacuate:* Evacuate your pets and all family members who are not essential to preparing the home. Anyone with medical or physical limitations and the young and the elderly should be evacuated immediately.

Wear Protective Clothing

- *Remove combustibles:* Clear items that will burn from around the house, including wood piles, lawn furniture, barbecue grills, tarpaulin coverings, etc. Move them outside of your defensible space.
- *Close/protect openings:* Close outside attic, eaves and basement vents, windows, doors, pet doors, etc. Remove flammable drapes and curtains. Close all shutters,

blinds or heavy non-combustible window coverings to reduce radiant heat.

- *Close inside doors/open damper:* Close all doors inside the house to prevent draft. Open the damper on your fireplace, but close the fireplace screen.
- *Shut off gas:* Shut off any natural gas, propane or fuel oil supplies at the source.
- *Water:* Connect garden hoses. Fill any pools, hot tubs, garbage cans, tubs or other large containers with water.
- *Pumps*: If you have gas-powered pumps for water, make sure they are fueled and ready.
- *Ladder:* Place a ladder against the house in clear view.
- *Car:* Back your car into the driveway and roll up the windows.
- *Garage doors:* Disconnect any automatic garage door openers so that doors can still be opened by hand if the power goes out. Close all garage doors.
- *Valuables:* Place valuable papers, mementos and anything you can't live without inside the car in the garage, ready for quick departure. Any pets still with you should also be put in the car.

Preparing to Leave

- *Lights:* Turn on outside lights and leave a light on in every room to make the house more visible in heavy smoke.
- *Don't lock up:* Leave doors and windows closed but unlocked. It may be necessary for firefighters to gain quick entry into your home to fight fire. The entire area will be isolated and patrolled by the police and firefighting personnel.

What to do After a Wildfire

Check the roof immediately. Put out any roof fires, sparks or embers. Check the attic for hidden burning sparks. If you have a fire, get your neighbors to help fight it.

The water you put into your pool or hot tub and other containers wilt come in handy now. If the power is out, try connecting a hose to the outlet on your water heater.

For several hours after the fire, maintain a fire watch. Re-check for smoke and sparks throughout the house.

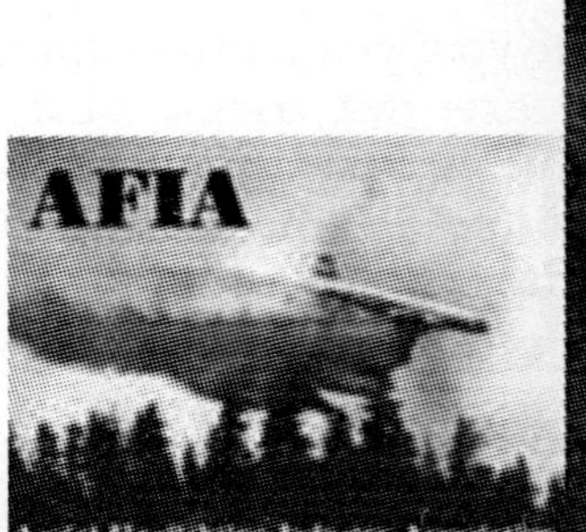

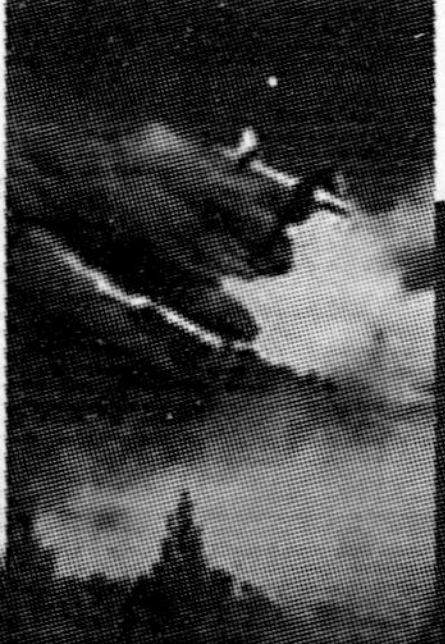
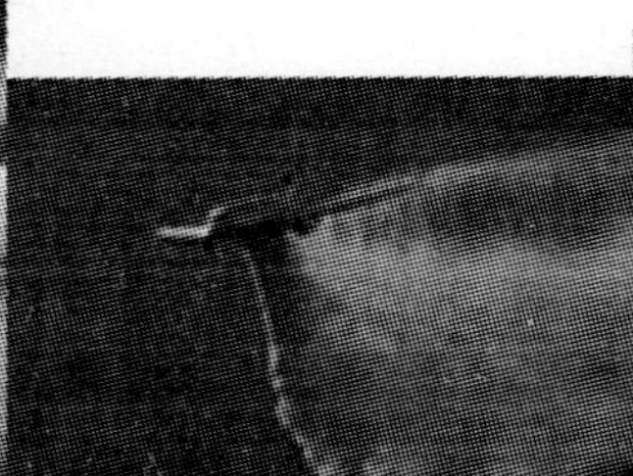
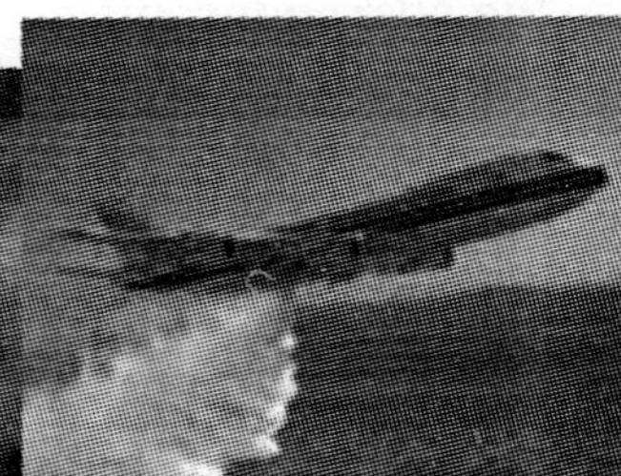

Fig. 25.2

AERIAL FIREFIGHTING OF WILDFIRES

Definition

Aerial firefighting is the use of aircraft and other aerial resources to combat wildfires.

Aircraft Used

The types of aircraft used include fixed-wing aircraft and helicopters. Smoke jumpers and rappellers are also classified as aerial firefighters, delivered to the fire by parachute from a variety of fixed-wing aircraft, or rappelling from helicopters. Chemicals used to fight fires may include water, water enhancers such as foams and gels, and specially-formulated fire retardants wide variety of terminology has been used in the popular media for the aircraft (and methods) used in aerial firefighting.

Air attack is an industry term used for the actual application of aerial resources, both fixed-wing and rotorcraft, on a fire, although colloquially, "air attack" is also a term used for the airborne manager in a spotter plane who is charged with directing the use of the aerial resources. Initial attack refers to the first-response of aerial assets to suppress a fire before it grows out of control; aviation assets can usually respond to a reported blaze much more quickly than ground-based resources can. Extended attack refers to the continued use of aerial and other resources on an out-of-control fire, primarily to assist ground units in the establishment of firelines in advance of the fire.

After the close of World War II, advances made in military aircraft technology during the war were quickly pressed into peacetime service to fight one of the oldest and most feared natural phenomena—wildfires. Until the 1950s, once a wildfire had spread across bone-dry forests or parched grasslands, there wasn't much that firefighters could do except watch it burn and try to rein in its swath of destruction. That unbalanced playing field was somewhat leveled with the introduction of the air tanker.

Ingenious (but ultimately impractical) early experiments in California focused on dumping water or fire-retardants onto forest fires from wooden beer kegs mounted in single engine airplanes, or even using a common garden hose to spray water from above into the inferno. In the early 1950s, public safety officials in California recognized the potential for aerial firefighting and teamed up with the U.S. Forest Service to develop a practical air tanker to combat forest fires.

By the mid-1950s, surplus World War II Stearman PT-17 and N3N military biplanes had been modified for use as air tankers and the development effort was shifted to larger military aircraft that could carry greater loads of fire retardant chemicals or water. The decision to retrofit existing military aircraft was a wise one based on several factors: surplus aircraft were readily available and relatively inexpensive; originally constructed to transport bombs or cargo over long distances, they were ideally suited to haul the heavy loads of fire retardant chemicals or water required for efficient aerial firefighting; designed for maneuverability and speed, they could withstand extreme stresses on their airframes; and they were sturdily built, which allowed for the installation of heavy water or retardant storage tanks.

The smallest aircraft used are the Single Engine Air Tankers (SEATs). These are agricultural sprayers that generally drop about 800 gallons of water or retardant. An example is the Airtractor AT-802F, which can deliver around 3000lt of water or fire retardant solution each drop. Medium aircraft include the S-2 Tracker (retrofitted with turboprop engines as the S-2T), Boeing B-17 Flying Fortresses, Grumman PBY Supercats and Privateers, F7F Tigercats, and Fairchild C-119 Boxcars were some of the early recruits in the aerial firefighting ranks. Later in the century, more modern military aircraft, such as Lockheed P-3 Orions, P-2V Neptune, DC-7 and C-130 Hercules, formed the backbone of the air tanker fleet and used as heavy tankers. Large commercial aircraft, such as the Douglas DC-6 and Ilyushin IL-76, have also been transformed into air tankers The largest aerial firefighters currently in use include two converted Martin Mars flying boats in British Columbia carrying 7,200 U.S. gallons of water or fire retardant each, and Tanker 910, a converted McDonnell Douglas DC-10 that can carry 12,000 gallons of water or retardant. The Russian Ministry of Emergency Situations operates convertible-to-cargo IL-76 airtankers (Airtankers or water bombers are fixed-wing aircraft fitted with tanks that can be filled on the ground at an air tanker base or, in the case of flying boats and amphibious aircraft, by skimming water from lakes, reservoirs, or large rivers) that can carry up to 15,000 gallons but have been operating with 11,000 gallon tanking systems, and a few of Beriev Be-200 amphibians. Evergreen International Aviation is developing a Boeing 747 aerial firefighter, known as the Evergreen Supertanker that can carry 24,000 gallons fed by a pressurized drop system Bombardier's Dash 8 Q Series aircraft are the basis for two new ventures. Cascade Aerospace has converted two pre-owned Q400s to act as part-time water bomber and part-time transport for France's Sécurité Civile while Neptune Aviation is converting a pre-owned Q300 as a prototype to augment their P2V aircraft. They also own Canadian CL-xx series, a handful of Grumman Trackers and some Russian Mil Mi-6 helicopters. Their pilots are usually recruited amongst the best pilots from "l'Armée de l'Air", usually from "Aéronavale" (Navy pilots on aircraft carriers) or acrobatic teams like "La Patrouille de France". It is a highly risked job that requires very skilled aerial fighters.

Similar in configuration to the World War II era PBY Catalina, the Canadair CL-215 Scooper, and Bombardier CL-415 Super-Scooper are designed and built specifically for firefighting. CL-215s have been employed with success in the USA.

Another amphibian is Russian Beriev Be-200. It can carry a maximum payload of about 3,170 gallons (12,000 litres) of water, making "scoops" in suitable stretches of water in 14 seconds.

The most unique aircraft engaged in aerial firefighting—and the only aircraft in the world specifically built for that purpose—is the Canadair CL-215. This plane was designed to meet the requirement for a firefighting amphibian that could replace the assortment of planes used as "water bombers" in the 1960s and also employed in forest fire detection and suppression. The plane also had a secondary role for search and rescue and utility work. Flying just 100 feet (30 meters) above a fire, the CL-215's belly-doors—much like the bomb bay doors on a military aircraft—open to drop 10,000 pounds (4,536 kilograms) of water or chemicals onto a fire. An amphibian by design, the CL-215 can take off (and land) from both airfields and open water using its retractable landing gear, with floats fitted to the end of its wings for greater stability on the water. When operating from an airfield, the CL-215's storage tanks can be quickly pressure-filled with water or fire-retardants in just about two minutes. The CL-215's unique capabilities become apparent when the twin-engine water bomber swoops down onto a lake and scoops up more than 1,400 gallons of water in just over ten seconds, then smoothly climbs back up to drop the water onto the wildfire. Twin scoops incorporated into a narrow hull allow the CL-215 to scoop up water from shallow lakes or rivers just 4.5 feet (1.4 meters) deep. Equipped with two 705-gallon (2,669-liter) main water tanks, positioned in the left and right center of the fuselage, the CL-215 is a very ruggedly constructed aircraft, designed not only to withstand its "dive bomber" tactics but also to endure corrosion from the water and retardant chemicals as well as the heat and pollutants from the fire itself. Durability and reliability were the driving requirements in the CL-215's design since the demands of a raging forest or wildfire may require dozens of fire bombing runs in a single day and a single

CL-215 in Yugoslavia has flown an amazing 225 water bombing runs in a 24-hour period.

Once over the fire, the water bomber pilot tries to attack his target with a dispersal pattern that suits the particular circumstances of the wildfire. Dumping water (or flame retardants) concurrently from both wing tanks focuses the water on a concentrated area in a deluge, while dumping the four tanks in sequence soaks a longer, slender swath of earth. On certain CL-215 models, water spray pipes and nozzles have been affixed to the bottom of the wings, allowing a fine mist to be sprayed over a much larger area.

The Beriev Be-200 is an amphibious multirole turbofan aircraft designed by the Berieva Aviatsionnyi Kompaniya (Beriev Aviation Company), with the Russian Irkutsk Aircraft Production Association (IAPO) responsible for the production engineering development phase of the program. The Be-200 was first developed for fire-fighting missions. It can start, take-off and land on water. The first prototype aircraft was delivered in June 2003 and has successfully completed 650 flight hours and carries Russian certification as a fire fighting aircraft. In a fire-fighting mission, the fully fuelled aircraft can fly 200km from the airfield to a water reservoir, make successive trips between the site of the fire and the reservoir (over a range of 10km from the fire zone to the reservoir), to drop a total of 310,000kg of water on the fire and make the 200km return flight to the airfield for refuelling. The aircraft is capable of scooping 12 tonnes of water in 14 seconds from seas with waves up to 1.2 m. The aircraft flies at speeds above a minimum drop speed of 220km/h to empty the water tanks over the site of the fire in 0.8 to 1.0 seconds.

Leadplanes

The Lead Plane function directs the activities of the airtankers by both verbal target descriptions and by physically leading the airtankers on the drop run. The O-2 Skymaster and OV-10 Bronco have both been used as spotter and lead plane platforms. The Beechcraft Baronwas long used as a lead plane or air attack ship, but most were retired in 2003; more common now is the Beechcraft King Air, used as an air attack ship and lead plane.

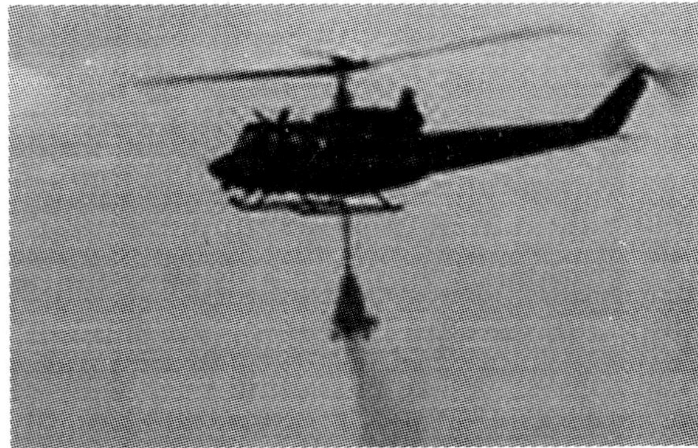

Fig. 25.3

HELICOPTERS

Helicopters may be fitted with tanks or carry buckets. Buckets are usually filled by submerging in lakes, rivers, reservoirs, or portable tanks. The most popular of the buckets is the flexible Bambi Bucket. Tanks may be filled on the ground or water may be siphoned from lakes or reservoirs through a hanging snorkel. Popular firefighting helicopters include variants of the Bell 204 and the Erickson S-64 Aircrane helitanker, which features a sea snorkel for filling while in flight. Modified helicopters, including the Sikorsky Black Hawk, are widely used in aerial firefighting to extract firefighters and victims from dangerous fire zones, and also to precisely apply water and fire-retardant chemicals to smaller fires in "mop-up" operations.

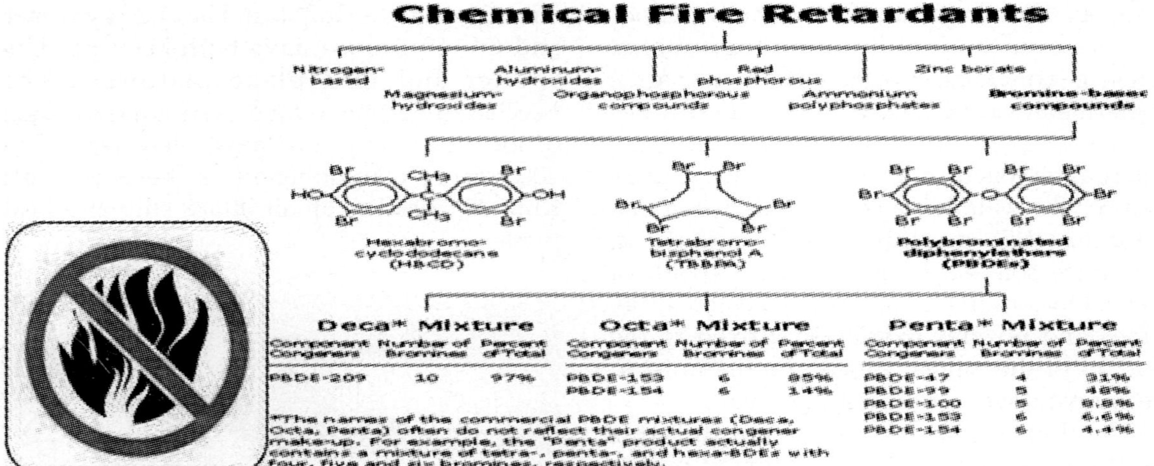

Fig. 25.4

FIRE RETARDANT

Borate salts were used in the past to fight wildfires but were found to sterilize the soil, were toxic to animals, and are now prohibited. Newer retardants use ammonium sulfate or ammoniumpolyphosphate with attapulgite clay thickener or diammonium phosphate with a guar gum derivative thickener. These are not only less toxic but act as fertilizers to help the regrowth of plants after the fire. Fire retardants often contain wetting agents, preservatives and rust inhibitors and are colored red with ferric oxide or fugitive color to mark where they have been dropped. Brand names of fire retardants for aerial application include Fire-Trol and Phos-Chek. Some water-dropping aircraft carry tanks of a guar gum derivative to thicken the water and reduce runoff.

Tactics

Helicopters can hover over the fire and accurately drop water or retardant. The S-64 Helitanker has microprocessor-controlled doors on its tank. The doors are controlled based on the area to be covered and wind conditions. Fixed-wing aircraft must make a pass and drop water or retardant like a bomber. Spotter (Air Tactical Group Supervisor) aircraft often orbit the fire at a higher altitude to coordinate the efforts of the smoke jumper, helicopter, media, and retardant-dropping aircraft; while lead planes fly low-level ahead of the airtankers to mark the trajectory for the drop, and ensure overall safety for both ground-based and aerial firefighters.

Water is often not dropped directly on flames because its effect is short-lived. Fire retardants are typically dropped ahead of the moving fire or along its edge and may remain effective for two or more days. This can create artificial firebreaks where the terrain is too rugged or remote for ground crews to cut a fireline.

Helicopters are also used to deliver firefighters or ignite backfires and controlled burns. A driptorch slung beneath the helicopter (helitorch) can be used for this purpose. Another device called a Delayed Aerial Ignition Device (DAID) can be used, which shoots a stream of flaming "ping-pong balls" into the forest. The small plastic spheres which contain potassium permanganate are individually injected with ethylene glycol or glycerine just before they are ejected from the aircraft. This method's delayed Redox exothermic reaction, results in vigorous fire soon after mixing the chemicals, poses less of a danger to the helicopter than transporting burning materials. The ping-pong ball system works best in continuous fuels or in areas where a mosaic burn pattern is desired.

Aerial firefighting is almost always used in conjunction with ground-based efforts, as aircraft are only one weapon in the firefighting arsenal. However, there have been cases of aircraft extinguishing fires long before ground crews were able to reach them.

26 Action Plan During An Earthquake

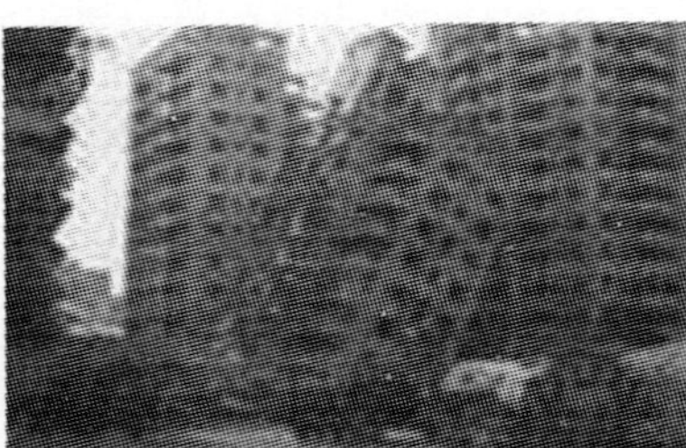

Fig. 26.1

INTRODUCTION

An earthquake is caused by sudden, violent shifting of massive rocks called plates under the earth's surface. This movement of the plates releases stress that accumulates along geologic faults. A fault is a deep crack that marks the boundary between two of these plates. Vibrations produced in the earth's crust when rocks in which elastic strain has been building up suddenly rupture, and then rebound. The vibrations can range from barely noticeable to catastrophically destructive. Earthquakes can release energy thousands of times greater than the world's first atomic bomb. Earthquake belts occur along faults around the world. Many run along coastal areas. The epicenter is the point on the surface where the earthquake is the strongest. It is estimated that there are 500,000 detectable earthquakes in the world each year. 100,000 of those can be felt, and 100 of them cause damage. Earthquakes strike suddenly, violently and without warning. Identifying potential hazards ahead of time and advance planning can reduce the dangers of serious injury or loss of life. Six kinds of shock waves are generated in the process. Two are classified as body waves—that is, they travel through the earth's interior—and the other four are surface waves. The waves are further differentiated by the kinds of motions they impart to rock particles. Primary or compressional waves (P waves) send particles oscillating back and forth in the same direction as the waves are travelling, whereas secondary or transverse shear waves (S waves) impart vibrations perpendicular to their direction of travel. P waves always travel at higher velocities than S waves, so whenever an earthquake occurs, P waves are the first to arrive and be recorded at geophysical research stations throughout the world.

The Global Seismographic Network and IRIS detect seismic activities worldwide and provide early warnings to all regions at risk. The intensity of an earthquake can be measured by the Richter scale. In 1935, Charles Richter first defined local magnitude of earthquakes and the Richter scale is commonly used today to describe earthquake intensity. Earthquakes below 4.0 on the Richter scale usually do not cause damage, and earthquakes below 2.0 usually can't be felt. Earthquakes over 5.0 on the scale can cause damage. A magnitude 6.0 earthquake is considered strong and a magnitude 7.0 is a major earthquake. Earthquakes are sometimes called temblors, quakes, shakers or seismic activity.

Earthquakes—The Modified Mercalli Scale and the Richter Scale

Scale	*Magnitude*	*Damage*	*Richter Value*
Mercalli 1-4	Instrumental to moderate	No damage	Richter 4.1–4.3
Mercalli 5	Rather strong	Damage negligible. Small, unstable objects displaced or upset; some dishes, glassware broken	Richter 4.4–4.8
Mercalli 6	Strong damage	Windows, dishes, glassware broken. Furniture moved or overturned. Weak plaster and masonry cracked	Richter 4.9–5.4
Mercalli 7	Very strong	Damage slight-moderate in well-built structures; considerable in poorly-built structures. Furniture and weak chimneys broken. Masonry damaged	Richter 5.5–6.1
Mercalli 8	Destructive	Structure damage considerable particularly to poorly built structures Chimneys, monuments, towers, elevated tanks may fail. Frame houses moved. Trees damaged. Cracks in wet ground and steep slopes	Richter 6.2–6.5
Mercalli 9	Ruinous	Structural damage severe; General damage to foundations. Serious damage to reservoirs. Underground pipes broken. Conspicuous cracks in ground	Richter 6.6–6.9
Mercalli 10	Disastrous	Most masonry and frame structures/foundations destroyed. Some well-built wooden structures and bridges destroyed. Serious damage to dams, dikes, embankments. Sand and mud shifting on beaches and flat land	Richter 7.0–7.3
Mercalli 11	Very disastrous	Few or no masonry structures remain standing. Bridges destroyed. Broad fissures in ground. Underground pipelines completely out of service. Rails bent. Widespread earth slumps and landslides	Richter 7.4–8.1
Mercalli 12	Catastrophic	Damage nearly total. Large rock masses displaced Lines of sight and level distorted	Richter > 8.1

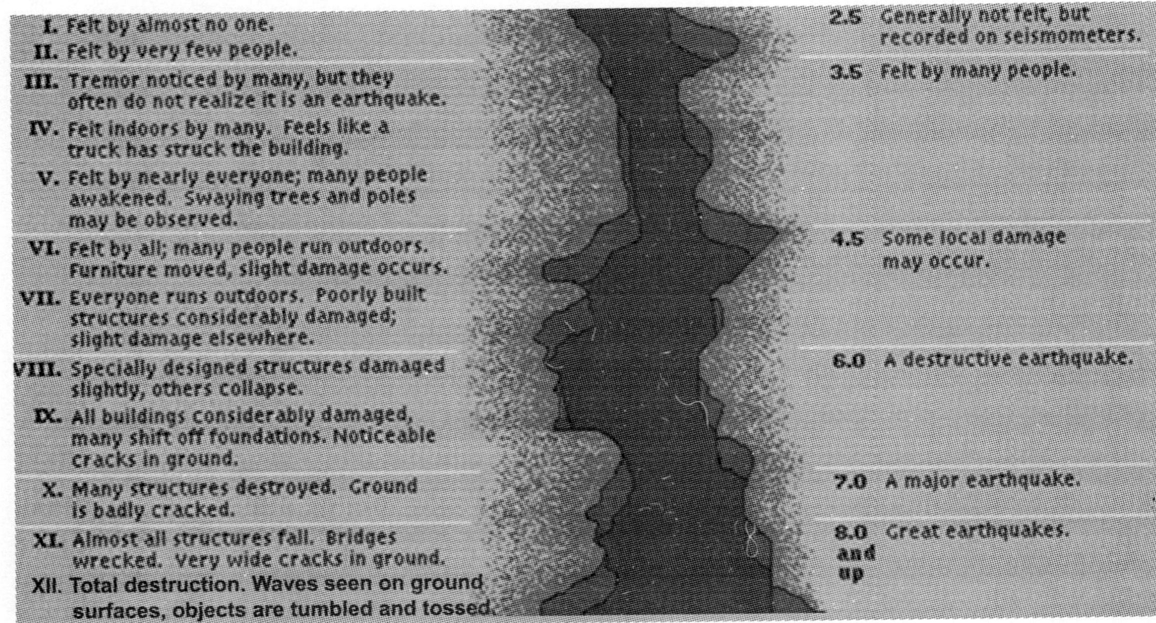

Fig. 26.2

BEFORE

- Check for hazards in the home.
- Fasten shelves securely to walls.
- Place large and heavy articles on the lower shelves.
- Store breakable items in low, closed cabinets with latches.
- Hang heavy items like pictures, mirrors away from beds, couches, lounging and sitting areas.
- Brace overhead light fixtures.
- Repair defective electric wiring and leaky gas connections.
- Repair all deep cracks in the walls, ceilings or foundations and expert help to diagnose and mend structural defects.
- Store weed killers, poisons, flammable products in secure closed cabinets with latches and on bottom shelves.
- Identify safe places in each room under sturdy furniture, against an inside wall and away from hazards like bookcases, glassware, picture frames, mirrors, etc.
- Locate safe places outdoors in the open, away from trees, buildings, telephone and electrical lines.
- Each member of the family must know how to turn off the gas and mains.
- Teach all members to contact emergency, fire, police department.
- Have supplies on hand.
- Flashlight with spare batteries.
- Portable radio.
- First aid kit.
- Emergency food and water supplies.
- Mechanical can opener.
- Cash and credit cards.
- Sturdy shoes.
- Helmets.

Develop an emergency plan for communication and meeting and reuniting if separated during a disaster. Have a family contact out of the state and make sure everyone in the family has his or her contact. It is often easier to make long distance calls in a disaster situation as local lines would be affected.

DURING EMERGENCY

- Take cover under a sturdy table and stay indoors.
- If outdoors move into a clearing away from buildings, electric lines and trees and stay there till quakes stop.
- If in a moving vehicle, stop and stay inside clear from trees, buildings, electric cables, bridges, tunnels. Once quaking stops, proceed slowly with caution, avoiding bridges and ramps that may be damaged or weakened by tremors.
- Be prepared for aftershocks
- Help injured and trapped persons
- Listen to the radio for latest emergency bulletins and announcements
- Stay out of damaged buildings and return home only after it is cleared as safe by municipal authorities.
- Do not enter any room if it smells suspiciously. If possible, open a few windows, switch off the mains supply and leave quickly. Call the fire services or professional help.

MITIGATION

House/dwelling construction in earthquake prone regions must be modified suitably as follows:

- Concrete foundations for greater stability.
- Wooden columns treated with tar or pitch to protect against humidity, concreted into the ground with nails embedded in the wood at the base to give extra anchorage.
- Using concrete wall bases to prevent humidity affecting the wood and the canes in the walls.
- Careful jointing between columns and beams to improve structural integrity.
- Canes woven in a vertical fashion to provide greater stability.
- Lightweight metal sheet roofing to reduce danger of falling tiles.
- Nailing roofing material to roof beams; tying of beams and columns with roof wires.
- Incorporating roof eaves of sufficient width to ensure protection of walls from heavy rains.

27 Action Plan During a Volcanic Eruption

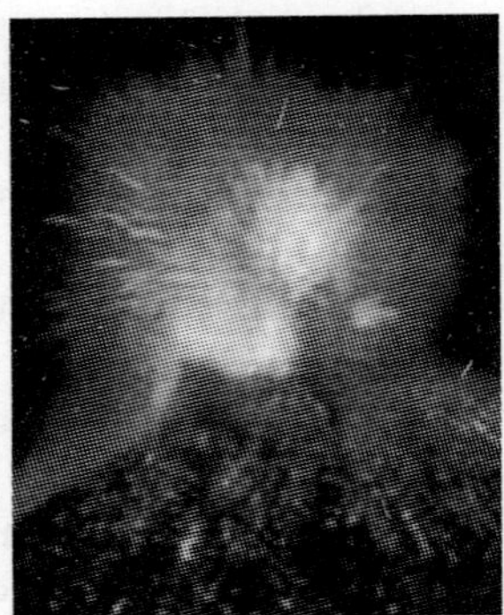

Fig. 27.1

INTRODUCTION

Volcanic eruptions are usually associated with ash fall. A sustained ash fall may keep people housebound for hours or even days. Volcanic ash is a great nuisance and gets everywhere in the house and office, including inside televisions, computers, cameras and other valuable equipment, where it can cause irreparable damage. Ash is different from ordinary house dust. It is sharp, crystalline structure causes it to scratch and abrade surfaces when it is removed by wiping or brushing. In wet weather the ash deposits are dampened down and the air can be clear, but in drier weather ash can easily be stirred up and remobilized by wind and traffic. As a result suspended dust levels become much higher and can be at levels potentially harmful to health. Rainfall and wind are effective in removing the ash and grass and other plants will eventually bind it to the soil, but with large ash falls this process is too slow and the ash must be cleaned up and taken away from populated areas. In addition, wind may also bring ash into areas which were previously clean so ash may be present in the environment for months or even years following an eruption. In fine-ash environments, wear goggles or corrective eyeglasses instead of contact lenses to protect eyes from irritation. Lightly water down the ash deposits before they are removed by shovelling, being careful not to excessively wet the deposits on roofs, causing excess loading and danger of collapse. Dry brushing can produce very high exposure levels and should be avoided. Use extra precaution on ladders and roofs. The ash makes surfaces much more slippery, consequently many people have died from falls while cleaning ash from their roofs. Be aware of the extra load caused by standing on an already overloaded roof - tread carefully. It is preferable to clean roofs before more than a few centimetres of ash has accumulated since most roofs cannot support more than four inches (10 cm) of wet ash. Where possible use a harness. Keep ash out of buildings, machinery, vehicles, downspouts, water supplies, and wastewater systems (for example, storm drains) as much as possible. The most effective method to prevent ash-induced damage to machinery is to shut down, close off or seal equipment until ash is removed from the immediate environment, though this may not be practical in all cases.

CLEANING UP

Coordinate clean-up activities with your neighbours and community-wide operations. After an ash fall, remove ash from roofs in a timely manner to prevent streets from being repetitively cleaned. Cut grass and hedges only after rain or light sprinkling and bag clippings. Seek advice from public officials regarding disposal of volcanic ash in your community. In most cases, ash should be separated from normal rubbish for collection for disposal at a designated location-mixing ash with normal rubbish can result in damage to collection vehicles and take up space in landfills. Dampen ash in yards and streets to reduce suspension of ash, however try to use water sparingly – do not soak the ash. Widespread use of water for clean-up may deplete public water supplies. Follow requests from public officials regarding water use during cleanup operations. Remove outdoor clothing before entering a building.

- Do not soak the ash as it will cake into a hard mass, making cleanup more difficult. On roofs the added weight of the water will increase the risk of roof collapse.
- Do not dump the ash in gardens or on the roadside.
- Do not wash the ash into the guttering, sewers or storm drains. (It can damage waste water treatment systems and clog pipes).
- Do not drive unless absolutely necessary, driving stirs up the ash. Furthermore, ash is harmful to vehicles.

Keep these items in your home in case of an ash fall:

- Dust masks and eye protection.
- Enough drinking water for at least 72 hours (one gallon per person per day).
- Enough non-perishable food for at least 72 hours for family and pets.
- Plastic wrap (to keep ash out of electronics).
- Battery-operated radio and extra batteries.
- Lanterns or torches (flashlights) and extra batteries.
- If cold, extra wood for a fireplace or stove.
- If cold, extra blankets and warm clothing.
- Extra stocks of medication for both family and pets.
- First aid kit.
- Cleaning supplies (broom, vacuum cleaner and bags/filters, shovels etc.).
- Small amount of money (ATM machines may not be working).
- Consider that you could be stuck in your vehicle, so store emergency supplies in your vehicle too.

Actions to be taken during preparedness

- Close doors and windows.
- Place damp towels at door thresholds and other draft sources. Tape draughty windows.
- Protect sensitive electronics and do not uncover until the environment is totally ash-free.
- Disconnect drainpipes/downspouts from gutters to stop drains clogging, but allowing ash and water to empty from gutters onto the ground.
- If you use a rainwater collection system for your water supply, disconnect the tank prior to ash falling.
- If you have chronic bronchitis, emphysema or asthma, stay inside and avoid unnecessary exposure to the ash.
- Ensure livestock have clean food and water.
- If you have children, know your school's emergency plan and have indoor games and activities ready.

What to Do if Volcanic Ash is Falling

- Don't panic—stay calm.
- Stay indoors.
- If outside, seek shelter (e.g. car or building).
- Use a mask, handkerchief or cloth over your nose and mouth.
- If warning is given before ash fall starts, go home from work.

- If at work when ash fall starts, stay indoors until the ash has settled.
- Do not tie up phone lines with non-emergency calls.
- Listen to your local radio for information on the eruption and cleanup plans.
- Do not wear contact lenses as these will result in corneal abrasion.
- If there is ash in your water, let it settle and then use the clear water. If there is a lot of ash in the water supply, do not use your dishwasher or washing machine. Water contaminated by ash will usually make drinking water unpalatable before it presents a health risk.
- You may eat vegetables from the garden, but wash them first.

VOLCANIC ERUPTIONS—THE VOLCANIC EXPLOSIVITY INDEX

A widely accepted measure of the size of an eruption is the volume of lava ejected as pumice and ash (tephra) during an explosive phase or the volume of lava extruded during an effusive phase. The Volcanic Explosivity Index (VEI) was devised by Chris Newhall of the U.S. Geological Survey and Steve Self at the University of Hawaii in 1982 to provide a relative measure of the explosiveness of volcanic eruptions. Eruption volumes are commonly expressed in cubic kilometers (km^3). One km^3 is roughly equivalent to 0.24 cubic mile. A related measure of size is the "Volcanic Explosivity Index", or VEI. This scale is similar to the Richter scale used for indicating earthquakes size. Like the "Richter magnitude" scale, the VEI scale is logarithmic such that each unit increase in VEI (from 2 to 3, for example) corresponds to a tenfold increase in the volume of material erupted onto the surface. Descriptive phrases such as "small" or "moderate eruption" are only loosely tied to the VEI scale or the volume of explosively erupted lava.

Category	*Category Description*
0	Non-Explosive (Hawaiian) Plume: < 100 m/Volume: > 1000 m3
1	Gentle (Hawaiian—Strombolian) Plume: 100–1000 m/Volume: >10,000 m3
2	Explosive (Strombolian—Vulcanian) Plume: 1– 5 km/Volume: > 1,000,000 m3
3	Severe (Vulcanian) Plume: 3–15 km/Volume: > 10,000,000 m3
4	Cataclysmic (Vulcanian - Plinian) Plume: 10–25 km/Volume: > 100,000,000 m3
5	Paroxysmal (Plinian) Plume: >25 km/Volume: > 1 km3
6	Colossal (Plinian—Ultraplinian) Plume: > 25 km/Volume: > 10 km3
7	No Adjectival Description Plume: > 25 km/Volume: > 100 km3
8	No Adjectival Description Plume: > 25 km/Volume: > 1,000 km3

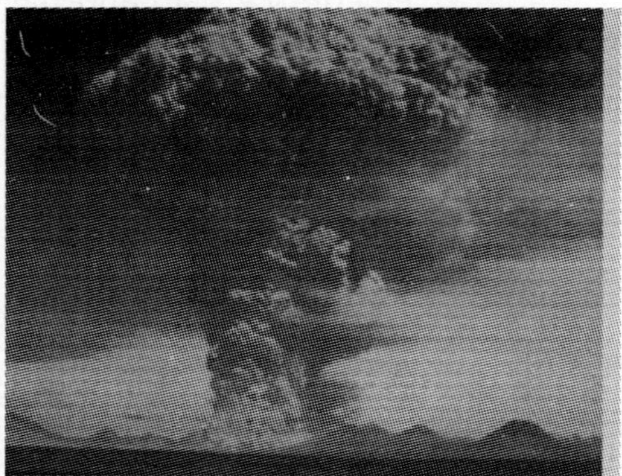
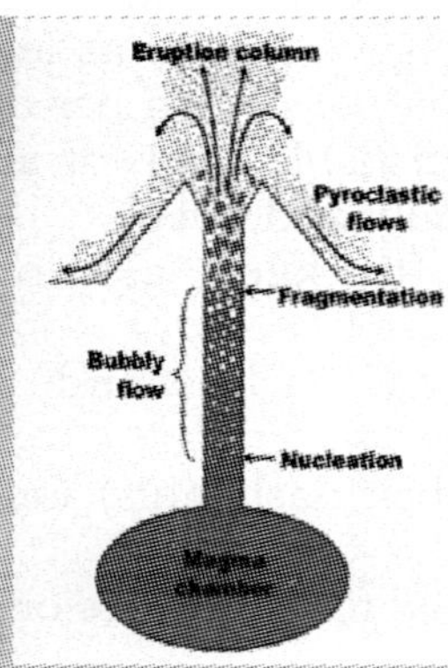

Fig. 27.2

28 Action Plan During Extreme Cold Weather

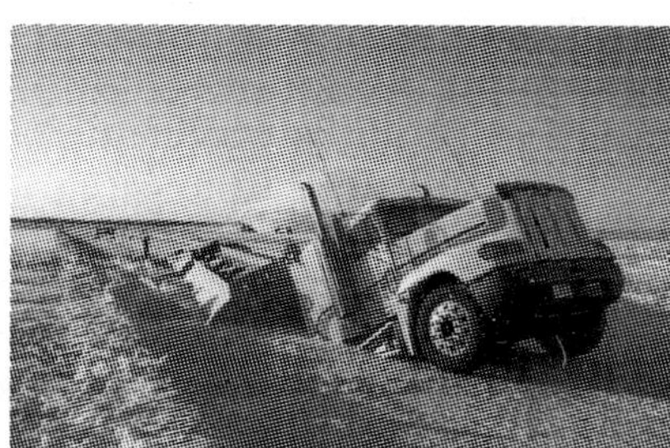

Fig. 28.1

INTRODUCTION

A winter storm is an event in which the dominant varieties of precipitations are forms that only occur at cold temperatures such as snow or sleet, or a rainstorm where ground temperatures are cold enough to allow ice to form (i.e. freezing rain). In temperate continental climates, these storms are not necessarily restricted to the winter season, but may occur in the late autumn and early spring as well. Very rarely, they may form in summer. In many locations in the Northern Hemisphere, the most powerful winter storms usually occur in March and, in regions where temperatures are cold enough, in April too.

Snowstorms are storms where large amounts of snow fall. Snow is less dense than water, by a factor of approximately 10 at temperatures slightly below freezing, and even more at much lower temperatures. Therefore, conditions that would produce 2 cm of rain could produce as much as 20 cm of snow. In places where snow is uncommon, 5 cm of snow is enough to create serious disruptions to traffic due to slick roads. In places where snowfall is common, such small snowfalls are rarely disruptive, because winter tyres are routinely used, but large snowstorms in excess of 15 cm could be quite dangerous as unplowed roads would become impassible. Snowstorms exceeding 30 cm can cause caving in of roofs of homes and, coated in ice, telephone and power lines can sag and break, resulting in power outages. Standing dead trees can also be brought down by the weight of the snow, especially if it is wet or very dense. Even a few centimetres of dry snow can form drifts many feet high under windy conditions.

Snowstorms are usually considered less dangerous than ice storms. However, the snow brings secondary dangers. Snowstorms in mountains can produce cornices (an overhanging edge of snow formed by wind blowing snow over a ridge or the crest of a mountain) and avalanches. Heavy showers of freezing rain occur when a layer of warm air hovers over a region, but the ambient temperature is near 0°C, and the ground temperature is sub-freezing. A storm in which only roads freeze is called a freezing rain storm and one resulting in widespread icing of plants and crops is called ice storm – a farmer's nightmare.

A severe snowstorm with strong winds and heavy blowing snow is known as a blizzard or winter hurricane. They are formed when a high pressure system, also known as a ridge, interacts with a low pressure system. This results in the advection of air from the high pressure zone into the low pressure area. A winter storm must have winds of 40 km/h or more, have snow or blowing snow, visibility less than 200 m and wind chil below 0°C lasting for 3 hours or more before it can be termed a blizzard.When there are blizzard conditions but no snow falling, it is called a ground blizzard because all the snow is already present at the surface of the earth and is simply being blown by high winds. Ground blizzards require large expanses of open and relatively flat land with a sufficient amount of accumulated and loosely packed, powdery snow.

Whiteouts occur mostly in the Arctic and Antarctic during the spring, when snow is still deep on the ground and there is lots of daylight and surprisingly calm weather and excellent visibility. Whiteouts occur when rays of sunlight are bounced in all directions between bright white clouds, especially a thin layer of overcast and bright snow or ice. Clean snow and ice reflects nearly 85% of incoming light. Falling snowflakes, suspended fog droplets or ice particles in the air would make conditions even worse. In a true whiteout, neither shadows, nearby objects, landmarks, nor clouds are discernible. All sense of direction, depth perception and even of balance may be lost. Land and sky seem to blend, and the horizon disappears into a white nothingness. Whiteouts trick pilots and travelers into believing down is up and thinking far is near.

Extreme winter cold often causes poorly insulated water pipelines and mains to freeze. Even some poorly-protected indoor plumbing ruptures as water expands within them, causing much damage to property and the generation of electrical power may fail due to the freezing of water necessary for the generation of hydroelectricity. Some metals may become brittle at low temperatures and crack. Motor vehicles may stall as antifreeze is rendered ineffective and motor oil gels. The air during a cold wave is typically denser and any cold air that a fire draws in and it is likely to cause a more intense fire because the colder, denser air contains more oxygen and firefighting becomes a problem.

A Winter Storm Warning is issued if at least 10-15 or more centimetres of snow or 7 or more centimetres of snow with a large accumulation of ice is forecast. A Winter Storm Watch is issued in an area 24 to 36 hours before a storm with a potential for heavy snow (15 cm or more) or significant ice accumulations. A Heavy snow warning is a weather advisory issued during times when a high rate of snowfall of 15 cm or more in 12 hours, or 20 cm or more in 24 hours is forecast. An ice storm warning is issued any time more than 6 mm of ice is expected to accumulate in an area (in some areas, the criterion is 13 mm. A cold wave is a rapid fall in temperature within a 24 hour period requiring substantially increased protection to agriculture, industry, commerce, and social activities.

Factors in Cold Weather Injuries

Weather, type of operations, clothing, physique and psychological factors.

Types of cold injuries are chilblain, immersion syndrome, frostbite, snowblindness, dehydration and hypothermia.

Signs and symptoms: Redness or discolorization of skin, swelling of affected area, and lack of sensation/acute pain.

Treatment: Re-warm with body heat, avoid massaging the affected part/exposure to direct heat of fire or stove/rubbing with snow or soaking in cold water. Avoid walking on injured feet, keep dry, avoid alcohol intake and seek early medical aid.

During a Winter Storm

- Listen to your radio, television, for weather reports and emergency information.
- Eat regularly and drink ample fluids, but avoid caffeine and alcohol.
- Conserve fuel, if necessary, by keeping your residence cooler than normal. Temporarily close off heat to some rooms.
- If the pipes freeze, remove any insulation or layers of newspapers and wrap pipes in rags. Completely open all faucets and pour hot water over the pipes, starting where they were most exposed to the cold (or where the cold was most likely to penetrate).
- Maintain ventilation when using kerosene heaters to avoid build-up of toxic fumes. Refuel kerosene heaters outside and keep them at least three feet from flammable objects.

If You are Outdoors

- Avoid overexertion when shoveling snow. Overexertion can trigger a heart attack, a major cause of death in winters. If you must shovel snow, warm up before going outside.
- Cover your mouth. Protect your lungs from extremely cold air by covering your mouth with a muffler when outdoors. Try not to speak unless absolutely necessary.
- Keep dry. Change wet clothing frequently to prevent a loss of body heat. Wet clothing loses all of its insulating value and transmits heat rapidly.
- Watch for signs of frostbite. These include loss of feeling and white or pale appearance in extremities such as fingers, toes, ear lobes, and the tip of the nose. If symptoms are detected, get medical help immediately.
- Watch for signs of hypothermia. These include uncontrollable shivering, memory loss, disorientation, incoherence, slurred speech, drowsiness, and apparent exhaustion.
- If symptoms of hypothermia are detected get the victim to a warm location remove wet clothing put the person in dry clothing and wrap their entire body in a blanket. Warm the center of the body first give warm, non-alcoholic or non-caffeinated beverages if the victim is conscious.
- Get medical help as soon as possible.

If You are Driving

Drive only if it is absolutely necessary. If you must drive, consider the following:

- Travel in the day, do not travel alone, and keep others informed of your schedule.
- Stay on main roads; avoid back road shortcuts.

If a blizzard traps you in the car:

- Pull off the highway. Turn on hazard lights and hang a distress flag from the radio antenna or window.
- Remain in your vehicle where rescuers are most likely to find you. Do not set out on foot unless you can see a building close by where you know you can take shelter. Be careful; distances are distorted by blowing snow. A building may seem close, but be too far to walk to in deep snow.
- Run the engine and heater for about 10 minutes each hour to keep warm. When the engine is running, open a downwind window slightly for ventilation and periodically clear snow from the exhaust pipe. This will protect you from possible carbon monoxide poisoning.
- Exercise to maintain body heat, but avoid overexertion. In extreme cold, use road maps, seat covers, and floor mats for insulation. Huddle with passengers and use your coat for a blanket.
- Take turns sleeping. One person should be awake at all times to look out for rescue crews.

- Drink fluids to avoid dehydration.
- Be careful not to waste battery power. Balance electrical energy needs (the use of lights, heat and radio) with supply.
- Turn on the inside light at night so that work crews or rescuers can see you.

If stranded in a remote area, stomp large block letters in an open area spelling out 'HELP' or 'SOS' and line with rocks or tree limbs to attract the attention of rescue personnel who may be surveying the area from the air.

- Leave the car and proceed on foot, if necessary, once the blizzard has passed.

If At Home

Add the following supplies to your disaster supplies kit:

- Rock salt to melt ice on walkways
- Sand to improve traction
- Snow shovels and other snow removal equipment.
- Prepare your home and family for possible isolation by having sufficient heating fuel as regular fuel sources may be cut off. Store a good supply of dry, seasoned wood for your fireplace or wood-burning stove.
- Winterize your home to extend the life of your fuel supply by insulating walls and attics, caulking and weather-stripping doors and windows, and installing storm windows or covering windows with plastic.
- Winterize your house, barn, shed or any other structure that may provide shelter for your family, neighbors, livestock or equipment. Clear rain gutters; repair roof leaks and cut away tree branches that could fall on a house or other structures during a storm.
- Insulate pipes with insulation material or newspapers and plastic and allow taps and faucets to drip a little during cold weather to avoid freezing.
- Keep fire extinguishers on hand, and make sure everyone in your house knows how to use them. House fires pose an additional risk, as more people turn to alternate heating sources without taking the necessary safety precautions.
- Learn how to shut off water valves (in case a pipe bursts).
- Know ahead of time what you should do to help elderly or disabled friends, neighbors or employees. Hire a contractor to check the structural ability of the roof to sustain unusually heavy weight from the accumulation of snow or water, if drains on flat roofs do not work.

Prepare Your Car

Check or have a mechanic check the following items on your car:

- Antifreeze levels—ensure they are sufficient to avoid freezing.
- Battery and ignition system—should be in top condition and battery terminals should be clean.
- Brakes—check for wear and fluid levels.
- Exhaust system—check for leaks and crimped pipes and repair or replace as necessary. Carbon monoxide is deadly and usually gives no warning.
- Fuel and air filters—replace and keep water out of the system by using additives and maintaining a full tank of petrol.
- Heater and defroster—ensure they work properly.
- Lights and flashing hazard lights—check for serviceability.
- Oil-check for level and weight. Heavier oils congeal more at low temperatures and do not lubricate as well.
- Thermostat—ensure it works properly.
- Windshield wiper equipment—repair any problems and maintain proper washer fluid level.

- Install good winter tyres. Make sure the tyres have adequate tread. All-weather radials are usually adequate for most winter conditions. However, some jurisdictions require that to drive on their roads, vehicles must be equipped with chains or snow tires with studs.
- Maintain at least a half tank of gas during the winter season.
- Place a winter emergency kit in each car that includes a shovel, windshield scraper and a small broom, flashlight, battery powered radio, extra batteries, water, snack food, matches, extra hats, socks and mittens.
- First aid kit with pocket knife.
- Necessary medications.
- Blanket(s).
- Tow chain or rope.
- Road salt and sand.
- Booster cables.
- Emergency flares.
- Fluorescent distress flag.
- *Dress for the weather:* Wear several layers of loose fitting, lightweight, warm clothing rather than one layer of heavy clothing. The outer garments should be tightly woven and water repellent. Wear mittens, which are warmer than gloves. Wear a hat and cover your mouth with a scarf to protect your lungs.

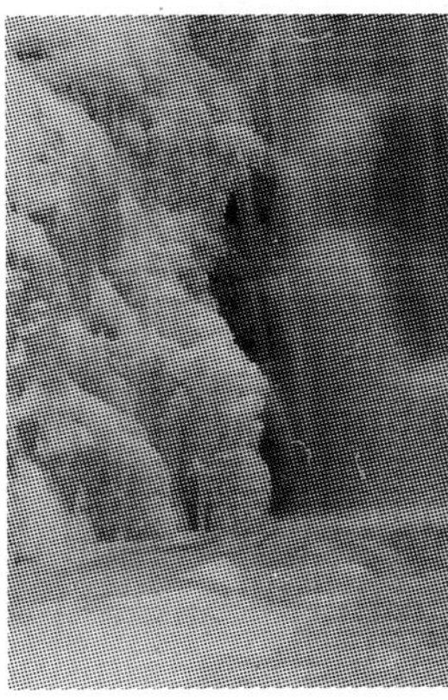

Fig. 28.2

AVALANCHES

Introduction

Avalanches have always occurred in the mountainous regions of the world. With the growth of winter-time recreations, fatalities have been on the rise since the 1950s. Avalanches claim over 150 lives each year worldwide and hundreds more are injured or trapped following an avalanche. Internationally, the Alpine countries of France, Austria, Switzerland, and Italy experience the greatest number of avalanches and loss of life annually. The United States ranks fifth worldwide in avalanche danger.

Snow avalanches are active geological agents of erosion and have been a source of natural disasters as long as man has dwelled in the mountains. A common feature of mountainous terrain throughout the temperate and arctic regions of the earth, they may occur wherever snow is deposited on slopes steeper than about 30 degrees. Small avalanches, or sluffs, run in uncounted numbers each winter, while the larger avalanches, which may encompass slopes a mile or more wide and millions of tons of snow, fall infrequently but inflict most of the destruction.

The fundamental classification of avalanches is based on conditions prevailing at the point of origin, or the release zone. There are three main kinds of avalanches: dry snow avalanches, wet snow avalanches, and slab avalanches. Dry snow avalanches are mixtures of powdery snow and air and can move at speeds up to 100mph. A wet snow avalanche is, of course, a mound of wet snow that typically moves slower than dry snow avalanches. Slab avalanches contain large slabs of snow that breaks off and falls apart as it slides. Each is subdivided according to whether snow involved is dry, damp or wet, whether the slide originates in a surface layer or involves the whole snow cover (slides to the ground), and whether the motion is on the ground, in the air, or mixed. Loose snow avalanches form in snow with little internal cohesion among individual snow crystals. When such snow lies in a state of unstable equilibrium on a slope steeper than its natural angle of repose, a slight disturbance sets progressively more and more snow in downhill motion. If enough momentum is generated, the sliding snow may run out onto level ground, or even ascend an opposite valley wall. Such an avalanche originates at a point, growing wider as it sweeps up more snow in its descent. The demarcation between sliding and undisturbed snow is diffuse, especially in dry snow. Avalanches are caused by events that makes the snow unstable e.g. earth tremors, heavy winds, and explosions Avalanches that occur in dry snow at below freezing temperatures can be either as sluffs (loose snow) or slabs. The vast majority of avalanche fatalities are caused by dry slab avalanches. Trigger of one of these snowfalls occurs at a "starting zone". The avalanche continues downslope along the "track" and ultimately the avalanche fans out and settles in the "runout zone". Avalanches run in the same paths year after year, the danger zones often being well known in normal circumstances. Exceptional weather at intervals of many years may produce exceptional avalanches which overrun their normal paths and even break new ones where none existed for centuries. Unwise timber removal in alpine terrain can also create avalanches where none existed before. Given exceptional snow conditions, even short slopes like the walls of a ravine can become dangerous. Snow avalanche may fall anywhere that enough snow is deposited in the right circumstances on an inclined surface. These right circumstances sometimes consist of abnormally large snowfalls, but not always so. Avalanches find their genesis in snow cover structural weaknesses which are often induced by internal changes. A large overburden of snow alone may not result in avalanching if it is anchored to a solid underlayer. On the other hand, even a shallow snow layer can slide from the mountainside if poorly bonded. The snow avalanche is a complex problem in mechanical stability which can best be understood in terms of the physical processes taking place in the changeable winter snow and the dependence of these on temperature. The wide variety of snow avalanche origin, nature of motion, and size reflects the highly changeable nature of snow.

Three processes commonly leave snow in a state of unstable equilibrium on a slope steeper than its natural angle of repose:

1. Deposition of stellar or dendritic crystals with little or no wind.
2. Reduction of internal cohesion among crystals by metamorphism, and
3. Reduction of internal cohesion by intrusion of liquid water.

Though very numerous, most dry loose snow avalanches are small, and few achieve sufficient size to cause damage. With advent of spring melting, wet loose snow avalanches also are common. Most of the latter, too, are small, but they are more likely to develop occasional destructive size, especially when confined to gulleys.

Slab avalanches originate in snow with sufficient internal cohesion to enable a snow layer, or layers, to react mechanically as a single entity. The degree of this required cohesion may range from very slight in fresh, new snow (soft slab) to very high in hard, wind drifted snow (hard slab), according to circumstances of layer attachment to the external environment. A slab avalanche breaks free along a characteristic fracture line, a sharp division of sliding from stable snow whose face stands perpendicular to the slope. The entire surface of unstable snow is set in motion at the same time. A slab release may take place across an entire mountainside, with the fracture racing from slope to slope to release adjacent or even distant slide paths. The mechanical conditions leading to slab avalanche formation are found in a wide variety of snow types, both new and old, dry and wet. They may be induced by the nature of snow deposition (wind drifting is the prime agent of slab formation), or by internal metamorphism. Slab avalanches are often dangerous and unpredictable in behavior. Providing most of the winter avalanche hazard, they axe the primary object of avalanche defense and control measures. Avalanches composed of dry snow usually generate a dust cloud as part of the sliding snow is whirled into the air. Such slides, called powder snow avalanches, most frequently originate as soft slabs. Under favorable circumstances, enough snow crystals are mixed with the air to form an aerosol which behaves as a sharply bounded body of dense gas rushing down the slope ahead of the sliding snow. This wind blast can achieve high velocities to inflict heavy and capricious destruction well beyond the normal bounds of the avalanche path.

Wet snow avalanches move more slowly than dry ones and seldom are accompanied by dust clouds. Their higher snow density can lend them enormous destructive force in spite of lower velocities. As wet slides reach their deposition zones, the interaction of sliding and stagnated snow produces characteristic channeling.

Direct action avalanches fall as the immediate result of a single snow storm. They usually involve only the fresh snow. Climax avalanches are caused by a series of snow storms or a culmination of weather influences. Their fall is not necessarily associated with a given current storm or weather situation.

The Mechanism of Avalanche Release

Most avalanches of dangerous size originate on slope angles between 30 degrees and 45 degrees. They seldom occur below 30 degrees and hardly ever below 25 degrees. Above 45 degrees to 50 degrees sluffs and small avalanches are common, but snow seldom accumulates to sufficient depths to generate large slides.

Though internal metamorphism or stress development may sometimes initiate snow rupture, avalanches are often dislodged by external triggers. An overload of new snow may dislodge an existing slab. Falling cornices or chunks of snow from trees are common natural triggers, similar in action to the sunballs or snow wheels which frequently initiate wet slides. In the absence of external triggers; unstable snow may revert to stability with passage of time and no avalanche occurs. Artificial triggers in the form of mechanical disturbance may be intentionally introduced for control purposes. Unintentional triggers are a major cause of accidents; most skiers who fall victim to an avalanche trigger the slide which traps them.

The primary instability develops when the component of force parallel to the slope due to the weight of the slab exceeds the shear strength of the bond to the underlayer (sliding surface). The situation is mechanically complex due to irregular attachment of the slab to stable snow or other anchorages at the head, toe and sides. In general, slab avalanche release occurs when one of these attachments is broken by a trigger; redistributed stresses then exceed the strength of the other bonds and an avalanche falls. Only part of the slab attachments may be weak, while others are strong. In this case a trigger will initiate fracturing in the snow but the slab remains in place and no avalanche falls.

Snow settles as destructive metamorphism proceeds, and on an inclined surface it also creeps downhill under the influence of gravity by internal plastic deformation and slip on the ground. Creep velocity varies with temperature., snow type, snow depth, slope inclination and profile., and ground cover. These variations from one zone of the snow cover to another develop creep stresses. The zones of creep tension are favorable locations for slab avalanche fracture lines; these commonly occur on convex profiles or at the head of open slopes where the snow cover first finds anchorage (trees, ridge top, etc.). A snow slab under tension may not only break free when triggered but shatter into blocks as well when the stress is relieved. This release may achieve almost explosive violence. Creep stresses are in large measure responsible for the dangerous and unpredictable character of slab avalanches.

Forecasting Snow Avalanches

Although the general features of snow instability are known many details of avalanche formation are not clearly understood. Forecasting snow avalanches is therefore largely an empirical art based on accumulated experience. Known physical and mechanical principles of snow behavior provide a qualitative understanding of avalanche origin, but quantitative extension of these principles to specific situations is difficult for nature presents too many variables to allow exact calculation of snow stress and strength variations with time. The precise time a given slope will avalanche cannot be predicted, but the general degrees of instability in a given area can be estimated with reasonable accuracy.

There are two basic methods of anticipating avalanche hazard. One is the examination of snow cover structure for patterns of weakness, particularly those leading to slab avalanches. This method finds its greatest success in forecasting climax slab avalanches caused by structural weaknesses which may be evolved over a period of time and by a variety of weather conditions. The second method is analysis of meteorological factors affecting snow depositions. The latter is now successful in forecasting direct action soft slab avalanches which run in fresh surface snow layers where structure is poorly differentiated. In practice the two methods overlap and both are used. Emphasis on one or the other depends on local climate, snow type, and avalanche characteristics. Both apply principally to winter avalanches in dry snow; forecasting wet spring avalanches depends on knowledge of heat input to the snow surface as well as elements of the foregoing methods.

Snow cover structure is investigated directly by digging pits and examining the exposed stratigraphy. Snow temperature, density, strength properties, and crystal type are all important for determining stability. Time variations in these properties are examined by a succession of pits in a given study area, the result being plotted in a time profile. Indirect evidence on snow structure can be gathered by instruments probing from the surface. The most useful of these is the ran penetrometer which measures snow strength variations with depth by means of a pointed rod driven by a falling weight. Periodic observations at representative study plots (usually on level ground) are compared with snow profiles from actual avalanche fracture lines to determine and anticipate stability trends.

Observation of contributory weather factors before and during a snow storm provides the basis for forecasting a hazard situation. The depth and surface character of the existing snow base, established by previous storms, must be known. A deep snow cover favours avalanching by smoothing the terrain, while certain surface conditions such as a crust offer a good sliding surface. The new snow depth, type, and density also offer clues to stability. New snow densities above about 0.12 g/cm^{-3} are a warning sign. (Very low new snow densities, 0.05 g/cm^{-3} or less, are usually associated with dry loose snow avalanches). Settlement in the new snow is a stabilizing factor.

Rising temperature during a storm accompanied by rising new snow density tends to cause avalanching while falling temperatures have the opposite effect. New snow precipitation intensity is a significant factor, for it represents the rate at which the slopes are being overloaded. Values above 2.5 mm of water per hour warn of impending hazard. In practice this factor may not be measured directly; instead, new snow density and snowfall intensity are observed. The wind is also critically important, for soft slab avalanches seldom occur unless sustained average wind velocity exceeds 6 to 7 m/sec^{-1}. The most reliable indicator of developing avalanche hazard is a sustained period of coincident high wind and high precipitation intensity.

Rapid temperature rise-quickly alters snow behavior, while the water itself reduces snow strength. Liquid water accumulating at an impervious crust provides an especially good lubricating layer for slab release. The most extensive wet snow avalanching occurs during winter rains or the first prolonged melt period in spring, when liquid water intrudes into previously subfreezing snow. Snow melt by solar radiation is the commonest source of wet snow avalanching and this is amenable to quantitative prediction. It is essential that the total snow surface energy balance be considered in estimating amount of melt, for longwave radiation, vapor exchange and sensible heat from the air all play an important part. A warm, windy, overcast day may produce more melting (and avalanche activity) than sunshine and cloudless skies.

Accuracy of formal forecasting procedures is enhanced by frequent field checks of snow stability. For this purpose small, accessible avalanche paths are sometimes chosen as sites for test skiing where snow conditions are checked by actually trying to set the snow in motion. This technique is particularly useful in detecting incipient soft slab formation during storms. It is less effective (and more dangerous) on hard slabs formed by heavy wind drifting. Tests of the latter are usually restricted to blasting with high explosives.

Avalanche Control Techniques

Avalanche hazard can be mitigated or eliminated by the application of operational and engineering techniques. There are two fundamental methods of avalanche control: modification of terrain, and modification of the snow cover.

Terrain modification may deflect the sliding snow away from fixed facilities to be protected, or actually prevent the avalanche release. Examples of deflecting structures are snowsheds used to protect railways and highways. These must be strong enough to support the dynamic load of sliding snow; hence most modern snowsheds are built of reinforced concrete. Where sheds are impractical, the sliding snow can be diverted laterally by wedges, pylons, or diversion walls.

In favorable terrain the snow may be arrested by snow dams or catchment basins. Avalanches are also arrested in the outrun, or transition zone, of their paths by braking mounds conical earthen or masonry mounds four meters or more high which are arranged in a pattern to break up the flowing snow into crosscurrents which internally dissipate its kinetic energy. All of the passive deflection structures act principally on snow sliding on the ground which may exert impact forces up to 50 tons/m^2. They have less effect on the dust cloud accompanying a powder snow avalanche.

Active avalanche defense by terrain modification is achieved with supporting structures in the avalanche release zone. These are large walls, fences, or nets arranged to retain snow and prevent avalanches from falling. Their size and spacing are designed to (1) terrace the mountainside into discrete zones, each of which has snow deposited to a surface slope less than the mean, (2) break up the continuity of the snow surface and prevent slab formation, and (3) support snow on the mountainside in small, manageable sections. These supporting structures, mostly massive fences in modern design, must be strong enough to support creep pressures reaching tons per square meter, while at the same time being light enough for economical transport and erection high on a mountainside. Another type of defense used in the release zone is the wind baffle, a wall or panel arranged to induce irregular wind drifting which breaks the continuity of snow slabs. They are not designed to withstand large creep pressures and are less effective than supporting structures.

Avalanche control by snow modification does not give the high degree of protection afforded by terrain modification but is much cheaper. It commonly is used to reduce the hazard to mobile entities, such as skiers or highway traffic, which may be removed during periods of danger. The commonest technique is artificial release, which brings down avalanches at a chosen safe time and inhibits formation of large avalanches by relieving slopes of their snow burden piecemeal in small ones. Slides on small paths are sometimes intentionally released by skiing, but the preferred method is the detonation of a high explosive on the snow surface close to the expected fracture line. One kilogram of TNT or its equivalent is considered the minimum reliable charge. The charge may be placed by hand, but this can be difficult and is sometimes dangerous. Artillery shells, armed with superquick point detonating fuses, are much more efficient, for a number of targets can quickly and safely be engaged from a single gun emplacement. Principal disadvantages of artillery are limitations to military or government use and possible damage from shrapnel dispersion. Mortars, light howitzers, and recoilless rifles have all been successfully used for avalanche control; the 75mm recoilless rifle is the most practical weapon for this purpose. Where frequent artificial release is undertaken to protect a ski area or highway, a fixed artillery emplacement permits increased efficiency by blind firing during storms or at night. Artificial release cannot be effectively employed at random. It must be based on accurate appraisal of snow and weather conditions, and careful selection of targets.

Another snow modification technique is the application of mechanical disturbance to break up slab formation (especially soft slabs) and induce stabilization through age hardening. Skier traffic is the commonest available disturbance, while deliberate packing of the snow by foot or ski is sometimes used. Depth hoar can be satisfactorily stabilized only by intensive foot packing. Mechanical aids, such as oversnow vehicles, can seldom be used at the slope angles existing in avalanche release zones.

Techniques to Help Survive An Avalanche

Several times every winter, one reads about skiers, snowboarders or snowmobilers who have been caught in avalanches. Some survive, in part because they are properly equipped with beacons, probes and knowledge. Others don't! If you're heading into mountains where there could be slides, take time to learn about avalanche safety. The majority of avalanches victims are caught in are triggered by themselves or others in their party.

Despite advances in medicine and search and rescue the death rate from avalanches remains fairly constant at around 25-30 per year or around 60% of victims on extraction. This is largely due to the average response time of the search and rescue services which is 45 minutes, taken to process the emergency call, warm the motor of a helicopter, fly to and locate the scene of the accident then deploy the search and rescue services. Two thirds of avalanche victims succumb in that critical half hour. A Swiss study on avalanche mortality published in 1992 indicates that approximately 90 percent of persons buried in avalanches survive if recovered in the first 15 minutes. Chances for a live recovery at the 35-minute mark fall to 30 percent and after two hours the survival rate is three percent. However, there are exceptions to every statistic and people have been found alive in certain circumstances 5-6 hours after being buried and in a few documented cases people have been recovered still alive after 24 hours.

Avalanche search and rescue gear can be broken down into three groups: avalanche avoidance, avalanche survival and search and rescue. Given that avalanches prove fatal to 50% of victims that are completely buried even when equipped with avalanche transceivers the emphasis should be on avalanche avoidance.

Phases

Survival Phase: In the first 15 minutes 93% of avalanche victims are still alive, indeed most of the deaths occur during the fall either by hitting rocks or trees or being carried over cliffs or by being crushed or suffocated by the weight of snow. Wet snow avalanches, characteristic of spring, are most likely to suffocate or crush skiers during this phase but it is less common for skiers to be caught these.

Asphyxiation Phase: In this half hour period, two thirds of victims will die from asphyxiation. Apart from wet snow avalanches the snow encasing victims contains a significant amount of oxygen and is permeable. If a victim has protected or can clear airways and can breath (that is the weight of snow is not compressing the lungs or thorax) they can usually breath. During this period the surrounding air will either be exhausted or the victims respiration will condense and freeze slowly rendering the surrounding snow impermeable.

Waiting Phase: Between 45 minutes and rescue the victim will probably have found an air pocket and is in a phase of relative security which will allow them to survive for a considerable period. Death is either from slow asphyxia or hypothermia. With an adequate air supply hypothermia is slowed down.

Rescue Phase: Between being rescued and arrival and recovering in hospital the risk of hypothermia is great. Hypothermia begins

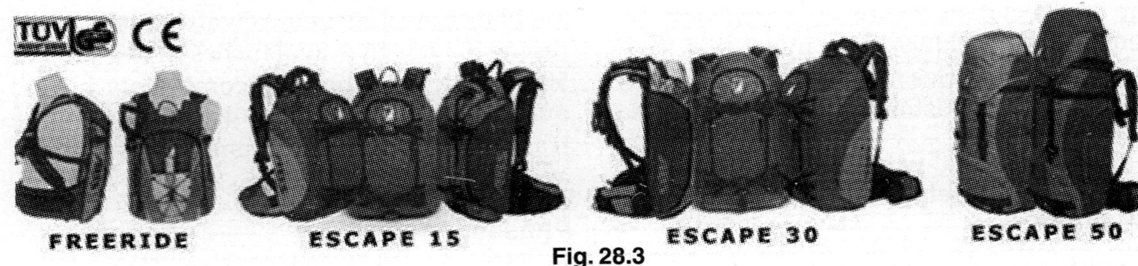

Fig. 28.3

when the body temperature drops below 35°C (body temperature is around 37°C) and it is extremely rare for a victim to survive once their body temperature drops to 29°C. The survival phase is critical, when the body is cooled it will divert blood from the extremities to the vital organs, when the body is warmed blood will return to the extremities but at too low a temperature this will cool the vital organs causing death by thermal shock.

Rescue Devices

RECCO Equipment System: This is a passive search device employing harmonic radar system consisting of reflectors and detectors that enables rapid directional pinpointing of victims. A small circuit board is sewn into clothing or glued onto the boots. It has the advantage that the circuit doesn't need batteries and can't be forgotten or turned off. To be effective the rider should always wear two reflectors on both sides of the body. However the system requires special equipment and although this is available in many ski resorts the rescue services must first transport it to the avalanche site. This delay is critical and therefore the system should not be considered by riders going far from the pistes.

ABS AIRBAG SYSTEM

The closer you are to the surface the greater your chance of survival. The ABS Airbag system consists of a special ruck-sack equipped with a gas canister and two large sacks situated on either side. If there is an avalanche a handle on the left shoulder must be pulled, the canister fills the two sacks with gas providing the skier with both some impact protection and buoyancy. The handle can be easily removed in ski lifts or restaurants to avoid accidental release. The system relies on a certain presence of mind of the user. The system is also bulky, it is popular with ski guides who work largely lift served off-piste within stations but is heavy for ski mountaineering use. The system is being continually improved.

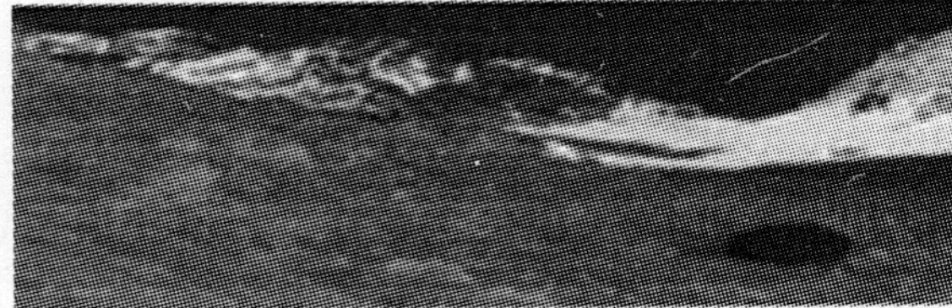
Fig. 28.4

THE AVALANCHE BALL

This is a development of the avalanche cords that skiers used before the development of avalanche transceiver. The actual ball is a small, spring loaded canvas ball that sits in a sack at the top of the skiers rucksack. If there is an avalanche a cord is pulled, releasing the ball which is connected to a skier by a cord Like a cord, it floats to the surface giving an immediate visual clue as to the location of the wearer. This is one of the most important factors governing speedy rescue and

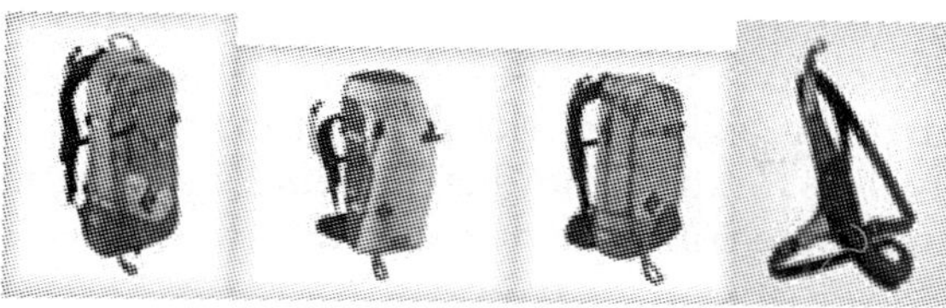

Fig. 28.5

eventual survival. The biggest disadvantage is that the ball may come to rest on the surface some meters away from the victim. However the connecting cord is thin and light and will cut through compact snow so the cord can be pulled tight until the search is directly above the victim. It is important to remember that the ball will not aid floatation so you still need a buddy to rescue you.

THE AVALUNG

Most victims who survive the initial slide suffocate in the period 15 to 45 minutes after being buried. There is considerable air in an avalanche, at least closer to the surface. However if the victim isn't lucky to find himself in an air pocket the water vapour in his breath freezes in the surrounding snow. This quickly builds up an impermeable layer around the victim trapping CO_2 and asphyxiating the victim. The AvaLung is an air filtration system. Oxygen enters from the front, the wearer breathes this through a tube and CO_2 is expelled from the back. It serves to prolong the time someone can be buried without suffocating. There is still the danger of hypothermia so quick rescue is still vital. There are a couple of drawbacks. The AvaLung is worn outside skier's clothing and attention has to be paid to make sure the tube isn't compressed, say by rucksack straps. The skier also has to ride with the tube in front of their mouth. The unit is ultralightweight <300 grams.

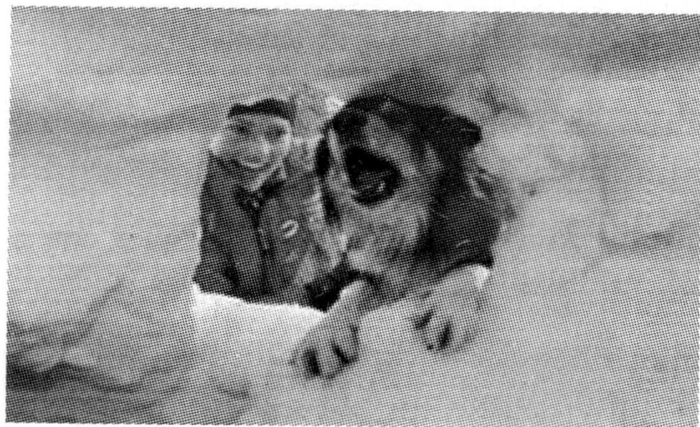

Fig. 28.6

SNIFFER DOGS

For years, snow related rescue operations were best described as chaotic and it wasn't until the late 1930's that the Swiss Army started training search dogs in Avalanche Rescue. Since that time trainers have refined their training techniques and now many avalanche victims can owe their lives to dogs trained in avalanche rescue. The trained search dog works a snowfield rapidly, searching for "pools" of human scent rising up through the snow pack. When the dog finds a potential scent source he will bury his head into the snow trying to locate the source. If the human smell intensifies, he begins to dig trying to get closer to the source. If the scent becomes weaker, a trained dog will start to work outwards from the area to attempt to either pinpoint an area of stronger buried source or rule the scent out as surface odor left by human searchers. When someone is buried in an avalanche, speed in locating the individual is of the essence.. A well-trained avalanche rescue dog is a model of efficiency in that one dog is equivalent to approximately 20-foot searchers and can search the same area in an eighth of the time. A trained Avalanche Dog can search one hectare in approximately 30 minutes, where it takes 20 foot searchers 4 hours to search the same area with probe poles (covering about 2.5% of the total area that the dog could cover). During a Fine search, one dog can cover the same hectare in 1-2 hours where it would take 20 searchers 20 hours to cover the same area (only accomplishing 10% of what a dog could cover). Surface conditions, snow conditions, capabilities of the particular dog and scent diffusion all play an important role in how deep the victim can actually be buried and still be located. There have been confirmed reports, in optimal conditions, of a dog in Austria locating a body at approximately 12 meters. In the U.S. there has been a confirmed find at 10 meters. However, this type of success is few and far between. Realistically one can expect an experienced dog to be able to locate victims between 2-4 meters without a lot of difficulty in most scenting conditions.

CONCLUSION

The basic message is that to survive an avalanche you have to be rescued within 15 minutes. Your life depends on carrying and being proficient in the use of avalanche transceivers and having snow probes and shovels. In ideal conditions it will take around 5 minutes to locate a victim with a transceiver and 10 to 15 minutes to dig them out from the average depth of burial which is 1 meter.

While the avalanche is taking place try to follow the skier who is trapped and point to the place where they disappeared under the snow. Look for other clues below this point for where they may have finished up, a ski or stick pointing out the snow may be a good place to start a search. They may also have stopped on a flatter part of the slope, above or below an outcrop, rock or tree. A 60 degree angle from the point where the skier vanished is considered a *sweet zone*, the avalanche victim will most likely to lie within this area. The effective range of an avalanche transceivers is around a fifth of the maximum range, 10 meters for digital and 20 meters for analogue, so any help in locating the rough area to search is welcome.

If there is more than one searcher someone should take charge. Rescuers should proceed directly to the avalanche zone, riding off to the side should be avoided as this may provoke a secondary avalanche. Any equipment not of immediate use in the search should be placed at this point to avoid littering the search area with rucksacks, skis etc not associated with the rescue. These may confused rescue dogs if they are needed later.

When the helicopter(s) arrive make a Y signal by holding both arms above your head to indicate that you are the party requesting assistance. Telephone or radio calls should be made away from any avalanche transceivers to avoid interference with the search. The effective number of searchers with transceivers is between 3 to 6, depending on the size of the area avalanched. Other people could begin a probe or audio search around any visual clues spotted on the surface.

It is important to set all avalanche transreceivers to search mode. This includes any bystanders who may have witnessed the avalanche.

Summary of Avalanche Mitigation

Short term protection measures:

- Avalanche forecasting and warnings.
- Artificial release of avalanches with pyrotechnics.
- Closure of roads and railways.
- Evacuation of people at risk.
- Sniffer dog rescue services.
- Explorers are strongly advised to not only know how to identify avalanche hazard areas but also to carry a avalanche beacon/ transceiver and a shovel in case of emergency.

Long term measures:
- Hazard mapping and land use planning.
- Construction measures like:
  Supporting structures at starting zones
  Deviation dams along avalanche paths
  Retaining dams at deposition zone of avalanches.
  Silivicultural measures and reforestation.

Cold Injuries

Tissue temperature in cold weather is regulated by two factors, the external temperature and the internal heat flow. All cold injuries described below are intimately connected with the degree of peripheral circulation. As peripheral circulation is reduced to prevent heat loss to the core these conditions are more likely to occur. Cold weather-related injuries can be divided into two general categories. These are those that occur without the freezing of body tissue (chilblains and trench foot) and those that occur with the freezing of body tissue (frostbite).

Factors influencing cold injuries:
- Low ambient temperature.
- Wind chil—increases rate of freezing dramatically.
- Moisture—wet skin freezes at a higher temp than dry.
- Insulation.
- Contact with metal or supercooled liquids (white gas).
- Exposed skin.
- Vasodilation.
- Vasoconstriction.
- Previous cold injuries.
- Constricting garments.
- Local pressure.
- Cramped position.
- Body type.
- Dehydration.
- Women do better in cold than men (greater subcutaneous body fat).
- Caloric intake.
- Diabetes, some medications.
- Alcohol.
- Caffeine, nicotine.

Cold-induced Vasodilation

When a hand or foot is cooled to 59 degrees F, maximal vasoconstriction and minimal blood flow occur. If cooling continues to 50 degrees F, vasoconstriction is interrupted by periods of vasodilation with an increase in blood and heat flow. This "hunting" response recurs in 5-10 minute cycles to provide some protection from cold. Prolonged, repeated exposure increases this response and offers some degree of acclimatization. E.g., Eskimos have a strong response with short intervals in between.

Pathophysiology of Tissue Freezing

As tissue begins to freeze, ice crystals are formed within the cells. As intracellular fluids freeze, extracellular fluid enters the cell and there is an increase in the levels of extracellular salts due to the water transfer. Cells may rupture due to the increased water and/or from tearing by the ice crystals. There occurs cellular dehydration, protein denaturation, inhibition of DNA synthesis, abnormal cell wall permeability with resultant osmotic changes, damage to capillaries, and pH changes. Rewarming causes cell swelling, erythrocyte and platelet aggregation, endothelial cell damage, thrombosis, tissue edema, increased compartment space pressure, bleb formation, localized ischemia, and tissue death.

Underlying responses to these injuries include generation of oxygen free radicals, production of prostaglandins and thromboxane A2, release of proteolytic enzymes, and generalized inflammation. Tissue injury is greatest when cooling is slow, cold exposure is prolonged, rate of rewarming is slow, and, especially, when tissue is partially thawed and refreezes.

Hence rubbing tissues vigorously or massaging *causes cell damage from the ice crystals.* As the ice melts there is an influx of salts into the tissue further damaging the cell membranes. Cell destruction results in tissue death and loss of tissue. Tissues do not freeze if the temperature is above 32 degrees F. Freezing occurs at below 28 degrees F because of the salt content in body fluids. Distal areas of the body and areas with a high surface to volume ratio are the most susceptible e.g., ears, nose, fingers and toes.

- Surface frostbite generally involves destruction of skin layers resulting in blistering and minor tissue loss. Blisters are formed from the cellular fluid released when cells rupture.
- Deep frostbite can involve muscle and bone (Table 28.1).

Cold Response

- Circulation is reduced to the area to prevent heat loss.
- The area is usually pale and cold.
- The affected area has blunted sensation or is numb.

Frostnip

- Freezing of top layers of skin tissue.
- It is generally reversible.
- Skin is white and waxy, top layer feels hard and rubbery but deeper tissue is still soft.
- Numbness present.
- Most typically seen on cheeks, earlobes, fingers, and toes.

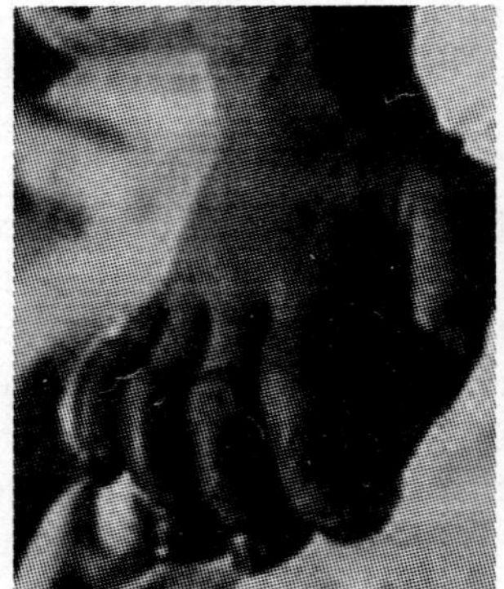

Fig. 28.7

Treatment

- Rewarm the area gently, generally by blowing warm air on it or placing the area against a warm body part (partner's stomach or armpit).
- *Do not rub the area:* This can damage the effected tissue by + having ice crystals tear the cell.

FROSTBITE

Frostbite occurs when there is freezing of the affected area and it is the most serious of the cold weather-related injuries. Frostbite usually affects the hands, feet, nose, or ears; though other parts of the body may also be affected. This type of injury results from decreased blood flow and heat delivery to

Table 28.1

Cold response		*Mild frostnip*	*Superficial frostbite*	*Deep frostbite*
Sensation	Painful	May have sensation	Numb	Numb
Feels	Normal	Normal	Soft	Hard
Color	Red	White	White	White

body tissues resulting in damaging ice crystal formation.

Frostbite injuries can be classified as either superficial, involving only the skin and subcutaneous tissues or deep depending on the depth of injury. Superficial frostbite injuries involve the skin and subcutaneous tissues, while deep frostbite injuries extend beyond the subcutaneous tissues and involve the tendons, muscles, nerves, and even bone. Superficial frostbite injuries have a better prognosis than deep injuries.

The symptoms of frostbite may progress from pain/burning to numbness and eventual complete loss of sensation. Depending on the extent and time of injury, the affected area may appear pale, red, bluish/gray or black with the presence of clear or purplish colored blisters. The skin and underlying tissue may feel hard to the touch with advanced injury.

The prognosis for frostbite injuries depends on the extent of injury and whether or not there are any resultant complications from the initial injury, such as infection. It may be weeks to several months before it is possible to determine exactly how much tissue damage has occurred, and what if any tissue needs to be removed/amputated. Sometimes cold sensitivity or numbness of the affected area persists.

- Skin is white and somewhat rubbery without blanching or evidence of capillary refill after mild pressure or, if deep, has a "wooden" feel all the way through
- Superficial frostbite includes all layers of skin
- Numbness, possible anesthesia present
- Deep frostbite can include freezing of muscle and/or bone, it is very difficult to rewarm the appendage without some damage occurring

Degree of Injury

- *First-degree injury:* Erythema, edema, waxy appearance, hard white plaques, and sensory deficit.
- *Second-degree injury:* Erythema, edema, and formation of blisters filled with clear or milky fluid and which have high thromboxane content (These blisters form within 24 hours of injury).
- *Third-degree injury:* Presence of blood-filled blisters, which progress to a black eschar over a matter of weeks.
- *Fourth-degree injury:* Full-thickness damage affecting muscles, tendons, and bone, with resultant tissue loss.

Treatment

- Superficial frostbite may be rewarmed as frostnip if only a small area is involved.
- If deep frostbite, rewarming must be initiated as detailed below.

Rewarming of Frostbite

- Rewarming is accomplished by immersion of the effected part into a water bath of 105-110 degreesF(40–42°C). *No hotter or additional damage will result. Avoid dry heat.* This is the temperature which is warm to your skin. Monitor the tempera-ture carefully with a thermometer. Remove constricting clothing. Place the appendage in the water and continue to monitor the water temperature. This temperature will drop so that additional warm water will need to be added to maintain the 105 - 110 degrees. *Do not* add this warm water directly to the injury. The water will need to be circulated fairly constantly to maintain even temperature. The effected appendage should be immersed for 25 to 40 minutes. Thawing is complete when the part is pliable and color (tissue flush) and sensation has returned. Once the area is rewarmed, there can be significant pain. Discontinue the warm water bath when thawing is complete.

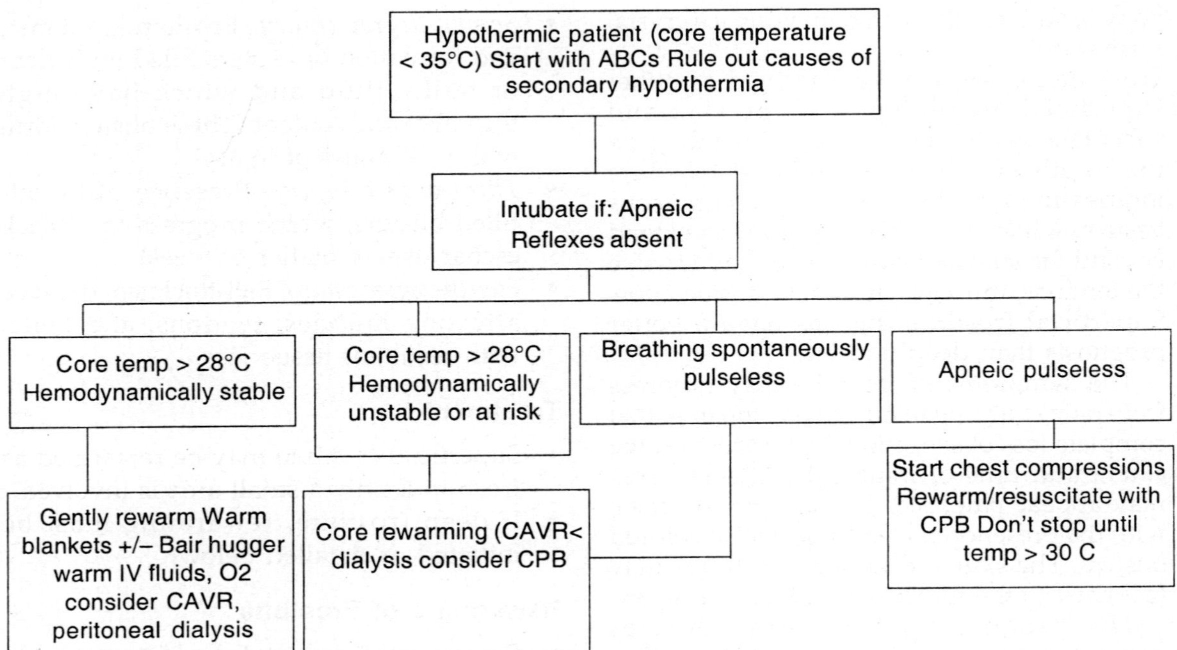

Management of the hypothermic patient CAVR, continuous arteriovenous rewarming; CPB, cardiopulmonary bypass

- *Do not use dry heat to rewarm. It cannot be effectively maintained at 105–110 degrees F and can cause burns further damaging the tissues.*
- Once rewarming is complete the injured area should be wrapped in sterile gauze and protected from movement and further cold.
- *Once a body part has been rewarmed it must be immobilized and it is essential that the part is kept from refreezing as* refreezing after rewarming causes extensive tissue damage and may result in loss of tissue. If you cannot *guarantee* that the tissue will stay warm, *do not rewarm it*. Mountaineers have walked out on frozen feet to have them rewarmed after getting out with no tissue loss. Once the tissue is frozen the major harm has been done. Keeping it frozen will not cause significant additional damage.
- For deep frostbite, daily water therapy in a 40°C (104°F) whirlpool bath will be performed in order to remove any dead tissue.

Special Considerations for Frostbite

- If the person is hypothermic and frostbitten, the first concern is core rewarming. Do not rewarm the frostbitten areas until the core temp approaches 96 degrees F or 35°C.
- No alcohol – vasodilation may increase fluid buildup.
- No smoking – nicotine is a vasoconstrictor may increase chances for developing frostbite.
- Liquids such as white gas can "supercool" in the winter (drop below their freezing

point but not freeze). White gas also evaporates quickly into the air. Spilling supercooled white gas on exposed skin leads to instant frostbite from evaporative cooling. Always were gloves when handling fuel.

- Touching metal with bare skin can cause the moisture on your skin to freeze to the metal and when you pull away, you may leave a layer of skin behind. Don't touch metal with bare skin.
- Give anti tetanus prophylaxis.
- Role of Heparin, oral anticoagulants, low molecular weight dextran, tPA and pentoxyphylline is controversial.
- Topical aloe vera may be useful.
- Technetium 99m scanning 5 days after injury may assist in defining deep involvement.
- Medical/surgical sympathectomy and also hyperbaric oxygen can be tried.
- A common saying among surgeons who have treated people with frostbite is "frostbite in January, amputate in July." It often takes months before the final separation between healthy and dead tissue may be determined. If surgery is performed too early, the risks of removing tissue that may eventually recover or leaving behind tissue that may eventually die are great.
- Long-term sequelae include paresthesias and sensory deficits, hyperhidrosis or anhidrosis, cracking skin and loss of nails, abnormal color changes indicative of vasospasm, cold sensitivity, joint stiffness, tremor, premature closure of epiphyses in children, osteoporosis, intrinsic muscle atrophy, and phantom pain of amputated extremities.

TRENCH FOOT—IMMERSION FOOT

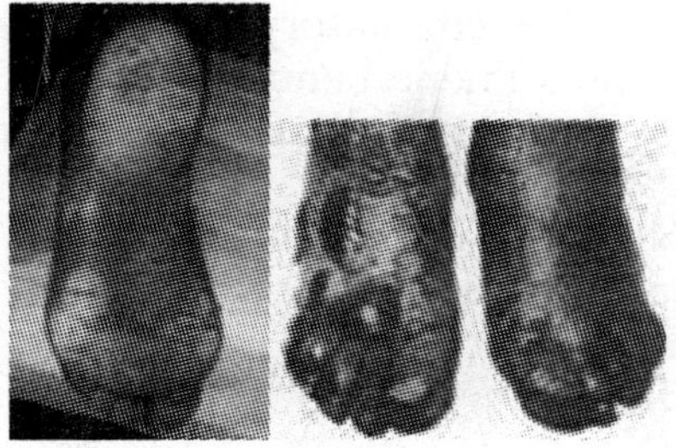

Fig. 28.8

Trench foot (immersion injury) was named after the condition suffered by many soldiers in the trenches during World War I. Trench foot develops after prolonged exposure (12-24h) to a wet, cold environment and is typically a more serious condition than chilblains. It can occur at temperatures as high as 60 degrees F if the feet are constantly wet. This can happen with wet feet in winter conditions or wet feet in much warmed conditions (ex. sea kayaking). The mechanism of injury is as follows: wet feet loses heat 25x faster than dry, therefore the body uses vasoconstriction to shut down peripheral circulation in the foot to prevent heat loss. Skin tissue begins to die because of lack of oxygen and nutrients and due to buildup of toxic products. The skin is initially reddened with numbness, tingling pain, and itching then becomes pale and mottled and finally dark purple, grey or blue. The effected tissue generally dies and sloughs off. In severe cases trench foot can involve the toes, heels, or the entire foot. If circulation is impaired for > 6 hours there will be permanent damage to tissue. If circulation is impaired for > 24 hours the victim may lose the entire foot. Trench Foot causes permanent damage to the circulatory system making the person more prone to cold related injuries in that area. A similar phenomenon can occur when hands are kept wet for long periods of time such as kayaking with wet gloves or pogies. The damage to the circulatory system is known as Raynaud's Phenomenon.

The symptoms of trench foot include:

- Pain,.
- Numbness, and swelling.

The affected area may appear:

- Red.
- Blotchy.
- Pale.
- Bluish or even black with advanced injury.

As with chilblains, blisters and open sores can also develop. With severe trench foot, the development of gangrene can occur. A hyperemic or vasodilatory phase follows lasting 5-10 days. The usual recovery period from uncomplicated trench foot can be for several weeks and, as with chilblains, subsequent cold sensitivity of the affected area may also occur.

Treatment and Prevention of Trench foot

- Includes careful washing and drying of the feet, gentle rewarming and slight elevation. Since the tissue is not frozen as in severe frostbite it is *more* susceptible to damage by walking on it. Cases of trench foot should not walk out; they should be evacuated by litter. Pain and itching are common complaints. Give Ibuprofen or other pain medication.
- Prevention is the best approach to dealing with trench foot. Keep feet dry by wearing appropriate footwear. Check your feet regularly to see if they are wet. If your feet get wet (through sweating or immersion), stop and dry your feet and put on dry socks. Periodic air drying, elevation, and massage will also help. Change socks at least once a day and do not sleep with wet socks. Be careful of tight socks which can further impair peripheral circulation. Foot powder with aluminum hydroxide can help. High altitude mountaineers will put antiperspirant on their feet for a week before the trip. The active ingredient, aluminum hydroxide will keep your feet from sweating for up to a month. Vapor barrier socks may increase the possibility of trenchfoot. When you are active and you are wearing a vapor barrier sock, you must carefully monitor how you sweat. If you are someone who sweats a lot with activity, your foot and polypropylene liner sock may be totally soaked before the body stops sweating.
- Dress warmly using multiple layers and adequately cover body areas prone to injury.
- Try to have an extra change of dry clothing so you can remove any wet clothing if necessary.
- Always keep your hands and feet dry and avoid wearing tight fitting clothing on these areas as it may decrease the circulation.
- Most importantly, however, move indoors to a warmer environment when you begin to feel cold.

There may be quite a bit of pain when the injured area is rewarmed. Paracetamol or Ibuprofen may be used to help with the discomfort. If stronger pain medications are required, contact a healthcare provider.

Other treatments for cold-related injuries include local wound care for blisters and open sores. Keep the wounds clean and dry and avoid rupturing blisters. Topical aloe vera cream is recommended.

CHILBLAINS

- Caused by repeated exposure of bare skin to dry air with temperatures below 60 degrees.
- Chilblains is a common type of cold weather-related injury that can develop several hours after exposure to extreme cold. Chilblains are itchy, painful, reddish,

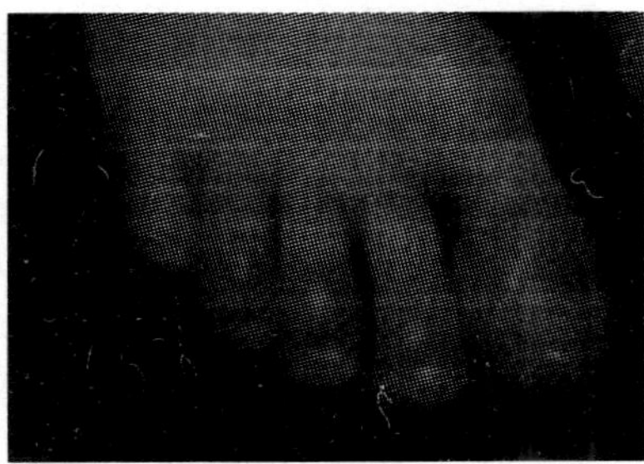

Fig. 28.9

or purplish areas of swelling that usually affect the fingers, toes, nose or ears; though other areas of the body may also be involved. In some individuals, blisters or small open sores may also form. Chilblains usually last for several days, and the affected area usually heals after several weeks. Though the affected area may remain sensitive to the cold in the future, there is usually no permanent damage. It is not uncommon for a recurrence of chilblains in susceptible individuals.

- Women and young children are the most susceptible.
- Those with increased vascular tone appear to have a predisposition to developing chilblains. Those with collagen vascular disease, hyperviscosity of blood and Raynaud's disease also have a greater risk.
- The cold exposure causes damage to the peripheral capillary beds and vasculitis. The redness and itching tend to recur annually during the cold season.

Avoiding Frostbite and Cold Related Injuries

- "Buddy system" – keep a regular watch on each other's faces, cheeks, ears for signs of frostnip/frostbite.
- Keep a regular "self check" for cold areas, wet feet, numbness or anesthesia.
- *If at any time you discover a cold injury, stop and rewarm the area (unless doing so places you at greater risk).*

Eye Injuries

a. Freezing of cornea
  - Caused by forcing the eyes open during strong winds without goggles.
  - Treatment is very controlled, rapid rewarming e.g. placing a warm hand or compress over the closed eye. After rewarming the eyes must be completely covered with patches for 24 - 48 hours.

b. Eyelashes freezing together
  - Put hand over eye until ice melts, then can open the eye

c. Snowblindness
  - Sunburn of the eyes
  - Prevention by wearing good sunglasses with side shields or goggles. Eye protection from sun is just as necessary on cloudy or overcast days as it is in full sunlight when you are on snow. Snow blindness can even occur during a snow storm if the cloud cover is thin.

Symptoms

- Occur 8-12 hours after exposure.
- Eyes feel dry and irritated, then feel as if they are full of sand, moving or blinking becomes extremely painful, exposure to light hurts the eyes, eyelids may swell, eye redness,and excessive tearing.

Treatment

- Cold compresses and dark environment.
- Do not rub eyes.

POLAR MEDICINE

The Arctic and Antarctic circles lie at latitudes 66'33' North and South respectively where, at least on one day in a year, the sun does not rise or set. While both poles of the earth

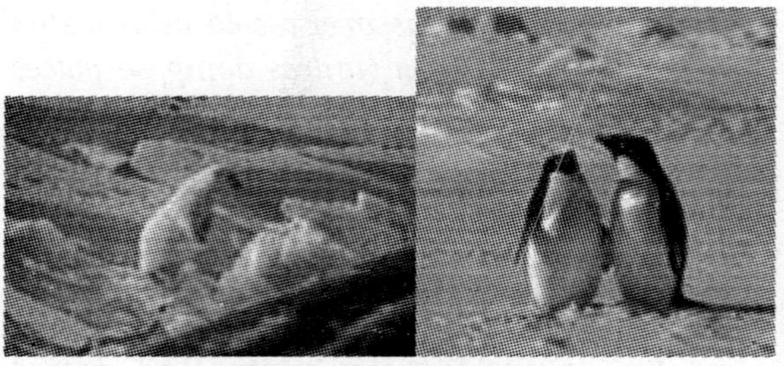

Fig. 28.10

share common attributes of cold, dark and severe weather, the two ends are vastly different. The Arctic is a sea surrounded by land while the Antarctic is a land mass surrounded by the ocean, hence colder and drier. The average winter temperature in the South Pole is almost 40ºC colder than the North. It is a frozen desert much of it a plateau above 10,000 feet above sea level. Very high latitudes provide the most remote settings that are so unusual that they have been termed as the "Fourth World". The geographical location and the remoteness, isolation, hostility and unforgiving nature of the environment makes polar medicine very challenging. Physiological differences are no different from other branches of medicine unlike hyperbaric work and the principles of trauma care, environmental and occupational medicine are similar but doctors need to be more self reliant, a better generalist and depend less on investigations and develop greater clinical judgement. A broad based knowledge and wide range of practical skills are vital to provide good polar medical care, mostly without the luxury of anesthesiologists, dermatologists and psychiatrists. Modern developments in communications and information technology have made the polar physician less isolated. Most of the health problems here are related to cold, altitude and trauma.

29 Action Plan During a Pandemic

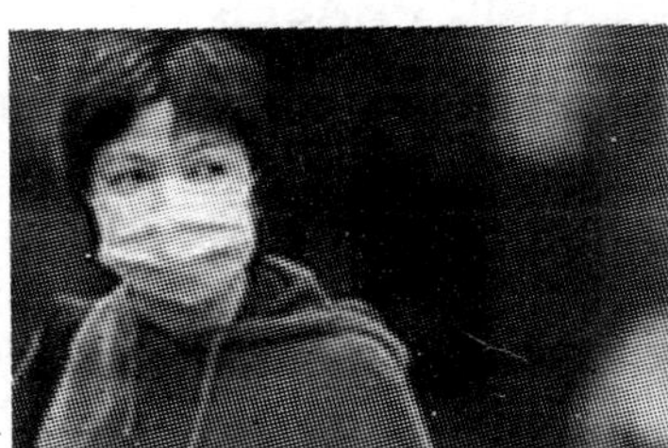
Fig. 29.1

INTRODUCTION

The threat of a pandemic is real. If the threat manifests itself, millions of lives will be lost. Such widespread death would be catastrophic, but the tragedy would be even worse if society ignores. The goals of the Government's response to any pandemic are:

a. To limit the spread of a pandemic.
b. Mitigate disease, suffering, and death.
c. Sustain infrastructure and lessen the impact on the economy and the functioning of society.

Without mitigating interventions, even a less severe pandemic would likely result in dramatic increases in the number of hospitalizations and deaths. In addition, an

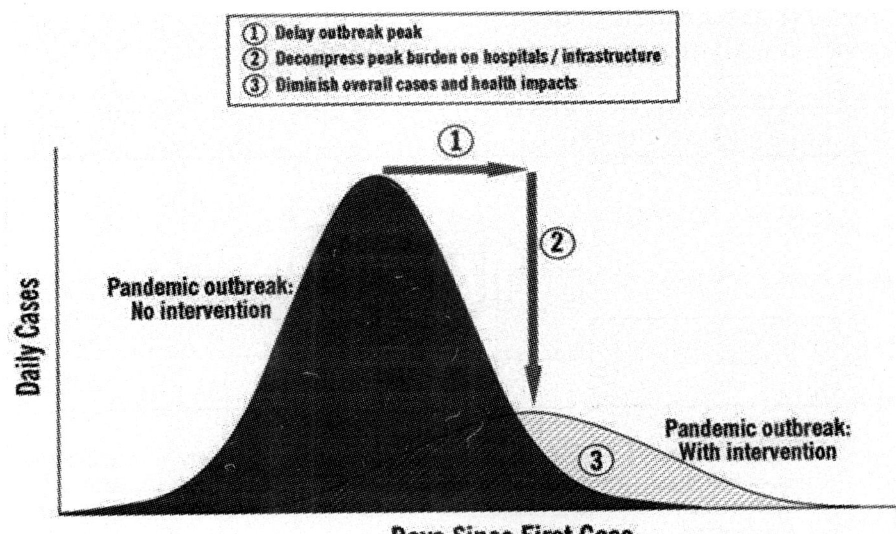

Fig. 29.2: Goals of community mitigation

unmitigated severe pandemic would overwhelm a nation's critical health care services and impose significant stress on a nation's infrastructure.

The two principal strategies for containing serious human outbreaks of infectious diseases are:

1. Therapeutic countermeasures (e.g., vaccines and antiviral medications at the very outset of the pandemic); and
2. Public health interventions (e.g., infection control, social separation, and quarantine).

With current technology it will take at least 6 months from the onset of an outbreak, and possibly longer, for the first doses of vaccine to be available. Furthermore, there is no guarantee that medical countermeasures will be efficacious. Experimental vaccines may not be effective against a mutated strain. Given limited supplies of vaccines, antiviral drugs, and ventilators, non-pharmaceutical interventions are likely to dominate the public health response to any pandemic, at least in the near term. Community strategies that do not involve vaccines or medications (also called non-pharmaceutical interventions) may, therefore, serve as a first line of defense to help delay or mitigate the spread of the pandemic. Public health interventions, while incapable of completely stopping the transmission of the virus, will be able to slow the pandemic. By reducing the rate of spread of the disease, public health countermeasures can buy time for the development of medical countermeasures while also helping to ensure that the health-care system does not become overwhelmed by a surge of patients.

WHO PANDEMIC PHASES

In the 2009 revision of the phase descriptions, WHO has retained the use of a six-phased approach for easy incorporation of new recommendations and approaches into existing national preparedness and response plans. The grouping and description of pandemic phases have been revised to make them easier to understand, more precise, and based upon observable phenomena. Phases 1–3 correlate with preparedness, including capacity development and response planning activities, while Phases 4–6 clearly signal the need for response and mitigation efforts. Furthermore, periods after the first pandemic wave are elaborated to facilitate post pandemic recovery activities.

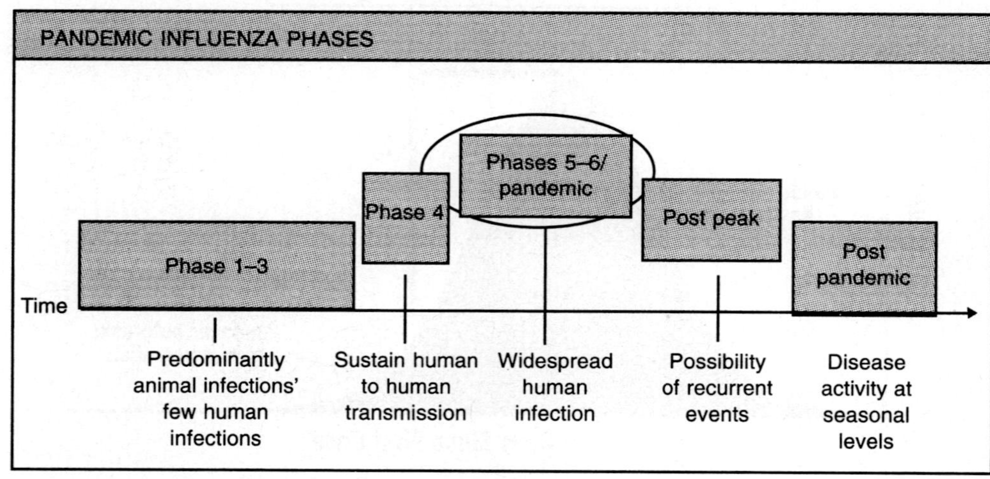

Fig. 29.3

The current WHO phase of pandemic alert is 6 (Fig. 29.2).

Phase 6, the pandemic phase, is characterized by community level outbreaks in at least one other country in a different WHO region and designation of this phase will indicate that a global pandemic is under way.

During the *post-peak period*, pandemic disease levels in most countries with adequate surveillance will have dropped below peak observed levels. The post-peak period signifies that pandemic activity appears to be decreasing; however, it is uncertain if additional waves will occur and countries will need to be prepared for a second wave.

Previous pandemics have been characterized by waves of activity spread over months. Once the level of disease activity drops, a critical communications task will be to balance this information with the possibility of another wave. Pandemic waves can be separated by months and an immediate "at-ease" signal may be premature.

In the *post-pandemic period*, disease activity will have returned to levels normally seen for seasonal infections. At this stage, it is important to maintain surveillance and update pandemic preparedness and response plans accordingly. An intensive phase of recovery and evaluation may be required.

Pre-pandemic Planning: The Pandemic Severity Index

Appropriate matching of the intensity of intervention to the severity of a pandemic is important to maximize the available public health benefit that may result from using an early, targeted, and layered strategy while minimizing untoward secondary effects. The concept of a Pandemic Severity Index based primarily on case fatality ratio is a measurement that is useful in estimating the severity of a pandemic on a population level and which may be available early in a pandemic for small clusters and outbreaks. It is designed to enable better prediction of the impact of a pandemic and to provide local decision-makers with recommendations that are matched to the severity of future pandemics. Excess mortality rate may also be available early and may supplement and inform the determination of the Pandemic Severity Index. Pandemic severity is described within five discrete categories of increasing severity (Category 1 to Category 5).It presumes a 30% illness rate in the community and an unmitigated pandemic without any interventions or mitigation efforts:

- Category 1: Case Fatality rate <0.1%.
- Category 2: Case Fatality Rate 0.1 to <0.5%.
- Category 3: Case Fatality Rate 0.5 to <1.0%.
- Category 4: Case Fatality Rate 1.0 to <2.0%.
- Category 5: Case Fatality Rate > 2.0%.

Future pandemics will be assigned to one of five discrete categories of increasing severity (Category 1 to Category 5). The Pandemic Severity Index provides communities a tool for scenario-based contingency planning to guide local pre-pandemic preparedness efforts. Accordingly, communities facing the imminent arrival of pandemic disease will be able to use the pandemic severity assessment to define which pandemic mitigation interventions are indicated for implementation. Other epidemiologic features that are relevant in overall analysis of mitigation plans include total illness rate, age-specific illness and mortality rates, the reproductive number, intergeneration time, and incubation period. However, it is unlikely that estimates will be available for most of these parameters during the early stages of a pandemic; thus, they are not as useful from a planning perspective. Also, though many factors may influence the outcome of an event, it is reasonable to maintain a single criterion for classification of severity for the purposes of guiding contingency planning. If additional epidemiologic characteristics become well established during the course of the next pandemic through collection and analysis of surveillance data, then local jurisdictions may develop a subset of scenarios, depending upon, for example, age-specific mortality rates.

Incremental increases in case fatality ratio result in proportionally greater mortality in comparison to increasing illness rates, which result in proportionally much smaller increases in mortality. However, it is possible that at the onset of an emerging pandemic, very limited information about cases and deaths will be known. Efforts now to develop decision algorithms based on partial data and efforts to improve global surveillance systems for various epidemics is needed.

Use of Nonpharmaceutical Interventions (NPIs) by Pandemic Severity Category

At the time of an emerging pandemic, depending on the location of the first detected cases, there may be scant information about the number of cases and deaths resulting from infection with the virus. Although surveillance efforts may initially only detect the "herald" cases, public health officials may choose to err on the side of caution and implement interventions based on currently available data and iteratively adjust as more accurate and complete data become available. These strategies that do not involve vaccines or medications (also called non-pharmaceutical interventions) may serve as a first line of defense to help delay or mitigate the spread of the pandemic. These include social distancing strategies to reduce contact between people and the pandemic mitigation measures include the following:

1. Isolation and treatment (as appropriate) with antiviral medications of all persons with confirmed or probable pandemic disease features. Isolation may occur in the home or healthcare setting, depending on the severity of the individual's illness and/or the current capacity of the healthcare infrastructure.
2. Voluntary home quarantine of members of households with confirmed or probable disease and consideration of combining this intervention with the prophylactic use of antiviral medications, providing sufficient quantities of effective medications exist and that a feasible means of distributing them is in place.
3. Dismissal of students from schools (including public and private schools as well as colleges and universities) and school-based activities and closure of childcare programs, coupled with protecting children and teenagers through social distancing in the community to achieve reductions of out-of-school social contacts and community mixing.
4. Use of social distancing measures to reduce contact between adults in the community and workplace, including, for example, cancellation of large public gatherings and alteration of workplace environments and schedules to decrease social density and preserve a healthy workplace to the greatest extent possible without disrupting essential services. Enable institution of workplace leave policies that align incentives and facilitate adherence with the nonpharmaceutical interventions (NPIs).

Planning for use of these NPIs is based on the Pandemic Severity Index, which may allow more appropriate matching of the interventions to the magnitude of the pandemic. All interventions should be combined with infection control practices, such as good hand hygiene and cough etiquette. In addition, the use of personal protective equipment, such as surgical masks or respirators, may be appropriate. 12 weeks of intervention may be essential in the most severe scenarios. This approach to pre-pandemic planning will provide a baseline of readiness for community response even if the actual response is shorter. Recommendations for use of these measures for pandemics of lesser severity may include a subset of these same interventions and, possibly, suggestions that they be used for shorter durations, as in the case of the social distancing measures for children.

For Category 2 or Category 3 pandemics, planning for voluntary isolation of ill persons is recommended, whereas other measures (voluntary quarantine of household contacts, social distancing measures for children and adults) are to be implemented only if local decision-makers have determined that characteristics of the pandemic in their community warrant these additional mitigation measures. However, within these categories, pre-pandemic planning for social distancing measures for children should be undertaken with a focus on a duration of 4 weeks or less, distinct from the longer timeframe recommended for pandemics with a greater Pandemic Severity Index. For Category 1 pandemics, only voluntary isolation of ill persons is recommended on a community-wide basis, although local communities may still choose to tailor their response to Category 1-3 pandemics differently by applying NPIs on the basis of local epidemiologic parameters, risk assessment, availability of countermeasures, and consideration of local healthcare surge capacity. Thus, from a pre-pandemic planning perspective for Category 1, 2, and 3 pandemics, capabilities for both assessing local public health capacity and healthcare surge, delivering countermeasures, and implementing these measures in full and in combination should be assessed.

Voluntary Isolation of Ill Persons

The goal of this intervention is to reduce transmission by reducing contact between persons who are ill and those who are not. Ill individuals not requiring hospitalization would be requested to remain at home voluntarily for the infectious period, approximately 7-10 days after symptom onset. This would usually be in their homes, but could be in a home of a friend or relative. Voluntary isolation of ill children and adults at home is predicated on the assumption that many ill individuals who are not critically ill can and will need to be cared for in the home. In addition, this intervention may be combined with the use of antiviral medications for treatment (as appropriate), as long as such medications are effective and sufficient in quantity and that feasible plans and protocols for distribution are in place.

Requirements for success include prompt recognition of illness, appropriate use of hygiene and infection control practices in the home setting. measures to promote voluntary compliance (e.g., timely and effective risk communications); commitment of employers to support the recommendation that ill employees stay home; and support for the financial, social, physical, and mental health needs of patients and caregivers. In addition, ill individuals and their household members need clear, concise information about how to care for an ill individual in the home and when and where to seek medical care. Special consideration should be made for persons who live alone, as many of these individuals may be unable to care for themselves if ill.

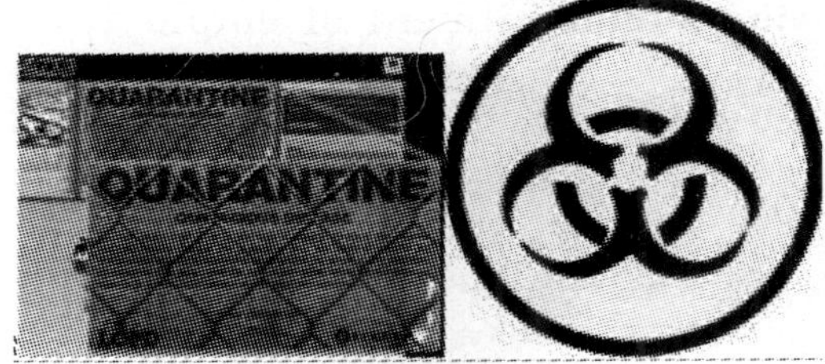

Fig. 29.4

Voluntary Quarantine of Household Members of Ill Persons

The goal of this intervention is to reduce community transmission from members of households in which there is a person ill with a pandemic disease. Members of households in which there is an ill person may be at increased risk of becoming infected with a pandemic virus. As determined on the basis of known characteristics of the disease, a significant proportion of these persons may shed virus and present a risk of infecting others in the community despite having asymptomatic or only minimally symptomatic illness that is not recognized as pandemic disease. Thus, members of households with ill individuals may be recommended to stay home for an incubation period (voluntary quarantine) following the time of symptom onset in the household member. If other family members become ill during this period, the recommendation is to extend the time of voluntary home quarantine for another incubation period, from the time that the last family member becomes ill. In addition, consideration may be given to combining this intervention with provision of antiviral medication to persons in quarantine if such medications are effective and sufficient in quantity and if a feasible means of distributing them is in place.

Requirements for success of this intervention include the prompt and accurate identification of an ill person in the household, voluntary compliance with quarantine by household members, commitment of employers to support the recommendation that employees living in a household with an ill individual stay home, the ability to provide needed support to households that are under voluntary quarantine, and guidance for infection control in the home.

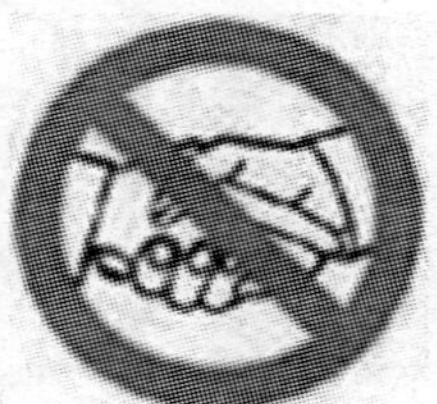

Fig. 29.5

Child Social Distancing

The goal of these interventions is to protect children and to decrease transmission among children in dense classroom and non-school settings and, thus, to decrease introduction into households and the community at large. Social distancing interventions for children include dismissal of students from classrooms and closure of childcare programs, coupled with protecting children and teenagers through social distancing in the community to achieve reductions of out-of-school social contacts and community mixing. Childcare facilities and schools represent an important point of epidemic amplification, while the children themselves, for reasons cited above, are thought to be efficient transmitters of disease in any setting. The common sense desire of parents to protect their children by limiting their contacts with others during a severe pandemic is congruent with public health priorities, and parents should be advised that they could protect their children by reducing their social contacts as much as possible.

However, it is acknowledged that maintaining the strict confinement of children during a pandemic would raise significant problems for many families and may cause psychosocial stress to children and adolescents. These considerations must be weighed against the severity of a given pandemic virus to the community at large and to children in particular. Risk of introduction of an infection into a group and subsequent transmission among group members is directly related to the functional number of individuals in the group. Although the available evidence currently does not permit the specification of a "safe" group size, activities that recreate the typical density and numbers of children in school classrooms are clearly to be avoided. Gatherings of children that are comparable to family-size units may be acceptable and could be important in facilitating social interaction and play behaviors for children and promoting emotional and psychosocial stability.

Children in group care with six or more children are 2.2 times as likely to have an upper respiratory tract illness as children reared at home or in small-group care (defined as fewer than six children). If a recommendation for social distancing of children is advised during a pandemic and families must nevertheless group their children for pragmatic reasons, it is recommended that group sizes be held to a minimum and that mixing between such groups be minimized (e.g., children should not move from group to group or have extended social contacts outside the designated group).

Requirements for success of these interventions include consistent implementation among all schools in a region being affected by an outbreak of a pandemic, community and parental commitment to keeping children from congregating out of school, alternative options for the education and social interaction of the children and support for parents and adolescents who need to stay home from work. Interim recommen-dations for pre-pandemic planning for this intervention include a three-tiered strategy:

1. No dismissal of students from schools or closure of childcare facilities in a Category 1 pandemic.
2. Short-term (up to 4 weeks) dismissal of students and closure of childcare facilities during a Category 2 or Category 3 pandemic; and
3. Prolonged (up to 12 weeks) dismissal of students and closure of childcare facilities during a severe influenza pandemic (Category 4 or Category 5).

Colleges and universities present unique challenges in terms of pre-pandemic planning because many aspects of student life and activity encompass factors that are common to both the child school environment (e.g., classroom/dormitory density) and the adult sphere (e.g., commuting longer distances for university attendance and participating in activities and behaviors associated with an older student population). Questions remain with regard to the optimal strategy for managing this population during the early stages of a pandemic.

At the onset of a pandemic, many parents may want their children who are attending college or university to return home from school. Immediately following the announcement of an outbreak, colleges and universities should prepare to manage or assist large numbers of students departing school and returning home within a short time span. Where possible, policies should be explored that are aligned with the travel of large numbers of students to reunite with family and the significant motivations behind this behavior. Pre-pandemic planning to identify those students likely to return home and those who may require assistance for imminent travel may allow more effective management of the situation. In addition, planning should be considered for those students who may be unable to return home during a pandemic.

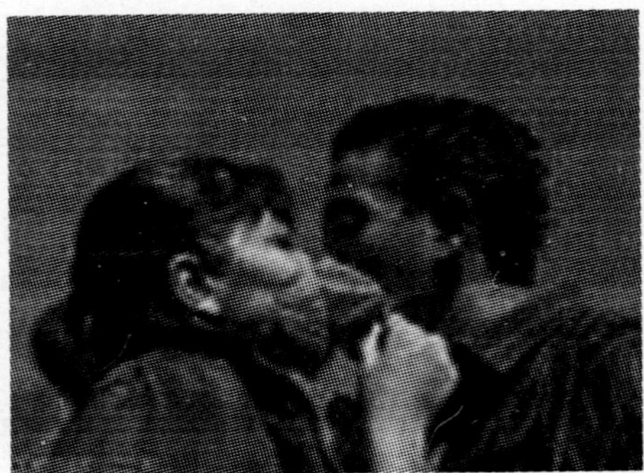

Fig. 29.6

Adult Social Distancing

Social distancing measures for adults include provisions for both workplaces and the community and may play an important role in slowing or limiting community transmission pressure. The goals of workplace measures are to reduce transmission within the workplace and thus into the community at large, to ensure a safe working environment and promote confidence in the workplace, and to maintain business continuity, especially for critical infrastructure. Workplace measures such as encouragement of teleworking and other alternatives to in-person meetings may be important in reducing social contacts and the accompanying increased risk of transmission. Similarly, modifications to work schedules, such as staggered shifts, may also reduce transmission risk.

Within the community, the goals of these interventions are to reduce community transmission pressures and thus slow or limit transmission. Cancellation or postponement of large gatherings, such as concerts or theatre showings, may reduce transmission risk. Modifications to mass transit policies to decrease passenger density may also reduce transmission risk, but such changes may require running additional trains and buses, which may be challenging due to transit employee absenteeism, equipment availability, and the transit authority's financial ability to operate nearly empty train cars or buses.

Requirements for success of these various measures include the commitment of employers to providing options and making changes in work environments to reduce contacts while maintaining operations; whereas, within communities, the support of political and business leaders as well as public support is critical.

Reverse Quarantine / Snow Days / Self-Shielding

Implementation of "snow days" - asking everyone to stay home - involves the entire community in a positive way, is acceptable to most people, and is relatively easy to implement. A "snow day" occurs when winter weather makes travel sufficiently hazardous that officials request that employees/students not report to work/school. In the context of a disease epidemic, a "snow day" would be declared to reduce public gatherings and limit contact among people. Snow days may be instituted for an initial 10-day period, with final decisions on duration based on an epidemiologic and social assessment of the situation. States and local authorities need to consider recommendations to the public for acquisition and storage of necessary provisions including type and quantity of supplies needed during snow days. Snow days can effectively reduce transmission without explicit activity restrictions (i.e., quarantine). Consideration would be given to personnel who maintain primary functions in the community (e.g. law enforcement personnel, transportation workers, utility workers [electricity, water, gas, telephone, sanitation]).

Compliance with snow days might be enhanced by "self-shielding" behavior (i.e., many people may stay home even in the absence of an official snow day. Reverse quarantine involves the sequestration of people to reduce the likelihood of their exposure to the contagion. Short-term, voluntary home curfew is known as shelter-in-place or self-shielding. Self-shielding refers to self-imposed exclusion from infected persons or those perceived to be infected (e.g., by staying home from work or school during an epidemic). There has been essentially no discussion of these measures in the context of pandemic influenza.

The self shielding construct was developed as a response to the threat of terrorist use of biological agents. The essential features are that people will remain at-home for a few days, or for a few weeks at most, and that the disease epidemic is thus aborted, prevented or minimized. Shielding can be undertaken by individuals, families or communities. It constitutes a positive action for the public, and engages them in plans and preparations before an incident. The shielding concept also offers advantages in insuring the continuation of some normalcy of finance, legal, and social institutions. The very planning to remain in the home and community will serve a positive mental health purpose during and following an incident. The period of incubation prior to development of an infectious stage of each disease and the period of disease will determine the required period for quarantine or the alternative of shielding. By one estimate this would range from 7 days for Anthrax to 28 days for Viral Hemorrhagic Fevers.

The purpose of shielding in responding to bio-terror attacks is to allow individuals, families and groups to undertake self-imposed exclusion from contact with the disease state, and infected persons, while encouraging those who are shielding to engage in appropriate routine activities. For those excluded from contact the important criteria will be to maintain a "shielded" status by ensuring no contact with anyone in the quarantine, isolation or asymptomatic groups, and that they self-monitor for signs of disease. In the case of smallpox this self-monitoring requires nothing more than monitoring their body temperature twice daily. If during the course of any 24 hour period the individual develops two successive fevers >101° F (38°C) they notify health department personnel and not have direct contact with other persons until they can be transported to an appropriate facility for further evaluation.

Triggers for Initiating Use of Non-pharmaceutical Interventions

The timing of initiation of various NPIs will influence their effectiveness. Implementing these measures prior to the pandemic may result in economic and social hardship without public health benefit and may result in compliance fatigue. Conversely, implementing these interventions after extensive spread of a pandemic influenza strain may limit the public health benefits of an early, targeted, and layered mitigation strategy. Identifying the optimal time for initiation of these interventions will be challenging, as implementation likely needs to be early enough to preclude the initial steep upslope in case numbers and long enough to cover the peak of the anticipated epidemic curve while avoiding intervention fatigue. The use of these measures is aligned with declaration by WHO of having entered the Pandemic Period Phase 6.

Mortality estimates alone are not suitable trigger points for action. This guidance suggests the primary activation trigger for initiating interventions be the arrival and transmission of pandemic virus. This trigger is best defined by a laboratory-confirmed cluster of infection with a novel virus and evidence of community transmission (i.e., epidemiologically linked cases from more than one household). Other factors that will inform decision-making by public health officials include the average number of new infections that a typical infectious person will produce during the course of his/her infection (*R0*) and the illness rate. For the recommendations in this interim guidance, trigger points for action assume an *R0* of 1.5-2.0 and an illness rate of 20 percent for adults and 40 percent for children. In this context, in all categories of pandemic severity, it is recommended that health authorities activate appropriate interventions when a laboratory-confirmed human pandemic case cluster is reported in their State or region (as appropriate) and there is evidence of community transmission.

Defining the proper geospatial-temporal boundary for this cluster is complex and should recognize that our connectedness as communities goes beyond spatial proximity and includes ease, speed, and volume of travel between geopolitical jurisdictions

From a pre-pandemic planning perspective, the steps between recognition of pandemic threat and the decision to activate a response are critical to successful implementation. Thus, a key component is the development of scenario-specific contingency plans for pandemic response that identify key personnel, critical resources, and processes. To emphasize the importance of this concept, this guidance section on triggers introduces the terminology of *Alert*, *Standby*, and *Activate*, which reflect key steps in escalation of response action. *Alert* includes notification of critical systems and personnel of their impending activation, *Standby* includes initiation of decision-making processes for imminent activation, including mobilization of resources and personnel, and *Activate* refers to implementation of the specified pandemic mitigation measures. Pre-pandemic planning for use of these interventions should be directed to lessening the transition time between *Alert*, *Standby*, and *Activate*. The speed of transmission may drive the amount of time decision-makers are allotted in each mode, as does the amount of time it takes to truly implement the intervention once a decision is made to activate.

These triggers for implementation of NPIs will be most useful early in a pandemic. For the most severe pandemics (Categories 4 and 5), *Alert* is implemented during WHO Phase 5 (confirmed human outbreak overseas), and *Standby* is initiated during WHO Phase 6 (widespread human outbreaks in multiple locations overseas). *Standby* is maintained through Stage 4 (first human case). The recommendation for that State or region is to *Activate* the appropriate NPIs when identification of a cluster and community transmission is made. Other States or regions *Activate* appropriate interventions when they identify laboratory-confirmed human pandemic disease case clusters with evidence of community transmission in their jurisdictions.

Determining the likely time frames for progression through *Alert*, *Standby*, and *Activate* postures is difficult. Predicting this progression would involve knowing:

1. The speed at which the pandemic is progressing; and
2. The segments of the population most likely to have severe illness.

These two factors are dependent on a complex interaction of multiple factors, including but not limited to the novelty of the virus, efficiency of transmission, seasonal effects, and the use of countermeasures. Thus it is not possible to use these two factors to forecast progression prior to recognition and characterization of a pandemic outbreak, and predictions within the context of an initial outbreak investigation are subject to significant limitations. Therefore, from a pre-pandemic planning perspective and given the potential for exponential spread of pandemic disease, it is prudent to plan for a process of rapid implementation of the recommended measures.

Once the pandemic strain is established , it may not be necessary to wait for documented pandemic strain infections to guide their implementation of interventions, especially for a strain that is associated with a high case fatality ratio or excess mortality rate. When a pandemic has demonstrated spread to several regions or when W.H.O. has declared that the world has entered Pandemic Phase 5 (substantial pandemic risk), it may be used to trigger implementation.

Duration of Implementation of Nonpharmaceutical Interventions

Duration of implementation of NPIs is significantly associated with overall mortality rates. Stopping or limiting the intensity of interventions while pandemic virus is still circulating within the community is temporally associated with recrudescent increases in mortality due to pneumonia and influenza in some communities. Total duration of implementation for the measures specified in this guidance will depend on the severity of the pandemic and the total duration of the pandemic wave in the community, which may average about 6-8 weeks in individual communities. However, because early implementation of pandemic mitigation interventions may reduce the virus's basic reproductive number, a *mitigated* pandemic wave may have lower amplitude but longer wavelength than an unmitigated pandemic wave. Communities should therefore be prepared to maintain these measures for up to 12 weeks in a Category 4 or 5 pandemic.

It is important to emphasize that as long as susceptible individuals are present in large numbers, spread may continue. Immunity to infection with a pandemic strain can only occur after natural infection or immunization with an effective vaccine. The significant determinants for movement of a pandemic wave through a community are immunity and herd effect, and there is likely to be a residual pool of susceptible individuals in the community at all times. Thus, while NPIs may limit or slow community transmission, persisting pandemic virus circulating in a community with a susceptible population is a risk factor for re-emergence of the pandemic. Monitoring of excess mortality, case fatality ratios, or other surrogate markers over time will be important for determining both the optimal duration of implementation and the need for resumption of these measures.

It is recommended for planning purposes that a total duration of 12 weeks for implementation of these measures be considered, particularly with regard to severe pandemics of Category 4 or 5 in which recrudescent disease may have significant impact. However, for less severe pandemics, a shorter period of implementation may be adequate to achieving public health benefit.

A three-tiered strategy for planning with respect to the duration of dismissal of children from schools, colleges and universities, and childcare programs is recommended:

- No dismissal of students from schools or closure of childcare facilities in a Category 1 pandemic.
- Short-term (up to 4 weeks) dismissal of students and closure of childcare facilities during a Category 2 or Category 3 pandemic.
- Prolonged (up to 12 weeks) dismissal

of students and closure of childcare facilities during a severe pandemic (Category 4 or Category 5 pandemic).

This planning recommendation acknowledges the uncertainty around the length of time a pandemic virus will circulate in a given community and around the potential for recrudescent disease when use of NPIs is limited or stopped. When cancellations and closures are indicated for the most severe pandemics, thoughtful pre-planning for their prolonged duration may allow continued use of this intervention.

Critical Issues for the Use of Nonpharmaceutical Interventions

A number of outstanding issues should be addressed to optimize the planning for use of these measures. These issues include the establishment of sensitive and timely surveillance, the planning and conducting of multi-level exercises to evaluate the feasibility of implementation, and the identification and establishment of appropriate monitoring and evaluation systems. Policy guidance in development regarding the use of antiviral medications for prophylaxis, community and workplace-specific use of personal protective equipment, and safe home management of ill persons must be fast-tracked and prioritized as part of future versions of the overall community mitigation strategy. As well, developing and delivering appropriate and effective risk communication content and a means for its effective delivery, soliciting active community support and involvement in strategic planning decisions, and assisting individuals and families in identifying their own preparedness needs are critical community factors in achieving success.

Establishing and maintaining sensitive and timely surveillance at national, State, and local levels is critical. Achieving this goal will require enhancing the capability of local physicians and public health authorities to rapidly identify suspect cases of the pandemic infection. This increased capability may be facilitated by the development of point-of-care testing and the appropriate laboratory capacity and ability to transmit specimens and data to reference laboratories.

In addition, establishing protocols for notification and establishing effective reporting and feedback systems to ensure information is shared appropriately with State and local decision-makers is a key requirement. The establishment of electronic mortality records may facilitate the rapid robust reporting of data elements to support the timely and appropriate implementation of NPIs. Similarly, establishing surveillance systems to monitor trends in disease in a community and to provide guidance on adjusting implementation of interventions and determining appropriate durations for intervention are critical component for implementation and will provide valuable data for decision-making around lifting interventions.

Critical issues remain with regard to ensuring both timely implementation and appropriate layering of interventions. Preliminary analysis of historical data and mathematical modeling suggest that the early, coordinated application of multiple interventions may be more effective in reducing transmission than the use of a single intervention. Multi-level exercises to evaluate the feasibility of implementation and identify critical enablers for use of these measures are required. In addition, early planning for appropriate monitoring and evaluation systems to provide assessment of the effectiveness of all proposed pandemic interventions is needed. Policies and plans are required to ensure the availability of rapid diagnostic testing to distinguish illness due to seasonal strains and other respiratory pathogens from illnesses due to pandemic strains. Accurate ascertainment of pandemic cases is needed early during the course of a pandemic to minimize unnecessary application of mitigation interventions and in later stages of the pandemic to ascertain persisting community transmission.

Policies and planning for distribution of antiviral medications for treatment (and prophylaxis) needs to account for local capabilities, availability of the antiviral medications, and systems for distribution that could leverage the combined capabilities of public health organizations, the private sector, community organizations, and local governments. As well, guidance for community- and workplace-specific use of personal protective equipment is required, as are policies and planning to support their use.

Clear and consistent guidance is required for planning for home care of ill individuals, such as when and where to seek medical care, how to safely care for an ill individual at home, and how to minimize disease transmission in the household. In addition, guidance is required for appropriate use of community resources, such as home healthcare services, telephone care, the emergency telephone system, emergency medical services, and triage services (nurse-advice lines, self-care guidance, and at-home monitoring systems) that could be deployed to provide resources for home care.

Community engagement is another critical issue for successful implementation and includes building a foundation of community preparedness to ensure compliance with pandemic mitigation measures. Community planners should use media and trusted sources in communities to (1) explain the concepts of pandemic preparedness, (2) explain what individuals and families can do to be better prepared; and (3) disseminate clear information about what the public may be asked to do in the case of a pandemic. In addition, developing and delivering effective risk communications in advance of and during a pandemic to guide the public in following official recommendations and to minimize fear and panic will be crucial to maintaining public trust.

Assessment of the Public on Feasibility of Implementation and Adherence

In an opinion poll, approximately 95 percent or more of the citizens and stakeholders supported encouraging ill persons to stay at home, and the same high percentage supported canceling large public gatherings and altering work patterns for the purpose of social distancing. A lower percentage (83-84 percent) supported encouraging the members of households with ill persons to stay at home, and a similar percentage favored closing schools and large day care facilities for an extended period. Overall, approximately two-thirds of both citizens and stakeholders (64-70 percent) supported all of the interventions. Based on the scenario of a severe pandemic, nearly half (44-48 percent) of the citizens and stakeholders supported implementation of the interventions when a pandemic first strikes. However, it is uncertain how the public might react when a pandemic occurs. Adherence rates may be higher during the early stages of a pandemic and adherence fatigue may increase in the later stages. It is difficult to predict how the public would respond to a severe pandemic in their community or how the public will tolerate measures that must be sustained for several months.

Planning to Minimize Consequences of Community Mitigation Strategy

Pandemic mitigation interventions will pose challenges for individuals and families, employers (both public and private), and local communities. Some cascading second- and third-order effects will arise as a consequence of the use of NPIs. However, until a pandemic-strain vaccine is widely available during a pandemic, these interventions are key measures to reduce disease transmission and protect the health of the citizens. The community mitigation strategy emphasizes care in the home and underscores the need for individual, family, and employer preparedness. Adherence to these interventions will test the resiliency of individuals, families, and employers.

The major areas of concern derive from the recommendation to dismiss children from school and closure of childcare programs. The concerns include (1) the economic impact to families; (2) the potential disruption to all employers, including businesses and governmental agencies; (3) access to essential goods and services; and (4) the disruption of school-related services (e.g., school meal programs). Other interventions, such as home isolation and voluntary home quarantine of members of households with ill persons, would also contribute to increased absenteeism from work and affect both business operations and employees. These issues are of particular concern for vulnerable populations who may be disproportionately impacted.

However, these and other consequences may occur in the absence of community-wide interventions because of spontaneous action by the public or as a result of closures of schools and workplaces related to absenteeism of students and employees. These consequences associated with the pandemic mitigation interventions must be weighed against the economic and social costs of an unmitigated pandemic.

Many families already employ a number of strategies to balance childcare and work responsibilities. Pandemic mitigation interventions, especially dismissal of students from school classes and childcare programs, will be even more challenging. These efforts will require the active planning and engagement of all sectors of society.

Impact of School Closure on the Workforce

Workplace absenteeism is the primary issue underlying many of the concerns related to the pandemic mitigation strategies. Absenteeism for child minding could last as long as 12 weeks for a severe pandemic. The potential loss of personal income or employment due to absenteeism related to prolonged cancellation of school classes and the need for child minding can lead to financial insecurity, fear, and worry. Workplace absenteeism, if severe enough, could also affect employers and contribute to some workplaces reducing or closing operations (either temporarily or permanently). Depending on the employers affected, this could limit the availability of essential goods and services provided by the private sector and the government, interrupting critical business supply chains, and potentially threatening the ability to sustain critical infrastructure. Workplace absenteeism and the resulting interruption of household income would test the resiliency of all families and individuals but would be particularly challenging for vulnerable populations. The potential impact on society underscores the need for preparedness of individuals, families, businesses, organizations, government agencies, and communities.

Impact of Voluntary Home Isolation and Voluntary Home Quarantine

Absenteeism due to illness is directly related to the rate of clinical illness in the population.

The proposed community interventions attempt to reduce disease transmission and illness rates. As illness rates are reduced, absenteeism related to illness and quarantine would be expected to decline, whereas absenteeism related to child minding would remain constant.

The feasibility of following pandemic mitigation interventions is of particular concern for vulnerable populations (e.g., people who are living alone, the poor or working poor, and the elderly [particularly those who are homebound], homeless, recent immigrants, disabled, institutionalized, or incarcerated). Additionally, the millions of frail elderly individuals who require life-sustaining supports to remain in the community would need additional consideration. Planning should begin now to include solutions to address the needs of the frail elderly. Communities will need to plan for how these vital supports can continue for this population as well as for other groups with unique physical and mental challenges in light of efforts to protect lives and limit the spread of disease.

Strategies to Minimize Impact of Workplace Absenteeism

Solutions or strategies for minimizing the impact of dismissal of students from school and closure of childcare programs and workplace absenteeism may include the following:

1. Employing child-minding strategies to permit continued employment.
2. Employing flexible work arrangements to allow persons who are minding children or in quarantine to continue to work.
3. Minimizing the impact on household income through income replacement; and
4. Ensuring job security.

In contrast to the unpredictable nature of workplace absenteeism related to illness (unpredictability of who will be affected and who will be absent from work), it may be easier to forecast who is likely to be impacted by the dismissal of students from school and/or the closure of childcare. Impacted families and individuals can be identified well in advance of an event. Accordingly, early planning and preparedness by employers, communities, individuals, and families is critical to minimizing the impact of this intervention on families and businesses.

In a severe pandemic, parents would be advised to protect their children by reducing out-of-school social contacts and mixing with other children. The safest arrangement would be to limit contact to immediate family members and for those family members to care for children in the home. However, if this is not feasible, families may be able to develop support systems with co-workers, friends, families, or neighbors, to meet ongoing childcare needs. For example, they could prepare a plan in which two to three families work together to supervise and provide care for a small group of infants and young children.

Interruption of School Meal Programs

An additional concern related to dismissal of students is the interruption of services provided by schools, including nutritional assistance through the school mid-day meal programs. This would alter the nature of services schools provide and require that essential support services, including nutritional assistance to vulnerable children, be sustained though alternative arrangements.

Strategies to Minimize the Impact of Interrupting School Meals

During a severe pandemic, it will be important for individuals and families to plan to have extra supplies on hand, as people may not be able to get to a store, stores may be out of supplies, and other services (e.g., community soup kitchens and food pantries) may be disrupted. Communities and families with school-age children who rely on school meal programs should anticipate and plan as best they can for a disruption of these services and school meal programs for up to 12 weeks.

This may be particularly challenging for families with children who already depend on a number of these programs. Plans to address community nutrition assistance needs during a pandemic have to be worked out like an alternate supply and delivery of food through commercial markets.

School Resources Available for Community Service

If students are dismissed from school but schools remain open, school- and education-related assets, including school buildings, school kitchens, school buses, and staff, may continue to remain operational and potentially be of value to the community in many other ways. In addition, faculty and staff may be able to continue to provide lessons and other services to students by television, radio, mail, Internet, telephone, or other media. Continued instruction is not only important for maintaining learning but also serves as a strategy to engage students in a constructive activity during the time that they are being asked to remain at home.

Testing and Exercising Community Mitigation Interventions

Because pandemics occur rarely, drills and exercises are required to test plans and to maintain response proficiency. Such real-world operational experience could yield invaluable empirical evidence regarding how readily particular pandemic mitigation measures might be implemented and how well they might work if applied on a larger scale and/or for longer duration. Drills and exercises permit individuals and organizations to carry out their normal duties and relate to each other under unusual circumstances in simulated environments that are far less costly and threatening than real events.

Discussion-based exercises (e.g., tabletop exercises) are a first step to help identify "gaps" in the plan, policies, protocols, processes, and procedures, included in planning for pandemic mitigation interventions. Such gaps should be filled before expensive, resource-intense, operations-based drills and exercises are conducted. For example, developing community communications plans to notify the public about the status of a pandemic, what protective actions should be taken, and where to seek medical advice during a pandemic, as well as planning for distribution of antiviral medications, determining the process for dismissal of students from schools and closure of childcare facilities, and planning for possible closure of mass gatherings should be decided before conducting a full-scale exercise.

As responders practice the plan through exercising, they learn which aspects of response do not go "as planned." After the exercise, responders debrief ("hot wash") and create an after-action-report to describe corrective actions to fix response problems, including who is responsible for fixing what by when (a "corrective action plan"). Proposed solutions should be re-tested to ensure that they adequately correct the response problem.

Research Needs

This agenda should include conducting studies to gain more knowledge of the epidemiology of pandemic infectious organisms, the effectiveness of community-based interventions, the use of medical countermeasures that complement community strategies, the modification of existing mathematical modeling to include adverse societal consequences, and the development of new modeling frameworks to assess the effectiveness of interventions. Key areas for further research include the following:

- *Enhancing epidemiologic and laboratory surveillance*: A high priority must be given to the development of more timely surveillance for laboratory-confirmed cases of human infections with pandemic potential viruses, methods to rapidly estimate the excess mortality rate during a pandemic, better use of existing electronic data sources, and the development of platforms that can be used to assess the effectiveness of pandemic interventions, including vaccines, antiviral medications, and NPIs.
- *Development of rapid diagnostics:* The development of sensitive and specific point-of-care rapid tests for viruses with pandemic potential may play an important role in pandemic preparedness. Laboratory diagnosis of influenza is critical for treatment, prophylaxis, surveillance, vaccine development and efficacy, and the timing of the initiation of pandemic mitigation strategies.
- *Measurement of effectiveness of personal protective equipment (PPE, e.g., surgical masks and respirators) in community settings:* Quantification of the effectiveness of PPE for infection prevention, the ability of community members to correctly use PPE, the relative benefit of fit-testing for respirator-use in community settings, the utility of PPE for children and the elderly for whom PPE is not currently designed, and the relative contribution of PPE to safety in the context of other NPIs should be undertaken.
- *Determination of markers to signal that it might be appropriate to end or lift pandemic mitigation interventions:* Pandemic mitigation measures may be employed in communities until sufficient vaccine is available to that population or until other parameters are reached. Retrospective and other studies could provide detailed information regarding these predictive factors.
- *Advancing the knowledge base on pharmaceutical interventions:* Antiviral medications and vaccines are integral components of pandemic mitigation strategies. Availability and use of medications can complement the effectiveness of voluntary isolation and quarantine and enhance compliance within communities. Therefore, the capacity to rapidly obtain data on antiviral and vaccine effectiveness, the development of resistance, and the assessment of distribution dynamics is important to successful implementation of pandemic mitigation strategies.
- *Determination, through prospective field studies, of the effectiveness of interventions required to achieve reduced transmission:* The evidence base for most of the interventions currently suggested for use is based on historic reviews, common sense, and biological plausibility. Given the socioeconomic ramifications of pandemic mitigation interventions, such as social distancing measures for children and adults, adherence with prolonged use of interventions is likely to be limited. Therefore, in addition to the assessment of effectiveness, studies should also be done to assess factors that promote compliance and the optimal duration of interventions.

- *Improved understanding of fundamental questions of viral transmission and epidemiology:* Prospective epidemiological studies to address gaps in understanding of infection epidemiology and transmission and the natural history of disease may guide the application of NPIs in the community.
- *Improved understanding of environmental factors that may influence influenza survival and transmissibility:* Studies to elucidate the impact of temperature, humidity, radiation, seasonality, and other factors and their relation to viral transmission in communities are needed to identify complementary mitigation interventions.
- *Improved measures of uncertainty with regard to parameter and model estimates for mathematical modeling of NPIs:* Development of improved metrics of uncertainty around interpretation of modeling outputs may more appropriately guide the incorporation of modeling results into development of policy for community use of these measures.
- *Characterize and determine the potential psychosocial sequelae of voluntary home quarantine and social distancing strategies:* Investigation of the use of home quarantine and social distancing strategies in simulations and in severe seasonal influenza outbreaks could determine key issues that might arise during a severe pandemic requiring long-term social distancing strategies and might suggest possible strategies to reduce untoward effects. Studies that focus on incidences of school closure that might be used for other disease outbreaks might help to better understand facilitators and barriers to adherence with public health recommendations.

CONCLUSIONS

The goals of planning for a pandemic are to save lives and to reduce adverse personal, social, and economic consequences of a pandemic; however, it is recognized that even the best plans may not completely protect everyone. Such planning must be done at the individual, local, tribal, State, Central, and international levels, as well as by businesses and employers and other organizations, in a coordinated manner. Interventions intended for mitigating a pandemic pose challenges for individuals and families, employers (both public and private), schools, childcare programs, colleges and universities, and local communities. Pre-pandemic, scenario-based planning offers an opportunity to better understand and weigh the benefits of possible interventions as well as identify strategies to maximize the number of people protected while reducing, to the greatest extent possible, the adverse social, logistical, and economic effects of proposed interventions.

The early use of combinations of NPIs that are strategically targeted, layered, and implemented in a coordinated manner across neighboring jurisdictions and tailored to the severity of the pandemic is a critical component of a comprehensive strategy to reduce community disease transmission and mitigate illness and death. The Pandemic Severity Index must be the criterion for categorizing the severity of a pandemic as this is designed to enable better forecasting of the impact of a pandemic and allows for fine-tuning the selection of the most appropriate tools and interventions, balancing the potential benefits against the expected costs and risks. Decision-makers may find the Pandemic Severity Index useful in a wide range of pandemic planning scenarios beyond pandemic mitigation, including, for example, in plans for assessing the role for pre-pandemic vaccine or estimating medical ventilator supply and other healthcare surge requirements.

This planning guidance should be viewed as a dynamic process that will be revisited and refined on a regular basis and informed by new knowledge gained from research, exercises, and practical experience. The array of public health measures available for pandemic mitigation is also evolving, and future versions of this document will need to incorporate the changing landscape. These include the role and further development of point-of-care rapid diagnostics, antiviral medications, pre-pandemic vaccines, face mask and respirator use in community settings, and home-care infection control management strategies. The development of sensitive and specific diagnostic tests for pandemic strains not only enables a more efficient use of antiviral medication for treatment and prophylaxis but also helps minimize the need for isolation and quarantine for persons with nonspecific respiratory infections. The increasing availability of antiviral medications will prompt new discussions about the role of antiviral prophylaxis for households and workers in critical infrastructure to further reduce transmission potential and to provide incentives to comply with voluntary home quarantine recommendations and for healthcare and other workers to report to work. Changes in the technology and availability of personal protective equipment will influence guidance on community use of face masks and respirators. Guidance for safe management of ill family members in the household should serve to decrease the risk of household transmission of infections and increase the effectiveness of pandemic mitigation interventions.

Planning and preparedness for implementing pandemic mitigation strategies is complex and requires participation by all levels of government and all segments of society. Pandemic mitigation strategies call for specific actions by individuals, families, businesses and employers, and organizations. Building a foundation of community and individual and family preparedness and developing and delivering effective risk communication for the public in advance of a pandemic is critical. If embraced earnestly, these efforts will result in enhanced ability to respond not only to any pandemic but also to multiple hazards and threats. While the challenge is formidable, the consequences of facing a severe pandemic unprepared will be intolerable. Just as communities plan and prepare for mitigating the effect of severe natural disasters (e.g., hurricanes), they should plan and prepare for mitigating the effect of a severe pandemic.

FURTHER READING

1. Institute of Medicine; Committee on Modeling Community Containment for Pandemic Influenza. Modeling Community Containment for Pandemic Influenza. A Letter Report. Washington D.C.: The National Academies Press; 2006, p.1.
2. U.S. Homeland Security Council. National Strategy for Pandemic Influenza Implementation Plan. 2006 [cited 2007 January 23]; ch type of public health intervention raises serious ethical and human rights concerns.

LEGAL AND ETHICAL CONSIDERATIONS IN PANDEMIC MITIGATION

Surveillance is the backbone of public health, providing the data necessary to understand an epidemic threat and to inform the public, provide early warning, describe transmission characteristics and incidence and prevalence, and assist a targeted response. Surveillance strategies include rapid diagnosis, screening, reporting, case management reporting, contact investigations, and the monitoring of trends. It is clear that surveillance is necessary to quickly identify and respond to a pandemic. The revised International Health Regulations (IHR) require member states to notify WHO of all events which may constitute a "public health emergency of international concern". Consequently, once a country identifies a signal suggesting human-to-human transmission, the country is expected to begin investigations immediately and simultaneously to notify WHO of the event. Surveillance thus comprises a crucial element of the early response to a forming pandemic.

But because governments must collect sensitive health information from patients, travellers, migrants, and other vulnerable populations, surveillance also poses privacy risks. The IHR requires states to keep data "confidential and processed anonymously as required by national law", but in a crisis it can sometimes be necessary to disclose certain information without any undue delay. In such a situation, when the immediate use of the information is necessary for an important public health purpose, disclosure can be warranted, but the identity of the affected person should be protected as much as possible. A breach of the right to privacy can result not only in economic harms, such us unemployment or loss of insurance or housing, but also in social and psychological harms. For that reason, if information is released outside of the public health system, it is particularly important to avoid the inclusion of any uniquely identifiable characteristics, such as names, government identification numbers, fingerprints, or phone numbers. Cases should stay anonymous or encrypted when reasonably feasible. In every situation the rights to privacy and personal autonomy require that only the minimum amount of information necessary to achieve the goal should be released and to as few people as possible. Dignity and respect for the person should be protected.

Screening and testing can pose serious threats to a person's privacy and bodily integrity. Ideally, public health officials should receive an individual's informed consent before performing any medical tests, and education programs can help convince many people to agree to voluntary testing, but there may be rare times when mandatory testing is necessary to advance the public good. In such cases, interference with the right to bodily integrity and with the right to refuse testing may be permissible when the mandatory testing policy is clearly necessary and effective in protecting the public health, when it is performed by competent public health officials, and when the least intrusive means are used. At a minimum, compulsory testing should be limited to individuals known or at least suspected to be infected and should be done in a fair and nondiscriminatory way. The people whose privacy and autonomy are being infringed should be informed of the reasons for the infringement. And in all cases compulsion should be the last resort and used only if voluntary or less restrictive means are ineffective.

Community Hygiene and Hospital Infection Control

Hygienic measures to prevent the spread of respiratory infections are broadly accepted and have been widely used in pandemics, although with uncertain benefits. These hygienic methods include hand-washing, disinfection, the use of personal protective equipment (PPE) such as masks, gloves, gowns, and eye protection, and respiratory hygiene, such as the use of proper etiquette for coughs, sneezes and spitting.

It is important that the public be informed of the need for hygienic measures, and that accurate information, including the uncertainty of the effectiveness of the recommended interventions, be provided. Furthermore, a consideration for personal dignity implies that individuals should be provided with adequate information to make informed decisions about their own health. Public education campaigns should be grounded in the science of risk communication, as the acceptability of health measures is vital to community adherence. The information disseminated through public education campaigns should be accurate, clear, uncomplicated, not sensationalistic or alarmist, and as reassuring as possible (SARS Commission, 2006). Past experience shows that one consistent response to epidemics has been to decrease social mixing and increase social distance by such means as community restrictions and voluntary social separation (WHO, 2005d; Stern and Markel, 2004). There is some limited evidence that school closings do reduce seasonal influenza transmission, and it is assumed—although but not proven—that other limits on social mixing also slow the spread of respiratory disease (World Health Organization Writing Group, 2006). Thus societies faced with pandemics have often closed public places (schools, childcare, workplaces, mass transit) and cancelled public events (sports, arts, conferences). As fear rises, the public itself may shun public gatherings. Predicting the effect of policies to increase social distance is difficult, as infected persons and their contacts may be displaced into other settings, and individuals may voluntarily separate in response to perceived risk.

Social separation, particularly for long durations, can cause loneliness and emotional detachment, disrupt social and economic life, and infringe individual rights. Community restrictions raise profound questions about the government's right to interfere in such areas as faith (by, for instance, limiting religious gatherings), family (with, for example, restrictions on funeral attendance), and protection of the vulnerable (e.g., by making it more difficult to visit vulnerable individuals and provide them with food, water, clothing, or medical care).

Legal and logistical questions that need to be addressed are:

- Who has the power and under what criteria to order closings, and for what period of time?
- What threshold of disease should trigger closings, and should thresholds be different for different entities?
- Under what circumstances should compensation for closings be paid?
- What should the penalties be for non-compliance?

One fear is that governments might put into effect restrictions on personal liberties that are unnecessary—implementing restrictions before they are needed, extending them past the end of the crisis, or enacting restrictions that do nothing to decrease disease transmission. In such situations, closings would not meet the appropriate standards for either necessity or proportionality. Furthermore, it is important to remember that the cost of restrictive policies will be borne most heavily by those with the fewest resources, so errant social-distancing actions have distributive-justice implications. A final worry is that governments might use social distancing in a discriminatory fashion, scapegoating ethnic or religious minorities, or that governments might use social distancing as a pretext to crack down on dissidents who assemble to protest.

Ideally, questions of government authority and accountability should be answered by policy decisions made in an open and transparent process that encourages input from all portions of society and that is carried out before a pandemic hits. Governments should explicitly define who has the power to order social distancing strategies and for what period of time. Governments should also clearly state the criteria under which such power is exercisable and delineate the legitimate bases for any differential treatment. Penalties should be proportional to offenses and not based on irrational fears or discriminatory beliefs.

On the other hand, one must recognize that detailed pandemic preparations will often not be the highest priorities for countries dealing with important and more immediate concerns. Furthermore, some countries lack the legal and governmental infrastructures to implement such an ideal plan as is outlined above. In such countries, completely determining issues of government authority and accountability prior to a pandemic may be extremely difficult. One should also note that pandemics are difficult to predict, and information acquired as a pandemic evolves may render some of what was previously believed about various social-distancing strategies obsolete.

At the very least, though, governments should dedicate themselves to non-discrimination and transparency before a pandemic occurs. It is important that governments implement social-distancing policies fairly and with as broad involvement in planning as possible. This will not only make it more likely that the appropriate ethical considerations have been taken into account, but it will also improve the likelihood that the public will accept social distancing as a means to slow disease transmission. And, since compliance with social-distancing instructions will be difficult to enforce, public acceptance will be critical to such a measure's success.

Workplace and School Closings

Workplace and school closings present particularly difficult ethical issues. Apart from the uncertainty of their effectiveness, the most important issues center on the subject of distributive justice. Workplaces are vital to the livelihoods of both employers and employees, so closing them can cause severe financial hardships. In extreme cases, lost profits caused by closings may push companies to go out of business, leading to job losses and other economic hardships. Even for people who have an economic safety net, these problems can have a significant effect, but for people living at a subsistence level the effect of lost income can be far worse. If workplaces stay closed for a significant amount of time, such people may be unable to pay for shelter, food, or medicine. Similar issues are raised by school closings, which may require parents to stay at home in order to care for young children.

Ideally, public health authorities should work cooperatively with businesses, schools, and communities prior to an emergency in an effort to establish mutually agreeable closure procedures. Though governments should retain the legal power to enforce closings if absolutely necessary, it would be preferable to subsidize lost profits and incomes as necessary in order to create incentives for complying with closure requests. The latter approach was used extensively in countries affected by SARS for people placed in quarantine Practical constraints may sometimes make this approach impossible. The governments of many countries have more pressing needs than addressing a potential pandemic. Furthermore, some countries may be financially unable to provide compensation for closure. In 1918 each of the waves of the pandemic lasted for several months, and most locations were hit by multiple waves. The amount of resources needed to compensate for lost income or profits for this amount of time will be out of the reach of many of the world's governments.

In light of these constraints, governments should at least make a serious effort to weigh the risks to health and welfare from workplace closings and other social-distancing measures against those risks of disease transmission that the closings might mitigate. In different locations the balance of risks may be resolved differently, depending on resources and the number of people living at or below a subsistence level. Countries should consider tactical closures if necessary, such as closing only those entities that most facilitate transmission. For example, schools have been identified as a primary driver of seasonal influenza, and some believe that closing schools will slow the spread of a pandemic. Countries might also consider using closings as a means to buy time for other preparations; closings could be put in place until the level of disease in a community exceeds a predetermined level and then relaxed, with the hope of slowing the initial spread of disease through the community.

Provision of Necessities

If people are instructed to avoid public places, such as markets, stores, and pharmacies, or if those places are required to close, there will be a need for people to procure food, medicine, and other necessities in some other way. Similarly, shutting down mass transit may prevent people from being able to get to those facilities that do remain open, and it could prevent some people from being able to seek medical care. Such a situation also raises distributive-justice concerns since those people with the least resources will be least likely to be able to procure additional resources before closings occur.

Ideally governments would set up networks for the distribution of necessary provisions to citizens' homes, with a particular focus on those most in need. Such distribution should be consistent and reliable, and it should provide necessities such as food and medicine for the duration of social-distancing measures. It should also be conducted in such a manner as to minimize interaction with potentially infectious people, and those people responsible for distributing provisions should use infection-control precautions to decrease the likelihood that they will spread disease. Transportation for medical care should be provided as needed by personnel who are apprised of the risks involved in transporting potentially infectious people; these personnel should be provided with protective equipment that will allow them to guard themselves from the disease and to avoid spreading it to others. Similarly, a program should be put in place for the removal of bodies from homes in a safe and efficient manner.

Resource constraints and logistical difficulties are likely to impede such a program in many areas. Many governments may lack the resources to provide food, medicine, and other necessities to its citizens during a pandemic. Even if the resources are available, the workforce needed to conduct distribution may be absent, especially at the height of a pandemic when a substantial number of people would be ill. Furthermore, there may not be enough people willing to interact closely with potentially infectious people to allow such a system to function. Shortages of personnel may be especially likely for medical transport and mortuary services.

At the very least, governments should do what they can to facilitate the provision of resources before an area is hit by disease. To the extent possible governments should give advance warning of disease and make

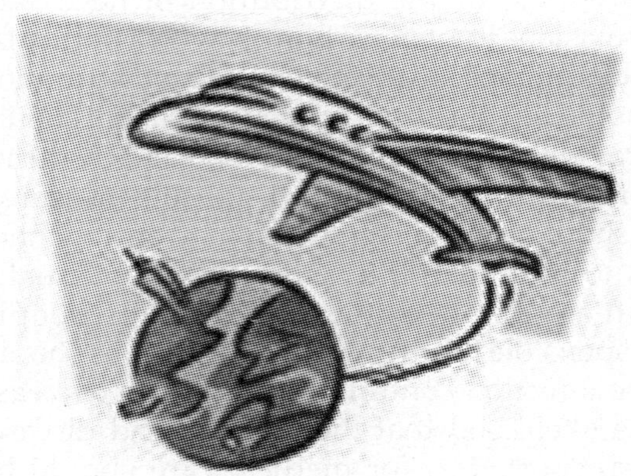

Fig. 29.7

recommendations about what food, medicine, and other supplies should be stockpiled and in what quantities. If they are able, governments should provide such necessities for people unable to afford them on their own. Governments should provide access to medical care to the greatest extent possible, perhaps by reassigning public safety officers to this purpose. Governments should also provide a means by which people who have recovered from influenza—and who thus presumably would be immune—could volunteer to assist others in the provision of necessities.

International Travel and Border Controls

Transnational public health law has become increasingly important in global health, as evidenced by the WHO's International Health Regulations and by national health agencies' proposed communicable disease regulations (HHS, 2005a). These legal initiatives reflect WHO recommendations for border controls (WHO, 2004; IOM, 2005). Transnational containment measures can be far-reaching: entry or exit screening, reporting, health-alert notices, collection and dissemination of passenger information, travel advisories or restrictions, and physical examination or management of sick or exposed individuals. These kinds of powers were exercised in Asia and North America during the SARS outbreaks, although their effectiveness has not been established. The IHR also authorizes a variety of sanitary measures at borders and on conveyances, including inspection, fumigation, disinfection, pest extermination, and destruction of infected or contaminated animals or goods (HHS, 2005b). Although border protection is permitted, it can severely disrupt travel, trade, and tourism, and it should be balanced against the global economic impact.

Controls placed on international travel can also infringe upon civil liberties. The freedom of movement is a basic right protected by national laws and international treaties, but it is subject to limits when necessary for the public's health. In particular, some of these limits can present serious risks to privacy. For example, containment measures may require the travel industry to collect and disclose passenger data (CDC, 2005b). Such infringements on privacy rights can be justified only if there is a genuine need to obtain high-quality surveillance data and if the infringements are carried out in accordance with the fair information practices described in the surveillance section above. To avoid discrimination and to ensure proportionality, public health officials should inform the affected individuals about the reasons for the infringement, the intended use of the information, and the extent to which third parties can have access to the data.

Given the transborder nature of travel advisories as well as the economic impact they can have on affected countries, it should be left to the WHO to issue transparent and clearly justified travel recommendations in accordance with the revised IHR. It is the responsibility of individual countries to communicate all relevant information on the emergence of a public health threat to the international community. This responsibility is related to the surveillance duties and to the issues that accompany them. Ultimately, it is the responsibility of the government to use whatever policy instruments it has available to ensure that it can comply with the requirements of the new IHR.

Isolation and Quarantine

Isolation and quarantine are two of the oldest disease-control methods in existence and would likely be used in at least some instances during a pandemic. While the terms "quarantine", "isolation", and "compulsory hospitalization" are often used interchangeably, they are, in fact, distinct. The modern definition of quarantine is the restriction of the activities of asymptomatic persons who have been exposed to a communicable disease, during or immediately prior to the period of communicability, to prevent disease transmission. In contrast, isolation is the separation, for the period of communicability, of known infected persons in such places and under such conditions as to prevent or limit the transmission of the infectious agent. Quarantine and isolation can be accomplished by various means, including confining people to their own homes, restricting travel out of an affected area, and keeping people at a designated facility. Whatever techniques are used, it is important to treat symptomatic, potentially infected, and non-exposed populations differently. For example, it would be inappropriate to place infected individuals in the same room as those who are only possibly exposed.

Quarantine and isolation are the most complex and controversial public health powers. Given that they involve a significant deprivation of an individual's liberty in the name of public health, quarantine and isolation expose the tension between the interests of society in protecting the health of its citizens and the civil liberties of individuals, such as privacy, non-discrimination, freedom of movement, and freedom from arbitrary detention. Although these civil liberties are protected by both universal and regional human rights declarations and conventions, large-scale public health threats can require extraordinary measures by the government. Coercive public health powers such as quarantine and isolation can be legitimately justified if the public health interests of society are carefully balanced against the freedom of the individual. To pass the balancing test, the benefits to the public should outweigh the burdens or harms that a quarantine may place on individuals. In addition each country should comply with the Siracusa principles, a set of internationally agreed-upon legal principles that establish the conditions under which restrictions on civil liberties are justified (United Nations Economic and Social Council, 1985). These principles hold that restrictions of liberty should be legal, proportionate, necessary, and accomplished by the least restrictive means that are reasonably available. Measures as coercive as quarantine and isolation should only be used when a disease is known through extensive scientific study to be contagious. It should be limited to people who have in fact been exposed to the disease. In cases of scientific uncertainty, however, resource and time restraints can make it necessary for the government to take action without performing medical testing on each individual. There may be situations, for example, in which the availability of accurate tests and competent medical staff is limited. But at a minimum the state's power should be exercised fairly. In a crisis situation, reasonable suspicion based on known contact with the pandemic virus can be sufficient to issue a quarantine or isolation order.

However, to ensure the legitimacy of the measures taken, the decision to use restrictive measures must be made in an open, fair, and legitimate manner. The public has a right to know the legitimate public health reasons for restricting liberty. Public health authorities should fully and honestly disclose their reasons for action and allow community participation. Such transparency will enhance public trust and the acceptance of the proposed containment measures.

Quarantine and isolation should be voluntary whenever possible, and, when that is impossible, they should be enforced by the least intrusive means available. Research in the aftermath of SARS showed that people understood and accepted the need for restrictive measures. Many perceived it as their civic duty and were willing to sacrifice their right to freedom of movement. However, if governments expect full voluntary compliance, the decisions need to be made in an open and fair manner, and society should ensure that those who are quarantined or isolated receive adequate care and do not suffer unfair economic burdens.

When the protection of a community's health requires that individual liberty and autonomy be restricted, the principle of reciprocity obliges society to provide those affected with the necessities of life. During quarantine, these necessities would include being housed in safe, humane conditions and receiving high-quality medical care and psychological support. Recent studies have confirmed that quarantine imposes some serious financial and psychological hardships on the affected individuals. About 30 percent of individuals quarantined for SARS, for example, suffered from posttraumatic stress disorder and depression.

Distributive justice requires that officials limit the extent to which the personal and economic burdens of a public health threat fall unfairly upon individual citizens. A lack of resources and amenities should be addressed in the most fair and equitable possible way. Governments as well as national and international organizations should stockpile medical supplies and food. A pandemic will require solidarity among nations and collaborative approaches that set aside traditional values of self-interest and territoriality.

CONCLUSION

Preparing for a pandemic forces society to face a number of difficult challenges, many of which transcend the issue of mere scientific effectiveness. Public health emergencies raise serious ethical issues which are central to society's commitment to freedom and social justice. Even when effective, public health interventions can have serious adverse consequences on economic and civil liberties. It is vital that individual rights are only sacrificed when absolutely necessary to protect the public's health. As such, laws must clearly establish the criteria under which governments can exercise emergency powers. These laws must also provide adequate due process and ensure that any infringements on individual rights are minimized.

It is crucial that society decide as soon as possible how it wants to respond to these ethical concerns so that in the event of a pandemic we are equipped— scientifically as well as ethically—to deal with its impact.

Given limited supplies of vaccines, antiviral drugs, and ventilators, non-pharmaceutical interventions are likely to dominate the public health response to any pandemic, at least in the near term. Law cannot anticipate the specifics of each public health emergency.

Thorny ethical and legal issues present barriers to pandemic mitigation like issues regarding personal freedom and public good that are implicit in social-distancing measures; the global implications of quarantine and travel restrictions; the need for consistency among various disease-control policies; and the definition of appropriate, measurable "triggers" for when to impose each potential countermeasure.

Strategies for containing smallpox epidemics resulting from bioterrorism based on explicit models of disease. While models cannot replace human judgment, they can better inform our choices, and while they cannot eliminate uncertainty, models can identify crucial gaps in knowledge. Collaboration with medical experts to produce disease scenarios and containment strategies (e.g. for smallpox) make these models more robust than would be possible either through pure computation or through expert opinion alone.

30 Action Plan During a Hazardous Material Accident (Hazmat)

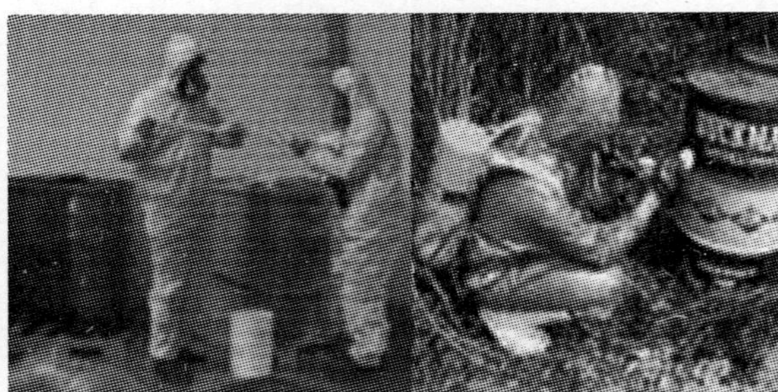

Fig. 30.1

A hazardous materials accident can occur anywhere. Communities located near chemical manufacturing plants are particularly at risk. However, hazardous materials are transported on our roadways, railways and waterways daily, so any area is considered vulnerable to an accident.

BEFORE

- Learn to detect the presence of a hazardous material. Many hazardous materials do not have a taste or an odor. Some materials can be detected because they cause physical reactions such as watering eyes or nausea. Some hazardous materials exist beneath the surface of the ground and can be recognized by an oil or foam-like appearance.
- Find out evacuation plans for your workplace and your children's schools.
- Be ready to evacuate. Plan several evacuation routes out of the area.
- Ask about industry and community warning systems.
- Have disaster supplies on hand like flashlight with spare batteries, portable, battery-operated radio and extra batteries, first aid kit and manual, emergency food and water, non electric(battery operated or manual) can opener, essential medicines, cash and credit cards and sturdy shoes.
- Develop an emergency communication plan.
- In case family members are separated from one another during a hazardous materials accident (this is a real possibility during the day when adults are at work and children are at school), develop a plan for reuniting after the disaster.
- Ask an out-of-state relative or friend to serve as the family contact. After a disaster, it's often easier to call long distance. Make sure everyone knows the name, address and phone number of the contact person.

DURING

If you hear a siren or other warning signal, turn on a radio or television for further emergency information.

IF CAUGHT AT THE SCENE OF AN ACCIDENT

If you see an accident, call the police or the local fire department to report the nature and location of the accident as soon as possible.

Move away from the accident scene and help keep others away. Do not walk into or touch any of the spilled substance. Try not to inhale gases, fumes and smoke. If possible, cover mouth with a moist cloth while leaving the area.

Stay away from accident victims until the hazardous material has been identified.

Try to stay upstream, uphill and upwind of the accident.

IF ASKED TO STAY INDOORS (IN-PLACE SHELTERING)

- Seal house so contaminants cannot enter.
- Close and lock windows and doors.
- Seal gaps under doorways and windows with wet towels and duct tape.
- Seal gaps around window and air conditioning units, bathroom and kitchen exhaust fans, and stove and dryer vents with duct tape and plastic sheeting, wax paper or aluminum wrap.
- Close fireplace dampers.
- Close off non essential rooms such as storage areas, laundry rooms and extra bedrooms.
- Turn off ventilation systems.

Assisting Accident Victims

Don't try to care for victims of a hazardous materials accident until the substance has been identified and authorities indicate it is safe to go near victims. Then you can move victims to fresh air and call for emergency medical care. Remove contaminated clothing and shoes and place them in a plastic bag. Cleanse victims who have come in contact with chemicals by immediately pouring cold water over the skin or eyes for at least 15 minutes, unless authorities instruct you not to use water on the particular chemical involved.

Bring Pets Inside

- Immediately after the in-place sheltering announcement is issued, fill up bathtubs or large containers for an additional water supply and turn off the intake valve to the house.
- If gas or vapors could have entered the building, take shallow breaths through a cloth or a towel.
- Avoid eating or drinking any food or water that may be contaminated.
- Monitor the Emergency Broadcast System station for further updates and remain in shelter until authorities indicate it is safe to come out.

Evacuation

- Authorities will decide if evacuation is necessary based primarily on the type and amount of chemical released and how long it is expected to affect an area. Other considerations are the length of time it should take to evacuate the area, weather conditions, and the time of day.
- Stay tuned to a radio or television for information on evacuation routes, temporary shelters, and procedures.
- Follow the routes recommended by the authorities—shortcuts may not be safe. Leave at once.
- If you have time, minimize contamination in the house by closing all windows, shutting all vents, and turning off attic fans.
- Take pre-assembled disaster supplies.
- Remember to help your neighbors who may require special assistance—infants, elderly people and people with disabilities.

AFTER

- Return home only when authorities say it is safe.

- Follow local instructions concerning the safety of food and water.
- Clean up and dispose of residue carefully. Follow instructions from emergency officials concerning clean-up methods.

DECONTAMINATION CORRIDOR

The following are recommendations to protect the first responders from the release area:

- Position the decontamination corridor upwind and uphill of the hot zone.
- The warm zone should include two decontamination corridors. One decontamination corridor is used to enter the warm zone and the other for exiting the warm zone into the cold zone. The decontamination zone for exiting should be upwind and uphill from the zone used to enter.
- Decontamination area workers should wear appropriate personal protective equipment (PPE).
- A solution of detergent and water (which should have a pH value of at least 8 but should not exceed a pH value of 10.5) should be available for use in decontamination procedures. Soft brushes should be available to remove contamination from the PPE.
- Labeled, durable 6-mil polyethylene bags should be available for disposal of contaminated PPE.

INDIVIDUAL DECONTAMINATION

The following methods can be used to decontaminate an individual:

Decontamination of First Responder

- Begin washing PPE of the first responder using soap and water solution and a soft brush. Always move in a downward motion (from head to toe). Make sure to get into all areas, especially folds in the clothing. Wash and rinse (using cold or warm water) until the contaminant is thoroughly removed.
- Remove PPE by rolling downward (from head to toe) and avoid pulling PPE off over the head. Remove the self contained breathing apparatus after other PPE has been removed.
- Place all PPE in labeled durable 6-mil polyethylene bags.

Decontamination of Patient/Victim

- Remove the patient/victim from the contaminated area and into the decontamination corridor.
- Remove all clothing (at least down to their undergarments) and place the clothing in a labeled durable 6-mil polyethylene bag.
- Thoroughly wash and rinse (using cold or warm water) the contaminated skin of the patient/victim using a soap and water solution. Be careful not to break the patient/victim's skin during the decontamination process, and cover all open wounds.
- Cover the patient/victim to prevent shock and loss of body heat.
- Move the patient/victim to an area where emergency medical treatment can be provided.
- Ensure that the patient/victim has an unobstructed airway. Evaluate respiratory function and pulse. If shortness of breath occurs or breathing is difficult (dyspnea), administer oxygen. Assist ventilation as required. Always use a barrier or bag-valve-mask device.
- Do not induce vomiting (emesis). Administer charcoal as a slurry (240 mL water/30 g charcoal). Usual dose: 25 to 100 g in adults/adolescents, 25 to 50 g in children (1 to 12 years), and 1 g/kg in infants less than 1 year old.

ENVIRONMENT/SPILLAGE DISPOSAL

The following methods can be used to decontaminate the environment/spillage disposal:

- Do not touch or walk through the spilled agent if at all possible. However, if you must, personnel should wear the appropriate PPE during environmental decontamination.
- Keep combustibles (e.g., wood, paper, and oil) away from the spilled agent.
- Use water spray to reduce vapors or divert vapor cloud drift. Avoid allowing water runoff to contact the spilled agent.
- Do not direct water at the spill or the source of the leak.
- If leaking occurs, stop the leak if it is possible to do so without risk to personnel.
- Prevent entry into waterways, sewers, basements, or confined areas.
- Ventilate the area.
- Agents can seep into the crevices of equipment making it dangerous to handle.

31 Action Plan During House and Building Fires

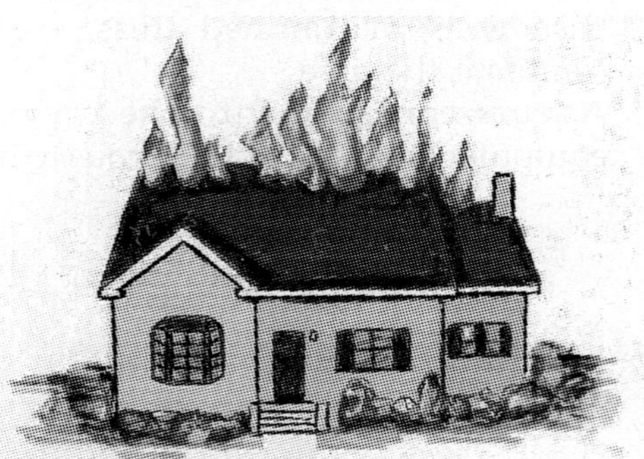

Fig. 31.1

A fire can engulf a structure in a matter of minutes. Understanding the basic characteristics of fire and learning the proper safety practices can be the key to surviving a house or building fire.

HOUSE FIRES

Heat and smoke from fire can be more dangerous than the flames. Inhaling the super-hot air can sear your lungs. Fire produces poisonous gases and fumes that you may not be able to smell. It makes you disoriented and drowsy and instead of being awakened by a fire, you may fall into a deeper sleep. The smoke from a house fire can be so thick that your house would be completely dark in 4 minutes, even with all the lights on! Asphyxiation is the leading cause of fire deaths, exceeding burns by a three-to-one ratio. Fires kill more people than all other natural disasters combined. House fires are often called "silent disasters" since they rarely generate the same publicity as floods, hurricanes and earthquakes. In only 3-1/2 minutes, the heat from a house fire can reach over 1100 degrees Fahrenheit. Death rate from fires is estimated at 14.9 deaths per million population making it the third leading cause of accidental death in the home; at least 80 percent of all fire deaths occur in residences.

Fire is a chemical reaction that needs three ingredients for it to occur:

- **Oxygen:** There cannot be a fire if there is no oxygen.
- **Heat:** Can come from friction, like when a match is struck—or from a spark like when two stones strike each other or an electrical arc.
- **Fuel:** Is anything that is combustible—like wood, paper or cloth.

Substances like petrol, paint thinner or aerosol sprays are fire accelerants. It only takes the fumes from these to cause fire. These fumes are invisible, heavier than air, and sometimes you cannot even smell them. Keeping these things anywhere near a pilot light or source of heat can have disastrous consequences.

Prevention

- *Inspect your home*: You may need someone experienced in home electrical wiring, plumbing (gas), heating, and air conditioning.
- *Electrical safety measures:* Look for improperly grounded plug points. Many modern appliances require a "three pin" (grounded) plug point, but people will

sometimes use an adapter to bypass this safety feature, or even disconnect the earthing point off an appliance cord. Check the power cords for your appliances. Look for missing grounding prongs on the plugs and damaged insulation, and replace or repair them if defects are found. Changing existing circuits to provide grounding is usually a job best left to a professional electrician. Look for overloaded circuit breakers, panel boxes, or fuse boxes. Check for breakers or fuses which may have circuits "piggy-backed" on them. These are rated for single circuit protection, but sometimes in outdated or undersized panel boxes, people will put two or even more wires in the terminal of a single breaker or fuse. Check the vent stacks on gas water heaters, furnaces, and clothes dryers. Check the automatic ignition systems or pilot lights on these fixtures, as well, particularly for any guards which are not properly installed, and for lint or dust buildup in the immediate area around them.

1. Notice flickering lights, or intermittent power surges. These conditions may be caused by outside influences, but if they occur often, they may indicate a bad connection or short in the circuit.
2. Note breakers which "trip", or fuses that "blow" frequently. This is almost always a sign of an overloaded circuit or other wiring problem, usually of a most serious nature.
3. Look at the individual breaker connections, especially in outdoor panel boxes, for corrosion, signs of thermal damage (smut or smokey residue near terminals) splices which are poorly taped or wire nutted, or abraded or damaged wire insulation.
4. Check the ground cable. A failure in the building grounding system and bonding can be dangerous in regard to electrical shock, as well as fire. Look for loose split bolts, clamps, or other connecting devices, and corrosion.
5. Be especially careful to notice any connections in wiring other than copper. Installed correctly, and with tight connections, aluminum wire is not excessively dangerous, but when connections are made to copper wires, an electrolytic reaction may occur, causing increased resistance in the connection which will generate excessive heat. If you are able to apply an antioxidant compound to aluminum connections, it will help decrease the risk of oxidation causing a short circuit at these locations.
6. Look into the possibility of installing a lightning protection system in your home if you live in an area where lightning is a frequent problem. The savings from reduced damages to appliances may offset the cost of this upgrade.

Kitchen Safety Measures

Always stay in the kitchen when using the range for cooking. If you are leaving for just a minute, turn off all the burners on the range. If you are going to the basement for a can of tomatoes, or running out to check the mail, going to the bathroom, answering the phone in another part of the house, simply turn off all the burners. After all, you are just leaving for a minute. You can immediately turn the pot or frying pan back on when you return. Doing this simple step will prevent one of the most common situations that cause house fires: unattended cooking. When cooking with oil, keep a lid or flat sheet close by. If flames appear, simply suffocate the fire with the lid and immediately turn off the stove or fryer to let it cool down. Do not try to move the pan.

Do not use water. The super-heated water will explode into steam, and can cause severe burns, and oil can splash and sputter and spread the fire. Don't cook when drinking alcohol, using drugs, or very tired. Eat something prepared, make a cold sandwich, and go to sleep. Cook your meal later, when you are fully conscious. Keep the range and hood clean. Grease fires are no fun. Keep your stove and oven clean, especially watching for grease accumulation. Check stove vent hoods, clean the filter regularly, and make sure that if it is equipped with an exterior vent, insects or birds do not build nests or otherwise impede the air flow through it. Check the natural gas/LP gas system in your home. You will want to look for loose fittings, leaking valves, faulty pilot lights, and debris or improperly stored flammable materials in areas near these appliances. Have the gas plumbing (pipes), valves, and regulators inspected by a professional any time you smell gas or suspect a leak. Propane has ignition temperatures of 920 to 1120 degrees F; whereas natural gas has ignition temperatures of 900 - 1170 degrees F. Propane gas is thinner than air (and settles to low areas generally); whereas, natural gas (methane) is lighter than air (and rises generally). Both are odorless in their natural state and both are suppose to have odorant added as a warning agent. You are four times more likely to be involved in a fire or explosion using Propane (LP Gas) vs Natural Gas (Methane). You are 13 times more likely to be severely injured or burned with Propane (LP Gas) vs. Natural Gas (Methane). You are more than 100 times more likely to be killed or severely injured if there is a product failure using Propane (LP Gas) vs. Natural Gas (Methane).

Safety Measures for Smokers

Don't sit down or lie down when smoking. Standing up will usually prevent you from falling asleep while smoking. Put out the cigarette thoroughly in an ash tray or water-damp sink and go to bed. Place the ashes from an ashtray in the sink and dampen them, then scoop them up and place them in the trash can away from the house.

Consider having fire alarms, smoke detectors and carbon monoxide sensors as well as a home sprinkler system installed, to extinguish fires when you are away and at home.

Air Conditioning and Heating Safety

Check the air conditioning and heating units in your home. These systems operate with electric motors and air moving equipment which requires periodic maintenance.

- Clean, or have your interior AC coils cleaned, and replace your return air filters regularly. This will prevent the fan motor from being overworked, and also save money on your energy bill. For window AC's, never use extension cords!
- Lubricate belt drive pulleys (where applicable), boss bearings on drive motors, and other equipment as needed.
- Have the resistance coils or furnace burners cleaned and serviced at the beginning of the heating season, since debris may accumulate there while the system is off during the summer.
- Listen to the system when it is operating. Squealing sounds, rumbling noises, or banging and tapping sounds may indicate loose parts or bearings which are seizing up.
- If you have access to a snap-on amp meter, you may check the amperage draw on the high amperage circuit to your heating coils to make sure they are in the normal operating range. Higher than normal amperage draw on a circuit indicates unusual resistance, and in an electrical circuit, resistance is what causes heat, and

ultimately, fires. Check the power cords for your appliances. Look for missing grounding prongs on the plugs and damaged insulation, and replace or repair them if defects are found.

- Keep the lint trap and outside vent clean in your clothes dryer. Some dryers have internal ductwork which may become clogged and require servicing, so if the dryer is operating poorly, have it checked. Lint or other material collecting near the heat coils in clothes dryers is extremely dangerous. Stay nearby while using the dryer. Have a smoke alarm and fire extinguisher nearby. If you must leave the area for a minute, turn off the dryer. After all, you are not going to be away long, and you can immediately turn the dryer on when you return.
- Be very careful with space heaters. Keep flammable materials (curtains, the couch) a safe distance (usually 3 feet) from portable heaters. Set heaters where they are not in the traffic flow of the room. As a rule, extension cords are not recommended with space heaters. Small, low wattage heaters may be an exception, but check the manufacturer's recommendations prior to using an extension cord with one. Be SAFE, just don't use extension cords. Use space heaters only on solid, firm surfaces. They should never be placed on tables, chairs or other places where they may tip over. Replace old space heaters with ones that will automatically turn off if tipped over.
- Maintain your fireplace correctly. Inspect the fire box (hearth) for cracks, damaged sheet metal (for inserts) and other hazards. Use glass fire doors or a wire mesh spark screen to prevent embers from popping out of the fireplace. Burn dry, seasoned wood to prevent creosote buildup in the chimney. Note that some woods, like cedar, pop excessively when burned, and should not be used in an open fireplace. Remove ash and unburned wood only when there are no embers or sparks in the fire box. Place ash in a metal (NOT plastic bucket) and place outside away from any buildings. Have your chimney inspected and cleaned at least once a year.
- Never store flammable liquids near ignition sources. Flammable liquids are divided into two classes: Flammable liquids(like petrol/kerosene) have a flash point below 100° F or 38° C and combustible liquids (like diesel fuel) have a flash point at or above 100° F or 38° C. Ignition sources can ignite vapors that have traveled quite a distance from the actual liquid. Ignition sources are anything which can cause something to burn or explode. These include: cigarette lighters or matches, pilot light on a gas appliance, electrical heaters, electrical switches and static electricity. Gasoline should always, be tightly sealed in an approved container, kept out of the house and out of the reach of children. Seal both the spout on the container and the vent. Never keep gasoline anywhere in the house. Keep it away from the ignition sources, in a detached garage or shed, keep it tightly sealed and away from children. Do not store any flammable liquid in a garage or utility room with that has a pilot light equipped appliance in use in it. Play safe, keep the minimal quantity of these items outdoors, or in a separate outbuilding. Be careful with candles, oil lamps, and other open flame illumination or decorations. Cover the flame with a wire cage to prevent something from falling or blowing onto the flame, and to prevent children and pets from coming in contact with the flame. Extinguish the fire when leaving the room, if even for a minute. After all, you'll be right back, and you can immediately

relight the candle. Use caution with holiday decorations, particularly Christmas trees. Natural Christmas trees are highly combustible when they become dry, and old, damaged, or low quality tree lights cause many fires when combined with an under watered or otherwise dry tree. Watch a video of a Christmas tree fire. It is amazing how fast it can destroy a room, and a home. Teach your children not to play with lighters or matches. Children are often the cause and victims of fires, and should not be allowed access to matches or cigarette lighters. Consider getting a lockable box, and keeping matches and lighters locked up. Do not pile up lawn clippings near a building. Fermenting lawn clippings can create heat, and catch on fire. Barn fires start this way from bales of hay with no electricity; house fires have been started from a pile of lawn clippings. Be careful using a grill on a deck. Decks are flammable. Place non-flammable pads under your grill. Have a fire extinguisher readily available. Stay with your grill while cooking. Turn off propane if leaving, if even for a minute. After all, you'll be right back and can turn on the propane again. Crate train dogs and other pets and use the crates when you are not home to prevent the pets from chewing on electrical cords, or urinating on electrical objects and starting a fire. After using matches quickly place in or run under water to extinguish any invisible flame or heat source that could cause a fire in the trash can. If you suspect or notice electrical problems or strange odors, don't hesitate to have them checked by a competent person. Never store oily rags, especially rags saturated with mineral spirits, paint thinners, or linseed oil. Under certain conditions, these materials may spontaneously combust (start on fire without any known source).

BUILDING FIRES

Accidental fire and explosion can strike anywhere. Fire fatalities tend to be distributed according to population density, i.e., those states with the largest populations tend also to have the greatest number of fire fatalities. Loss of life from fires has been significantly reduced because of improved technology for fire response and a better educated public—particularly regarding the life-saving advantages of using and maintaining smoke detectors. Someone dies in a fire every 40 minutes. Most often, victims are children or the elderly. Nearly 25 percent of the fires that kill young children are started by children playing with fire. Approximately 1,300 senior citizens die in fires annually. Approximately three-quarters of all fire fatalities occur in residential dwellings. Each year, fire causes crores of rupees worth of damage to homes. Fire is the fourth largest accidental killer, behind motor vehicle accidents, falls, and drownings. It is also the disaster that families are mostly likely to experience. Over 80 percent of all fire deaths occur where people sleep, such as in homes or hotels. Most fires occur when people are likely to be less alert such as between midnight and morning. Eighty-four percent of house and building fires are accidental, such as those caused by poor electrical wiring or careless behavior. However, 16 percent are set intentionally through arson or acts of terrorism. The leading cause of death in a fire is asphyxiation. Fire victims seldom see the flames. Fire consumes the oxygen in the air, thereby increasing the concentration of deadly carbon monoxide in the atmosphere. Inhaling carbon monoxide causes a loss of consciousness or death within minutes. A fire can engulf a structure in a matter of minutes. Understanding the basic characteristics of fire and learning the proper safety practices can be the key to surviving a house or building fire.

ACTION AND PREVENTION

a. Develop and practice an escape plan. Make sure all family members know what to do in a fire. Draw a floor plan with at least two ways of escaping every room. Get out as quickly and as safely as possible. Use the stairs to escape. When evacuating, stay low to the ground. If possible, cover mouth with a cloth to avoid inhaling smoke and gases. Close doors in each room after escaping to delay the spread of the fire. Teach your children proper evacuation techniques in case of a fire. Practice family fire drills and watch videos together on fire exercises and escape as one will have very little time in a real fire to make a safe getaway. Fix a meeting place outside (by the tree in the front yard, or at the mailbox or front gate) so that all know that everyone is safely outside. Never go back into a house on fire. Practice alerting other household members. It is a good idea to keep a bell and a flashlight in each bedroom for this purpose. Also practice evacuating the building blindfolded. In a real fire situation, the amount of smoke generated by a fire will most likely make it impossible to see. Feel all doors before opening them. If the door is hot, get out another way. Learn to stop, drop to the ground, and roll if clothes catch fire. If in a room with a closed door where smoke is pouring in around the bottom of the door or it feels hot, keep the door closed. Open a window to escape or for fresh air while awaiting rescue. Signal to rescuers outside by waving a makeshift flag. If there is no smoke at the bottom or top and the door is not hot, then open the door slowly. If there is too much smoke or fire in the hall, slam the door shut.
b. Post emergency numbers near telephones. However, be aware that if a fire threatens your home, you should not place the call to your emergency services from inside the home. It is better to get out first and call the fire department from a location outside the house.
c. Purchase collapsible ladders at hardware stores and practice using them. Install A-B-C type fire extinguishers in the home and teach family members how to use them.
d. Do not store combustible materials in closed areas or near a heat source. Keep the stove area clean and clear of combustibles such as bags, boxes, and other appliances. If a fire starts, put a lid over the burning pan or use a fire extinguisher. Be careful. Moving the pan can cause the fire to spread. Never pour water on grease fires. Heating devices such as portable heaters, wood stoves, and fireplaces demand safe operation. Use portable heaters in well-ventilated rooms only. Refuel kerosene heaters outdoors only.
e. Check electrical wiring. Replace wiring if frayed or cracked. Make sure wiring is not under rugs, over nails, or in high traffic areas. Do not overload outlets or extension cords. Outlets should have cover plates and no exposed wiring. Only purchase appliances and electrical devices that have a label indicating that they have been inspected by a testing laboratory such as ISI.
f. Give first aid where appropriate. Seriously injured or burned victims should be transported to professional medical help immediately.
g. Stay out of damaged buildings as they may have structural damages. Return home

only when local fire authorities say it is safe. Check that all wiring and utilities are safe. Discard food that has been exposed to heat, smoke, or soot. Contact insurance agent. Don't discard damaged goods until after an inventory has been taken. Save receipts for money spent relating to fire loss.

h. Smoke detectors more than double the chance of surviving a fire. Smoke detectors sense abnormal amounts of smoke or invisible combustion gases in the air. They can detect both smouldering and burning fires. At least one smoke detector should be installed on every level of a structure. Test the smoke detectors each month and replace the batteries at least once a year. Purchase smoke detectors labeled by the Indian Standards Institute.

Classification of Fires

- Class A fires are ordinary materials like burning paper, wood, cardboard, plastics etc.
- Class B fires involve flammable or combustible liquids such as gasoline, kerosene, and common organic solvents used in the laboratory.
- Class C fires involve energized electrical equipment, such as appliances, switches, panel boxes, power tools, hot plates and stirrers. Water can be a dangerous extinguishing medium for class C fires because of the risk of electrical shock unless a specialized water mist extinguisher is used.
- Class D fires involve combustible metals, such as magnesium, titanium, potassium and sodium as well as pyrophoric organometallic reagents such as alkyllithiums, grignards and diethylzinc. These materials burn at high temperatures and will react violently with water, air, and/or other chemicals and must be handled with care.
- Class K fires are kitchen fires.

Types of Fire Extinguishers and Their Uses

The two most common types of extinguishers in laboratories are pressurized dry chemical (Type BC or ABC) and carbon dioxide (CO_2) extinguishers. Water extinguishers are suitable for class A (paper, wood etc.) fires, but not for class B, C and D fires such as burning liquids, electrical fires or reactive metal fires. In these cases, the flames will be spread or the hazard made greater! Water mist extinguishers are suitable for class A and C fires.

1. Dry chemical extinguishers are useful for either class ABC or class BC fires (check the label) and are your best all around choice for common fire situations. They have an advantage over CO_2 and "clean agent" extinguishers in that they leave a blanket of non-flammable material on the extinguished material which reduces the likelihood of re-ignition. They also make a terrible mess—but if the choice is a fire or a mess, take the mess! There are two kinds of dry chemical extinguishers:
   - Type BC fire extinguishers contain sodium or potassium bicarbonate.
   - Type ABC fire extinguishers contain ammonium phosphate.

   Dry chemical extinguishers can be quite corrosive to metals such as aluminum and are also potentially abrasive. ABC extinguishers are much more corrosive than BC extinguishers because the ammonium phosphate agent can undergo hydrolysis to form phosphoric acid and because the molten agent flows into minute cracks. For this reason, dry chemical ABC extinguishers are not recommended for use on aircraft or electronics such as computers, MRI scanners, and scientific instruments. They may however be used when there are no other extinguishers available and there is imminent danger to property or personnel.

2. CO_2 (carbon dioxide) extinguishers are for class B and C fires. They don't work very well on class A fires because the material usually re-ignites. CO_2 extinguishers have an advantage over dry chemical in that they leave behind no harmful residue. That makes carbon dioxide (or Halotron I or FE-36) a good choice for an electrical fire involving a computer or other delicate instrument. Note that CO_2 is a bad choice for a flammable metal fires such as Grignard reagents, alkyl lithiums and sodium metal because CO_2 reacts with these materials. CO_2 extinguishers are not approved for class D fires! Carbon dioxide extinguishers do not have pressure gauges because carbon dioxide is a condensable gas. Thus, pressure does not tell you how much agent remains in the cylinder. Instead, the extinguisher should have a tare (empty) weight stamped on it. To determine the amount of carbon dioxide remaining in the extinguisher, subtract the tare weight from the current weight (Fig. 31.2).

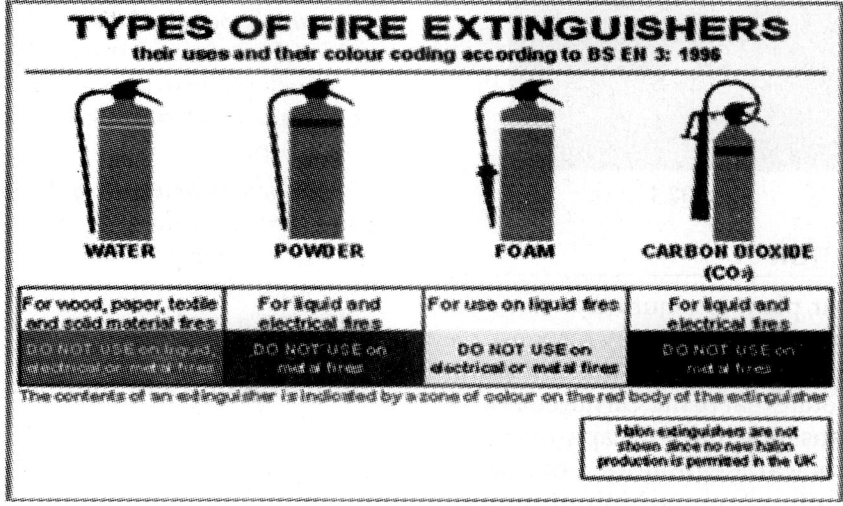

Fig. 31.2

32 Action Plan During a Nuclear Plant Emergency

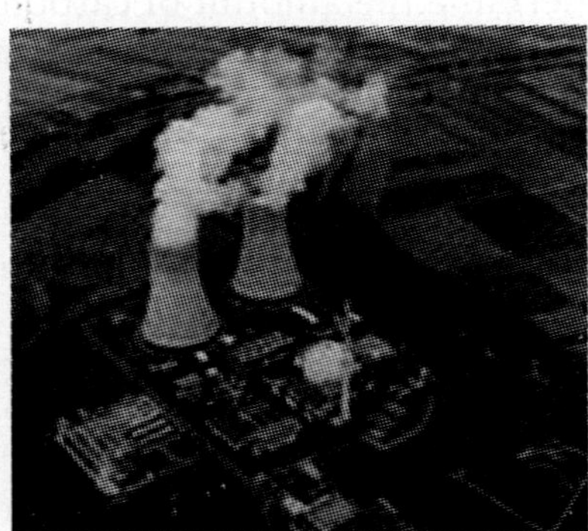

Fig. 32.1

INTRODUCTION

Every nuclear plant is required to have both an onsite and offsite emergency response plan as a condition of obtaining and maintaining a license to operate that plant. Onsite emergency response plans must have the approval of the National Nuclear Regulatory Commission (NRC). Offsite plans (which are closely coordinated with the utility's onsite emergency response plan) are evaluated by the Government and special laws establish the criterion for determining the adequacy of offsite planning and preparedness, i.e., plans and preparedness must be determined to adequately protect the public health and safety by providing reasonable assurance that appropriate measures can be taken offsite in the event of a radiological emergency.

Emergency planning zones (EPZ) are areas around a facility for which planning is needed to ensure prompt and effective action to protect the health and safety of the public if an accident or disaster does occur. The two EPZ for a radiological emergency preparedness program are:

Plume Exposure Pathway (1 mile EPZ): A 1 mile radius around the nuclear plant facility for which plans to prevent radiation exposure of the public from a radioactive plume is drawn up.

Ingestion Pathway (5 mile EPZ): A circular geographic zone of 5 mile radius of the nuclear plant to prevent public from ingesting food and water contaminated with radiation following a nuclear plant accident.

Although construction and operation of nuclear plants are closely monitored and regulated by the Government, an accident, though unlikely, is possible. The potential danger from an accident at a nuclear plant is exposure to radiation. This exposure could come from the release of radioactive material from the plant into the environment, usually characterized by a plume (cloud-like) formation. The area the radioactive release may affect is determined by the amount released from the plant, wind direction and speed and weather conditions (i.e., rain, snow, etc.) which would quickly drive the radioactive material to the ground, causing increased deposition of radionuclides.

If a release of radiation occurs, the levels of radioactivity will be monitored by authorities from Central and State governments to determine the potential danger and issue orders to protect the public.

Radiation is any form of energy propagated as rays, waves or energetic particles that travel through the air or a material medium. Radioactive materials are composed of atoms that are unstable. An unstable atom gives off its excess energy until it becomes stable. The energy emitted is radiation. The process by which an atom changes from an unstable state to a more stable state by emitting radiation is called radioactive decay or radioactivity.

People receive some natural or background radiation exposure each day from the sun, radioactive elements in the soil and rocks, household appliances (like television sets and microwave ovens), and medical and dental x-rays. Even the human body itself emits radiation. These levels of natural and background radiation is normal. The average citizen receives 36 millirems of radiation each year, 30 rems from natural sources and 6 rems from man-made activities (A rem is a unit of radiation exposure) (Fig. 32.2).

Radioactive materials, if handled improperly, or radiation accidentally released into the environment, can be dangerous because of the harmful effects of certain types of radiation to the body. The longer a person is exposed to radiation and the closer the person is to the radiation source, the greater is the risk.

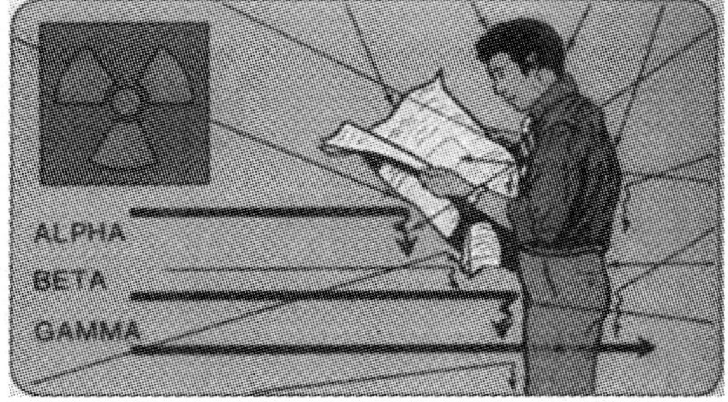

Fig. 32.2: Factors determining radiation received

Although radiation cannot be detected by the senses (sight, smell, etc.), it is easily detected by scientists with sophisticated instruments that can detect even the smallest levels of radiation.

PREPARING FOR AN EMERGENCY

Central, State and local officials work together to develop site-specific emergency response plans for nuclear power plant accidents. These plans are tested through exercises that include protective actions for schools and nursing homes.

The plans also delineates evacuation routes, reception centers for those seeking radiological monitoring and location of congregate care centers for temporary lodging.

State and local governments, with support from the Central government, develop plans that include a plume emergency planning zone with a radius of 1 miles from the plant, and an ingestion planning zone within a radius of 5 miles from the plant.

Residents within the 10 mile emergency planning zone are regularly disseminated emergency information materials (via brochures, the phone book, calendars, utility bills, etc.). These materials contain educational information on radiation, instructions for evacuation and sheltering, special arrangements for the handicapped, contacts for additional information, etc. Residents should be familiar with these emergency information materials.

Radiological emergency plans call for a prompt Alert and Notification System. If needed, this prompt Alert and Notification System will be activated quickly to inform the public of any potential threat from natural or man-made events. This system uses either sirens, tone alert radios, route alerting (the Paul Revere method), or a combination to notify the public to tune their radios or television to an Emergency Alert System (EAS) station.

The EAS stations will provide information and emergency instructions for the public to follow. If you are alerted, tune to your local media stations which includes radio stations, television stations, weather radio, ham channels, mobile phone alerts and the cable TV system.

Special plans must be made to assist and care for persons who are medically disabled or handicapped. If you or someone you know lives within ten miles of a nuclear facility, please notify and register with your local emergency management agency. Adequate assistance will be provided during an emergency.

In the most serious case, evacuations will be recommended based on particular plant conditions rather than waiting for the situation to deteriorate and an actual release of radionuclides to occur.

Emergency Classification Levels

Preparedness for commercial nuclear power plants includes a system for notifying the public if a problem occurs at a plant. The emergency classification level of the problem is defined by these four categories:

Notification of unusual event is the least serious of the four levels. The event poses no threat to you or to plant employees, but emergency officials are notified. No action by the public is necessary.

Alert is declared when an event has occurred that could reduce the plant's level of safety, but backup plant systems still work. Emergency agencies are notified and kept informed, but no action by the public is necessary.

Site area emergency is declared when an event involving major problems with the plant's safety systems has progressed to the point that a release of some radioactivity into the air or water is possible, but is not expected to exceed Environmental Protection Guidelines beyond the site boundary. Thus, no action by the public is necessary.

General emergency is the most serious of the four classifications and is declared when an event at the plant has caused a loss of safety systems. If such an event occurs, radiation could be released that would travel beyond the site boundary. State and local authorities will take action to protect the residents living near the plant. The alert and notification system will be sounded. People in the affected areas could be advised to evacuate promptly or, in some situations, to shelter in place. When the sirens are sounded, you should listen to your radio, television and tone alert radios for site-specific information and instructions.

If You Are Alerted

Remember that hearing a siren or tone alert radio does not mean you should evacuate. It means you should promptly turn to an EAS station to determine whether it is only a test or an actual emergency.

Tune to your local radio or television station for information. The warning siren could mean a nuclear power plant emergency or the sirens could be used as a warning for tornado, fire, flood, chemical spill, etc.

Check with Your Neighbors

Special rumor control numbers and information will be provided to the public for a nuclear plant emergency, either during the alert message, in the utilities' public information brochure, or both.

In a nuclear plant emergency, you may be advised to go indoors and, if so, to close all windows, doors, chimney dampers, other sources of outside air, and turn off forced air heating and cooling equipment, etc.

If You Are Advised to Evacuate the Area

- Stay calm and do not rush.
- Listen to emergency information.
- Close and lock windows and doors.
- Turn off air conditioning, vents, fans, and furnace.
- Close fire place dampers.
- Take a few items with you. Gather personal items you or your family might need.
- Flash light and extra batteries.
- Portable, battery operated radio and extra batteries.
- First aid kit and manual.
- Emergency food and water.
- Essential medicines.
- Cash and credit cards.

Use your own transportation or make arrangements to ride with a neighbor. Public transportation should be available for those who have not made arrangements. Keep car windows and air vents closed and listen to the local radio station.

Follow the evacuation routes provided. If you need a place to stay, congregate care information will be provided.

- If advised to remain at home.
- Bring pets inside.
- Close and lock windows and doors.
- Turn off air conditioning, vents, fans and furnace.
- Close fireplace dampers.
- Go to the basement or other underground area.
- Stay inside until authorities say it is safe.

When Coming in From Outdoors

- Shower and change clothing and shoes.
- Put items worn outdoors in a plastic bag and seal it.
- The thyroid gland is vulnerable to the uptake of radioactive iodine. If a radiological release occurs at a nuclear power plant, States may decide to provide the public with a stable iodine, potassium iodide, which saturates the thyroid and protects it from the uptake of radioactive iodine. Such a protective action is at the option of State, and in some cases, local government.
- Remember your neighbors may require special assistance—infants, elderly people, and people with disabilities.

School Evacuations

If an incident involving an actual or potential radiological release occurs, consideration is given to the safety of the children. If an emergency is declared, students in the 10-mile emergency planning zone will be relocated to designated facilities in a safe area. Usually, as a precautionary measure, school children are relocated prior to the evacuation of the general public.

For Farmers and Home Gardeners

If a radiological incident occurs at the nuclear facility, periodic information concerning the safety of farm and home grown products will be provided. Normal harvesting and processing may still be possible if time permits. Unharvested crops are hard to protect. Crops already harvested should be stored inside if possible. Wash and peel vegetables and fruits before use if they were not already harvested.

Livestock

- Provide as much shelter as possible. Take care of milk-producing animals.
- Provide plenty of food and water and make sure shelters are well-ventilated. Use stored feed and water, when possible.

Three Ways to Minimize Radiation Exposure

There are three factors that minimize radiation exposure to your body: Time, Distance and Shielding.

- *Time:* Most radioactivity loses its strength fairly quickly. Limiting the time spent near the source of radiation reduces the amount of radiation exposure you will receive. Following an accident, local authorities will monitor any release of radiation and determine the level of protective actions and when the threat has passed.
- *Distance:* The more distance between you and the source of the radiation, the less radiation you will receive. In the most serious nuclear power plant accident, local officials will likely call for an evacuation, thereby increasing the distance between you and the radiation.
- *Shielding:* Like distance, the more heavy, dense materials between you and the source of the radiation, the better. This is why local officials could advise you to remain indoors if an accident occurs. In some cases, the walls in your home or workplace would be sufficient shielding to protect you for a short period of time.

What you can do to stay informed

Attend public information meetings. You may also want to attend post-exercise meetings that include the media and the public. Contact local emergency management officials, who can provide information about radioactivity, safety precautions, and state, local, industry and federal plans. Ask about the hazards radiation may pose to your family, especially with respect to young children, pregnant women and the elderly. Ask where nuclear power plants are located.

Learn your community's warning systems. Learn emergency plans for schools, day care centers, nursing homes—anywhere family members might be. Be familiar with emergency information materials that are regularly disseminated to your home (via brochures, the phone book, calendars, utility bills, etc.) These materials contain educational information on radiation, instructions for evacuation and sheltering, special arrangements for the handicapped, contacts for additional information, etc.

33 Action Plan During a Dam Failure or Breach

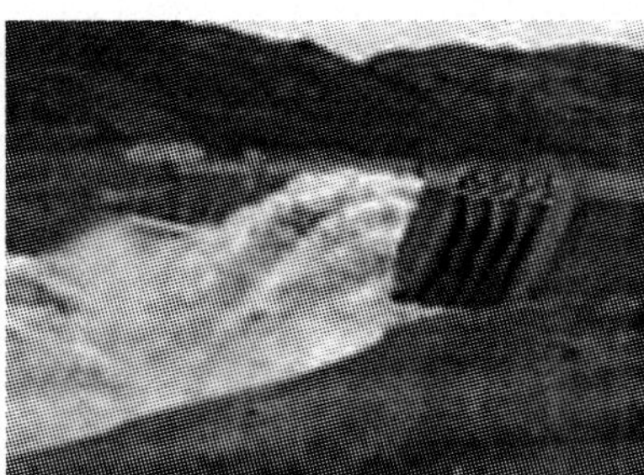

Fig. 33.1

INTRODUCTION

Natural and artificial barrages, impounding lakes or reservoirs possess a residual risk of potential failure. The public, and especially people living downstream a reservoir, have a more critical view on dams and their hazard potential. Even if it is statistical proven, that the risk getting hurt by a dam failure is much lower than the risk getting involved in a traffic accident, it is a legitimate request to get any information about it. This has been enabled by the legislation whereby analysis of a potential dam break including the flood routing is prescribed by law in many other countries of the world. If we consider a real dam, we have to ask how the potential breach formation would occur.

Dam Owner Responsibilities

Dam owners are responsible for safe design, operation, and maintenance of a dam. They are responsible to operate, maintain, and regularly inspect a dam so that it does not constitute a danger to human life or property. The owners of high or significant hazard dams are required to develop and maintain effective Emergency Action Plans and coordinate those plans with local officials. Dam owners are responsible to notify the Dam Safety Section and local authorities at adjacent and downstream communities of any condition that may threaten the safety of the dam. Dam owners must also perform timely maintenance and repair of the dam. During normal operations frequent, routine visual observations of the dam, outlet pipe, and emergency spillway and measurements of seepage rates, piezometer levels, and settlement monument movements must be made. The frequencies pg these inspections should be increased during major storm events, significant earthquakes and when the reservoir is full or nearly full.

Adverse Situations

The following are typical examples, but not necessarily all, adverse, unusual, or emergency conditions that may occur at a dam and should be watched for.

a. *Seepage:* Evidenced by cloudy discharges, increases from normal seepage rates, appearance of new seepages or sinkholes on the crest or slopes.
b. Instability of the dam or foundation evidenced by visible slumping or movement of the slopes, lowering of the crest, or appearance of new cracks.

c. *Erosion:* By wave action against of upstream face or across the top of the dam.
d. Dam overtopping by flood waters.

General Guidelines for Identifying Development of a Potential Dam Failure Situation

- The reservoir level reaches within three feet of the crest of dam and is projected to continue to rise.
- Based on the anticipated runoff from an arriving major storm, the reservoir level is projected to rise within three feet of the crest of dam.
- The spillway or outlet works is plugged and the reservoir level is projected to rise within three feet of the crest of dam.
- The reservoir level reaches within eighteen inches of the top of dam and is projected to continue to rise, or at any time the reservoir level is projected to rise above the crest of the dam.

Abnormal Instrumentation Readings

i. An unexpected drop in the reservoir level of two feet (>2) or more.
ii. Increased or decreased seepage rates may be fifty percent (50%) of normal flows previously established for the existing season and/or reservoir level.
iii. A significant change (two feet or more) of normal levels previously established for the existing season and/or reservoir level.
iv. Settlement monument movements of more than 6 inches vertical or horizontal per year.

Action Plan

- Have a description of the potential inundation area.
- Have an approximate number of residences and business houses to evacuate
- Have details of roads and highways requiring closure.
- Have inundation map(s).

Alert Methods

The failure mode depends firstly on the kind of dam. A realistic scenario could be found in the wide range, between a sudden and total dam break of an arch dam and a slow erosion process especially with respect to earth dams. A knowledge of historical dam break cases could help to find realistic scenarios. The final breach depth and width and the breach formation time are the most important parameters to calculate the outflow hydrographs. One should use not one definite value for each parameter but different values for peak discharge, outflow volume and time to peak. An occurrence probability can then be assigned to each of these values and obtain numerous hydrographs. During an earthquake, a sudden lowering of the reservoir water level or piping can lead to different breach formation mechanisms. In some cases the breaching of one of the two different dam sections can be combined with an flood wave due to a rainfall event. The resulting dam break scenarios and the calculated outflow hydrographs can then be summarized and analyzed to obtain outflow parameters and realistic occurrence probabilities.

In order to estimate the hazard potential of dams and to declare almost realistic flooding areas due to a dam breaking surge wave, a wide range of software are available. If the breach outflow hydrograph is available as well as the upstream boundary condition and a large number of other input data in addition, the dam break wave routing can be calculated, based on specific characteristics and details. In general the calculation of the flood wave propagation is possible using one dimensional or two dimensional numerical models. Since dams are located in mountain regions, the flow path of the surge wave is obviously downstream of the river valley. Two dimensional calculation schemes are necessary in the case of unknown flow paths in more even areas. These are indispensable in dyke break investigations or in the case of dams impounding settling ponds. The outflow through a dam breach is a two phase flow.

ASSESSING THE RISKS

Knowing your risk, making sure an Emergency Action Plan (EAP) is in place, and evacuating when directed by emergency response officials are the most important steps you can take to staying safe from a dam failure.

Know Your Risk

- Do you live downstream from a dam?
- Is the dam a high-hazard or significant-hazard potential dam?

Once you determine that you live downstream from a high-hazard or significant-hazard potential dam, find out who owns the dam, see if a current EAP is in place for the dam. An EAP is a formal document that identifies potential emergency conditions at a dam and specifies preplanned actions to be followed to reduce property damage and loss of life. An EAP specifies actions the dam owner should take to take care of problems at the dam. It also includes steps to assist the dam owner in issuing early warning and notification messages to responsible downstream emergency management authorities of the emergency.

If there is a dam failure or an imminent dam failure and you need to evacuate, know your evacuation route and get out of harm's way quickly. In general, evacuation planning and implementation are the responsibility of the state and local officials responsible for your safety. However, there may be situations where recreational facilities, campgrounds, or residences are located below a dam and local authorities will not be able to issue a timely warning. In this case, the dam owner should coordinate with local emergency management officials to determine who will warn you and in what priority. If you must prepare to evacuate, you should do the following:

- Secure your home. If you have time, bring in outdoor furniture. Move essential items to an upper floors.
- Turn off utilities at the main switches or valves if instructed to do so. Disconnect electrical appliances. Do not touch electrical equipment if you are wet or standing in water.

If you have to leave your home, remember these evacuation tips:

- Do not walk through moving water. Six inches of moving water can make you fall.
- If you have to walk in water, walk where the water is not moving. Use a stick to check the firmness of the ground in front of you.
- Do not drive into flooded areas. If floodwaters rise around your car, abandon the car and move to higher ground if you can do so safely. You and the vehicle can be quickly swept away.
- Listen for news reports to learn whether the community's water supply is safe to drink.
- Avoid floodwaters as these may be contaminated by oil, gasoline, or raw sewage. Water may also be electrically charged from underground or downed power lines.
- Avoid moving water.
- Be aware of areas where floodwaters have receded. Roads may have weakened and could collapse under the weight of a car.
- Stay away from downed power lines, and

report them to the power company.

- Return home only when authorities indicate it is safe.
- Stay out of any building if it is surrounded by floodwaters.
- Use extreme caution when entering buildings; there may be hidden damage, particularly to the foundations.
- Service damaged septic tanks, cesspools, pits, and leaching systems as soon as possible. Damaged sewage systems are serious health hazards.
- Clean and disinfect everything that is wet. Mud left from floodwater can contain sewage and chemicals.

34 Action Plan During Mining Disasters

> "Technology without hatred can be a blessing, technology with hatred is always a disaster".
>
> —*Simon Weisenthal*

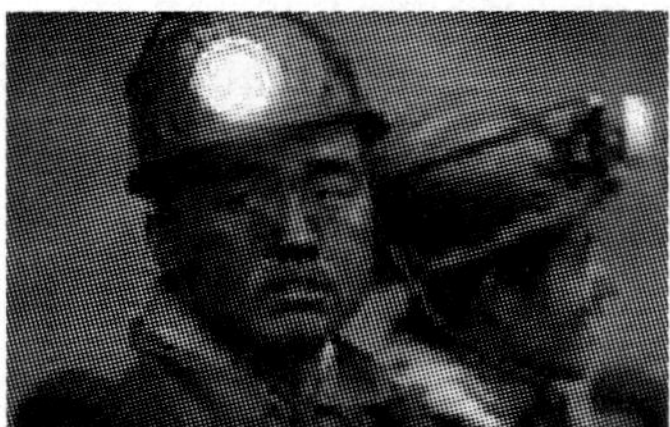

Fig. 34.1

INTRODUCTION

Mining has the highest fatal injury rate of any industry, and ground failures are a significant cause of those injuries and deaths. The reduction of ground failure fatalities and injuries is one of the National Institute for Occupational Safety and Health (NIOSH) Mining Program's strategic goals. Ground control conditions contribute significantly to fatalities in coal mining and, to a lesser extent, in metal and nonmetal mining. Ground failure fatalities range from 11 to 52 percent of the total number of coal mining fatalities per year, while the number of similar fatalities in the metal and nonmetal sectors ranged from 0 to 13 percent per year. Prevention, response, and self-rescue are all of high importance in mining operations to reduce the risk of mine disasters (fires, explosions, and inundations) and also to minimize the risk to, and enhance the effectiveness of emergency responders. Emerging hazards will arise as the production of resources enters into a higher level of geologic complexity. The strategic goal is in alignment with the major current challenges facing the mining industry including fire, explosion, inundation, and ground failure prevention. The overarching goal is to improve the miner's ability to self-rescue in the inherently dangerous mining environment.

The major barriers to accomplishing this integrated strategic goal include the following:

1. An incomplete understanding of the root causes of mine fires, explosions, and inundations;
2. The lack of totally effective engineering controls to prevent, detect, and mitigate mine disasters; and
3. The lack of education and training of the general mining workforce pertaining to methods to predict, prevent, and deal with a mine emergency.

The mining community must be able to maintain and improve mine escape, rescue, and emergency response capabilities through realistic training exercises, development and implementation of new or improved training aids and exploration, rescue, and escape technologies. Research is also necessary to enhance the effectiveness of emergency responders and reduce the risk to those individuals with better tools for the miner to self-rescue. Some glaring deficiencies in the existing protocols for incident management persist. The cell phone age has made it necessary for companies and government regulators to adjust communications procedures, as well as update mine rescue response.

Fire-resistant materials, early-warning devices, aggressive prevention of ignition sources (e.g., spontaneous combustion), fire suppression through improved ventilation, methane monitoring, rock dust evaluation, and degasification are essential. The addition of inert gas to smother mine fires has been practiced by industry since 1949. Prevention of mine inundation is related predominantly to design parameters of stoppings and bulkheads and the application of technology to identify voids and the potential for inundation in advance, for example, via accurate surveying control and geophysical methods. New technologies in such areas as through-the-ground communications systems, miner tracking systems, rescue chambers, new technologies for self-contained self-rescuers, greater oxygen supply on the belt of miners and in storage caches need to be introduced. In situ assessment of geologic conditions, monitoring of atmospheres behind seals, and reevaluation of mining methods would improve safety. Better underground-to-surface communications, communication between rescue teams and trapped miners, and permanently installed seismic systems that could be used on a day-to-day basis and based on real-time data and analysis are necessary. Some of the issues for developments are:

Coal mine operators are required to maintain an incombustible content of at least 65 percent in the entries and 80 percent in the returns. Research efforts have focused on coal dust explosibility and rendering the dust inert through the application of incombustible material. The hand-held Dust Explosibility Meter directly assesses the effectiveness of rock dusting, avoiding a two-week wait for laboratory analysis. Although it will not replace in-depth laboratory analysis, it will provide a more immediate determination of the adequacy of rock dusting and improves safety.

- Better methods of periodic or continuous monitoring of slope movement by evaluating recent advances in radar, photogrammetric, and other methods.
- Ground failure prevention research into blast-weakened materials.
- Minimizing risk to underground workers and potential damage to surface structures associated with mining-induced seismicity.
- The Mining Program should consider ways to improve sophisticated numerical techniques for modeling variously shaped openings in heterogeneous and discontinuous materials at different degrees of saturation.
- The Mining Program should be involved in developing best strategies for deep mining (>600 m).

With a few exceptions, ground failure prevention research within the Mining Program is limited to the reaction of the perimeter of excavations in the earth's crust. Such excavations are produced in the mining of coal, metal and nonmetal, and aggregate. Monitoring of highwalls and slopes in surface mines, avoiding inundations when mining is close to water impounding structures and abandoned mines, surface treatments to improve long-term stability of underground openings, monitoring roof conditions in underground stone mines, and reducing damage caused by conventional blasting and improved understanding of rock mass failure mechanics is required. This would be complemented by the development of better roof surface control technology leading to reduction of rock fall injuries in coal mines will nearly 50%. Better design-based control technology for multiple-seam coal mines is expected to reduce severe multiple-seam interactions by nearly 80%. New ground control technology for mines with low-strength roofs and more efficient standing support systems should minimize roof falls. Introduction of a sensor-based risk management system for roof falls in stone mines would reduce injuries caused by rock bursts. All these technologies can result in substantial safety improvement. Additional work is needed to reduce coal burst accidents in underground longwall operations, especially with the mine roof simulator and rock burst research. The simulator is a critical resource in testing new roof support ideas and has resulted in accelerated commercial development of more than 40 new roof support technologies. Seismic monitoring and basic research into strategies to reduce bursting potential will continue to serve the mining industry in the future. Investigations into blast patterns and rock damage caused by blasting, better understanding of ground falls and development of monitoring systems to detect the onset of instability and wall strain. Electromagnetic emissions and microseismic monitoring are likely to result in identifying rock burst failure mechanisms and warn of impending failure. Studies on the safe limits for roof spans and pillar dimensions and the effect of mine air temperature and humidity on pillar performance, deep-cover coal pillar recovery, high horizontal stress control, and multiple-seam mining should improve workplace protection by producing safer designs. Problems concerning bumps in deep coal mining remain a pressing problem. Development of surface treatments, specifically application of screens, along with methods of avoiding injury caused by installation of screens, and identification of geologic materials that deteriorate with time is directly related to improvements in workplace safety. Rock mass ratings and span widths and the use of fiber-reinforced shotcrete as a surface treatment to improve stability can improve workplace protection.

Slope Stability Hazard Recognition can improve safety near slopes in surface mines and near openings in large underground mines.

- ***Reducing injuries by improving shotcrete design criteria.*** Developing a set of design criteria for application of shotcrete as a means of rock support can reduce the prevalence of injuries and occasional fatalities caused by loose roof rock between primary supports.
- ***Improved pillar design in metal and industrial mineral mines to reduce ground control hazards.*** Recovery of pillars is commonly practiced in the national and international mining communities. Minimizing the size of support pillars in order to maximize resource recovery is worthwhile so long as it can be done safely.
- ***Voiding inundation: Developing guidelines for mining near bodies of water.*** Mining-induced seismicity (MIS) occurs in coal, metal, and nonmetal underground mining. MIS is a serious, potentially high-consequence event that can result in injuries to underground miners and possible failure of water-impounding surface structures. Failure of surface structures is a major concern for coal operations.
- ***Improved mine safety through optimized extraction.*** The extent of damage in the perimeter of mine openings created by conventional blasting is poorly understood. Such damage is

acknowledged as a primary cause of loose rock in underground roofs and ribs and on surface mine slopes. Fundamental research is needed to establish more effective guidelines for blasting practices that focus on reducing collateral damage.

- ***Multiple-seam mining design guidelines.*** A large number of underground coal mines are currently dealing with multiple-seam mining. It is therefore, a worthy topic for further research.
- ***Design of mine ventilation stoppings.*** Current mining law requires that stoppings withstand a transverse load of at least 39 pounds per square foot (psf). Air blast resulting from roof falls or mine explosions can produce overpressure in excess of 39 psf resulting in failure of the stoppings. Failure can precipitate more widespread consequences in the form of pollution of the mine atmosphere with toxic gases and/or catastrophic explosions and fires. This matter deserves further study to improve mine safety.
- ***Roof span and pillar layout guidelines for stone mines.*** A large number of underground limestone mines rely heavily on past practice for roof spans and pillar layout. This needs re evaluation.
- ***Reducing ground fall hazards in coal mines with low-strength roofs.*** Investigating the exacerbating influence of low-strength roofs in a specific geographic region can play a significant role in reducing injuries in the applicable underground environment.
- ***Highwall mining stability guidelines. This needs re evaluation.***
- ***Increasing roof fall forecast times with sensor-based monitoring techniques.*** Increasing fundamental knowledge of how roof falls behave and the development of warning systems is essential.
- ***Reducing ground fall hazards in metal mines with weak rock.*** Studies in ground fall in metal mines has improved mine safety.

MEDICAL PROBLEMS

Methane and Carbon Monoxide Poisoning

Explosions can be sparked by methane gas filling certain areas that are not properly ventilated. Coal-dust explosions, however, present a particular problem, because coal dust is something that is produced at every point in the mining process and accumulates, through the movement of air and the transportation of coal, on the floors, walls, and ceilings of the mine, all the way from the mine entrance to the deepest shafts. Therefore, when a small explosion occurs somewhere in the mine, it is followed by a chain reaction fuelled by the coal dust, and the resulting explosion envelops the entire mine infrastructure. Methane gas has caused tens of thousands of deaths among coal miners. And although methane awareness and safety is improving, it is still a deadly and justifiably feared hazard of the mining industry. The problem is that methane is unavoidable. When coal is mined, fissures and pores in the coal bed are exposed in which methane is lying. The gas is released into a confined area. It is not only highly flammable with the potential to violently explode in a ball of flame but one that is also an asphyxiant, capable of driving out oxygen and causing death by suffocation. A build up of hazardous gas in a mine is known as a damp. Methane build-ups are called "fire damps". Carbon monoxide accumulation, also called "white damp" adds to these dangers. When methane combusts, this highly toxic and flammable gas is generated as a by-product and spreads through a mine's labyrinth of tunnels and shafts. Coal dust also reacts badly to a methane explosion. As part of a violent chain reaction, it can burst into flames in a series of secondary explosions throughout a mine. The properties of methane make it as difficult to detect in a mine as elsewhere. It is colorless, odorless and non-toxic, so there are no obvious physical signs such as coughing or streaming eyes to warn of its proximity (although, as mentioned above, it will cause suffocation if it builds up in a badly ventilated space). Furthermore, it is difficult to assess how much methane is likely to be freed from a particular coal bed – factors such as coal type, the depth of the mine and the geologic age of the coal strata all play a part. Once present in the atmosphere of the mine, methane can be easily ignited. Modern mining equipment includes electric arcs, hammers and cutters that can all generate sparks and open flames – the very things that detonate a pocket of methane gas. This is why American federal standards stipulate that if there is 1.0 percent or more of methane in the working area, miners must immediately shut down all electrically powered tools and other mechanized equipment. Because of these environmental and working conditions, the risks of a methane gas explosion and the possibility of fatalities are greater in a coal mine than anywhere else. The testimony to this is the number of coal mining accidents throughout history and the amount of lives that have been lost. In order to prevent coal-dust explosions it is necessary to keep the dust out of the air by continuously sprinkling the area with water. Alternatively, rock dust, which is incombustible, can be mixed with the coal dust to prevent a chain reaction.

Ways of lowering methane explosion risk can include use of LEL (Low Explosive Level) sensors. These types of devices detect low explosive level gases. They alarm, vibrate, flash lights, etc when they detect a factory set level of gas. Basically LEL sensors let the minor know if he or she is inside a dangerous damp, though these devices have been known to false alarm from other hydrocarbon gases. Also, to alarm, the person operating the device must be inside the gas cloud, where as the laser gun can be used remotely before entering an area. LEL sensors must be bump tested daily and factory calibrated at least every 3-6 months to determine if sensors are still operating properly. Monthly calibration is recommended for coal mining applications.

BPA Laser Methane gas detector :Laser will not ignite methane or coal dust. The hand held device is lightweight with one-hand operation. It gives instant methane gas analysis 10-10,000 ppm-m (0.1 second response time) and is self calibrating, simple to operate, durable and shock and vibration resistant and has remote detection from up to 500 feet away (Fig. 34.2).

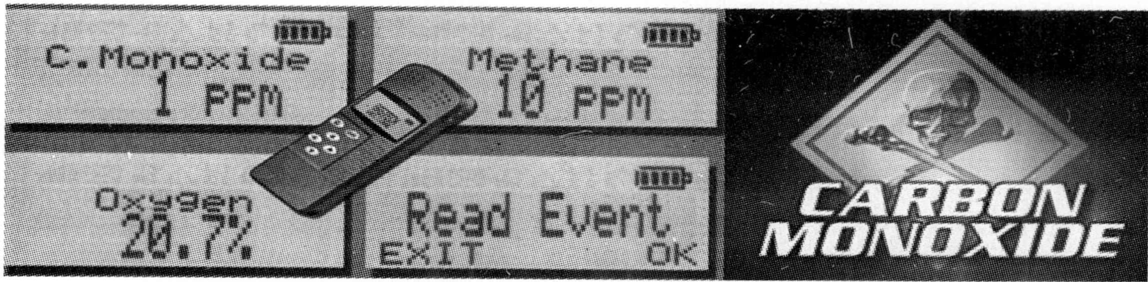

Fig. 34.2

Effects of Carbon Monoxide

- 50 ppm is the max permissible level in a 8 h period.
- 200 ppm= in 2-3 h can cause headache, nausea, giddiness.
- 400 ppm= after 1-2 h can cause frontal headache.
- 800 ppm= after 45 min can cause dizziness, nausea, convulsions.After 2 h is likely to result in coma and death.
- 1600 ppm= within 20 min these levels can cause giddiness, nausea and death < 1h.
- 3200 ppm= within 5-10 min these levels can cause giddiness, nausea, headache and death < 30 min.
- 5400= within 1-2 min can cause headache, giddiness, nausea and death <15 min.
- 12800 ppm= will be fatal in 1-3 min.
- Hyperbaric oxygen therapy is indicated if HbCO >30-35%.

CARBOXYHEMOGLOBIN SYMPTOMS

0–10% : No symptoms except shortness of breath after physical labour.

10–20% : Slight headache with feelings of pressure toward the front of the head. Shortness of breath with medium exertion.

20–30% : Bad headaches, feelings of emotional excitement, insecurity, increase in the number of mistakes made, loss of memory, and rapid tiring.

30–40%: Severe headache, weakness, vomiting, dizziness, loss of sight, confusion.

40–50%: Great confusion, hallucinations, difficulty in walking, difficulty in breathing, mental stupor.

50–60% : Unconsciousness, coma, periodic convulsions, difficulty in breathing, weak and fast pulse, pinkness or pallor of face.

60–70% : Deep coma, loss of sphincter control.

70–80% : Deep coma, loss of reflexes, weak pulse, shallow and irregular breathing, involuntary bodily movement.

Over 80%: Breathing stops and death follows rapidly.

Other medical problems relate to blast injuries, smoke inhalation, crush syndrome, compartment syndrome, hypo and hyperthermia.

35 Climate Change and Disasters

> "Climate change is expected to cause more severe and more frequent natural hazards. As our cities and coasts grow more vulnerable, these hazards can lead to disasters that are far worse than those we have seen to date."
>
> —*Ban Ki-moon, Secretary-General United Nations, 2007*

INTRODUCTION

Climate change is one of the most important challenges for social development and human security of our time. Since the beginning of this decade the issue has risen to become one of the highest priorities on national political agendas worldwide. Through educational campaigns and the media, global awareness of the risks posed by climate change has increased rapidly. Nearly all sectors of society – spanning from businesses to humanitarian aid organizations and schools– are now starting to understand the importance of integrating concerns of climate change into their daily operations as well as their programming and projects.

Climate change is altering the face of disaster risk, not only through increased weather-related risks and rising sea-level and temperature rise, but also through increases in societal vulnerabilities from stresses on water availability, agriculture and ecosystems. There is increased intensity and/or frequency of extreme climate events, shifting and distribution of existing hazards. Some regions in Asia and West Africa are facing hazards that they have not experienced in the past like considerable increase in the frequency and severity of flooding disasters. Man-made emissions of greenhouse gases and terrestrial carbon release has resulted in shorter winters, hotter nights, killer heat waves, floods and heavy rains, devastating droughts, and an increase in hurricane and tropical storm strength. The phenomenon has also been implicated in causing climate surprises, i.e. the emergence of historically unexpected and sudden climate change, partly due to increases in global average air and ocean temperatures, widespread melting of polar permafrost snow caps and rising sea levels. The rise in Arctic temperatures has resulted in permafrost meltdowns causing release of methane gas and glacier runoffs that is expected to cause a rise in sea level from 18 cm to 59 cm by the end of the 21st century. The intergovernmental panel on climate change established by the United Nations has forecasted an increase in the average world temperature by 1.0 to 3.5°C over the next 100 years. Global sea levels are set to increase by an average of 50 cm over the next century, flooding coastlines.

Warming of oceans by El Nino and La Nina. These can create a potential for more intense hurricanes and droughts, leading to large population shifts.

Disaster and climate change risks threaten to derail efforts to enhance economic growth and reduce poverty, if proactive action is not taken. These risks include:

- Direct threats: e.g. damages from extreme weather to infrastructure.
- Indirect threats: e.g. climate impacts on health impacting a non-health sector.
- Underperformance of investments: e.g. agricultural projects that fail when rainfall decreases.
- Addressing climate change takes the form of two main responses:
  A. Reducing greenhouse gas emissions and terrestrial carbon release that are responsible for changing the earth's climate (mitigation); and
  B. Adjusting to the experienced or expected changes (adaptation) like more frequent and severe extreme climate events, such as floods, droughts, hurricanes, typhoons, heat waves, and other climate-dependent hazards such as pest and disease outbreaks.

Adapting to climate change will require interventions that help society confront these natural hazards, as well as other changes that may be more insidious. Most of the impacts on humans will not be caused by climate change alone, but will be the result of a combination of factors, including numerous social, political, environmental and economic variables. Most importantly, the extent to which climate change will adversely affect societies is dependent on how vulnerable a given group of people is to these changes. Responding to climate change impacts requires sector-wide concerted action that spans everything from public health and urban planning to agriculture and water management. However, adaptation measures are typically not designed with such a wide array of stakeholders, and are unable to address the factors that underlie society's vulnerability to climate change. Due to the complexity of both the problem and the required response, adaptation initiatives tend to focus almost exclusively on how to adjust only to the experienced or expected impacts of climate change. This does not address the much more difficult question of how to tackle the factors that drive society's vulnerability to climate change, including poverty, gender, wealth inequality, cultural and ethnic marginalization and discrimination. This is because vulnerability is a complex, multi-faceted and situation-specific trait that can hardly be addressed adequately through top-down policies.

Integrated risk reduction measures and climate change adaptation is needed through the following priorities for action:

1. *Good governance,* planning, budgeting and implementing policies to avoid settlement in hazardous areas and ensure that hospitals, schools, and transportation are hazard resistant.
2. *Understand the risks* we face and take action based on that knowledge. We need to use risk knowledge to develop effective early warning systems.
3. *Raise awareness* and educate young and old alike so they can reduce their own vulnerability. Many countries are taking such steps through the media and in schools.
4. *Changing practices* and conditions that aggravate risk, such as environmental degradation and poverty. Protecting precious ecosystems, such as coral reefs and mangrove forests, allows them to act as natural storm barriers. Effective insurance and micro-finance initiatives

can help to transfer risks and provide additional resources.

5. *Prepare for the disasters* that will inevitably strike by having contingency plans in place and emergency funds established, as well as regularly conducting simulation exercises.

Managing disaster risks from climatic hazards has focused on reducing exposure and vulnerability of socio-economic systems to cyclone, storm, storm surge, flood, drought, heat wave, cold wave, etc. through prevention, mitigation, and preparedness actions, with an aim to reduce loss of lives, shelter, infrastructure and livelihoods.

Greater focus on reducing human-induced impacts on climate, segregating anthropogenic causes from natural climate variability, greater stakeholder participation in vulnerability assessments, prioritization of actions, capacity building, risk management, disaster risk reduction, and integration of adaptation into sectoral and national planning is essential to bring about a convergence between climate change adaptation and disaster risk management.

The success of the climate risk management approach, however, would depend, albeit heavily, upon the availability of climate information. Access to current and seasonal forecast information provide opportunities for more informed decision-making to reduce exposure to short-term climate risks. Knowledge of long-term trends associated with climate change provides opportunities to evaluate how decisions and investments made today can withstand future extremes. The shift in disaster management paradigm from reactive to proactive has greatly contributed to the reduce vulnerabilities and deaths by better and long term weather forecasting methods.

Risk assessment: A methodology to determine the nature and extent of risk by analysing potential hazards and evaluating existing conditions of vulnerability that could pose a potential threat or harm to people, property, livelihoods and the environment on which they depend. The process of conducting a risk assessment is based on a review of both the technical features of hazards such as their location, intensity, frequency and probability; and also the analysis of the physical, social, economic and environmental dimensions of vulnerability and exposure, while taking particular account of the coping capabilities pertinent to the risk scenarios. Risk assessment must address:

Climate change impact assessment: The practice of identifying and evaluating the detrimental and beneficial consequences of climate change on natural and human systems.

Adaptation: Adjustment in natural or human systems in response to actual or expected climatic stimuli or their effects, which moderates harm or exploits beneficial opportunities. Various types of adaptation can be distinguished:

a. Adaptation that takes place before impacts of climate change are observed. Also referred to as proactive adaptation.
b. Adaptation that does not constitute a conscious response to climatic stimuli but is triggered by ecological changes in natural systems and by market or welfare changes in human systems. Also referred to as spontaneous adaptation.
c. Adaptation that is the result of a deliberate policy decision, based on an awareness that conditions have changed or are about to change and that action is required to return to, maintain, or achieve a desired state.
d. Adaptation that is initiated and implemented by individuals, households or

private companies. Private adaptation is usually in rational self-interest.

e. Adaptation that is initiated and implemented by governments at all levels. Public adaptation is usually directed at collective needs.

f. Adaptation that takes place after impacts of climate change have been observed.

Adaptive capacity: The ability of a system to adjust to climate change (including climate variability and extremes) to moderate potential damages, to take advantage of opportunities, or to cope with the consequences.

Coping capacity: The means by which people or organizations use available resources and abilities to face adverse consequences that could lead to a disaster. In general, this involves managing resources, both in normal times as well as during crises or adverse conditions. The strengthening of coping capacities usually builds resilience to withstand the effects of natural and human-induced hazards.

There are a number of actions that can be taken to reduce vulnerability to natural hazards and adapt to climate change, which include the promotion of a culture of prevention and resilience, the development of institutions (policies, planning legislative, multi-stakeholder mechanisms, etc.) to actively contribute to these goals:

- Identification of risks (risk mapping, hazard and vulnerability assessments).
- Promotion of early warning systems.
- Building hazard-resistant structures in particular critical infrastructures, schools, and hospitals.
- Protection and development of hazard buffers (natural ecosystems such as forests, reefs, and mangroves); and
- Improving preparedness, response, and the development of pre-disaster recovery plan.

Vulnerability

Vulnerability is founded on a cluster of political and socioeconomic factors responsible for public health inequalities and social deprivation like poor housing, lack of education, social marginalization (and unable to influence decision makers), unemployment. Promoting health and protecting security are inseparable from social, economic and political factors and inextricably linked with promoting and protecting human rights. Vulnerability springs from a web of human actions, decisions and choices at various levels in society.. Vulnerability is a result of ignorance, a failure to educate, a lack of intervention or regulation by the government or a result of economic forces that forces people to become marginalized. Living in ignorance, in defective dwellings in exposed areas and destined by poverty to have limited choices and failure to learn from previous experiences to prevent losses in the future and not just apportion blame to builders, scientists, government or God! Governmental intervention to to devise mitigation measures may be viewed by suspicion by populations accustomed to and hardened by natural risks or more accustomed to political corruption.

Vulnerability is not the same as poverty, many scholars attempted to pick apart the concept to understand its most prominent drivers. Although poverty remains one of the most important factors determining degree of vulnerability, it is certainly not the only factor and not always the primary one. Furthermore, vulnerability is a relative term, referring to specific hazards. For example, while a family can be vulnerable to floods because they live near a river, they may not be vulnerable to earthquakes occurring in the same location if their home is designed to withstand strong tremors. In addition, people who are vulnerable to natural hazards are normally aware of this, and tend to have a series of response strategies, that may or may not be viable in all situations. It would be false to think that people who are vulnerable to climate change are 'helpless victims', but often there are significant challenges that stand in the way of overcoming their vulnerability.

Reducing Vulnerability

Vulnerability is sometimes described as the opposite of capacity to cope with hazards. To this end, strengthening coping capacity is promoted as a way to reduce vulnerability. To strengthen coping capacity, however, it is necessary to dig deeper than simply building storm shelters or setting up evacuation maps. Coping capacity is also dependent on factors such as social networks, alternative livelihood options and access to healthcare. But short-term coping solutions can have the adverse consequence of increased vulnerability in the long term. The typical example is selling off assets or borrowing money to cope with a drought, in order to manage for the year. However, if the drought persists, no assets will remain to sell and no crops will be produced to generate income to pay back the loan, the families will be worse off than in the first instance. In other examples, measures that reduce vulnerability of' one group might increase vulnerability of another group, for example by building a dam to address upstream water shortage during drought and thus depriving downstream users experiencing the same drought of a necessary resource. Thus, measures to reduce vulnerability must be carried out with awareness of their consequences in the long-term and on other potentially sensitive groups.

It is not surprising that vulnerability has gained such popularity; unlike any other concept, it addresses the social roots of risk. Because measures associated with reducing vulnerability are recognized as components of development, many international development organizations are carrying out activities to support vulnerability reduction, such as UNDP, Practical Action and CARE. But vulnerability reduction must also be driven by national and local governments, who have the power to influence how much control different groups in society have over their own circumstances by giving them voice, access to resources and say over their own assets. The vulnerability discourse is indeed expanding, and finding its way into numerous new disciplines. Although vulnerability is a useful concept for reflecting how socio-economic factors influence risk, it must not overshadow that climate change will also result in more extreme natural hazards – the other component of risk. Nevertheless, vulnerability does provide a useful link between climate change policy and development policy, where failures in development become more evident and more detrimental when climate change is added. Addressing factors that determine vulnerability will ultimately therefore also facilitate the process of adapting to climate change, and ensure that responses to the changed climate are long term and equitable.

Early Warning Long-lead location-specific disaster risk information would immensely help resource managers, disaster management practitioners, and the general public in taking pro-active response actions to an impending hazard high-performance computing system (HPC) was established at the regional facility at ADPC to downscale global climate forecast products to make them applicable at the local level in participating countries. The HPC is an IBM system in Power 5 Architecture (P5-575), running in a UNIX platform. With 128 processors over 8 nodes, it is able to compute with a clock speed of one teraflop. Storage capacity is 10TB, supplement-ed by a TS3310 external tape drive, which can handle up to

30 tapes of 800GB capacity at any time. The Weather Research Forecasting (WRF) modeling system of the U.S. National Center for Atmospheric Research is installed and customized over the Asian region for the generation of location-specific hydro-meteorological hazard information, which is done by incorporating appropriate, physical parameterization schemes and nesting techniques. To assess potential hazard risk parameters such as heavy rainfall, strong wind and coastal inundation associated with tropical disturbances, an attempt has been made to simulate the severe tropical cyclones and typhoons which occurred over the Indian seas and South China seas in 2007. The state-of-the art Weather Research Forecasting model was customized at ADPC HPC system and integrated upto 72 hours. Those hazards events are simulated with a horizontal resolution of 9 km with NCEP-GFS initial and boundary conditions. All the results are very encouraging in terms of track and distribution of rainfall for the purpose of disaster mitigation.

Disasters are becoming increasingly costly in terms of lives and destruction. There must be a paradigm shift in the way that organizations think about development work, but the goal is to be systematic about building up the resiliency of communities before a disaster hits. DRR activities can help reduce the toll on human lives and govern-ment budgets. In fact, research has shown that every $1 spent on disaster risk reduction activities saves nearly $7 in emergency response funds."

36 Disaster Risk Reduction (DRR)

> "Teamwork is a lot of people doing what I say."
>
> —*(Marketing Executive, Citrix Corporation)*

INTRODUCTION

Between 1980 and 2005, nearly 7500 natural disasters worldwide took the lives of over 2 million people and produced economic losses estimated at over 1.2 trillion US dollars. Of this, 90 per cent of the natural disasters, 72.5 per cent of casualties and 75 per cent of economic losses were caused by weather, climate, water-related hazards such as droughts, floods, windstorms, tropical cyclones, storm surges, extreme temperatures, land slides and wild fires, or by health epidemics and insect infestations directly linked to meteorological and hydrological conditions. The various hydrological or climate-related hazards in 2005, decreased to one-tenth of levels in the 1950's. This remarkable decline is a demonstration that preparedness and prevention, combined with effective emergency management and early warning systems, can significantly contribute to reducing impacts of hazards on human life. There is a need for a paradigm shift: from emergency response to disaster risk management, a more proactive, holistic and systematic approach.

ABOUT THE DISASTER RISK REDUCTION (DRR) PROGRAMME

World Meteorological Organization (WMO) established its DRR Programme in 2003 to strengthen and integrate disaster risk reduction processes related to meteorological, hydrological and climate services of its WMO operational and research networks in all countries, particularly those with least resources. Through this crosscutting programme, WMO is developing an organization-wide coordinating framework to achieve these objectives at the international, regional and national levels. Disaster risk management can be framed under three main areas:

Risk Identification, Risk Reduction and Risk Transfer

These should be supported by effective governance (e.g., legislation, policies, planning, legal frameworks, etc), as well as, institutional capacities at national to local levels, supplemented by effective information and knowledge sharing mechanisms among different stakeholders.

THE VISION OF THE DRR PROGRAMME

"To enhance the contributions of National Meteorological and Hydrological Services (NMHS), in a more cost-effective, systematic and sustainable manner, towards the protection of lives, livelihoods and property, through enhanced capabilities and cooperation in the

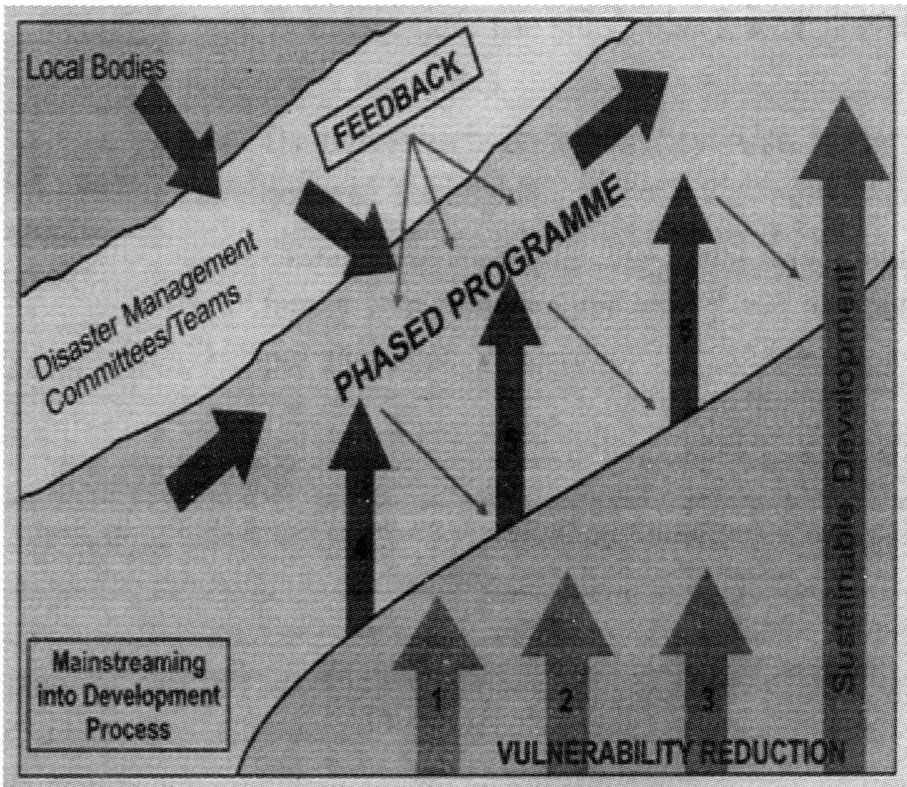

Fig. 36.1a

field of disaster risk reduction at national to international levels."

Strategic Goals

WMO strategic goals in disaster risk reduction are derived from key activity of the Hyogo Framework for Action (HFA). The strategic goals were approved by WMO Congress (the supreme governing body of WMO) in 2007:

- Development, improvement and sustainability of early warning systems, in particular related to scientific and technical infrastructures, systems and capabilities for research, observing, detecting, forecasting and warning of weather, water-, climate-related hazards.
- Development, improvement and sustainability of systems, methods, tools and applications of modern technologies such as geographic information systems for recording, analyzing and providing hazard information for risk assessment, sectoral planning and other informed decision-making.
- Development and delivery of warnings, specialized forecasts and other products and services that are timely, understandable to those at risk, and driven by requirements of disaster risk reduction decision processes and operations.
- Stimulate a culture of disaster preparedness through strengthening of capacities for better integration of NMHSs' products and services in disaster risk reduction, and continued public education and outreach campaigns.

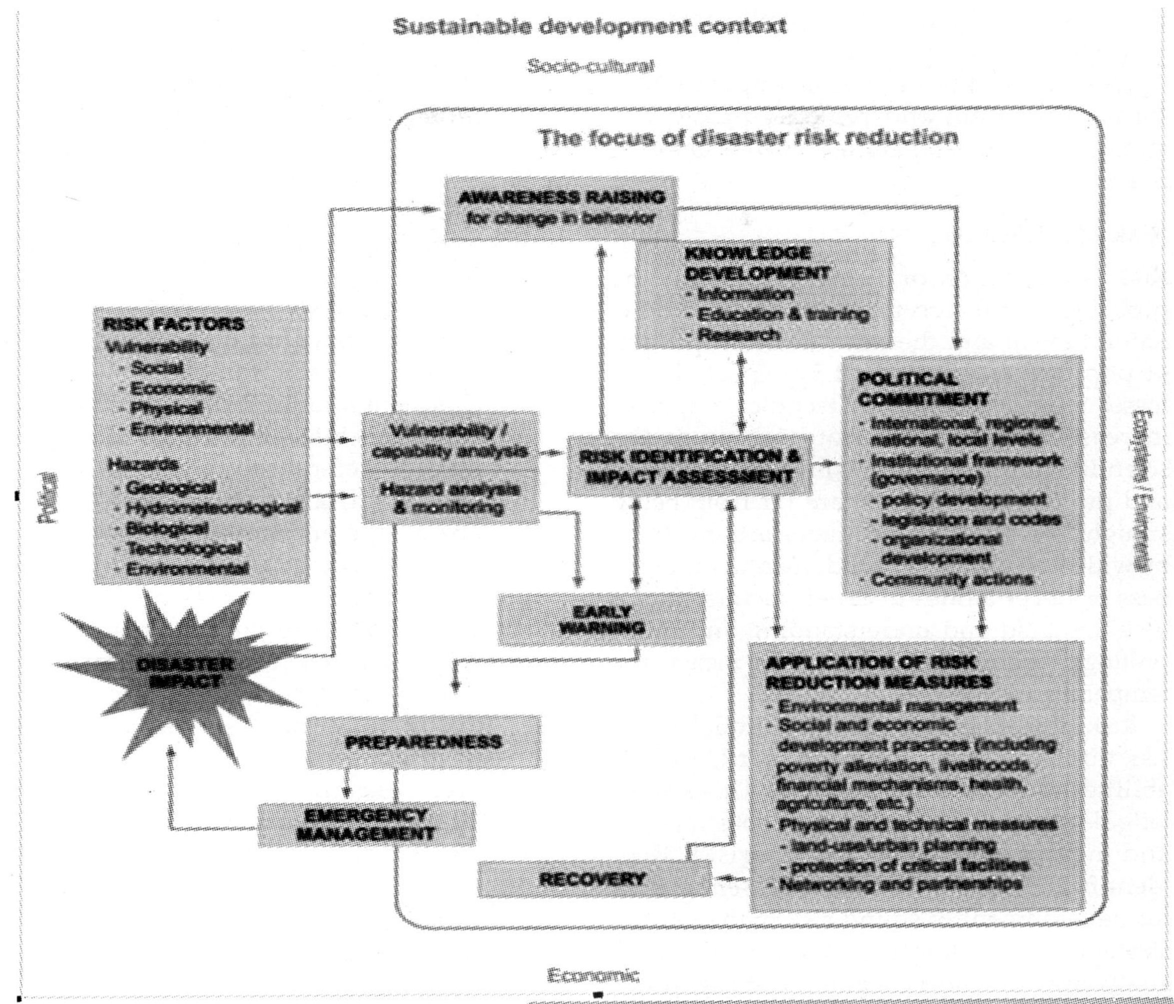

Fig. 36.1b

- Strengthen WMO and NMHSs cooperation and partnerships for implementation of disaster risk reduction in national, regional and international mechanisms and structures.

Implementation Plan

WMO's strategic goals in disaster risk reduction are being realized through an action plan, built upon the following five major thrusts:

1. Modernize NMHSs and observing networks.
2. Implement national operational multi-hazard early warning systems.
3. Strengthen hazard analysis and hydro-meteorological risk assessment tools.
4. Strengthen NMHSs cooperation with civil protection and disaster risk management agencies; and

5. Coordinate training and public outreach programmes.

This action plan is being implemented through national and regional projects to strengthen their capacities in disaster risk reduction

Risk Identification

Risk is a function of vulnerability and the probability of the occurrence of a hazardous natural event and the number or proportion of population exposed. It is expected that losses would decrease as technical capacity increased but this has not been so as the scientific ability to forecast natural hazards and protect against them are far from being straightforward. Risk estimates are thwarted by wide variations and fundamental randomness or uncertainties in causal factors cannot be eliminated and understanding and interpreting probabilities is not easy like measuring temperature or recording weight.

Risk identification involves quantification of risk through understanding hazard, vulnerabilities and exposure patterns. This knowledge is essential for development of strategies and measures for reducing the risks. Risk identification provides the first essential step for development of sound risk management strategies. A fundamental requirement is the availability of historical and real-time, systematic and consistent, observations of hydrometeorological parameters, complemented with other forecast products providing information on expected patterns of hazards from the next hour to longer time frames. This must be complemented with vulnerability and exposure information, tools and methodologies for hazard analysis, mapping as well as sectoral risk assessment and modeling.

Hazard events are characterized by magnitude, duration, location and timing. Calculating the probability of occurrence of hazard events in terms of these characteristics is the key in understanding fully the hazard component of disaster impacts. These defining characteristics provide a basis for extracting information on hazard frequency and severity from observational datasets. The fundamental requirement is the availability of, and access to, high quality historical meteorological and hydrological data that is provided by the NMHSs. This requires:

- Ongoing, systematic and consistent observations of hazard-relevant hydrometeorological parameters;
- Quality assurance and proper archiving of the data into temporally and geographically referenced, and consistently catalogued, observational datasets; and
- Ensuring that the data can be located and retrieved by users.

In a recent capacity analysis survey conducted by the World Meteorological Organization, in which 139 countries participated, nearly 90% of the participating countries indicated the need for strengthening their observing networks; capacity for maintenance of standard hazard databases and metadata; maintenance of sectoral disaster loss data; and, methodologies for risk modeling to support development planning in different economic sectors. Given the pervasive nature of hydrometeorological hazards and increasing levels of vulnerability, risk identification will require continuing and renewed commitment to maintaining the observing networks, basic data, and hazard forecasting capacities. WMO, through its various programmes, is developing guidelines for standardization of hazard monitoring databases, metadata, analysis and mapping. These guidelines are implemented for operational use of NMHSs through various national capacity development projects.

Risk Reduction

Risk reduction involves actions taken to reduce the overall risks associated with disasters. Such actions include short-, medium- and long-term sectoral planning, early warning systems, and emergency preparedness mechanisms.

Sectoral Planning

The economic and social impacts of weather, climate and water continue to grow year to year. Today, up to 30% of developed country's GDP is sensitive to meteorological, hydrological and climate conditions, while the sensitivity is even higher in developing and least developed countries. With the increasing risks associated with climate variability and change, the existing system for food, water, shelter, energy, etc could be significantly disrupted. Meteorological, hydrological and climate information underpins better informed decision making and planning for the protection of lives and livelihoods. NMHSs have the potential capacity to provide hazard information such as frequency, magnitude and trends that are required for the development of policy and legislation pertaining to disaster risk reduction such as mainstreaming of hydrometeorological risk assessment infrastructure and urban planning, costal zoning and land use planning. NMHSs are the primary authoritative source of hydrometeorological data, products and services that provide the basis for informed sectoral planning that insures community resilience to weather climate and water hazards.

Risk Transfer

Weather risk management markets enable distribution of the risk as follows:

i. Risks associated with extreme weather events (e.g. floods, droughts, earthquakes and tropical cyclones); and
ii. Accumulated risks linked to deviation of meteorological conditions from "normal" (e.g., late on-set, warmer or cooler than normal seasons).

Knowledge Sharing and Training

By mandate of its Convention, one of the objectives of the WMO is to encourage and support training of its Members to better fulfill their responsibilities for providing meteorological, hydrological and related products, information and services. To achieve this, WMO has established 30 Regional Training Centres around the world providing technical training for management and operation of NMHSs to enhance their abilities to provide better products and services, including services in support of disaster risk reduction operations and decision-making. These centres offer opportunities for customized training in disaster risk reduction.

Through its DRR Programme, WMO is developing a training strategy to provide joint training programmes at NMHS and their partners in areas related to utilization of meteorological, hydrological, and climate information to support risk assessment, sectoral planning, early warning systems and financial risk transfer mechanisms.

Governance and Organizational Coordination

The success of disaster risk management efforts is critically dependent on political commitment manifested through good governance. Good governance includes the adoption and promotion of robust and sound policies, legislation, coordination mechanisms and regulatory frameworks, and the creation of an enabling environment that is characterized by appropriate decision making processes to allow effective participation of stakeholders, complemented by the appropriate allocation of resources. In some countries, governments have started to integrate disaster risk reduction elements in their Poverty Reduction Strategies and other national development instruments. Countries are working to mainstream disaster risk reduction into development planning in sectors and at the local level. These efforts are supported through different international programmes and agencies' initiatives, such as the UNDP Institutional and Legislative Systems for Disaster Reduction (ILS) Programme and the World Bank's Global Facility for Disaster Reduction and Recovery (GFDRR).

HFA identifies legislation as a critical component of disaster risk reduction, and calls upon States to "adopt, or modify where necessary, legislation to support disaster risk reduction, including regulations and mechanisms that encourage compliance to codes and that promote incentives for understanding risk reduction and mitigation activities". Many developed countries have some kind of legislation to govern their disaster risk management activities, but they mostly focus on post-disaster response. Within the existing legislation, 55% of the countries lack clear legislation or policies on the role of NMHSs, which limits their contribution to disaster risk reduction at the national level. In some countries various coordination mechanisms are being established to address more effectively the decision process for disaster risk reduction. Examples of such coordination include:

- Governmental Inter-Ministerial Coordination Mechanisms, usually under the head of the government, to coordinate activities of various ministries related to disaster risk reduction.
- National Platforms for Disaster Risk Reduction involving different stakeholders (government institutions, private sector, NGOs, academic and research institutions, communities, etc.).
- Strengthening of the role of the Office of the UN Resident Coordinator for the coordination of disaster risk reduction activities among UN agencies and with governments.

Coordination mechanisms enable better identification of requirements, roles and responsibilities of various stakeholders in disaster risk reduction, and often lead to new partnerships to leverage capacities and resources of various agencies towards implementation of HFA. Development of legislation and regulatory frameworks, in many cases, has been instrumental for sustainability and reliability of disaster risk reduction coordination mechanisms.

Early Warning Systems and Emergency Preparedness

The second priority for action of the HFA stresses the need for "identifying, assessing and monitoring disaster risk and enhancing early warnings" as pre-conditions for natural disaster risk reduction. Effective early warning systems should include:

1. Strong political commitment from the government, supported by DRR plans, legislation and coordination mechanisms.
2. Coordination among national services for sharing of information, data, and issuance of warnings that take vulnerabilities and exposure of elements into account.
3. Communication and dissemination system that ensures warnings are received at community levels through clear protocols and procedures that are regularly tested, evaluated and maintained.
4. Emergency preparedness, including education to appropriately use weather-, water- and climate-related information and early warnings. This is realized through local to national contingency and/or emergency response plans with clear indication of actions, roles and responsibilities which are regularly updated and practiced through drills and simulation exercises. Feedback mechanisms between national to local governments, national services and the community, to facilitate evaluation and improvement of the warning system The WMO and NMHSs are key to the

availability of well-functioning early warning systems. Such systems should, with a multi-hazard approach, deliver accurate reliable and understandable warnings, in a timely fashion to authorities, emergency operations and the population at risk to enable preventive actions to reduce the impacts of potential disasters.

DRR Definitions

Acceptable risk: The level of loss a society or community considers acceptable given existing social, economic, political, cultural, technical and environmental conditions

Capacity: A combination of all the strengths and resources available within a community, society or organization that can reduce the level of risk, or the effects of a disaster.

Disaster: A serious disruption of the functioning of a community or a society causing widespread human, material, economic or environmental losses which exceed the ability of the affected community or society to cope using its own resources.

Exposure: Exposure is the total value of elements at-risk. It is expressed as the number of human lives, and value of the properties, that can potentially be affected by hazards. Exposure is a function of the geographic location of the elements

Hazard: Potentially damaging physical event that may cause the loss of life or injury, property damage, social and economic disruption or environmental degradation. Hazards can include latent conditions that may represent future threats and can have different origins. Each hazard is characterised by its location, intensity, and probability.

Hazard analysis: Identification, studies and monitoring of any hazard to determine its potential, origin, characteristics and behaviour.

Hydrometeorological hazards: Natural processes or phenomena of atmospheric, hydrological or oceanographic nature, which may cause the loss of life or injury, property damage, social and economic disruption or environmental degradation.

Intensity physical parameters describing the severity of the hazard.

Natural hazards: Natural processes or phenomena occurring in the biosphere that may constitute a damaging event.

Probability: Likelihood of an event happening. Probability is statistically higher for low-intensity hazards. Probability reflects the future frequency of occurrence of hazard event, and cannot be drawn using historical statistics alone. For hydro-meteorological hazards, probability assessments need to reflect trends related to ongoing evolutions (i.e. climate change, deforestation, etc.).

Resilience: Capacity to recover the normal functioning and development after being hit by a disaster. A high resilience reduces indirect impacts of disasters, such as business and services interruptions in the aftermath of a disaster.

Risk: Probable impacts, expressed in terms of expected loss of lives, people injured, property, livelihoods, economic activity disrupted or environmental damage.

Risk assessment/analysis: A methodology to determine the nature an extent of risk by analyzing potential hazards and evaluating existing conditions of vulnerability that could pose a potential threat or harm to people, property, livelihoods and the environment on which they depend.

Risk identification: The process used to determine what can happen, why and how events arise.

Risk management: The systematic management of administrative decisions, organization, operational skills and capacities to implement policies, strategies and coping capacities of the society and communities to lessen the impacts of natural hazards and related environmental and technological disasters. This comprises all forms of activities, including structural and non-structural measures to avoid (prevention) or to limit (mitigation and preparedness) adverse effects of hazards.

Risk reduction: The conceptual framework of elements considered with the possibilities to minimize vulnerabilities and disaster risks throughout a society, to avoid (prevention) or to limit (mitigation and preparedness) the adverse impacts of hazards, within the broad context of sustainable development.

Risk transfer: Insurance and reinsurance both for physical damage and business interruption, coverage that would provide cash compensation immediately after a disaster.

Vulnerability: Physical, social, economic and environmental factors which increase the susceptibility to be impacted by hazards. Vulnerability engages resistance and resilience.

37 Community Based Disaster Management

"The local community is taken as the primary focus of attention (in disaster reduction) since that is the common unit which is affected by disaster and, more importantly, responds to deal with the event."

—*Russell Dynes*

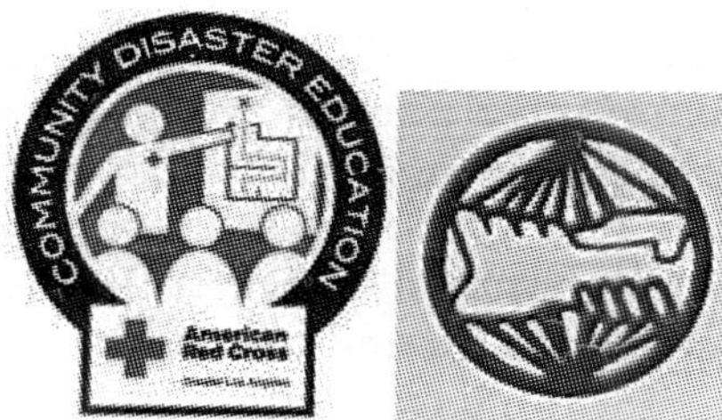

Fig. 37.1

INTRODUCTION

Community participation has been recognized as the additional element in disaster management necessary to reverse the worldwide trend of exponential increase in disaster occurrence of and loss from small- and medium-scale disasters, build a culture of safety, and ensure sustainable development for all. Major benefits of the community based risk assessment, mitigation planning and implementation processes underscored include building confidence, pride in being able to make a difference, and enhanced capabilities to pursue disaster preparedness, mitigation as well as bigger development responsibilities at the local level. Additionally, individual and community ownership, commitment and concerted actions in disaster mitigation, including resource mobilization produce a wide range of appropriate, innovative and do-able mitigation solutions, which are cost-effective and sustainable. Good practices in the community based approaches to disaster mitigation highlight key success factors such as applying best practice methodologies of community development to community based disaster mitigation, tapping traditional organizational structures and mechanisms (including formal and informal community leaders), and capability building activities with the community disaster committees and volunteers. The importance of various forms and channels of public awareness and education using local dialects, values and culture and partnerships of the community with various stakeholders such as community based organizations, community leaders, local government units, higher level government, NGOs, less vulnerable groups, and donors were also noted.

Whether a disaster is major or minor, of national or local proportion, it is the people at the community or village level who suffer its adverse effects. They use coping and survival strategies to face and respond to the situation long before outside help from NGOs or the government arrives. They are interested to protect themselves from the damage and harm.

The necessity of community participation for sustainable disaster reduction has to be translated into actions in keeping with the shift in perspective from the prevailing emergency management framework to disaster risk management to reverse the trend of exponential increase in disaster occurrence of and loss from small- and medium-scale disasters. These highlighted the need for proactive disaster management activities and the significant role of local communities. The community-based approach also corrected the defects of the top-down approach in development planning and disaster management which failed to address local needs, ignored the potential of indigenous resources and capacities, and may have even increased people's vulnerabilities.

Experiences in developing regions and countries now affirm the gains of community based disaster management. in managing and reducing disaster risk. A network for risk reduction and sustainable development, gives priority to minimizing the impact of natural and other threats by strengthening the environmental, social, and economic resilience of vulnerable communities.

THE PIONEERING EFFORT

The Asian Disaster Preparedness Center (ADPC) started the Asian Urban Disaster Mitigation Program (AUDMP) in 1995 in collaboration with the USAID Office of Foreign Disaster Assistance embarked on efforts to reduce the disaster vulnerability of urban populations. Four AUDMP projects with a participatory approach were taken up during the session on Community Based Approaches to Disaster Mitigation, viz. Urban Flood Mitigation in Bangladesh, Mitigating Flood Risk in Cambodian Communities, Earthquake Disaster Mitigation in Nepal and Landslide Disaster Reduction in Sri Lanka with Community Based Disaster Management (CBDM) as a core strategy for disaster reduction and sustainable development. The concepts, approaches, interventions, methodologies, tools and practical tips/considerations for communities to improve safety and achieve livelihood security, together with sustainable economic, social and physical development, by community participation was considered the crucial and pivotal element.

The top-down mitigation programs had serious flaws such as failure to involve people since community participation was often limited to provision of labor in self-help projects, failure to address vulnerability as a complex relationship between people and their social, physical and economic environment, and the susceptibility to political manipulation by powerful groups. community based approach to disaster mitigation. The new approach stated that:

- The principal responsibility and authority for the development of the program rested with the community-based organization (CBO).
- Problems faced by the community had to be correctly defined and the responsive mitigation measures and strategies for recovery worked out by the community members themselves as they could now express their real needs and priorities to the CBOs.
- Existence of CBOs would permit rapid and effective response to emergencies.
- The principal resource during disasters are the victims themselves and their local knowledge and expertise would enable programs with small financial inputs but

significant results.

- A community was defined as a group of individuals and households living in the same disaster prone location and having the same hazard exposure, sharing the same objectives and goals in disaster risk reduction. The community members may have varying perception of disaster risk depending on social class, education, age, gender, etc., and the community risk assessment and disaster risk reduction planning processes would help unite the community in understanding aspects of the risks and collectively evolve preparedness, mitigation and prevention actions.

Community based disaster management (CBDM) is now anchored in the disaster risk reduction framework, and it covers a broad range of interventions, measures, activities, projects and programs to reduce disaster risks, primarily designed by people in at-risk localities and based on their urgent needs and capacities.

AIMS AND DEFINITIONS

The aims of CBDM are to:

1. Reduce vulnerabilities and increase capacities of vulnerable groups and communities to cope with, prevent or minimize loss and damage to life, property, and the environment.
2. Minimize human suffering and
3. Hasten recovery.

Through CBDM vulnerable groups and communities can be transformed to disaster resilient communities, which can withstand and recover from stresses and shocks from the natural/physical and socio-economic political environment like the bamboo, which sways with the battering of strong winds but stays rooted and weathers the catastrophe.

Key indicators are safety, livelihood security and sustainable economic, social and physical development (general well-being, health, education, amenities, natural and physical environment, etc.).

With the shifting of paradigms from reactive emergency management to disaster risk reduction, there is more stress on proactive pre-disaster interventions, which are usually categorized as prevention, mitigation, and preparedness. While natural hazards may not be prevented, human-induced hazards such as those associated with industries, technological failures, pollution, and civil strife can be prevented.

Prevention covers measures to provide permanent protection from disasters or reduce the intensity/frequency of a hazardous event so that it does not become a disaster. These include safety standards in industries, poverty alleviation and assets redistribution schemes, and provision of basic needs and services such as preventive health care and education.

Mitigation reduces and limits the destructive and disruptive effects of hazards on the elements at risk.

APPROACH

1. Physical measures: Engineering works like bridges, protective dikes, embankments, and safe building design to the disaster mitigation.
2. Non-structural interventions such as community risk assessment, community risk reduction planning, public awareness, food security programs, group savings, cooperatives, crop insurance, strengthening community disaster management organizations and advocacy on disasters and
3. Development issues, legislation and land use zoning. Mitigation and prevention interventions are directly linked to development planning as disaster mitigation is intrinsic to sustainable development.

Preparedness involves measures taken in anticipation of a disaster to ensure that appropriate and effective actions are taken during the emergency such as setting up the systems for early warning, coordinative and institutional arrangements, evacuation and emergency operations management, public awareness, disaster and evacuation drills, and stockpiling. Emergency responses are measures undertaken to ensure survival and prevent further deterioration of the situation. These include search and rescue, immediate repair and restoration of critical facilities and utilities, conduct of damage needs and capacity assessment, food and non-food relief assistance, medical assistance, evacuation center management and networking.

Recovery covers rehabilitation and reconstruction and can be undertaken within the framework of mitigation and vulnerability reduction, and not just bringing back the situation to pre-disaster levels. The Chinese characters for the word crisis is composed of two characters that mean 'danger and opportunity'. Disaster mitigation and risk reduction offers the greatest opportunity for the integration of disaster management into the development programming process.

Alternative Perspectives

Disasters/conflicts are often viewed as isolated events or aberrations in the normal path of development and linkages with conditions in society during normal times are not analyzed.

Technical/Law and Order solutions tend to be top-down dictated and often inflexible and invariably having minimal participation of the local population who are viewed as mere victims.

Implementing agencies are often less accountable and their processes lacking transparency. Most interventions are made after the event occurs. The objective of the interventions are to return to the pre disaster situation. Disasters are linked to unresolved problems arising from the very processes of development. Relationships/structures within a society are considered to determine why certain groups of people are more vulnerable to disasters than others.

The New Strategy

"Development is the process through which people increase their capacities for producing things they need and for managing their political and social lives as they desire, and at the same time (especially in disaster-prone areas) reduce their immediate and long-term vulnerabilities to events which threaten their economic and socio-political existence."

—*Anderson and Woodrow*

Participation of people paramount in intervention strategies; people treated as partners in development and builds on people's capacities to protect themselves against hazards.

Ensuring accountability and transparency emphasized in implementation.

Mitigation of disasters/conflict viewed as a fundamental aim.

Disasters/conflicts are viewed as opportunities for social transformation.

The new strategy got its inspiration from Ms Arnstein's typology of eight levels on a ladder for the type of citizen (community) participation to aspire and work for. Each rung of the ladder corresponds to the extent of the citizens' power in determining plans and programs as under:

Manipulation and therapy of "participants" by the government or 'powerholders' are actually forms of non-participation (levels 1 and 2, respectively).

Level 3 (being informed).

Level 4 (being consulted).

Level 5 (placation) are forms of "tokenism" by the "haves" towards the "have-nots", where the have-nots have a voice in the process but still do not make decisions.

Citizen power increases in the last three levels (6, 7 and 8) through citizen participation – partnership, delegated power and finally achieving citizen control.

The challenge posed to the targetted communities and organizations is to innovate and explore appropriate models and schemes based on their local contexts and organizational mandates.

Community Organization

Before the community can be mobilized for disaster mitigation, they have to be organized first. Steps followed for the disaster management/mitigation are patterned after the basic methodology in community organizing for community development. This methodology covers consciousness raising, organization building and mobilization. The approach is systematized as follows:

1. Site entry and rapport building—a process whereby the facilitator establishes rapport and constructive relationship with the people. Mutual respect and trust are the key elements that characterize effective integration.
2. Community situational analysis—the process of gathering all relevant data about the community such as physical characteristics, demographic features, economic and socio-political aspects of the community.
3. Identification of priority sectors—the process of identifying the target groups or sector of the project or those most in need/most at risk.
4. Identification of natural leaders or "progressive members"—the process of selecting natural leader or "progressive members" of the identified priority group(s) or tapping existing structures/organizations in the community. The core group serves as catalyst or prime mover in the formation of the group.
5. Feedback/validation of results of community situation analysis—the purpose is to inform the people about the whole situation of the community and to fill in the gaps.
6. Further analysis of priority problem/need/aspiration—the process whereby the community discusses and analyzes their problem and transforms it into community goals or aspirations.
7. Planning of the solution/action—the process whereby the community plans how to solve their problems.
8. Organization of the group—the role and responsibilities of each member vis-à-vis the community's activities and tasks are identified and agreed upon. Skills improvement is provided to the community organization and they are encouraged to forge links with other institutions.

In general, the goal of CBDM is to transform the vulnerable or at-risk communities into disaster resilient communities, specifically through CBD mitigation (CBDMit). Although steps may vary from community contexts and organizational mandates, the process and requisites for disaster risk reduction can be generalized as follows:

1. *Initiating the process:* Linkage and building rapport with community.
2. *Community profiling:* Initial understanding of the disaster situation and orientation by CBDM and CBDMit.
3. *Community risk assessment:* Participatory assessment of hazards, vulnerabilities, capacities and also the community's perception of the risks.
4. *Formulation of initial disaster risk reduction plan:* Identification of appropriate mitigation and preparedness measures including public awareness, training and education.

5. Formation of community disaster response organization—Community organizing and mobilization, capability building in CBDMit and preparedness.
6. Implementation of short- medium- and long-term risk reduction measures, activities, projects and programs, implementation strategies and mechanisms; organizational/institutional strengthening.
7. Monitoring and evaluation: Making continuous improvements in the disaster risk reduction plan, documentation and dissemination of good practices for replication.

Notwithstanding the order, the community volunteers, disaster management committee, and disaster response organization are the necessary interface or the channel for outsiders such as NGOs or government agencies to assist/support the community at-large. The community groups and organizations in disaster management are essential in sustaining the risk reduction process for the community to meet intended aims and targets.

Within this 7-step process, the formation and strengthening of community disaster response organization or community disaster management volunteer's team is the key to mobilizing communities for sustainable disaster risk reduction. In many of the experiences of the AUDMP projects, this step comes even before the risk assessment/ mapping and identification of mitigation solutions/action planning. Local authorities such as leaders of communes, villages and village groups, temple committee members, monks and village elders are tapped in order to reach the maximum members of the community and arrive at a consensus and also prioritize mitigation solutions. Opportunities presented by community gatherings at special events or traditional ceremonies are utilized to gather ideas and suggestions on mitigation solutions and also request contributions in cash or kind. Mitigation project proposals (not exceeding Rs.50,000 per project) are presented by the communities which included proposed mitigation measures and local contributions in terms of labor, materials and finance. These may be water control structures necessary for livelihood, including repairing dams and dikes; cleaning of irrigation ditches, culverts and water gates; and improving access by raising road levels or constructing small bridges to reduce flood vulnerability to mitigate, prepare for and respond to a disaster in a self-reliant and cooperative manner. It involves:

1. Selecting project sites, targeting the most vulnerable communities.
2. Selecting community members as volunteers and training them to work with communities in reducing vulnerabilities.
3. Organizing communities and establishing village-level Disaster Management Committees (DMC) as a coordinating body.
4. Identifying, estimating and ranking local disaster risks through risk mapping.
5. Building consensus on mitigation solutions.
6. mobilizing resources and implementing the community's mitigation solutions.
7. Drawing lessons from implementation, sharing lessons and learning from similar experiences to evolve a broad range of mitigation measures, processes and requisites, tools and methodologies.
8. Replication and overall improvement of the CBDMit and preparedness system.

The Core Values of CBDMit

- *People's participation:* Community members

are the main actors and propellers; they also directly share the benefits of disaster risk reduction. This must include the vulnerable sections like the elderly, the differently abled, children and women because of their care giving and social function roles.

- *Risk reduction measures are community-specific* and are identified after an analysis of the community's disaster risk (hazards, vulnerabilities and capacities and perceptions of disaster risk)
- *Existing capacities and coping mechanisms are recognized* – CBDMit builds upon and strengthens existing capacities and coping strategies
- *The aim is to reduce vulnerabilities by strengthening capacities; the goal is building disaster resilient communities.*
- *Links disaster risk reduction with development*
  - Addresses existing vulnerable conditions and the causes of those vulnerabilities.
  - *Outsiders have a supporting and facilitating role.*
  - *Participatory process and content*: Involvement of community members, particularly the most vulnerable sectors and groups in the whole process of risk assessment, identification of mitigation and preparedness measures, decision making and implementation as the community directly benefits from the risk reduction and development process.
- *Responsive*: Based on the community's felt and urgent needs; considers the community's perception and prioritization of disaster risks and risk reduction measures so that the community can claim ownership.
- *Integrated*: Pre, during and post-disaster measures are planned and implemented as necessary by the community; there is linkage of the community with other communities, organizations and government units/agencies at various levels, especially for vulnerabilities which the local community cannot address by itself.
- *Proactive*: Stress on pre-disaster measures for prevention, mitigation and preparedness.
- *Comprehensive*: Structural (hard, physical) and non-structural (soft, health, education, livelihood, organization, advocacy, etc.) mitigation measures are undertaken; short-, medium-term and long-term measures to address vulnerabilities.
- *Multi-sectoral and multi-disciplinary*: Considers the roles and participation of all stakeholders in the community; combines indigenous/local knowledge and resources with science and technology and support from outsiders; addresses concerns of various stakeholders while upholding the basic interest of the most vulnerable sectors and groups.
- *Empowering*: People's options and capacities are increased; there is greater access to and control of resources and basic social services through concerted action; more meaningful participation in decision making which affects their lives; more control over their natural and physical environment; participation in disaster mitigation and risk reduction develops the confidence of community members to participate in other development endeavors.
  - *Developmental*: Contributes to addressing and reducing the complex relation of conditions, factors and processes of vulnerabilities present in society.

Sustainability is a function of the convergence of the various elements and parameters above, and the presence of an organizational mechanism, the Disaster

Management Committee (DMC) or grassroots disaster response organization, to see the risk reduction process through. Replication follows from the immediate results and benefits and success stories show and tell that CBDM works!

Where the initiative comes from is not so important. What matters is that after initiating the process, the community participates in the study of their disaster risks, action planning and decision making on mitigation and preparedness solutions and also during the implementation stage. Community participation can be sustained if the risk reduction project responds to their immediate needs and they are involved in the process.

- The goal is to reduce people's vulnerability by increasing their capacities to prepare for, to cope with and to mitigate the adverse effects of disasters. Aware and organized communities can pressurize their government to implement policies and programs recognizing people's needs and interests and promoting a safer environment.
- People affected by disasters are active actors in rebuilding their lives and livelihood. People's existing capacities are recognized and further strengthened.
- It addresses the root causes of people's vulnerabilities and contributes to transforming or else removing structures generating inequity and underdevelopment.
- People's participation is essential in all phases of disaster management and contributes to building their capacities. Assessment of disaster threat situations is a continuous process before, during and after disaster events and involves all community members and considering class, gender, age, culture, location, etc.
- Premium on building organizational capacity of the most-vulnerable communities through formation of grassroots disaster response organizations.
- The less vulnerable sectors are mobilized into a partnership with the vulnerable sectors in disaster management and development work in order to identify relevant, realistic and do-able mitigation and preparedness solutions. Relevance and community participation then creates ownership and, with even small successes achieved, sustainability of the CBDMit process can be ensured.
  - The grassroots disaster management/response organizations (community based organizations, groups or volunteers) are the key to mobilize the community at large. These groups are the focal point for local leadership and responsibility in CBDM. Within these grassroots disaster management organizations/committees, the importance of grassroots leaders who would take pains to educate and motivate the individuals of their community to prepare for and mitigate disasters has to be underscored. These leaders work with the grassroots disaster management organizations to open up the minds of the community members to develop more creative and appropriate ways to reduce disaster risk.
  - Communities are no longer just recipients/beneficiaries but are now partners in the disaster risk reduction and local development process. Capacity building and public awareness activities enables communities to increase participation and eventually, to sustain even on their own the CBDMit and preparedness activities.
  - Aside from raising awareness on hazard exposure and its consequences, and the appropriate preparedness and

mitigation measures to be undertaken, public awareness focuses on information dissemination, gaining consensus, building interest and commitment to the actual community risk reduction assessment, action planning and implementation process through its various stages.

- Assessments formed the basis for the identification and prioritization of structural mitigation measures at the household and community level such as the raising of homesteads, tube wells, roads, community place, cluster village raising, as well as construction of new dams, drainage, and roads, distribution of new tube wells and installation of new latrines above flood level.
- Placing CBDM on the political agenda by raising awareness through posters, billboards in vulnerable wards, signboards on rickshaws, newsletters, bulletins, actual demonstrations, cultural events, ideas sharing workshop, cross visits, street plays are among the various forms and venues used. The government's role is integral in CBDMit as a facilitator, enabler, and partner. The decentralization of power and responsibility to provide basic development services from the national center to lower government units has augured well for CBDM/CBDMit to be integrated into the formal disaster management, development planning and urban management system. Although largely dependent on the local official's political will and development orientation, AUDMP experiences show that sustainable CBDMit can be achieved with proactive local government support. When CBDMit is incorporated into the agenda, plans and programs of local government units, institutionalization and mainstreaming can be facilitated. The process also helps reduce the vulnerability of cities to landslide, flood, erosion, subsidence, pollution, and contamination of water supplies. Focus is also on developing tools and skills to incorporate into urban development planning. Some of the communities have identified the hazards and vulnerabilities associated with their locations and have formulated action plans to mitigate adverse impacts. Women and senior citizens actively participate in decision-making. The communities' openness for supports from the outside, provides opportunities to improve livelihood options through skills development programs. Community credit and savings projects pool funds to meet future needs. Mitigation measures include development of community forest, community forest fire break and construction of community drainage systems. The CBDM/CBDMit process and content leads to more partnerships, mobilization and self-reliance, and control and access to power, resources, basic services and decision making to solve community problems. It is a power sharing and voice gaining process of the community.
- Negative feedback from cases where inadequate involvement of community members in the DMCs decision making has resulted in problems with project development and design, mobilization of funds and labor for projects, and consequent delays in timetable can prove to be eye openers.
- Tools for hazard assessment include aspects of the nature and behavior of hazards, hazard mapping, seasonal

calendar studies and getting historical profile through community elders. Tools for vulnerability assessment include the vulnerability mapping (hazard map showing elements at risk), institutional and social network analysis for designing structural mitigation works that can prove useful in identifying problems and raising awareness. Some organizations and communities refer to this as the hazard and resource map. Community hazard and resource maps also help in generating outside support.

– Participatory methods have been used even with low literacy groups with the use of a lot of visualization such as drawings, tables and locally available materials such as seeds, leaves, and rocks. Higher technology methods are also employed like the use of GPS for the initial hazard and resource mapping. The digitized hazard and resource maps are then publicized using materials such as posters and comics to arrive at consensus based problem identification and ranking solutions.

Construction of a hanging bridge, a health center, protecting the mangroves from being converted into commercial fishponds are a few examples where the community provided the labor while Red Cross and other agencies have provided the materials for the projects. Technical help in engineering design have been provided by the municipal government and, since the projects had been identified by the community as being urgent, they worked very hard to see the construction projects to completion, and then manage and sustain the project with their own resources.

Replication and Sustainability

Replication follows from immediate results/ benefits and success stories which show and tell that CBDMit works. Within and beyond the project areas, the indication that local initiatives can be sustained is the replication of the mitigation solutions. Initial and even small successes provide the springboard to sustain disaster preparedness and mitigation, even without a project with outside funding. Increased confidence and trust in concerted action can lead the community to address bigger problems.

Success Stories

Rapid population growth, unplanned development, constructions that do not meet the building code requirements and a general lack of awareness about safety make some areas increasingly vulnerable to earthquakes. The design of an earthquake preparedness curriculum and production of proposals to retrofit most at-risk buildings by pilot structural interventions through community participation has been implemented in Nepal and other seismic zones. Trained masons have been drawn from other cities to train locals by conducting evening classes for 3 months. The local masons then identified the structures and schools that needed quake-proofing. Community workshops were convened for ideas exchange on how the community and outside organizations could work together. A model prototype of earthquake resistant technology was exhibited and shake table demonstration helped convince the community of their utility. Community leaders were involved in the risk assessments and labor for the retrofitting project was provided by the locals. Funds and materials were also generated by the communities themselves. Even school children helped in carrying material like bamboo and sticks. The project had such impact such that homeowners within and outside the community were influenced to construct their houses using seismic-resistant features and duplicate the school retrofitting process. As they completed their project, their community became closer and cohesive and the members had a tremendous sense of ownership of the project. Because all family members were involved, all houses were reconstructed in record time at half the normal cost when compared to other rehabilitation interventions made when the external agency did everything with very little learning scope for the locals. Every villager took pride in what had been achieved in his or her community and the project served to build community solidarity and bring people together. In other places, micro-projects in the by community based flood mitigation programs (CBFMP) reduced the communities' physical vulnerability to flood. They also improved livelihood in terms of enhanced safety, ease of access and economic benefits. For example, the construction of an emergency evacuation route enhanced the safety of villagers and their livestock. Raising of roads and construction of bridges provided reliable transportation routed and increased accessibility, allowing students to travel to school and traders to transport their agricultural produce to local markets. New, enlarged or rebuilt culverts increased the community's control over water flow, enabling them to increase their rice crop yield, and for some communities, even harvest a second rice crop.

Ownership Leads to Better Management and Sustainability

The results of the community based approaches to disaster mitigation are vulnerability reduction solutions which are more relevant and in tune with what people need and want. Because community members have been involved in the whole process of problem identification to ranking/prioritizing solutions, they have ownership of the project. Popular and appropriate methods and channels in public awareness and information dissemination ensure that community members are included in the information and decision making loop. Schemes for project implementation take into account preferences of the community, example when the community prefers the construction of safe areas for individual families close to their homes rather than a collective shelter. Since they have ownership of the project and its results, they would naturally manage, maintain and sustain it better. Community participation builds their confidence, skills and ability to cooperate. This enables them to tackle other challenges and bigger problems both in the individual, household and community level. This AUDMP experience demonstrates the cascading effects which even structural measures for physical safety have on the household and the community's social and economic life.

Impact Measurement

In urban management, general impact indicators revolves around changes in the following dimensions: social and economic well-being of local population, the physical configuration and quality of the environment; and, local institutional/organizational capacity. A framework for the measurement of impact of CBDMit and the risk reduction process is increased in capacities and reduced vulnerabilities.

CONCLUSION

Recognizing and considering the interests (which in other instances translates into demands) of the various stakeholders in the community risk reduction process must ensure the interests of vulnerable sectors/ groups. Synchronizing efforts and strategies of the multi-stakeholders in the risk reduction process is important. There is a need for more public awareness and capability building activities in the initial stages to overcome barriers such as ignorance, fatalism, and pessimism. Community organizing and mobilizing takes times. Capacity building and strengthening grassroots disaster management organizations is a gradual and phased process as mobilizing volunteers and manpower to undertake and sustain community mobilization for risk reduction takes awhile. There is also a need for continued development of tools, instruments, applicable technologies and mechanisms to put in place mitigation, in both urban and rural communities. Big funding requirements are sometimes needed, especially for materials used in structural measures and various schemes to mobilize resources from donors (external and internal) have to be initiated. When the political environment is not enabling, non-structural mitigation such as lobby and advocacy work can have more confrontational approaches. Community Based Approaches to Disaster Mitigation circumvents this through a local consensus approach. After all, when disasters occur it is our community that is affected first, and it is vital that they be prepared because there is always a gap between the actual disaster event and the time external assistance arrives.

FURTHER READING

Community based approach to disaster mitigation by lorna P Victoria, Director, Center for disaster preparedness.

38 Guidelines for Relief Workers During Disasters

> "Calamity is a man's true touchstone."
>
> —*Anon*

The following information will be useful for relief workers deputed to disaster areas:

DISEASE SPECTRUM AND PREVENTION

Malaria

Malaria occurs in most parts of the world. Ways to prevent malaria include the following:

- Taking a prescription antimalarial drug.
- Using insect repellent and wearing long pants and sleeves to prevent mosquito bites.
- Sleeping in air-conditioned or well-screened rooms or using bed nets.

No antimalarial drug is 100% protective, so it is important to use all three ways to prevent malaria.

All of the following antimalarial drugs are equal options for preventing malaria: atovaquone/proguanil (Malarone®), chloroquine, doxycycline, or mefloquine. Each drug has its own side effects, contraindications, and precautions. You will need to talk to your doctor to decide which of these drugs would be best for you, depending on your current health, medical history, drug allergies, and specific needs.

Malaria is always a serious disease and may be a deadly illness. If you become ill with a fever or flu-like illness either while in disaster affected areas or after you return home (for up to 1 year), you should seek immediate medical attention and should tell the doctor that you have recently been abroad.

Dengue

Dengue is a common infection in many third world countries. Dengue is a disease caused by a virus transmitted to people by the bite of an infected mosquito. Some important information to know about dengue as you travel are:

- No vaccine or medications are available to prevent dengue.
- The best way to reduce your risk of dengue is to protect yourself from mosquito bites (see the section below called "Protection Against Insects and Animals").
- The mosquitoes that spread dengue usually bite at dusk and dawn but may bite at any time during the day.
- Symptoms and signs are high fever, chills, headache and muscle pain. Additionally, a faint rash on the trunk and upper arms may appear on the second to third day of illness.
- There are no specific medicines to treat dengue, so treatment is supportive with fever-reducing medicines and fluids.
- You can help control mosquito populations by draining all standing water that you find in open containers left outdoors.

HIV

Many countries have a high prevalence of HIV infection. To reduce the risk of HIV and other sexually transmitted diseases, always use latex condoms. Healthcare workers should also take the following additional precautions:

- Wear gloves for touching blood and body fluids, mucous membranes, or broken skin and for handling items or surfaces soiled with blood or body fluids.
- Use masks and protective eyewear or face shields to prevent exposure of the mouth, nose, and eyes during procedures that are likely to generate droplets of blood or body fluids.
- Wear gowns or aprons during procedures that are likely to generate splashes of blood or body fluids.

Tuberculosis (TB)

Rates of tuberculosis is also very high in many countries.

- If you anticipate giving medical care or working closely with ill or injured victims, a tuberculin skin test (ideally, a two-step test) is recommended prior to travel and then 6-8 weeks after return.
- If exposure to known TB patients will occur, traveling with personal respiratory protective devices (e.g., N-95 respirators), along with training, is recommended.

Anthrax

Anthrax is primarily transmitted by direct contact with infected animals or with contaminated products from infected animals. Cases of cutaneous and inhalation anthrax have been reported among the local population.

- Symptoms of anthrax can occur within 7 days of infection. Symptoms include: fever (>100° F) and chills or night sweats; cough; chest discomfort; shortness of breath; fatigue; muscle aches; sore throat followed by difficulty swallowing; enlarged lymph nodes; headache; nausea; loss of appetite; abdominal discomfort, vomiting, or diarrhea; a sore, especially on your face, arms, or hands that starts as a raised bump and develops into a painless ulcer with a black area in the center.
- If you develop any of these symptoms, see a healthcare provider immediately.

Baggage

There will be almost no infrastructure support available on arrival in disaster affected regions. Relief workers, volunteers, and other travelers will need to be self-sufficient.

Pack basic supplies, including:

- Food and water sufficient for the length of your stay.
- Insect protection: Insect repellent and a bed net.
- *Medications:* Antimalarial pills, medications for the treatment of travelers' diarrhea (e.g., loperamide and an antibiotic), personal prescriptions (including extras), any preferred over-the-counter medications, and copies of all your prescriptions.
- An extra set of prescription eyeglasses and/or contacts.
- Water purification tablets (iodine or chlorine), bleach, or a water purifier.
- Persons with pre-existing health conditions should consider wearing an alert-bracelet and make sure this information is on a contact card in their wallet or travel documents. A contact card should include the following information:
  - Name and contact information of family member or close contact.
  - Name and contact information of health-care provider.

  - Pre-existing health conditions and treatment.
- Personal protective equipment (PPE): safety glasses or goggles, work boots, leather gloves for physical labor, rubber gloves for handling blood or body fluids, surgical masks, hard hat, ear plugs, N-95 respirators for those who are fit-tested.
- Due to severe damage to health facilities and shortages of medical supplies, carry a first aid kit for your own protection. Minimum suggested contents:
  - Bandages (roller, adhesive, triangular).
  - Sterile gauze pads.
  - Disposable gloves.
  - Scissors.
  - Tweezers.
  - Cold compress.
  - Antiseptic wipes.
  - Antibiotic ointment.
  - Hydrocortisone ointment.
  - Commercial suture/syringe kits to be used by a local health-care provider. These items will require a letter from the prescribing physician on letterhead stationery. Pack these items in checked baggage, since they may be considered sharp objects and confiscated by airport or airline security if packed in carry-on bags.

Wash your hands often with soap and clean water or use an alcohol-based hand cleaner (with at least 60% alcohol). Clean your hands especially before you eat or prepare food.

Safe Food and Drinks

- Eat foods that are packaged or that are freshly cooked and served hot.
- Do not eat raw and undercooked meats and seafood or unpeeled fruits and vegetables.
- Drink only bottled, boiled, or chemically treated water and bottled or canned carbonated beverages. When using bottled drinks, make sure that the seal has not been broken.
- Avoid tap water, fountain drinks, and ice cubes.
- To disinfect your own water: Boil for 1 minute or filter the water and add 2 drops of household bleach or 1/2 an iodine tablet per liter of water.
- Use bottled, boiled, or chemically treated water to wash dishes, brush your teeth, wash and prepare food, or make ice.

Protection Against Insects

Insect-borne diseases such as malaria and dengue are best avoided. Prevent insect bites by:

- Using insect repellent (bug spray) that contains one of the following active ingredients: DEET, picaridin (KBR 3023), Oil of Lemon Eucalyptus/PMD, or IR3535. Always follow the instructions on the label when you use the repellent.
- In general, repellents protect longer against mosquito bites when they have a higher concentration (percentage) of the active ingredient. However, concentrations above 50% do not offer a marked increase in protection time. Products with less than 10% of an active ingredient may offer only limited protection, often no longer than 1-2 hours.
- Wearing lightweight long-sleeved shirts, long pants, and a hat outdoors. For greater protection, clothing may also be sprayed with repellent containing permethrin or another EPA-registered repellent. (*Remember:* Don't use permethrin on skin.)
- Remaining indoors in a screened area or using insect repellent frequently on uncovered skin during the peak biting period for malaria (dusk and dawn) and dengue (any time of day).
- Sleeping in beds covered by a bed net (preferably treated with permethrin), if

not sleeping in an air-conditioned or well-screened room.
- Spraying rooms with products effective against flying insects, such as those containing pyrethroid.

Protection Against Animals

- Contact with animals can spread diseases like rabies or cause serious injury or illness. Displaced animals may revert to the wild and go about in packs. They will also be hungry and may be searching for food and may be more likely to bite.
- It is important to prevent animal bites and scratches.
- Stay away from all animals, including dogs and cats. Even animals that look like healthy pets can have rabies or other diseases.
- If you are bitten or scratched, wash the wound well with soap and clean water and *seek medical care right away*. If you have a povidone-iodine solution (such as Betadine®), use that to clean the wound after washing it.
- Resist the urge to rescue animals with the intent to bring them home. Dogs and cats may be infected with rabies but not show signs until several days or weeks after you first encounter them.
- When you return home, be sure to tell your doctor or health department if you were bitten or scratched during travel.

Injuries

The risk of injury after an earthquake is high. Hazards such as electrocution from downed power lines and structural damage to buildings and roads all pose a risk. Accidents and violence are documented risks for humanitarian workers and cause more deaths than disease and natural causes.

- The majority of the roads may not be paved and terrain may be predominately mountainous and show extensive deforestation and soil erosion, making travel over roadways especially hazardous. Exercise extreme care when traveling on roads particularly in rural areas.
- There may be extensive structural damage to buildings. Avoid unstable structures if possible.
- Other potential hazards to be aware of in collapsed buildings include standing water from water system breaks, natural gas leaks, airborne smoke and dusk, hazardous materials such as ammonia or leaking fuels, exposure to germs from sewer line breaks, and exposed wiring.
- Use personal protection equipment, such as hard hats and steel-toed boots, if in areas with damaged buildings.

Exposure to Human Remains

Human remains may contain blood-borne viruses and diarrhea-causing bacteria. Relief workers who are handling remains should take precautions to avoid being exposed to these organisms:

- Protect your face from splashes of body fluids and fecal material by using a plastic face shield or a combination of eye protection and surgical mask. In extreme situations, a cloth tied over the nose and mouth can be used to block splashes.
- Protect your hands from direct contact with body fluids and from injuries that break the skin by using a combination of a cut-proof inner layer glove and a latex (or similar) outer layer.
- Wash your hands with soap and water or with an alcohol-based hand cleaner immediately after you remove the gloves.
- Protect your feet and ankles against sharp debris by wearing foot wear that covers the entire foot and has thick soles.
- Give prompt care—including immediate cleansing with soap and water, and a teta-

nus booster if indicated—to anyone who is injured during work with human remains.

Psychological/Emotional Difficulties

As a first responder or relief worker, you may encounter extremely stressful situations, such as witnessing a tremendous loss of life, serious injuries, missing and separated families, and destruction of whole areas. It is important to recognize that these experiences may cause you psychological or emotional difficulties.

Normal Reactions to a Disaster Event

- Profound sadness, grief, and anger are common.
- You may not want to leave the scene until the work is finished.
- You will likely try to override stress and fatigue with dedication and commitment.
- You may deny the need for rest and recovery time.

Ways to Help Manage Your Stress

- Limit on-duty work time to no more than 12 hours per day.
- Rotate work assignments between high stress and lower stress functions.
- Drink plenty of water and eat healthy snacks and other energy foods.
- Take frequent, brief breaks from the scene when you are able.
- Keep an object of comfort with you such as a family photo, favorite music, or religious material.
- Stay in touch with family and friends.
- Pair up with another responder so that you can monitor one another's stress.

After You Come Home

If you are not feeling well, you should see your doctor and mention that you have recently returned from response and relief work abroad. Also tell your doctor if you were bitten or scratched by an animal while traveling.

Symptoms of malaria can develop up to one year after travel, so be alert for fever or flu-like symptoms.

Approximately one-third of aid workers report depression shortly after returning home, and more than half of returned aid workers have reported feeling predominantly negative emotions on returning home, even though many reported that their time overseas was positive and fulfilling. You might want to see a professional counselor to help you adjust back into your home environment.

39 The Disaster Quiz

> "The stabbing horror of life is not contained in calamities and disasters, because these things wake one up and one gets very familiar and intimate with them and finally they become tame again."
>
> —*Henry Miller*

ANSWER TRUE OR FALSE

1. In case of disaster, send out an immediate appeal for international medical personnel.
   T/F
2. When a disaster occurs, people in other countries should not react immediately, organizing the collection and dispatch of whatever can be obtained by way of medicines, clothing, equipment, etc.
   T/F
3. A few weeks after a disaster occurs, things are usually back to normal and most of the major services are restored.
   T/F
4. Disasters cause fewer deaths in rich countries than in poor countries.
   T/F
5. Disasters brings out the worst in human behavior.
   T/F
6. When disaster strikes, outbreaks of infectious diseases are inevitable due to the presence of unattended dead bodies.
   T/F
7. Mass hunger can be avoided after a disaster strikes.
   T/F
8. Following a disaster, it is best to house people as close as possible to their own dwellings rather than in settlement camps.
   T/F
9. In case of limited food supplies following a disaster, priority should be given to the young and the old.
   T/F
10. When disaster strikes, each individual should take care of his own family and belongings first.
    T/F
11. The intensity of two recent earthquakes in Armenia and San Francisco was the same, but in Armenia, several thousand dies whereas, in San Francisco only sixty people died. This was mainly due to the difference in earthquake-proof construction.
    T/F
12. The Sahelian drought is caused by a combination of climactic and man-made factors.
    T/F

ANSWERS

1. **False:** Local health services are normally able to cope in case of disasters with the advantage of speaking the local language, being familiar with the health service infrastructure and problems. Foreign teams may provide specialized skills and equipment, but they have to be housed and fed.
2. **True:** A fast international response to disasters is not necessarily the best solution. An evaluation of the most urgent needs should first be made so that communication channels do not become blocked by inessential items or outdated medicaments and food products.
3. **False:** Whilst disaster may disappear from the news headlines, the impact may last for years with permanent damage to water supplies and health services, as reconstruction and rehabilitation are time consuming and costly.
4. **True:** Poverty leads to poor living conditions and the poor are more vulnerable in case of disasters. The richer countries have the resources with which to rebuild their lives and usually better prepared.
5. **False:** While some sensation-seeking scribes might encourage us to believe that looting and other forms of selfish behavior are common following disasters, on the contrary, it has been shown that disaster situations bring out the best in people and solidarity is strengthened.
6. **False:** Dead bodies do not cause epidemics or disease transmission during the first 72 hours. Decomposition after this time can contaminate water supplies. The first priority after a disaster must be to provide care for the injured.
7. **True:** Disasters such as earthquakes do not damage crops, although drought, hurricanes and floods do. If adequate storage and rationing of foods are organized, there should not be any serious hunger problem. When international assistance is called, tools and seeds are often more important than food.
8. **True:** Keeping people as close to their homes as possible is best and settlement camps must be the last resort since they create other problems. International assistance must seek building materials and tools.
9. **False:** Careful rationing must be organized so that everyone is fed. Those involved in salvage work and reconstruction are particularly in need of a regular food supply.
10. **False:** Team work is the most efficient way of dealing with the aftermath of a disaster. Training of teams prior to a disaster is important taking care that each person knows his or her responsibilities for proper management of the situation.
11. **True:** Strict adherence to the building code in earthquake prone areas significantly diminishes the loss of human life.
12. **True:** Overgrazing, failure to plant trees and mismanagement of land use leading to soil erosion, in addition to local climatic factors, led to an advancement of the desert in Sahel.

(Test created by Dorothy Hoffmann and Gilbert Padey, WHO, Geneva, Switzerland)

40 Medicare During Disasters

> "I beg you take courage; the brave soul can mend even disaster"
>
> —*Catherine II*

THE COMPONENTS OF DISASTER MEDICINE DELIVERY SYSTEM

The 3 Rs of any disaster management protocol are:

- Readiness.
- Response; and
- Recovery.

At the Scene Recognition of the emergency and aid by first responders/bystanders.

Initiation of the disaster response system.

Double cordoning of the area to render the scene safe and also to prevent looting and tampering with evidence.

Establishing an effective, all-weather communication network.

Establishing clear approach and exit routes.

Resuscitation and stabilization of victims.

Transportation with life support and expert pre-hospital care.

Siting parking bays for vehicles.

Mobilizing equipments like cranes, earth moving machinery, refrigerated containers, arc cutting gear.

Organizing video coverage of site and victims.

Hospital emergency care.

Operation theatre interventions.

ICU/ITU care.

Planning, education and evaluation.

Research (Clinical and public health aspects).

41 Casualty Evacuation (Casevac)

> "There is no calamity that right words will not begin to redress."
>
> —*Ralph Waldo Emerson*

INTRODUCTION

In the history of disasters, it is probable that more casualties have died as a result of inadequate and delayed medical treatment following trauma than as a direct result of the trauma itself. Trauma is the chief cause of death from the first week of life to the fourth decade and also the fourth most common cause overall. Globally, trauma accounts for 1-2% of any country's GNP. Its effects are protean, affecting not only the victim but also their relatives and society as a whole. While rapid casualty evacuation (Casevac) is a universally accepted criterion in assessing the effectiveness of a casualty treatment system, it cannot be an alternative to immediate treatment. The link between effective triage, early treatment and survival rates is no longer disputed. The concept of the Golden Hour following trauma is established, when not only life-threatening symptoms must be tackled and relieved, but the onset of potentially fatal problems must be preempted. It is estimated that 40% of trauma deaths are preventable. The statistics of wartime medicine over the past 20 years has demonstrated that survival depends on the length of the interval between trauma and medical aid. The concept of traditional first-aid is essentially reactive. It does little more than address the most obvious symptoms. This is largely unsatisfactory and has led to a revision of the earlier practice of scoop and run to one of stabilize at site. Trauma deaths occur in a trimodal distribution with respect to time. The three peaks of occurrence are immediate, early and late. Immediate deaths are due to massive head injury, brainstem injury and major injuries to the cardiovascular system like heart and large blood vessel laceration, and are not amenable to medical or surgical therapy. Half of all trauma deaths belong to this category and patients are not salvageable, with death occurring within the first few hours. Major torso trauma and closed head injuries account for a majority of immediate deaths and are treatable in modern trauma centers. When associated with multiple organ failure, the death rate is close to 20%. The second peak due to haemorrhage, subdural haematomas, hemopneumothorax, visceral injuries like lacerations of the liver and spleen, or fractures occurs within 1 to 4 hours of injury, accounting for 30% of deaths that can be prevented by appropriate and timely medical care. The third peak, or late trauma death, occurs about two weeks following injury, mainly due to complications like sepsis, multi organ failure and severe brain injuries. Early resuscitation prevents these delayed lethal complications. What is disputable in disaster situations is the type and extent of pre-hospital medicare that must be afforded to casualties.

It would be pertinent to note here that the term polytrauma is used to indicate that there is more than one casualty, i.e., multiple patient situations as in disasters, whereas the term multitrauma is used to describe a patient with more than one injury.

42 Trauma Prevention and Prehospital Care

> "There is no calamity that right words will not begin to redress."
>
> —*Ralph Waldo Emerson*

INTRODUCTION

Trauma ranks as the No. 3 killer of modern society. Up to 30% of prehospital deaths may be preventable. Even in areas with highly structured emergency care, the norm for ambulance response to a road crash is ten minutes. Many people will die if nothing is done to correct the slow response time to hypoxia. The application of first aid techniques, in particular the proper positioning of the victim prior to the arrival of the emergency response teams, can mean the difference between life and death in a road crash. The British Red Cross published in 2004 a report: *Anyone can save a life: Road safety and road accidents* recommending developing greater first aid knowledge amongst the general population be they drivers, car-users or pedestrians involved in, or bystanders to, road accidents. There are notable disparities in mortality rates for injured patients around the world. For example, one study looked at the mortality rates for all seriously injured adults in three cities, in countries at different economic levels. The mortality rate (including both pre-hospital and in-hospital deaths) rose from 35% in a high-income setting to 55% in a middle income setting, to 63% in a low-income setting.

A trauma system is an organized, coordinated effort in a defined geographic area that can deliver the full range of care to all injured patients and is integrated with the local public health system. The true value of a trauma system is derived from the seamless transition between each phase of care, integrating and coordinating existing resources to achieve improved patient outcomes. Success of a trauma system is largely determined by the degree to which it is supported by public policy. The different components must provide cost-effective services for injury prevention and patient care capable of delivering the full spectrum of care to an injured patient from the time of the injury through transport to an acute care facility and to rehabilitative care.

4 E's of Injury Prevention

1. Education: The cornerstone supporting change in behaviour to target groups.
2. Enforcement: Legislations seat belts, strict drunk driving laws.
3. Engineering: Initially expensive, greatest long term benefits, airbags. Highway design and safety.
4. Economics (incentives): Discounted premiums for helmet wearing.

At the center of this system is the continuum of care, which includes injury prevention, pre-hospital care, acute care facilities, and post-hospital care. Trauma systems must be based on the unique requirements of the population served, such as rural, inner-city and urban communities.

The infrastructure of a trauma care system includes eight key elements: leadership, professional resources, education and advocacy, information, finances, research, technology, and disaster preparedness and response.

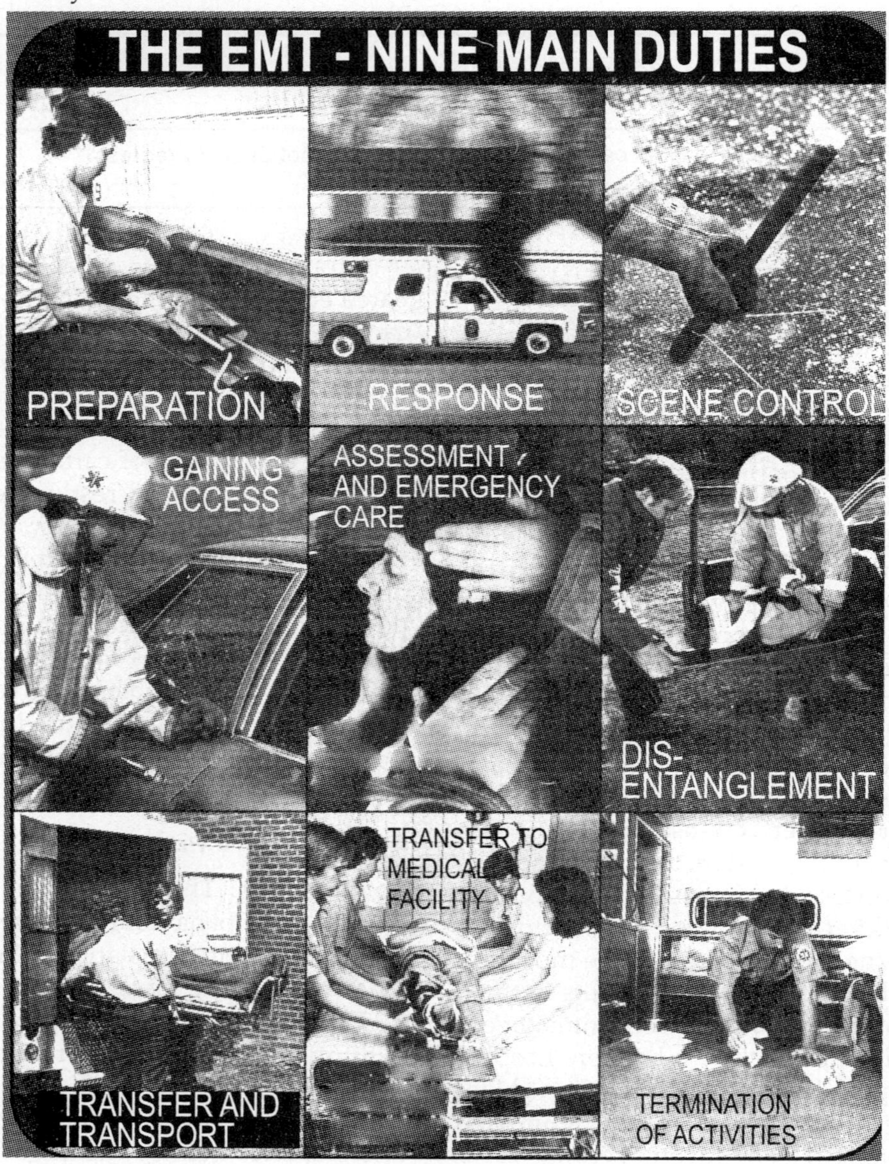

Fig. 42.1

43 Fundamental Components of Trauma Care

"If I can see Heaven, I will soon be there!"

TRAUMA MANAGEMENT PHILOSOPHY

The Advanced trauma life support (ATLS) is an immediate and phased approach to a trauma patient. It enables the first responders (doctors and nurses team) to:

- Identify and manage life threatening injury first.
- Then reassess and manage other injuries.

Approach

Primary survey:	
What is killing the patient? Resuscitation: Treat what is killing the patient	Best done on the spot
Secondary survey: Head-to-toe post resuscitation examination of the victim to identify all other injuries and Develop a definitive care plan	Best done in a static health care facility

Elements of Primary Survey

A: Airway assessment while protecting cervical spine.

B: Breathing and ventilation assessment-look, feel and listen approach especially for tension pneumothorax, open pneumothorax, massive hemothorax, flail chest, pulmonary contusion and cardiac tamponade. Look for bruises and wounds over the neck and chest wall, distended neck veins, dyspnea/abnormal breathing patterns, chest asymmetry. Feel for position of trachea, tenderness over ribs and wounds hidden at the back. Percuss the apex, axillae and bases and auscultate for presence or absence of breath sounds.

C: Circulation assessment and control of bleeding.

D: Dysfunction of the central nervous system.

E: Environmental considerations and exposure of the victim and also evacuation of the victim to appropriate care facility.

Injury Prevention

- Each state should have a core injury prevention program that provides assistance to local areas, with information and materials coordinated via a central repository or clearinghouse.
- A trauma registry data will help with problem identification and program evaluation and will be fully coordinated with the EMS and public health systems.
- A comprehensive study of the epidemiology of injuries and trauma must be conducted and predictive models regarding injury occurrence developed.
- Injury prevention legislation must be enacted, where compelling evidence exists.

- Injury prevention efforts must be conducted on a collaborative basis, with input from and the involvement of multiple stakeholders and constituency groups.
- Injury prevention must be recognized as a legitimate public and governmental activity, similar to other safety programs such as fire prevention. Proper funding will be secured for injury prevention, with a greater portion of public health budget allocated for injury prevention.
- Injury prevention efforts must be seen as a legitimate health care cost that is directly reimbursable to providers.
- Injury prevention programs, and their availability to the general public, must be required by lead agencies who designate all levels of trauma centers and by the public health systems.
- Injury prevention must be integrated into existing health delivery systems, such as pediatric and rural health clinics, and prevention materials must be readily available at places where families usually receive care.
- EMS and first responders must be integrated within the health care system, with links to prevention and acute care, with greater focus on promoting overall community health.
- Trauma care must be coordinated and integrated using standard protocols and triage. Triage criteria must be redesigned to ensure more accurate assessment, which facilitates direction and placement of patients to the most appropriate care setting for definitive care.
- Transport vehicles (air and ground) must be strategically placed rather than facility based and used appropriately to facilitate rapid access and response, especially in areas that are least accessible.
- A national 911 system, covering both wireless and wireline telephone systems, must be developed and implemented, with standard, seamless protocols that are evidence-based and that address bystander interface. Access to prehospital trauma care in rural areas must be greatly enhanced through development of consistent standards and more efficient deployment of limited resources.
- Enhanced communications among all components of the trauma care team during the pre-hospital phase must speed up deployment of resources, produce more appropriate triaging, and result in better patient outcomes.

Acute Care Facilities

A distributed system of acute care facilities and trauma care systems must be implemented across the country.

- Research must be conducted to determine the effectiveness of the current tiered resource allocation guidelines.
- The appropriate volume of patients with specific injuries that are needed at the highest echelon of care must be studied and clearly identified so that research and treatment options can be continually explored.
- Trauma systems must be linked on a regional basis through databases and technology to ensure efficient and effective patient care nationwide.
- There must be consistent standards for rural and urban trauma services, with the goal of every community having access to a consistent level of trauma care.
- All injury care providers within a community must be recognized as part of the system and provide data to a system-wide database, whereby injury care can be monitored throughout the system.
- Most facilities, whether small community hospitals or large tertiary care centers, must

have a designated role to play in the trauma system and the capacity to manage injured patients to one degree or another.
- Facilities in the system must have multi-casualty capabilities.
- The appropriate match of resources must be identified for injured patients with special needs, such as elderly, remote rural, or pediatric patients.
- Innovative treatment methods must be explored, including utilization of mobile trauma units for rural areas.

Table 43.1: Interhospital transfer criteria when the patient's needs exceed available resources

Clinical circumstances
Central Nervous System
• Head Injury
– Penetrating injury or depressed skull fracture
– Open injury with or without CSF leak
– GCS score <14 or GCS deterioration;
– Lateralizing Signs
– Spinal Cord Injury or Major Vertebral Injury
Chest
• Widened mediastinum or signs suggesting great vessel injury
• Major chest wall injury or pulmonary contusion
• Cardiac injury
• Patients who may require prolonged ventilation
Pelvis/Abdomen
• Unstable pelvic-ring—disruption
• Pelvic-ring disruption with shock and evidence of continuing hemorrhage
• Open pelvic injury
Extremity
• Severe open fractures
• Traumatic amputation with potential for replantation
• Complex articular fractures
• Major crush injury
• Ischemia
Multisystem Injury
• Head injury with face, chest, abdominal, or pelvic injury
• Injury to more than two body regions
• Major burns or burns with associated injuries
• Multiple, proximal long-bone fractures
Comorbid Factors
• Age >55 years
• Children
• Cardiac or respiratory disease
• Insulin-dependent diabetics, morbid obesity. pregnancy
• Immunosuppression
Secondary Deterioration (Late sequelae)
• Mechanical ventilation required
• Sepsis
• Single or multiple organ system failure (deterioration in central nervous, cardiac, pulmonary, hepatic, renal, or coagulation systems)
• Major tissue necrosis

Post-Hospital Trauma Care (Mobile Medical Response)

There is a pressing need to strengthen the quality and availability of pre-hospital trauma care systems throughout the world. To achieve this goal, leading experts in the field have proposed a collaborative effort to define a minimum acceptable level of pre-hospital care that could save lives, including the definition of core strategies, relevant equipment, and needed supplies and organizational structures. The World Health Organization (WHO) has been a central coordinator for this collaborative effort to achieve consensus around a simple but sustainable set of interventions that should constitute the "decent minimum" of pre-hospital trauma care that all countries should aspire to provide. Achieving this goal could save many lives and prevent countless disabilities worldwide.

- Long-term care coverage must be available, affordable, and encouraged to help address post-hospital care needs.
- Post-hospital care must focus on helping patients achieve greater independence, a higher degree of functionality, and a faster return to productivity.
- Functional recovery must go beyond traditional rehabilitation and include psychological support.

- Home-based care and monitoring must be used to manage costs and speed recovery, especially in areas lacking access to care.
- Appropriate support groups must be established and encouraged.
- Trauma registry data must include post-hospital care and rehabilitation so that the value and cost-effectiveness of the full cycle of trauma care can be more readily assessed.
- Research concerning the effectiveness of post hospital care must be supported. Problems in Pre Hospital Care

Problems in Pre Hospital Care

- Paramedics operate with less patient information in a much less controlled environment.
- Philosophy of prehospital care varies between countries. In USA basic resuscitation is performed at the scene as a 'scoop and run' management whereas in France, mobile intensive care units often attend the scene of an accident as a 'stay and play' management protocol.
- Potential problems at scene of accident like hostility of environment, lack of familiarity with surroundings and intrusive onlookers
- Assess safety for EMS staff and casualties. The accident site must be rendered as safe as possible before assessing any casualties
- Determination of the nature of accident and likely mechanism of injuries like the number, direction and types of vehicles involved, degree of intrusion of damages vehicles and whether occupants were wearing seatbelts and other personal safety devices.

Indications of Potential Significant Trauma

- Penetrating injury to chest and abdomen.
- Two or more proximal long bone fractures.
- Burns involving more than 15% of body surface area.
- Burns to face and airway.
- Evidence of high-energy impact.
- Fall more than 6m.
- Crash speed greater than 20 mph.
- Inward deformity of car of more than 0.6m.
- Rearward displacement of front axle.
- Ejection of passenger from vehicle.
- Rollover of vehicle.
- Death of another car occupant.
- Pedestrian hit at greater than 20 mph.

Abnormal Physiological Variables

- Glasgow coma score 9-11.
- HR >120.
- Systolic blood pressure < 90 in adult or age specific BP.
- Respiratory rate < 10 or > 29, Age < 5 or > 55.
- Cardiac or respiratory disease, immune suppression.
- Pregnancy, bleeding disorder, DM, cirrhosis or morbid obesity.
- Non extremity GSW.
- Multi casualty with 5 or more patients.
- Evidence of paralysis.
- Major burns/smoke inhalation.
- Amputation proximal to wrist or ankle.

Pre Hospital Resuscitation

- Should follow same principles as that in hospital. Resuscitation goals would be to secure a systolic blood pressure > 80 torr (mean 50-60 torr), heart rate <120 bpm, SpO_2>95%, utrine output >0.5 ml/kg/h, Hgb>8.0 g/dl, base deficit >–5, lactate <1.6 mmol/l and mental state permitting obeying commands level.
- Will need to be adapted to circumstances.
- Airway management can be difficult but it can often be maintained with basic measures.

- Intubation without anaesthesia and rapid sequence induction is ill advised as this can induce vomiting and raised intracranial pressure.
- The cervical spine should be immobilized with a hard collar.
- Oxygen should be given.
- Haemorrhage should be controlled with direct pressure.
- If casualty is entrapped, ensure good venous access before releasing from vehicle.
- Fluid resuscitation should be give to a systolic blood pressure of 90 mmHg. Role of hypertonic saline is doubtful.
- If venous access difficult consider 'scoop and run' rather than delay transfer.
- Analgesia can be achieved with ketamine 0.6 mg/kg oral, 0.5-1.0 mg kg I/V.
- Extrication requires close co-ordination between medical and fire services.
- Casualty should be 'packaged for transport'—this will require hard collar, head blocks, limb splints, scoop stretcher or vacuum mattress.
- Trauma patients are more susceptible to infections demanding a tight vigilance and a high degree of suspicion to diagnose and treat septic situations. Prophylactic antibiotherapy (ATB) is given to some trauma patients in pre hospital settings, especially those with open fractures, perforated wounds and also those who have had emergency invasive procedures.

Comprehensive Trauma Care System: Key Infrastructure Elements

Leadership

- A National Trauma System Leadership Council must be developed to advocate for system development in a facilitative manner, serve as the locus for policy development and support, and coordinate the work of central agencies and professional organizations with injury-related programs.
- All states must establish a Lead Agency to coordinate and administer trauma system development.
- A best practices study must be conducted to identify the optimal components and configuration for local and state lead agencies.
- The effectiveness of trauma system elements must be continually examined.
- State legislators and bureaucrats must be informed about the need for an identified and adequately funded lead agency for trauma systems in their region.

Professional Resources

- Professional resources in the system must be patient focused, team-oriented and physician led.
- New categories of providers and the use of physician extenders must address the need for additional resources.
- Creative opportunities for recruitment and retention of personnel must be explored.
- Reimbursement for all types of providers must be appropriate and sufficient so as to encourage participation in trauma care.
- Incentives for attracting trauma specialization, including addressing the burden of liability, must be explored.
- Ongoing professional education opportunities must be available and accessible.
- Volunteers must supplement career resources and enlisted to promote injury prevention as well as deliver care.

Education and Advocacy

- A compelling educational campaign must be launched to position trauma and injury as a disease rather than a random occurrence and to increase public awareness of the need for injury prevention and the value of trauma care.
- Targeted educational programs must be developed to inform policy makers about

the value of community-based trauma care in order to promote passage of legislation to support trauma system activities, including injury prevention.

- Trauma care providers and advocates must form or integrate into coalitions with trade associations, large corporations (such as Johnson and Johnson's work with the *Safe Kids* campaign) and payers to conduct public education programs about injury and injury prevention and to advocate for legislation to support injury prevention and trauma system activities.
- Health insurers must have a clear appreciation of the cost effectiveness of injury prevention and provide incentives for safe behavior.
- Communication, education, and training approaches for the public and key constituency groups must be thoroughly coordinated yet distinctly segmented and targeted to achieve maximum impact.
- The number of injuries and trauma cases must be reduced through education and training of clinicians, management and administrative personnel, volunteers, community support groups, potential "bystanders", and other key constituency groups.
- Trauma and injury prevention education and training must be increased for all healthcare professionals, beginning at school, under and post-graduate levels and continuing throughout their careers, appropriate to the level of their involvement in health risk assessment, primary care, or injury care.
- Advocacy efforts must facilitate passage of new laws designed to reduce injuries and trauma cases (based on evidence) and stronger enforcement of existing laws.
- Good Samaritans must not be subject to harassment by the law enforcement and legal system.
- Tort reform must be enacted to facilitate greater access to trauma services and facilities.
- There must be increased awareness of the vulnerability of the older, pediatric and pregnant population.

Prehospital Trauma Life Support (PHTLS)

This modality is recognized around the world as the leading continuing education program for prehospital emergency trauma care. PHTLS promotes excellence in trauma patient management through global education of all providers involved in the delivery of prehospital care. The program is based on a prehospital trauma care philosophy, stressing the treatment of the multi-system trauma patient as a unique entity with specific needs. This may require an approach to the trauma patient that varies from traditional treatment modalities. PHTLS promotes critical thinking as the foundation for providing quality care. It is based on the belief that, given a good fund of knowledge and key principles, EMS providers are capable of making reasoned decisions regarding patient care. The PHTLS course is continuously updated and revised to keep up with the advances in the field, ATLS Guidelines and feedback from PHTLS participants.

Developed by the National Association of Emergency Medical Technicians in cooperation with the American College of Surgeons Committee on Trauma it follows the principles of trauma care developed by the Committee on Trauma. The Committee provides the medical direction and content oversight for the PHTLS program.

- Basic and advanced training to reflect the current ATLS guidelines.
- A consistent approach for every body region includes content on anatomy and physiology, pathophysiology, and assessment and management.

- Airway, Thoracic, and Spinal Skills presented in an illustrated, step-by-step format as Specific Skills.
- Case Scenarios with end-of-chapter solutions and Review Questions included for every chapter to promote critical thinking and assess knowledge.
- A separate chapter on the Military provides special trauma considerations and protocols.
- More than 20 video presentations of the airway and spinal skills used in PHTLS is now included with every book. It also contains information to download onto a PDA.
- Injury Prevention, the Golden Principles of Pre hospital Trauma Care, and Triage, Transport, and Trauma Systems.
- Head Trauma, Shock, Patient Assessment and Management, Airway Management and Ventilation, and Trauma in the Elderly.
- Evidence-based prehospital trauma care.
- Concerns and needs of prolonged transportation.
- Commonly used drugs for pharmacologically assisted intubation provides general guidelines on the topic.
- User-friendly algorithms: assessment; airway management; indications for spinal immobilization; shock management; management of traumatic brain injury; and management of musculoskeletal trauma.
- Photos and video clips for alternative techniques such as face to face intubation, two-person standing longboard application, and two-person rapid extrication.

Basic Life Support Education

- Although the Basic Life Support (BLS) ability of a medical student is a crucial competence, poor BLS training programs have been documented worldwide. Various studies recommend inclusion of Basic Life Support studies in the First Year of Curriculum. 1st Year Physiology does teach CPR and First Aid forms a part of lectures in PSM and Casualty Clinics during Internship, However only 6% of the students/junior doctors performed correct CPR. The current standard for cardiopulmonary resuscitation (CPR) and automated external defibrillator (AED) retraining for laypersons is a four-hour course every two years. Though a large majorities of volunteers retained both CPR and AED core skills through 17 months after initial training, others have documented substantial skill deterioration during this time period. Furthermore, individual testing and retraining for CPR and AED skills were usually accomplished in less than 10 minutes per volunteer.
- BLS course consisting of both theoretical and practical training with proper examination system should be started in the 1st Year itself. During the 3rd Semester of the curriculum, students should be taught the Essentials of PreHospital trauma care and, during the internship a refresher course consisting of complete pre hospital trauma care as well as Advanced Life Support course should be organized.

Information Management

- A national database and uniform data standards must be used to facilitate hospital operations and provide regional and national information regarding availability of pre and post-hospital care.
- Trauma care must be designated as a specific research area for epidemiological study. Predictive models must be developed regarding outcomes and used in making funding and resource deployment decisions.
- Pre-hospital and functional outcomes must be tracked and used in a Total Quality Management initiative to improve

policies, procedures, and processes throughout the trauma continuum.

- Information related to the complete cycle of trauma-from prevention to post-hospital care-must be collected, analyzed, and made available to facilitate improvements in injury prevention, response times, patient care, and rehabilitation.
- Information systems should be usable for multi-center studies.
- A standardized training course must be used to enable trauma registrars to collect and categorize data in a consistent, comparable manner.
- Clear evidence must exist to document the contribution of an injury management system (prevention and treatment) to a community's overall health, and additional research must demonstrate which components of a trauma system provide the most value.
- Tools must be developed and region-specific injury data made available to assist communities in making decisions about their specific needs related to trauma system development, particularly which components will best meet community health needs.
- The culture of quality improvement must shift from using data to blame individuals to using the data to improve performance of the system.
- Access to and appropriate protection of patient records and quality improvement data must be addressed through legislative and regulatory changes at state and central levels.
- Efforts to enhance patient confidentiality should be balanced with the need for strong research.

Finances

- Trauma systems must be recognized as a public good and therefore valued and adequately funded not only for the clinical care they actually deliver, but also for the level of readiness required to meet the needs of all injured persons.
- The appropriate level of readiness in a community must be determined by a broad-based group of community members, including citizens, local employers, trauma and health care providers, and payers.
- There must exist a "rural modifier" or weightage to the medicare fee schedule for rural EMS providers.
- There must be a budgeting procedure to ensure dedicated funding for trauma system infrastructure costs.
- An open dialogue with managed care organizations, public and private, and other payers will facilitate greater mutual understanding of the costs of providing health care, ultimately leading to equitable payment mechanisms, which may include "carve outs" or risk sharing.
- An ongoing dialogue and review regarding the cost-effectiveness of trauma care systems must be done.
- A system must exist for reimbursing providers for uncompensated trauma care without cost shifting to non-governmental payers.
- The public must be encouraged to obtain long-term care coverage to augment other forms of payment for post-hospital care.
- Alternative payment mechanisms must be examined, tested, and piloted, especially in rural areas.
- Additional funding sources, such as seized drug/unaccounted money/issue and sale of health stamps must be explored.

In terms of treatment, there are many low-cost improvements that could be made to enhance the care of injured persons. In 2004, WHO published the *Guidelines for essential trauma care* to promote such low-cost improvements. These guidelines seek to set achievable standards for trauma treatment services which can be made available to almost every injured person in the world. The guide defines the resources that would be necessary for such care including human (training and staffing) and physical resources (infrastructure, equipment and supplies).

Research

- The Centre must establish a National Institute for Injury under the ministry of Health.
- Central agencies involved in or funding trauma research must be coordinated through a formal institutional process.
- There has to be formal efforts to interest young professionals in trauma research and initiate sponsored training programs in all types of research.
- Types of research conducted should include fundamental basic research, crash investigation research, evidence-based medicine, best practices, clinical trials, clinical guidelines, and health services and systems research.

Technology

- Automotive telematics systems and GPS in motor vehicles and even helmets can be used to locate crashes, monitor vital signs, and determine injury severity. GPS will also provide real-time route navigation for ambulances.
- Access technologies such as ACN and wireless E 9-1-1 must be fully developed.
- Various technological innovations must be used to provide services remotely.
- Monitoring devices must be used in a variety of settings, including computer chip implants to monitor patients and the use of monitoring devices in a patient's home, which would support injury prevention and rapid response.
- Computer chips can enable automatic transfer of sophisticated crash information and permit injury research databases to be utilized to evaluate and improve auto design.
- An artificial neural network can determine the most appropriate site for patient care, given the extent of a patient's injury.
- Access numbers must be consolidated to eliminate confusion and streamline access nationwide.
- Patient simulation technology must be used for provider education.
- Medical input must be sought early in the design phase of future technologies to ensure that these developments are coordinated with the health care system and result in improved patient outcome.
- Dedicated resources must be available for technology analysis.

BIBLIOGRAPHY

1. Coats TJ, Davies. Prehospital care for road traffic casualties. *Br Med J* 2002; 324: 1135-1138.
2. Fowler R, Pepe PE. Prehospital care of the patient with major trauma. *Emerg Med Clin North Am* 2002; 20: 953-974.
3. Kwan I, Bunn F, Roberts I. Timing and volume of fluid administration for patients with bleeding following trauma. *Cochrane Database Syst Rev* 2001(1): CD002245.

44 Disaster Preparedness and Response

Conventional and Unconventional

- Trauma systems must form an integral part of regional and state disaster plans and integrated with efforts of the public health system to provide disaster preparedness.
- Trauma and EMS systems must be integrated with other resources through the incident command system and coordinate in advance with other regional resources such as law enforcement and public health.
- There must exist targeted education covering all weapons of mass destruction (identification and response) for all providers.
- Hospital-based decontamination must be available in addition to more traditional field decontamination.
- A nationwide network of hospital and community surveillance systems will enable rapid identification of all major health threats, including those related to weapons of mass destruction. EMS electronic data systems have to be an integral part of this surveillance system.
- Emergency communications systems must connect all levels of the response infrastructure and developed with redundancy to assure backup when needed.
- The public health infrastructure must be reinforced to enable it to more effectively respond to emerging threats.
- Medical command centers must be an integral part of disaster incident command or incident management systems, to assure the most appropriate medical response.
- There must be an optimal resources document for the role of trauma systems in disaster preparation and response.

Psychological Support

Apart from the physical trauma, every road incident with injuries has psychological consequences. Victims of a road crash need to regain an acceptable physical quality of life as well as heal emotional scars. For severe injuries and in case of fatalities psychological support is essential for both the person having been involved in the road crash and for the family/relatives of the injured or killed. Stress-related emotions can overwhelm people's capacity to overcome personal grief and begin rebuilding their lives. If ignored, these psychological symptoms can progress into more severe disorders. Psychological support can help prevent this from occurring.

The key components of psychological assistance for victims are ongoing interaction and presence with the aim of build up feelings of security and hope. This strengthens the affected person's coping capacities and reinforces support from family members and friends. Psychological support deals with basic human feelings and needs - shock, loss, bereavement, and powerlessness. These feelings are common to everyone, but coping mechanisms vary with different cultures.

Support groups are established to help solve common problems, allow for emotional ventilation, improve communication skills, develop social networks, and build trust, empathy, and understanding. The *European Federation of Road Traffic Victims* is an example of a large network, but many local community groups offer great support too.

Telemedicine in Trauma

Advances in technology have made it possible for telemedicine to be used in multiple areas of medicine, including trauma care. Teleradiology and teleconsultation are becoming standard operating procedure for many rural facilities.

Future uses of telemedicine include teleproctoring and telepresence surgery. The medicolegal and financial impact of telemedicine remains to be determined. The potential influence of telemedicine in the care of future trauma patients is likely to be important and may alter patterns of referral, consultation, and treatment.

Advances in radio communication, electronics, and computer technology have greatly improved care of the trauma patient over the past several decades. In fact, it is unusual for prehospital providers not to communicate with medical personnel at the hospital base station long before a trauma or emergency patient arrives in the resuscitation suite. Such prehospital reports are usually the basis for activating the trauma team and making preparations for the care of the patient, not only in the emergency department, but also in the radiology department, operating room, and the ICU. Unfortunately, in remote locations, the usual modes of communication, such as very high frequency radio and cellular telephone, may be ineffective or unavailable.

Utilisation of Teleconferencing

Currently, one third of rural hospitals in the US have limited capability to link with at least one tertiary care facility. In addition to providing teleradiology services, emergency medicine practitioners at this tertiary care facility are immediately available for consultation with physicians, nurse practitioners, and physicians' assistants at small rural hospitals. Early experience with this system has documented many areas of improved patient care, including early triage of seriously ill patients, a decreased rate of transfer of patients who did not require treatment at a tertiary care facility, and more effective utilisation of ground and air ambulance services. A similar experience has been reported from several rural treatment facilities in UK.

Multisite teleconferencing for the purpose of providing education to a variety of medical professionals has become routine. To date, most of these conferences have been sponsored by pharmaceutical companies or instrument manufacturers and contain a significant marketing component. However, these industry-sponsored sessions have shown the potential for high-quality education programs via available satellite communications systems.

Most of the available telemedicine systems are distinctly "low tech" and slow. At present, most teleconferencing is dependent on communication via a conventional phone line, a T-1 line (a 24-channel, high-capacity circuit for data, voice, and video transmission), or in rare cases an OC3 fibreoptic cable connection (a 243-channel, high-capacity fibreoptic circuit for data, voice, and video transmission). Unfortunately, the T-1 communications link is inadequate for high-resolution, real-time clinical interactions. A conventional telephone line and modem provide data transmission at a maximum rate of 64 kb/sec. A T-1 line will provide maximum data transmission rates of from 1.5 to 2.0 megabytes (Mb) per second, and a fibreoptic OC3 line is capable of supporting rates of up to 155 Mb/sec under optimal circumstances. Unfortunately, these rates of data transmission are seldom achieved in routine daily use. A good example of the problems inherent with current telemedicine systems is the interpretation of clinical radiographic films. Using a currently available teleradiology system and a T-1 line takes approximately 11 minutes to transmit a digital mammogram, which contains only 128 Mb of data. Transmission of a more complex imaging study, such as MRI that contains as much as 1 gigabyte of data, will require 1 1/2 hours!

These time requirements are clearly unacceptable for most clinical activities, particularly in an emergency or trauma setting. In contrast, the same digital mammogram and MRI data would require only 6.4 seconds and 52 seconds, respectively, using an OC3 line. Transmission of the same data sets over an OC48 line would require only 0.4 seconds and 3.3 seconds, respectively. High-speed land lines, such as OC3 fibreoptic cables, are not widely available at this time. Current availability is limited primarily to large urban areas. Unfortunately, patients receiving care in rural hospitals who could benefit most from teleconferencing are not likely to be eligible for these services due to lack of fibreoptic infrastructure.

As technology continues to improve, substantial efforts have been directed toward development of telepresence as an adjunct to having physicians on site, or in some instances, as replacement for on-site physician expertise. Telepresence may be described as the ability to perform a "virtual examination or intervention" for a patient over a distance, made possible by telecommunication technology. While the potential for telepresence to improve patient care is obvious, caution must be exercised, since this concept remains in its developmental infancy. To date, the greatest obstacle to routine use of telemedicine and, particularly, telepresence interventions such as operations has been the lack of cost-effective, dependable, broad-bandwidth communication and data links as discussed earlier. Wider availability of high-speed fibreoptic land lines and satellite up-link and down-link services will greatly facilitate further development of telemedicine and telepresence interaction.

An area of telemedicine that has already proved moderately successful with present technology is that of trauma management for patients in remote or inaccessible rural medical facilities.

Matrix of Essential Knowledge, Skills, Equipment and Supplies for Pre Hospital Providers

- Basic and advanced first aid.
- Prehospital trauma care knowledge and skills.
- Alerting and ability to call for help.
- Scene survey.
- Assess scene safety (physical and environmental hazards).
- Establish need for additional help.
- Assess cause of injury.
- Provider safety.
- Receive training in universal precautions
- Limit exposure to HIV, hepatitis B and Cusing available supplies.
- Limit exposure to airborne pathogens.
- Patient assessment.
- Initial assessment.
- Evaluate adequacy of airway.
- Evaluate adequacy of breathing.
- Evaluate extent of external bleeding.
- Recognize level of consciousness.
- Recognize when injuries are not survivable.
- Establish priorities for immediate care.
- Conduct triage for multiple patients.
- Recognize at-risk patients and arrange transport.
- Detailed assessment.

- Assess head injury.
- Assess spinal injury.
- Assess chest injury.
- Assess abdominal injury.
- Assess extremity injury.
- Assess neurological function.
- Assess patient for psychological trauma.
- Recognize presence of life-threatening or limb-threatening injury.
- Evaluate level of discomfort.
- Recognize hypothermia.
- Assess evidence of shock.
- Assess wounds for potential mortality and disability.
- Assess degree of burns (depth and extent).
- Formulate differential diagnosis of cause of shock.
- Recognize platysmal penetration.
- Interventions.
- Scene management.
- Manage rescue situation.
- Manage safe rescue to prevent further neurovascular damage.
- Manage crowds, traffic and other threats.
- Avoid secondary collisions and injury.
- Manage transport of patient.
- Document incident.

Airway and breathing
- Remove foreign bodies from airway (e.g. using suctioning and Heimlich manoeuvre).
- Restore open airway using manual manoeuvres (e.g. chin lift, jaw thrust).
- Restore open airway using recovery position.
- Provide respiratory support (mouth-to-mouth resuscitation).
- Use suction devices.
- Insert oropharyngeal or nasopharyngeal airway/combitube.
- Provide respiratory support (use pocket mask for mouth-to-mask ventilation).
- Assist ventilation using bag–valve–mask device (BVM).
- Administer oxygen.
- Use airway adjuncts (i.e. blind insertion devices).
- Use three-way dressing.
- Use endotracheal intubation.
- Use oesophageal detection device.
- Perform needle cricothyroidotomy.
- Perform surgical cricothyroidotomy.
- Perform gastric decompression.
- Perform needle thoracostomy for thoracic decompression.
- Perform tube thoracostomy.

Circulation, hypothermia and shock
- Control external haemorrhage through direct pressure.
- Elevate victim's legs if there is evidence of shock.
- Immobilize the patient to ease pain,reduce bleeding and complications.
- Splint fractures for haemorrhage control and pain control.
- Prevent heat loss with a blanket or other material.
- Use external rewarming for hypothermia (e.g., blankets).
- Measure and record blood pressure and pulse rate.
- Monitor body temperature.
- Apply arterial tourniquet (in extreme situations).
- Understand parameters of fluid resuscitation.
- Wrap pelvic fractures for haemorrhage control.
- Establish peripheral percutaneous intravenous access.
- Administer intravenous fluid replacement.
- Establish peripheral venous cutdown access.
- Establish intraosseous access for children < 5 years
- Transfusion knowledge and skills.

Wounds
- Nonsurgical management of wounds (e.g. dressings).

- Use deep interfacial packing for severe wounds (e.g. landmine injuries).
- Administer tetanus prophylaxis (toxoid).
- Administer anti tetanus immunoglobulin.
- Use minor surgical management of wounds (e.g. cleaning, suturing).

Burns
- Cool the burn area with water.
- Cover the skin with clean dressings.
- Control risk of hypothermia.
- Cover the skin with sterile dressings.
- Use intravenous therapy for burn > 15% body surface area.

Injuries to extremities and fractures
- Use basic immobilization for fractured extremities.
- Use available material for splints.
- Use spine board.
- Use skin traction.
- Use closed reduction.

Head and spinal injuries
- Use spinal precautions when extricating or moving patients.
- Use selective immobilization (e.g. C-collar, backboard).
- Properly manage immobilized patient to prevent complications.
- Maintain normotension and oxygenation to prevent secondary brain injury I.
- Monitor neurological function.

Pain management
- Manage pain without medicine using ice, elevation, immobilization.
- Manage pain with non-narcotic analgesics and Entonox.
- Manage pain with narcotic analgesics and Inj ketamine.

Medicines
- Apply topical antibiotic dressing, disinfectants or antiseptics as appropriate.
- Administer vaccines and antibiotics (e.g."CODE RED". The Disaster Manual tetanus prophylaxis).
- Administer other medicines.
- Equipment and supplies.

Communications
- Wireless communication (e.g. radio, mobile phone).

Protection
- Non-sterile single-use gloves in size medium-large.
- Eye protection (plastic or glass goggles with side shields).
- Light-reflective clothing (e.g. waistcoat) for identification and protection.
- Flags or other traffic control devices.
- Torch plus spare batteries and bulb or reflector or candle.
- Soap or bactericidal foam for hand washing.
- Cleaning solution.
- Towel.
- Protective clothing,gowns or aprons.
- Disinfectant solution for equipment.
- Plastic bags for non-biohazard waste.
- Waterproof matches.
- Incineration bags for biological waste.
- Fire extinguisher.
- Sharps container.

Extrication
- Basic extrication equipment (e.g. machetes, crowbars, car jacks).
- Other extrication equipment (e.g. shears, saw, rope, shovel, protective clothing).
- Short-board for extrication.
- Specialized extrication equipment (e.g. cutters, spreaders, rams).

Immobilization and patient transfer
- Long, rigid wood, metal or plastic board
- Boards for limb splints.
- Stretcher (wooden,plastic or cloth device)
- Head immobilization device.
- Cervical collar.

Airway and breathing management
- Face shield.

- Pocket mask (e.g. for mouth-to-mask breathing).
- Bag–valve–mask.
- Nasopharyngeal and/or oropharyngeal airways (for infants,children and adults).
- Nasal cannula and associated tubing.
- Tongue depressor.
- Fixed oxygen equipment and administration equipment.
- Non-rebreather face mask.
- Suction device (manual or powered).
- Yankauer or other rigid suction tip.
- Blind insertion device.
- Laryngoscope handle and blades.
- Endotracheal tube and connector.
- Introducing stylet/bougie.
- Splinter forceps.
- Oesophageal detector device.
- Magill forceps.
- Needle and syringe.
- Needle for thoracostomy.

Haemorrhage control and skin injuries
- Potable water.
- Bandages.
- Elastic bandages.
- Gauze rolls.
- Compresses.
- Absorbent cotton wool.
- Adhesive tape.
- Oral rehydration solution.
- Blankets.
- Adhesive dressing bandage (wound plaster).
- Bandaging.
- Arterial tourniquet.
- Needles and syringes.
- Sterile compresses.
- Intravenous infusion set (lines and cannulas).
- Intraosseous needle or equivalent.

Burns
- Vaseline or paraffin gauze
- Sterile dressing.
- Dressing for burns.

Diagnosis and monitoring
- Clock or watch with second hand.
- Stethoscope.
- Blood-pressure measuring device.
- Penlight.
- Torch (flashlight).
- Thermometer.
- Pulse oximeter.
- Electronic cardiac monitoring device.

Medicines
- Oxygen.
- Topical antibiotic dressing.
- Diazepam (or equivalent).
- Controlled substances lockbox.
- Morphine sulfate.
- Acetylsalicylic acid.
- Ibuprofen (or equivalent).
- Paracetamol (acetaminophen).
- 50% dextrose solution.
- Crystalloid solutions (normal saline).
- Colloids-Polygeline and hydroxyl ethyl starch.
- Water for injection.

Miscellaneous
- List of local emergency contacts.
- Knife, scissors.
- Flask for drinking water or bottles of water.
- Container for supplies and equipment (e.g. shoulder bag,backpack or box).
- Rescue blanket (silver/silver or silver/gold).
- Shovel.
- Triage tags.
- Lubricating jelly.

Writing materials
- Pencil.
- Permanent marker.
- Notepad.
- Charts for documenting patient care and incident.

45 Disaster Associated Mortality and Morbidity

> "The man does better who runs from disaster than he who is caught by it."
>
> —*Homer*

The *various etiological factors* causing mortality and morbidity after a disaster situation are as following:

- *Injuries:* Depending upon the type of disaster, deaths exceeding injuries in landslides, avalanches, volcanic eruptions, tidal waves, floods and earthquakes. While injuries exceed deaths in explosions, typhoons, hurricanes, fires, famines, tornadoes and epidemics.
- *Emotional stress:* Disaster victims often exhibit disaster-shock syndromes consisting of successive stages of shock, suggestibility, euphoria and frustration. Each of these stages can vary considerably in extent and duration.
- *Disease epidemics:* They can be the cause or result of disaster. Water borne infections like cholera and typhoid, vector borne illness like plague and malaria, or those spread by person-to-person contact like hepatitis-A and shigellosis or respiratory borne like measles and influenza. Global eradication of certain diseases, high immunity levels due to immunization programs and availability of newer generation antibiotics and drugs has led to a significant reduction in the threat of epidemics following disasters. Energetic immunization programs following disasters are rarely indicated as a specific post-disaster effort except in biological warfare.
- *Increase in indigenous disease:* A disaster is often followed by an increase in the prevalence of diseases indigenous to the area due to disruption of medical and other health care facilities and programs.

46 Triage During Disasters

The act of triage is the ultimate humanitarian nightmare. Racing against time with limited resources, relief workers make split-second decisions: who gets treatment; who gets food; who lives; who dies. This impossible dilemma understandably haunts humanitarians like Dr. James Orbinski, who accepted the 1999 Nobel Peace Prize on behalf of Médecins Sans Frontières (MSF) as their President, and was a field doctor during the Somali famine, the Rwandan genocide, among other catastrophes.

MILESTONES IN THE HISTORY OF MEDICAL TRIAGE

The history of triage is the history of battlefield medicine. The lessons of battlefield medicine helped create our civilian trauma systems and triage tools are best understood within the context of the type of system they serve. As conditions and resources in the field change so must the trauma systems responsible for them.

There was no organized approach prior to 1700's. Rank trumped injury severity and friends and family were essential to ensure survival of victims.

1792: Baron Dominique Jean Larrey, surgeon-in-chief to Napoleon's Imperial Guard, articulates the first triage rule: "Those who are dangerously wounded should receive the first attention, without regard to rank or distinction. They who are injured in a less degree may wait until their brethren in arms, who are badly mutilated, have been operated on and dressed, otherwise the latter would not survive many hours; rarely, until the succeeding day." Outlined mission as rescue casualties, begin treatment immediately, transport to first line of hospitals, triage based on injury not rank and lastly to remove the dead for burial. Flying Ambulance created in 1797 for casualty transportation and served as a morale booster to troops as it reinforced the notion of Esprit de corps and introduced the "24-hour Principle" for casualty treatment. Baron Pierre Francois Percy started a rival Casualty Transport System to transport surgeons and equipment to the battle field, and establish a mobile hospital. When compared, Larrey's vs. Percy's System the former proved safer, more mobile, more flexible, more effective, emphasized rapid transport and treatment and also emphasized tiered approach.

1846: John Wilson, a British naval surgeon, notes that lifesaving surgery could only be performed on those most in need and likely to survive if treatment is withheld from those who are unlikely to survive their injuries and deferred for those with minor injuries.

1862-1864: Battle of Bull Run: Jul 1861 revealed dysfunction of medical corps due to too few ambulances, improperly organized casualty evacuation system resulting in casualties not evacuated for days. Surgeon General William

Hammond appointed in April 1862 and Jonathan Letterman, medical director of the Army of the Potomac, introduces triage along with frontline medical care during the US Civil War, which was reported to significantly decrease mortality among Union troops.3 Tiered Evacuation System evolved with Field Dressing (Aid) Station, Field Hospital (MASH Unit) and large referral hospital.

1914–1918: WWII sees larger numbers of casualties than any previous conflict due to the introduction of modern weapons of war. The philosophy of triage evolves further to doing the "greatest good for the greatest number," a measure beyond simply withholding treatment from those unlikely to survive even with treatment.

1900s: Through WWII and the wars in Korea, Vietnam, and Iraq, military triage shifted primarily to prioritization for air-medical evacuation to forward medical stations.

Mid-1900s: Civilian EDs begin to use triage to prioritize patients for assessment and treatment.

1983: Frykberg introduces the concept of "critical mortality" following US Marine barracks attack in Beirut. That same year the START triage system is developed and widely adopted for use in primary triage for civilian disasters.

2000s: Triage is widely used in various fields of medicine within the western world to prioritize access to limited resources ranging from ED treatment to MRIs, cardiac surgery, and cancer treatments. However, rationing is rarely a feature of the protocols. Threat of terrorist attacks, SARS, and threat of an infiuenza pandemic begin to shift the focus from primary and secondary triage to tertiary triage decisions involving critical care with publication of the first proposed critical care triage protocols.

In casualty management sorting of a large number of injured personnel is the 1st stage in establishing order. Triage the derived from "trier" French meaning to sort.

Definition

Triage is simply a sorting PROCESS that when applied *creates a situation* that allows for "doing the greatest good for the greatest number". Accordingly, mass-casualty triage does not always direct care to the most critically injured, but rather to those deemed most likely to survive with emergent aid.

Triage sets the stage for treatment and eventuates in transport of the injured. Triage is not to be considered with finality and triage categories change based upon the following:

Triage, the sorting of patients according to the severity of their injuries and the need for urgent surgery was a concept developed by Dr. Larrey, a military surgeon in Napoleon's army. Triage in civilian practice first became a serious issue with the development of dialysis for chronic renal failure in the 1960s and the problem of the allocation of this scarce and very expensive treatment. With new developments in organ transplantation and technology it continues to be an issue today. Two models of triage exist- egalitarian and utilitarian. Egalitarian triage is widely and successfully practiced in battlefield medicine, as well as in the emergency room and the ICU. Utilitarian triage has been sporadically practiced and typically collapses under the pressure of public scrutiny. Unfortunately, the two models tend to be conflated, confusing our understanding of the past and confounding our ability to plan for the future

Triage Considerations

- Number of injured.
- Available resources.
- Nature and extent of injury(s).
- State of hostile threat.

- Extent of resources.
- Condition of patient.
- Getting better.
- Getting worse.
- Transport availability.

If you have only one patient, that patient is Priority 1 Immediate regardless of anything else and there is no real need for triage. Once this number increases, the need for triage arises.

Guiding Principles of Triage

Substantive

- Individual liberty.
- Protection of the public from harm.
- Proportionality.
- Privacy.
- Duty to provide care.
- Reciprocity.
- Equity.
- Trust.
- Solidarity.
- Stewardship.

Procedural

- Reasonable.
- Open and transparent.
- Inclusive.
- Responsive.
- Accountable.

A CRITICAL CARE SURGE

A *critical care surge* refers to any increase in the number of critically ill or injured patients beyond the baseline rate a hospital or critical care unit usually experiences. Minor surges are a normal part of a hospital's day-to-day pattern of activity. For example, it is not unusual to see the number of visits to the ED increase during long summer weekends. Such surges are typically small, in the range of 15% to 20% above usual capacity, and they are often predictable. Moderate surges, such as those due to seasonal influenza or summer heat waves, are known to occur regularly, but their exact timing is less predictable. Large surges, which are typically caused by disasters, tend to occur infrequently and with little or no advance warning. Such events may demand up to double the resources required for day-to-day activities. Finally, it may be helpful to distinguish between large surges and megasurges, such as those seen during influenza pandemics and following large-scale natural disasters (e.g., tsunamis) and terrorist attacks. Megasurges may demand more than 200% of usual resources, which would overwhelm most healthcare systems. The types of illnesses and injuries patients present with as well as the timing of patients' arrivals are also key factors. *Surge capacity* refers to the ability to respond to an increased number of patients, whereas *surge capability* is defined as the ability to address unusual or specialized medical needs of an increased number of patients. Thus, while a relatively small surge of patients with typical illnesses or injuries will not overwhelm a system, the same number of patients all requiring specialized services (e.g. burn management) may overwhelm that same system. Although the absolute number of patients matters, even more important is the time over which those patients present to the hospital. A hospital is less likely to be overwhelmed if a moderate number of patients present at an even rate over 8 or 12 hours than if the same number of patients present over 2 to 3 hours. It is important to take all factors into consideration when planning how resources will be allocated during a surge. Those factors include the potential size of the surge, specialized resources that are likely to be required, and the anticipated rate of patient flow. If specific resources are likely to be depleted, it is crucial to begin implementing allocation processes early in the disaster to optimize resource availability.

Problems with Triage Tools

- No one size fits all solution as there is no perfect 'Traumanometer' that measures dose of trauma and resources needed to treat it.
- The system influences the outcome and mature systems have better outcomes.
- The incident influences the outcome. Mass Casualty Incidents (MCI) require simpler triage tools.
- The needs of the population changes.

TRIAGE CATEGORIES

- *Immediate:* Threat to life/limb. A lightly injured is immediate if he can be returned to duty with immediate simple management.
- *Urgent:* Patient is at risk if treatment or transportation is delayed unreasonably.
- *Delayed:* No risk to life or consequence if more definitive care is not rendered quickly.
- *Expectant:* Regardless of the level of care rendered, patient is likely to expire. Tough call to make for unit personnel.

The OBJECTIVES of doing Triage
Rapid sorting of the more serious patients from those less serious to facilitate the rapid care of the more serious patients and brings order to chaos thus facilitating the care of all patients.

The PROCESS?
Sorting into categories for evacuation and treatment.

The DECISIONS involved?
- How will the patients be sorted – who goes in which category?
- What will be done to/with the patients when sorted?
- What factors AFFECT/CHANGE the decisions?
- Resources.
- Circumstances.

Factors in Military Triage

- Continuing risk to medical care providers
- Resource limited.
- Adverse environment.
- "Reverse" Triage Situation; when care provided first to those who when treated can be quickly returned to duty.
- Triage of casualties should occur at every echelon.
- Military triage decisions are influenced by:
  - Numbers of patients and their medical problems.
  - Numbers of expendable and non-expendable medical supplies and capabilities of medical treatment facilities.
  - Numbers and capabilities of medical personnel.
- Military triage decisions are influenced by(cont):
  - Numbers and capabilities of evacuation assets.
  - Tactical situation.
  - Weather.
  - Echelon based.
  - Triage of casualties should occur at every echelon.

The Echelon System

- First echelon: Combat Medic Aid Station
  - First physician.
  - Treat/Street.
  - Emergent Procedures.
  - No holding capacity.
  - Supports 300–500 troops.
  - Kingpin of system.
- Second echelon
  - Medical Company.
  - Primary triage.
  - 72-hour holding.
  - May be attached to FAST.

- OR Capable.
- Supports 3-9 Aid Stations.

- Third echelon
  - Combat support hospital/MASH.
  - Advanced Care.
  - Mobile.
  - Rapid evacuation.
  - Fourth echelon.
  - Outside combat zone.
  - Full spectrum of hospitals with Rehab.
  - Definitive care.
  - No short term mobility.
  - Increased use of Air Transport.
  - Direct transport of most seriously injured patients and bypass within echelon system.

Surgical Prioritization Involves

- *Recognizing:* Which patients require surgery to save life/limb/sight.
- *Knowing:* Numbers of OR's, doctors, nurses, expendables, blood (Resources) each operation requires.
- *Resources appreciation:* (manpower, equip, expendables, blood etc) required to provide post-op care.
- How long each operation will take (Time as a resource).

The resources that each operation will consume (Must consider manpower as a consumable resource).

- Probability of successful surgery.

The Goal of Surgical Prioritization

Selection of cases with the highest probability of success that consume the least amount of resources. Make a decision and go with it! Once a MASCAL situation has been declared don't wait for the situation to evolve further before making a decision. Making decisions is more important than what decisions are made.

Triage Categories used in ICRC Hospitals

Category I: Priority for Surgery: Patients who need urgent surgery and who have a good chance of satisfactory recovery.
Category II: No Surgery. Patients with wounds so slight that they do not need surgery AND patients who are so severely injured that they are unlikely to survive.
Category III: Can wait for surgery patients who need surgery but not urgently.

EXAMPLES OF "CRITICAL" (RED) CASUALTIES

- Upper airway obstruction.
- Life-threatening bleeding.
- Tension pneumothorax.
- Contamination with a hazardous substance.
- Second or third degree facial bums (when the total body surface area burned is less than 50%) which may rapidly lead to upper airway obstruction.
- Stridor (crowing or raspy inspiratory sounds—suggests upper airway obstruction.
- Severe, rapidly progressing allergic symptoms such as: rash, generalized or facial swelling, wheezing, stridor or breathing difficulty, and weak, thready pulse.
- Severe sore throat when accompanied by drooling, muffled voice, inability to swallow, or difficulty opening the jaw-suggests a serious infection in the airway which may quickly lead to its obstruction.
- Complicated obstetrical delivery (e.g. breech position, or compressed umbilical cord).
- Cardiac rhythm abnormality if accompanied by the sudden onset of circulatory shock, decreased mental alertness, or pain, burning, pressure or tightness in the chest, upper abdomen, upper extremity, neck, jaw or back—suggests a heart attack.

- Untreated poisoning (after initial treatment such as the administration of syrup of ipecac, some cases may be retriaged to a lower priority category).
- Hypoglycemia, insulin shock, or insulin reaction (severe decrease in blood sugar which may occur in diabetics).
- Respiratory distress (blue skin color, asymmetrical chest motion or sounds, noisy breathing, nasal flaring, tightening of the neck muscles during breathing efforts, or retraction of the skin between the ribs, about the collar bones or above or below the breastbone).
- Circulatory shock.
- Rapidly deteriorating level of consciousness.
- Rapidly progressive nervous system disorder (paralysis, weakness, numbness, tingling, incoordination, confusion, or visual disturbance).
- Seizure during pregnancy (suggests eclampsia or toxemia).
- Status epilepticus (more than two seizures without regaining full consciousness in between).
- Penetrating wounds of the chest, abdomen, pelvis, rectum, vagina, head or neck.
- Embedded radioactive foreign bodies.
- Sunstroke or fever greater than 105° F.
- Coma.
- Untreated cervical spine injuries (after these are properly immobilized, their priority for care may decrease).

EXAMPLES OF "CATASTROPHIC" (BLUE) CASUALTIES

- Cardiac arrest (especially resulting from trauma or blood loss). Respiratory arrest when not due to drugs or upper airway obstruction.
- Sudden onset of severe abdominal pain and circulatory shock in an elderly subject who has a pulsating abdominal mass – suggests a ruptured abdominal aneurysm.
- Massive brain injuries (indicated by massive head trauma, dilated-fixed pupils, absence of all reflexes, extrusion of brain matter).
- Second and/or third degree burns exceeding a total of 50% of the body surface (especially in elderly persons with serious underlying medical disorders such as emphysema,. diabetes, or cirrhosis of the liver).
- Penetrating wounds of the trunk with coma and no detectable blood pressure.
- Penetrating gunshot wounds of the head with coma. Cardiogenic shock.

EXAMPLES OF "URGENT" (YELLOW) CASUALTIES

- Circulatory shock which has responded adequately to initial treatment with one liter of IV fluid.
- Interference with circulation due to a fracture or dislocation.
- Severe bleeding controlled by a tourniquet.
- Compartment syndrome (swelling due to an injury, usually a fractured elbow or shin, which interferes with capillary blood flow to the muscle tissue; usually characterized by severe pain which is aggravated by movement of the joints beyond the injury and, *sometimes*, by a sensory or pulse deficit).
- Dislocations of the hip, elbow, or knee- which may compress arteries or nerves, or may be difficult to reduce if treatment is delayed.
- Open dislocations and fractures.
- Acute urinary retention (especially in chronically paralyzed patients).
- Second or third degree bums (not including the face or airway, and totaling less than 50% of the body surface).
- Uncomplicated bends (decompression sickness, caisson's disease).

- Apparently complete recovery after resuscitation from drowning. Electrical burns.
- Non-severe bleeding from the genitalia, digestive tract or lungs in the absence of circulatory shock.
- Uncomplicated obstetrical delivery or impending delivery (some might even consider this belonging to category Green).
- Severe headache not related to an injury, with decreased alertness, or with confusion, fever, or a stiff neck (inability of the patient to touch his chin to his chest) suggests meningitis or an infection or bleeding in the brain.
- Uncomplicated hypothermia (rectal temperature less than 95°F). Swelling of a digit or the genitalia due to a constricting object or band.
- Sustained blood pressure exceeding 200 mm systolic or 120 mm diastolic, especially in pregnancy.
- Severe abdominal pain with abdominal wall rigidity or localized tenderness – suggests internal bleeding or infection such as that due to a perforated stomach ulcer or a ruptured appendix.
- Pelvic fractures in the absence of circulatory shock.
- Smoke inhalation in the absence of respiratory distress. Uncomplicated gunshot or stab wound to an extremity. Multiple fractures in the absence of shock.
- Immobilized, uncomplicated cervical spine injuries.
- Traumatic crush injuries or amputation of an extremity in the absence of serious bleeding or circulatory shock (except crush injuries of a fingertip, which may be in category Green).
- Fever with severe joint pain, or fever in a child or infant who refuses to use an extremity—suggests a severe infection of a joint. Sudden onset of confusion, disorientation, combativeness, or psychotic behavior (when not due to injury, hypoglycemia, poisoning or overdose, shock, or oxygen deficiency).
- First onset of severe, incapacitating headache—suggests meningitis, brain infection, or bleeding in the brain.
- Sudden onset, but not rapidly progressive, localized sensory loss or abnormality, partial or complete paralysis, or sustained loss of balance.
- Sudden, partial or complete, temporary or sustained, but not progressively deteriorating abnormality of vision.
- Penetrating wound of the eyeball.
- Rectal temperature greater than 104° F in a child.
- Fever in a child who is unusually lethargic or refuses to eat or play. Rectal temperature greater than 100° F in an infant less than 3 months old.
- Oral temperature greater than 103° F in an adult. Uncomplicated femoral (thigh) fractures.
- Vaginal bleeding in pregnancy.
- Vaginal bleeding accompanied by lightheadedness, fainting, or severe back, abdominal, or shoulder pain.
- Sudden onset of severe testicular pain - suggests a twisting of the testicular cord which has cut off the blood supply.
- Soft tissue infections of the face, especially about the eye or nose can travel to the brain if not treated.
- Soft tissue infections or animal (especially human) bites of the hand can cause, within hours, permanent damage to the hand. Wounds of the external genitalia (in the absence of shock or continued bleeding).
- First onset of seizures (in the absence of status epilepticus, hypoglycemia, poisoning or overdose, injury, cardiac rhythm disturbance, or oxygen deficiency).
- Vomiting more than twice after a head injury.

- Repeated vomiting or diarrhea in a child who is abnormally lethargic, has a weak cry, dry tongue or inability to make tears – suggests serious illness or dehydration.
- Repeated vomiting in a diabetic – suggests diabetes is out of control.
- Serious surface injury to the face or head (in the absence of uncontrolled bleeding, airway problems, circulatory shock, decreased mental alertness, confusion, vomiting or non-immobilized cervical spine injury).
- Large, dirty, or crushed soft tissue wounds.

EXAMPLES OF 'MINOR" (GREEN) CASUALTIES

- Closed dislocations of the jaw, kneecap, or finger (especially if they have been reduced).
- Closed, uncomplicated fractures of the upper extremity, lower leg, foot, kneecap, ankle or face.
- Uncomplicated, clean lacerations (including those involving tendons or peripheral nerves).
- Fingertip amputations with loss or crushing of the amputated part (which precludes sewing it back on).
- Burns in adults totaling less than 20% of the body surface area (when they do not involve the face, airway, groin or anal area, eye, feet or hands).
- First degree burns not affecting the airway or eye. Frostbite.
- Sprains, strains and moderate bruises.
- Dental pain in the absence of facial infection.
- Psychiatric or emotional disorders (when not due to physical injury or disorder and not involving suicidal or homicidal tendencies).
- Uncomplicated abrasions.
- Nosebleeds that can be stopped by direct pressure (firm pinching of the soft part of the nose).

Varieties of Triage

A. *Primary triage:* Primary triage occurs in the field. It is often performed by paramedics and based on very simple criteria that can be rapidly assessed. If, for example, a patient requires intubation due to acute respiratory distress, in all likelihood providers will perform that procedure if the scene is safe, they have the time, there is no risk to the providers (ie, highly transmissible infection), and they have accurate tools to determine if the patient will survive higher levels of care in the ED or ICU. Intubation and other procedures may also require related treatment, such as manual ventilation during transport.

B. *Secondary triage:* Secondary triage is typically performed by emergency physicians or surgeons immediately upon a patient's arrival at the hospital. They prioritize patients by assigning them to treatment areas for initial interventions. Efficient flow of critically injured or ill patients through this part of the system to definitive care is critical. Here treatment decisions may be more accurate than in the field, but they will remain limited until further information about the event or predicted outcomes can be ascertained. The goal is to provide critical initial ABC (airway, breathing, circulation) interventions rather than full resuscitation. After initial interventions, tertiary triage will assign patients to definitive care in surgery or intensive care, and only judiciously to radiology, for ongoing management.

C. *Tertiary triage:* Tertiary triage should be conducted by surgeons or intensivists in keeping with the best practices for triage officers discussed later in this chapter. At each stage of the triage process accuracy can be increased by measuring physiologic parameters and introducing structured physical examination. This third stage of triage is of primary relevance to critical care physicians because the situation and the patients' characteristics call for definitive critical care management. In disasters where most injuries are not life threatening or where few critically injured patients survive long enough to present to the hospital there will be less need to conduct tertiary triage. Using triage to ration resources should be done only when the system is overwhelmed and the resources are or will be insufficient to meet the demand. Critical care resources that may be depleted in a disaster include ventilators, medications, monitors, and trained personnel. Although the specific resources required vary with the nature of the disaster, some resources, such as ventilators, are key to the provision of critical care and lack a reasonable substitute. Further, it is important to remember that only a single pool of critical care resources exists to serve the needs of those directly affected by the disaster and all other patients with critical illnesses or injuries unrelated to the major incident.

EVACUATION PRIORITIES

Priority I: Urgent Evacuation Within 2 Hours.
Priority Ia: Urgent Surgical Evacuation To Nearest Surgical Facility Within 2 Hours.
Priority II: Priority Evacuation Within 4 Hours.
Priority III: Routine Evacuation Within 24 Hours.
Priority IV: Convenience.

Tagging During Triage

Upon completion of the initial assessment by medical or paramedical personnel, each patient will be labelled with a device called a triage tag This will identify the patient and any assessment findings and will identify the priority of the patient's need for medical treatment and transport from the emergency scene.

Patients are tagged for easy recognition by other rescuers arriving on the scene. Tagging is done using a variety of methods. Colored surveyors' tape or colored paper tags may be used. Upon completion of the initial assessment by medical or paramedical personnel, each patient will be labelled with a device called a triage tag. This will identify the patient and any assessment findings and will identify the priority of the patient's need for medical treatment and transport from the emergency scene. Triage tags may take a variety of forms. Some countries use a nationally standardized triage tag, while in other countries commercially available triage tags are used, and these will vary by jurisdictional choice. The most commonly used commercial systems include the METTAG, the SMARTTAG, and the CRUCIFORM systems. More advanced tagging systems incorporate special markers to indicate whether or not patients have been contaminated by hazardous materials, and also tear off strips for tracking the movement of patients through the process. Some of these tracking systems are beginning to incorporate the use of handheld computers, and in some cases, bar code scanners. At its most primitive, however, patients may be simply marked with coloured tape, or with marker pens, when triage tags are either unavailable or insufficient (Figs. 46.1 and 46.2).

The Four Colors of Triage

- Delayed care/can delay up to three hours–GREEN.
- Urgent care/can delay up to one hour–YELLOW.

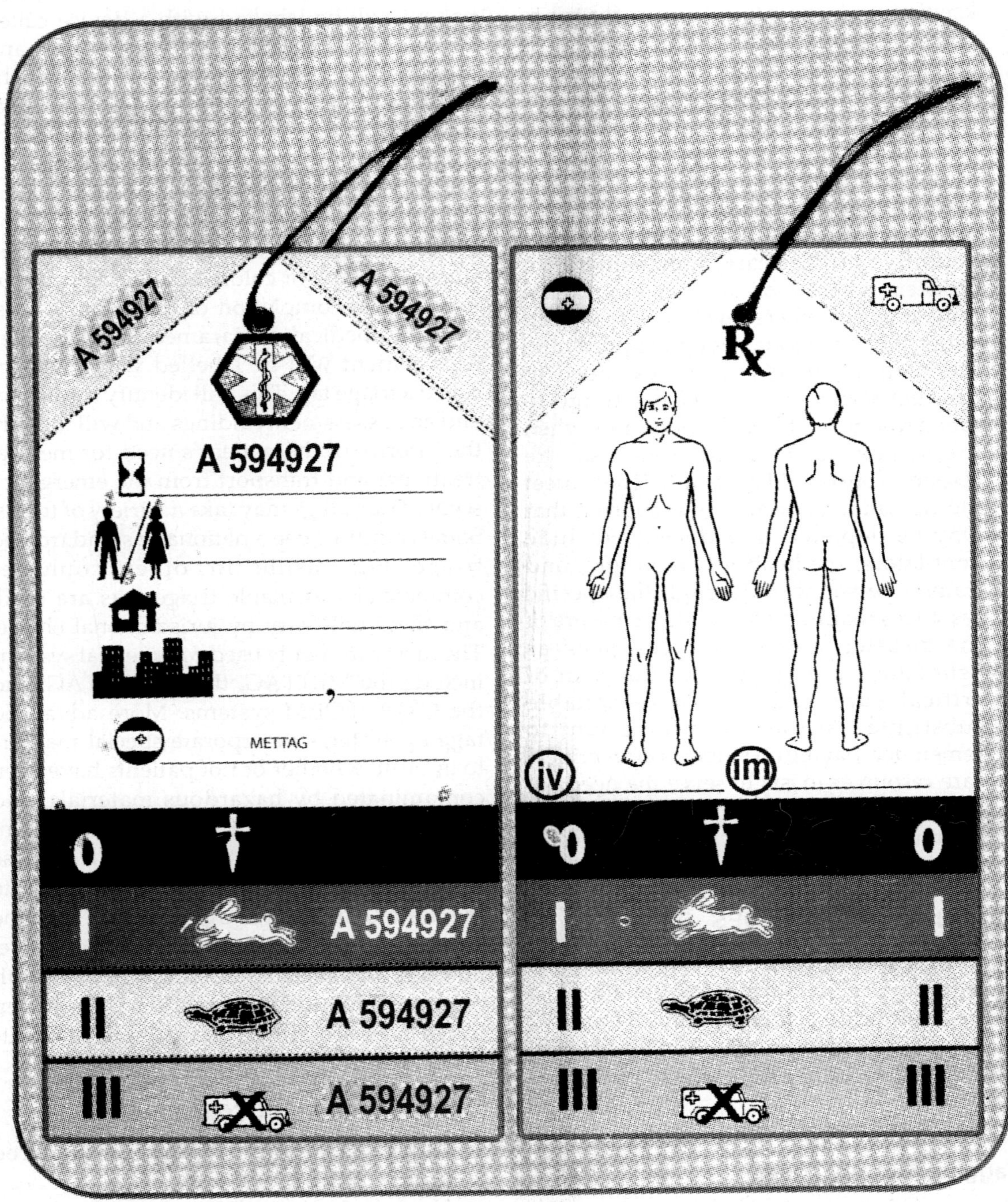

Fig. 46.1: Typical triage tags used to identify highest priority, second priority and lowest priority patients

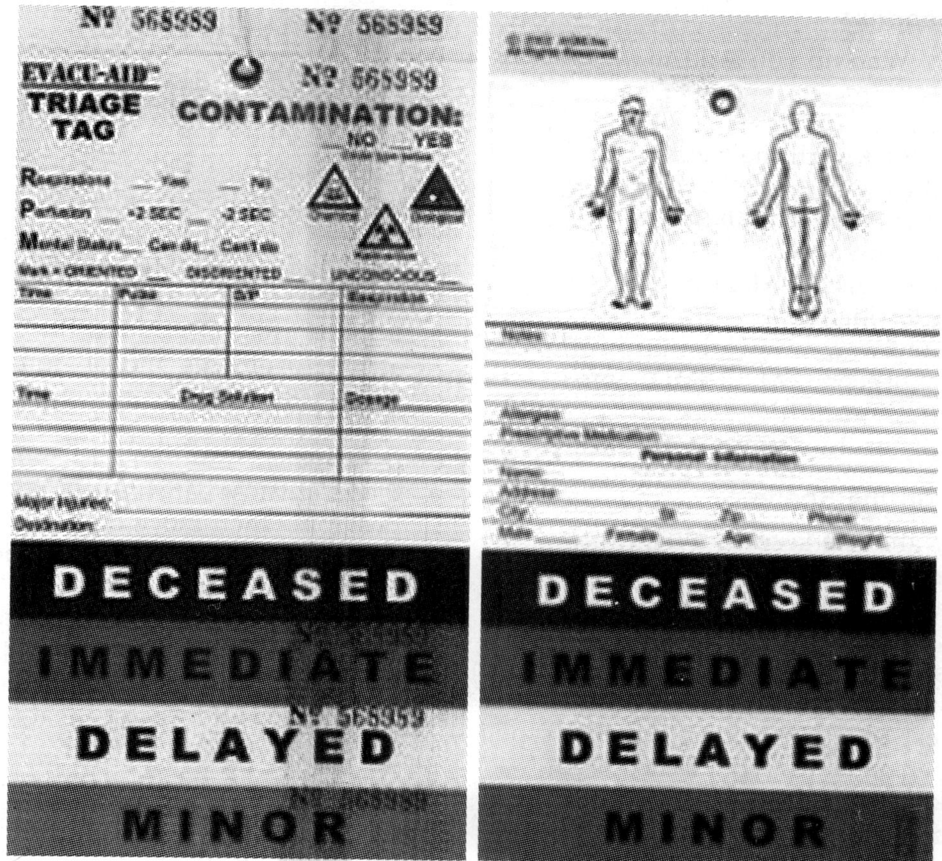

Fig. 46.2

- Immediate care / life-threatening–RED
- Victim is dead / no care required–BLUE

Reverse Triage

In addition to the standard practices of triage as mentioned above, there are conditions where sometimes the less wounded are treated in preference to the more severely wounded. This may arise in a situation such as war where the military setting may require soldiers be returned to combat as quickly as possible, or disaster situations where medical resources are limited in order to conserve resources for those likely to survive but requiring advanced medical care. Other possible scenarios where this could arise include situations where significant numbers of medical personnel are among the affected patients where it may be advantageous to ensure that they survive to continue providing care in the coming days especially if medical resources are already stretched. In cold water drowning incidents, it is common to use reverse triage because drowning victims in cold water can survive longer than in warm water if given immediate BLS and often those who are rescued and able to breathe on their own will improve with minimal or no help.

Field Response

- What / Who do you send to the disaster site?
- Equipment.
- Type – Stick with the basics.
- Dressings.
- Backboards/litter with straps.
- Tourniquets.
- Airways / suction devices.
- Quantity (lots).
- Personnel.
- Type (Surgeon, EM...) (MD, Nurse, PA, EMT-P...).
- Quantity.

Actions on the Scene

- Safety and site security FIRST.
- Survey the scene.
- Estimate number and type of casualties quickly.
- Transmit brief initial report to Med Tx Facility.
- Request additional equipment (#/type) and personnel (#/type) as required.
- Quickly choose a casualty collection point based upon:
  - Proximity to patients.
  - Proximity to potential helicopter landing site.
- *Safety:* Distance from potential hazards, secure.
- *Geography:* Large enough and appropriate for conduct of Geographic Triage). Separate sites for Immediate (next to transportation), Delayed, Minimal, Expectant, Deceased (out of sight of other victims).
- Collect all ambulatory patients at CCP by instructing them to walk to CCP. These patients are mostly in the minimal category although some may be delayed. What they are NOT is in the Immediate / Expectant (except in some burn cases) / Dead categories. Put one of the "walking wounded" in charge of ambulatory patients if limited manpower at scene.
- Most important responsibility is to maintain accountability and keep patients from leaving CCP.
- If more than one medical responder divide the scene into areas of responsibility and proceed to rapidly assess / treat / triage all remaining patients who were unable to walk to the CCP.
- Initially treat ONLY readily correctable airway problems and obvious external, potentially life-threatening, bleeding.
- No treatment for pulseless /apneic patients.
- Place comatose patients in lateral decubitus position – then move on.
- Apply triage tag to identify location in CCP where patient is to be taken.
- Have non-medical bystanders and uninjured or minimally injured patients at the scene act as litter bearers (at least one experienced litter bearer / team) and move patients to CCP.
- Triage Officer at CCP sorts ("triages") patients into separate geographic location based on tags.
- Performs rapid reassessment and changes triage category as required.
- Move rapidly from one patient to next– only identify and if possible quickly treat life threats.
- Identify ALL patients.
- Avoid becoming involved in prolonged procedures.
- Avoid becoming distracted by distraught, minimally injured patients.
- Pay attention to administrative concerns– Keep track of ALL patients.

Transportation Considerations / Decisions

- Do you put all immediate patients on the first available ambulance?

- Do you send one of your health care providers if there is no medical care on the transport?
- To what facility do you send the ambulance?
- Travel time.
- Level I, II, III trauma center?
- Do you wait for a helicopter?
- How secure is the route of travel?

Medical Treatment Facility Actions

- Maintain communication with the response team.
- Identify the scope of the problem.
- Identify the need for additional resources at the scene.
- Medical.
- Security.
- Administrative.
- Transportation—ground/Air.
- Arrange for helicopter transportation as appropriate.
- Notify higher HQ and other medical facilities of the situation and request that they standby.
- Activate medical treatment facility disaster response plan.
- Call in additional staff / keep staff in hospital at end of shift.
- Clear receiving area of all stable patients and set up additional beds as required.
- Cancel any non-emergent surgery.
- Clear OR's ASAP.
- Prepare hospital beds.
  Request higher echelons preposition ambulance at your medical treatment facility.
- When ability to provide medical care is overwhelmed—Bringing organization to the disaster site is the most important action.
- Avoid the overwhelming impulse to rush in and being to take care of first patient you come upon.
- Make sure that you do not become a casualty yourself.
- Remember—All the resources that you have to deal with a disaster did not come with you to the scene.
- Supervising medical care and ensuring the proper evacuation order and disposition of patients may not be glamorous but it will ultimately be the most important.
- Keeping track of the disposition of patients may seem like a waste of manpower but its not – trust me.

DELAYED DEAD

Some exceptions

Breathing

- Correctable on the scene, i.e. tension pneumothorax which when treated may turn patient from IMMEDIATE to DELAYED.
- Uncorrectable on the scene, i.e., large pulmonary contusion/flail chest with hypoxia–Needs *urgent evacuation.*
- Immediate.
- Circulation.
- Exsanguinating hemorrhage.
- External—usually correctable with a tourniquet and/or direct pressure at which point patient becomes DELAYED.
- Internal—*urgent evacuation.*
- Cardiac tamponade.
- Even when treated with pericardiocentesis patient remains IMMEDIATE because underlying cause is wound to the heart.

Disability

- Closed head injury with deteriorating mental status.
- URGENT EVACUATION required.
- Delayed: All injuries that require surgery but for which a delay of 4-8 hours will not cause loss of life/limb/sight.

- Penetrating abdominal wounds—hemodynamically stable.
- All fractures requiring ORIF—hemodynamically stable.
- Spinal cord injury – hemodynamically stable.
- Minimal: Minor soft tissue wounds not requiring surgical intervention
- Non-displaced, min. angulated, closed fractures of the upper extremities or digits
- *Expectant:* When resources are adequate no patients are made expectant. The creation of this category presumes inadequate resources and the types of patients included in this category is largely dependent on the ratio of resources/ patients – the lower the ratio, the more patients in this category.
- *Examples:* > 50% TBSA 2nd and 3rd degree burns, Unresponsive patient with an open head wound and exposed brain, Documented exposure to > 500 RADs and immediate signs of radiation sickness.

The accuracy of field triage can be thought of as the degree of match between the severity of injury and the level of care. Sensitivity and specificity of screening tests are useful indicators of accuracy. Maximally sensitive triage would mean that all patients with injuries appropriate for a Level I or Level II trauma center would be sent to such centers. Maximally specific triage would mean that no patients who could be treated at a Level III or Level IV center or community ED would be transported to a Level I or Level II center. Triage that succeeded in transporting only patients with high injury severity to a Level I or Level II center would maximize the positive predictive value (PPV) of the process, and triage the process, and triage that succeeded in transporting only patients with low injury severity to a Level III, IV, or community ED would maximize the negative predictive value (NPV) accuracy of field triage can be thought of as the degree of match between the severity of injury and the level of care. Sensitivity and specificity of screening tests are useful indicators of accuracy. Maximally sensitive triage would mean that all patients with injuries appropriate for a Level I or Level II trauma center would be sent to such centers. Maximally specific triage would mean that no patients who could be treated at a Level III or Level IV center or community ED would be transported to a Level I or Level II center. Triage that succeeded in transporting only patients with high injury severity to a Level I or Level II center would maximize the positive predictive value (PPV) of the process, and triage that succeeded in transporting only patients with low injury severity to a Level III, IV, or community ED would maximize the negative predictive value (NPV) rather than minimizing overtriage. Target levels for undertriage rates within a trauma system range from 0 to 5% of patients requiring Level I or Level II trauma-center care, depending on the criteria used to determine the undertriage rate (e.g., death and ISS). Target levels of overtriage vary (approximate range: 25%–50%). As Field triage continues to evolve on the basis of new research findings, overtriage rates might be reduced while maintaining low undertriage rates.

Triage Protocols

In general, triage protocols classify patients into 1 of 3 categories signified by standardized color codes:

1. Those who will survive whether they receive care or not (green and yellow).
2. Those who will benefit significantly from interventions (red) and
3. Those who are likely to die despite maximal medical effort (blue or black).

Triage protocols used in a disaster have two aspects that, using an Internet analogy, may be referred to as the front end and the back end. The front end is the user-friendly aspect of the protocol that the triage officer displays in dealing with casualties. The back end of the protocol is the algorithm used to determine the category in which a patient is placed and the cut-off point for treatment based on resource availability.

Many standardized protocols have been developed for use in specific triage situations. The notable exception is triage protocols that apply to mass casualty critical care or disasters.

Until recently, the few existing disaster triage protocols, like the START (Simple Triage and Rapid Treatment) protocol, were designed almost exclusively for primary triage. Protocols for primary and secondary triage vary more based on the type of disaster than do protocols for tertiary triage. For example, specific primary and secondary triage protocols have been developed for chemical, radiation, and crush injuries resulting from earthquakes. Primary and secondary triage protocols lend themselves to specialization because they are used at the scene of a major incident or at hospitals when casualties first arrive. In contrast, tertiary triage must apply to all patients who need critical care; it is not limited to casualties of the disaster. Although tertiary triage protocols may not be specialized by type of disaster, they must be significantly more complex to predict outcomes among a more diverse pool of patients.

The Ontario Protocol

The first protocol for triage of critical care resources, known as the Ontario protocol, was published in 2006. Although initially developed for use in an influenza pandemic, this protocol can potentially be used for any event in which critical care resources may be overwhelmed. Among those who have adopted or are in the process of modifying the Ontario protocol for local use are New York State; British Columbia; the European Society of Intensive Care Medicine; and a task force for mass critical care that includes representatives from the American College of Chest Physicians, the Society of Critical Care Medicine, the American Association of Critical Care Nurses, the American Association of Respiratory Care, and the American Society of Health System Pharmacists.

The Ontario protocol consists of 3 elements: Inclusion criteria, exclusion criteria and minimum qualifications for survival (MQS), which place a ceiling on resource expenditures for each patient. The exclusion criteria and MQS both utilize the Sequential Organ Failure Assessment (SOFA) score to identify patients likely to benefit from treatment as well as those who are too sick to.

Other protocols, such as the Pandemic Medical Early Warning Score (PMEWS) and that developed by Talmor et al. have been proposed for use specifically in a pandemic, but each has significant limitations. For example, PMEWS was principally designed for secondary rather then tertiary triage and is intended to identify patients who are at high risk of complications rather than those who are most likely to benefit from the limited resources available. Intended for secondary triage in the ED, Talmor's protocol also aims to identify patients at risk of complications. Neither protocol provides insight into which patients are unlikely to survive with treatment. Thus, both scoring systems would result in high rates of overtriage and extensive use of resources on patients who will not survive. Finally, because both protocols apply only to patients with influenza seeking access to critical care, they are of limited utility in general critical care triage. These scoring systems may be useful, however, as a disease-specific component within a general triage algorithm. At present no ideal tertiary triage algorithm exists for use in critical care. The ideal tertiary care triage protocol must be easy to use, not require laboratory tests, have good inter-rater reliability, determine priorities accurately, and apply to patients with a wide variety of critical illnesses and injuries. Although the end product (front end) must be simple, the development process itself is complex and time-consuming. Moreover, the triage protocol itself is only one aspect of conducting triage. Systems and processes must be in place to allow effective triage.

Systems and Processes of Triage

In a mass casualty incident, triage is performed on the local level, but to ensure effectiveness, each triage station must act as an interdependent element of a much larger, coordinated effort. Planning and preparation should be undertaken well before disaster strikes. The process starts with coordination between individual hospitals and continues up to the state level, where all is integrated into a comprehensive command and control system (i.e., incident management system). Planning at the highest level includes the development of an overall triage protocol to be followed during a mass casualty incident. If a disaster occurs, the triage protocol must be quickly activated. This requires information about both the demand for and the supply of resources at the local, regional, and state levels so that scarcities can be identified. Because individual hospitals do not normally have access to such information, they cannot initiate triage unilaterally. To ensure uniformity, the job of analyzing available resources and determining their adequacy is performed by a central triage committee that is integrated into the state incident management system. Gathering the essential information and then activating the protocol requires timely and efficient communication between local and regional healthcare officials and the central triage committee. The central triage committee is also responsible for monitoring triage outcomes to identify possible undertriage or overtriage and for adjusting treatment cut-off thresholds in response to changes in supply and demand.

Trauma Triage

Care Flight Triage Algorithm

In 2001, Nocera and Garner developed the Care Flight Triage algorithm with the intent of providing responders in Australia with a primary MCI triage tool to standardize disaster response in the country. Care Flight Triage relies only on qualitative observations and requires no quantitative vital sign measurements. This algorithm assesses the ability to obey commands, the presence of respirations, and the palpability of the radial pulse. It differs from START in that there is no respiratory rate assessment, and the level of consciousness is assessed first. The authors of Care Flight Triage state that it may be performed within 15 seconds and that it is appropriate for triaging children as well as adults. The use of Care Flight Triage has been reported in the evacuation of patients following the nightclub bombings in Bali in 2002.

Sacco Triage Method

In addition to the above triage algorithms, Sacco *et al.* developed the STM for prioritizing patients during a MCI. According to available resources, the STM is not an algorithm—it is a mathematical model that orders the treatment of patients based on their probability of survival, potential for deterioration, and available resources. To develop this model, Sacco and colleagues first estimated the probability of survival for a set of physiological scores that on ventilatory rate, pulse rate, and best motor response. The survivorship scores were derived empirically from a statewide trauma registry database containing records from > 76,000 blunt trauma patients deterioration was estimated by expert consensus for patients who remained at the scene for different periods of time. Based on the physiological score and the probability of deterioration, STM relies on a mathematical model that involves linear programming to determine the order in which victims are to be transported and treated given the resources at hand. Currently, the STM is the only empirically derived triage method, and it also is the only system that changes the prioritization of patients in a real-time manner based on available resources. Using STM also requires software support, personnel for data entry, communication to incident command or central dispatch, and resource availability information. Resource constraints and the requirement for software and hardware support may limit the usability of the STM. In addition, the proprietary nature of the system makes it less accessible to economically disadvantaged areas. There are no published reports using the STM or addressing its real-world applicability.

Continuous Integrated Triage

This was developed by the Founding Chairperson, Maurice A. Ramirez, of the American Board of Disaster Medicine by applying the lessons learned at the Louis Armstrong International Airport in New Orleans, Louisiana following the 2005 Hurricane Katrina to Mass Casualty Triage at hospitals and healthcare institutions.

Continuous integrated triage is an approach to triage in mass casualty situations. It is both efficient and sensitive to psychosocial and disaster behavioral health issues that effect the number of patients seeking care (surge), the manner in which a hospital or healthcare facility deals with that surge (surge capacity), and the overarching medical needs of the event.

Continuous integrated triage combines three forms of triage with progressive specificity to most rapidly identify those patients in greatest need of care. It balances the needs of the individual patients against the available resources and the needs of other patients. Continuous integrated triage employs:

- Group (Global) Triage (i.e., M.A.S.S. Triage).
- Physiologic (Individual) Triage (i.e., START or Simple Triage and Rapid Treatment).
- Hospital Triage (i.e., E.S.I. or Emergency Severity Index).

Using a Group (Global) Triage method (i.e. M.A.S.S. Triage), patients are divided into ambulatory (green) and non-ambulatory (red, yellow and black) triage categories.

Ambulatory patients are directed to self decontamination showers and then progress to the Green Triage holding area for re-triage using a Hospital Based Triage method and treatment.

Patients who are not responsive are immediately re-triaged using a Physiological (Individual) Triage method (i.e., S.T.A.R.T. or JumpS.T.A.R.T.) modified to include behavioral triage considerations prior to decontamination. Those found in respiratory arrest or pulseless are tagged deceased and not moved due to legal considerations.

Unresponsive patients with critical vital signs undergo assisted decontamination while receiving only immediately life sustaining interventions then re-triaged again using a Physiological (Individual) Triage method (i.e., S.T.A.R.T. or JumpS.T.A.R.T.) modified to include behavioral triage considerations.

Next, unresponsive patients with stable vital signs undergo assisted decontamination.

After decon these patients too are re-triaged using a Physiological (Individual) Triage method (i.e., S.T.A.R.T. or JumpS.T.A.R.T.) modified to include behavioral triage considerations.

Finally, non-ambulatory responsive patients undergo assisted decontamination followed by re-triage using a Physiological (Individual) Triage method (i.e., S.T.A.R.T. or JumpS.T.A.R.T.) modified to include behavioral triage considerations.

Following assisted decontamination, patients found to be Alert, Oriented, Responsive and able to Follow Commands but non-ambulatory are triaged to the Yellow Triage holding area for re-triage using a Hospital Based Triage method and treatment.

Following assisted decontamination, unresponsive patients are triaged to either the Critical (red) or Expectant (black) treatment areas based on whether or not there are sufficient resources available at that moment in time to treat the patient without denying care to two or more other patients.

Secondary Triage Instruments

Because of the evolving nature of some injuries and the deterioration that can occur if treatment is delayed, two secondary triage instruments, SAVE Triage and Triage Sort have been developed to provide prehospital personnel with more detailed guidelines for assigning treatment priorities. The SAVE Triage instrument is designed for MCIs in which providers with limited medical resources reach patients at the disaster site but evacuation to definitive care will be prolonged. It provides detailed guidelines to aid in prioritization of patients for treatment at the disaster scene once they have been assigned an initial treatment priority using the START algorithm. Triage Sort also is a secondary triage algorithm—it is designed to be used in conjunction with Triage Sieve during incidents in which there are many patients to prioritize for evacuation and treatment, but where resources have not been overwhelmed. The use of advanced triage may become necessary when medical professionals decide that the medical resources available are not sufficient to treat all the people who need help. The treatment being prioritized can include the time spent on medical care, or drugs or other limited resources. This has happened in disasters such as volcanic eruptions, thunderstorms, and rail accidents. In these cases some percentage of patients will die regardless of medical care because of the severity of their injuries. Others would live if given immediate medical care, but would die without it. In these extreme situations, any medical care given to people who will die anyway can be considered to be care withdrawn from others who might have survived (or perhaps suffered less severe disability from their injuries) had they been treated instead. It becomes the task of the disaster medical authorities to set aside some victims as hopeless, to avoid trying to save one life at the expense of several others. If immediate treatment is successful, the patient may improve (although this may be temporary) and this improvement may allow the patient to be categorized to a lower priority in the short term. Triage should be a continuous process and categories should be checked regularly to ensure that the priority remains correct. A trauma score is invariably taken when the victim first comes into hospital and subsequent trauma scores taken to see any changes in the victim's physiological parameters. If a record is maintained, the receiving hospital doctor can see a trauma score time series from the start of the incident, which may allow definitive treatment earlier.

START

The **S**imple **T**riage **A**nd **R**apid Treatment (**START**) system was developed jointly by Newport Beach (CA) Fire and Marine Dept. and Hoag Hospital in Newport Beach, California for use by emergency services. It has been field-proven in mass casualty incidents such as train wrecks and bus accidents, though it was developed for use by community emergency response teams (CERTs) and firefighters after earthquakes. It allows first responders to triage multiple victims in 30 seconds or less, based on three primary observations: **R**espiration, **P**erfusion, and **M**ental Status (**RPM**). S.T.A.R.T. (Simple Triage and Rapid Treatment) is a simple triage system that can be performed by lightly-trained lay and emergency personnel in emergencies. It is not intended to supersede or instruct medical personnel or techniques. It may serve as an instructive example, and has been taught to California emergency workers for use in earthquakes. It has proved itself in several mass casualty incidents such as train wrecks and bus accidents, though it was developed for use by community emergency response teams (CERTs) and firefighters after earthquakes.

The **START** system is designed to assist rescuers to find the most seriously injured patients. As more rescue personnel arrive on the scene, the patients will be re-triaged for further evaluation, treatment, stabilization, and transportation. This system allows first responders to open blocked airways and stop severe bleeding quickly.

The First Step in START: Get up and Walk!

The first step in START is to tell all the people who can get up and walk to move to a specific area. If patients can get up and walk, they are probably not at risk of immediate death.

In order to make the situation more manageable, those victims who can walk are asked to move away from the immediate rescue scene to a specific designated safe area. These patients are now designated as walking wounded P3. If a patient complains of pain on attempting to walk or move, do not force him or her to move.

The patients who are left in place are the ones on whom you must now concentrate.

The Second Step in START: Begin Where You Stand

Begin the second step of START by moving from where you stand. Move in an orderly and systematic manner through the remaining victims, stopping at each person for a quick assessment and tagging. The stop at each patient should never take more than one minute.

Remember: Your job is to find and tag the patients—those who require immediate attention. Examine each patient, correct life-threatening airways and breathing problems, tag the patient with a red tag and MOVE ON!

How To Evaluate Patients Using RPM

The **START** system is based on three observations: RPM—Respiration, Perfusion and Mental Status. Each patient must be evaluated quickly, in a systematic manner, starting with Respiration (breathing).

Breathing

It all STARTS Here.

If the patient is breathing, you then need to determine the breathing rate. Patients with breathing rates greater than 30 per minute are tagged. These patients are showing one of the primary signs of shock and need immediate care. If the patient is breathing and the breathing rate is less than 30 per minute, move on to the circulation and mental status observations in order to complete your 30-second survey. If the patient is not breathing, quickly clear the mouth of foreign matter. Use a head-tilt maneuver to open the airway. In this type of multiple- or mass-casualty situation, you may have to ignore the usual cervical spine guidelines when you are opening airways during the triage process.

Special Note

The treatment of cervical spine injuries in multiple or mass casualty situations is different from anything that you've been taught before. This is the only time in emergency care when there may not be time to properly stabilize every injured patient's spine.

Open the airway, position the patient to maintain the airway and—if the patient breathes—tag the patient. Patients who need help maintaining an open airway are tagged. If you are in doubt as to the patient's ability to breathe, tag the patient. If the patient is not breathing and does not start to breathe with simple airway maneuvers, the patient should be tagged.

Circulation

Is Oxygen Getting Around?

The second step of the RPM series of triage tests is circulation of the patient. The best field method for checking circulation (to see if the heart is able to circulate blood adequately) is to check the radial pulse. It is a medium sized artery and may not be easily felt in the wrist. The radial pulse is located on the palm side of the wrist, between the midline and the radius bone (forearm bone on the thumb side). To check the radial pulse, place your index and middle fingers on the bump in the wrist at the base of the thumb. Then slide it into the notch on the palm side of the wrist. You must keep your fingers there for five to ten seconds, to check for a pulse. If the radial pulse is absent or irregular the patient is tagged.

If the radial pulse is present, move to the final observation of the RPM series: mental status.

Mental Status

Open Your Eyes:

The last part of the RPM series of triage tests is the mental status of the patient. This observation is done on patients who have adequate breathing and adequate circulation. Test the patient's mental status by having the patient follow simple commands like:

"Open your eyes." "Close your eyes," "Squeeze my hand." Patients who can follow these simple commands and have adequate breathing and adequate circulation are tagged. A patient who is unresponsive or cannot follow this type of simple command is tagged. (These patients are "unresponsive" to verbal stimuli).

START and Patients

This system is designed to assist rescuers to find the most seriously injured patients. As more rescue personnel arrive on the scene, the patients will be re-triaged for further evaluation, treatment, stabilization, and transportation. A patient may be re-triaged as many times and as often as time allows. Remember that injured patients do not stay in the same condition. The process of shock may continue and some conditions will become more serious as time goes by. As time and resources permit, go back and recheck the condition of all patients to catch changes in condition that may require upgrading.

Working at a Multiple- or Mass-Casualty Incident

You may or may not be the first person to arrive on the scene of a multiple- or mass-casualty incident. If other rescuers are already at the scene when you arrive, be sure to report to the incident commander before going to work. Many events are happening at the same time and the incident commander will know where your help and skills can best be used. By virtue of training and local protocols, the incident commander is that person who is in charge of the rescue operation.

In addition to initially sizing up an incident, clearly and accurately reporting the situation, and conducting the initial START triage, the first responder will probably also be called on to participate in many other ways during multiple- and mass-casualty incidents.

As more highly trained rescue and emergency personnel arrive on the scene, accurately report your findings to the person in charge by using a format similar to that used in the initial arrival report. Note the following:

- Approximate number of patients.
- Numbers that you've triaged into the four levels.
- Additional assistance required.
- Other important information.

After you have reported this information, you may be assigned to use your skills and knowledge to provide patient care, traffic control, fire protection, or patient movement. You may also be assigned to provide emergency care to patients, to help move patients, or to assist with ambulance or helicopter transportation.

In every situation involving casualty sorting, the goal is to find, stabilize and move Priority One patients first.

Triage in Hazardous Materials Incidents

Hazardous materials (Hazmat) incidents involving chemicals occur every day, exposing many people to injury or contamination. During a hazardous materials incident, responders must protect themselves from injury and contamination.

Remember: A hazardous materials placard indicates a potential problem. But not all hazardous materials problems will be placarded. Be sure to find the proper response to the problem before beginning patient treatment.

The single most important step when handling any hazardous materials incident is to identify the substance(s) involved. Federal law requires that hazardous materials placards be displayed on all vehicles that contain large quantities of hazardous materials. Manufacturers and transporters should display the appropriate placard, along with a four-digit identification number, for better identification of the hazardous substance. These numbers are used by professional agencies to identify the substance and to obtain emergency information.

If there is Any Suspicion of a Hazardous Materials Spill—Stay Away!

The Department of Transportation lists and codes the most common hazardous materials and also the proper emergency actions to control the scene. It also describes the emergency care of ill or injured patients.

Unless you have received training in handling hazardous materials and can take the necessary precautions to protect yourself, you should keep far away from the contaminated area or "hot zone".

Once the appropriate protection of the rescuers has been accomplished, triage in hazardous materials incidents has one major function—to identify victims who have sustained an acute injury as a result of exposure to hazardous materials. These patients should be removed from the contaminated area, decontaminated by trained personnel, given any necessary emergency care, and transported to a hospital.

Remember: Contaminated patients will contaminate unprotected rescuers!

Emergency treatment of patients who have been exposed to hazardous materials is usually aimed at supportive care, since there are very few specific antidotes or treatments for most hazardous materials injuries. Because most fatalities and serious injuries sustained in hazardous materials incidents result from breathing problems, constant reevaluation of the patients in Priorities Two and Three is necessary so that a patient whose condition worsens can be moved to a higher triage level.

Summary

Every responder must understand the principles and operations behind your casualty sorting system. The START system is an excellent and easily understood triage or casualty sorting method.

Responders should be involved in periodic community disaster drills so that their skills and capabilities can be tested and improved.

You Should Know

- The responder's role at multiple- or mass-casualty incidents.
- How to use the START system.
- How to recognize a hazardous materials placard.

You Should Practice

- Using the START system during a simulated multiple- or mass-casualty incident. The START Triage Method doesn't work well in no/low light or excess noise.

JumpSTART Pediatric MCI Triage (Fig. 46.3)

- Developed by Lou Romig MD, a pediatric emergency/EMS physician.
- Now in widespread use throughout the US and Canada.
- Being taught in numerous countries around the world.
- Incorporated into national-level courses and EMS/disaster textbooks.
- Initially ages 1-8 years chosen.
- Less than one year of age is less likely to be ambulatory.
- The pertinent pediatric physiology (specifically, the airway) approaches that of adults by approximately eight years of age.

JumpSTART: Breathing?

- If breathing spontaneously, go on to the next step, assessing respiratory rate.
- If apneic or with very irregular breathing, open the airway using standard positioning techniques.
- If positioning results in resumption of spontaneous respirations, tag the patient immediate and move on.

The "JumpSTART" Part

- If no breathing after airway opening, check for peripheral pulse. If no pulse, tag patient deceased/non salvageable and move on.
- If there is a peripheral pulse, give 5 mouth to barrier ventilations. If apnea persists, tag patient deceased/nonsalvageable and move on.
- If breathing resumes after the "jumpstart", tag patient immediate and move on.

JumpSTART: Respiratory Rate

- If respiratory rate is 15-45/min, proceed to assess perfusion.
- If respiratory rate is <15 or >45/min or irregular, tag patient as immediate and move on. JumpSTART: Perfusion.
- If peripheral pulse is palpable, proceed to assess mental status.

Jump START Pediatric MCI Triage

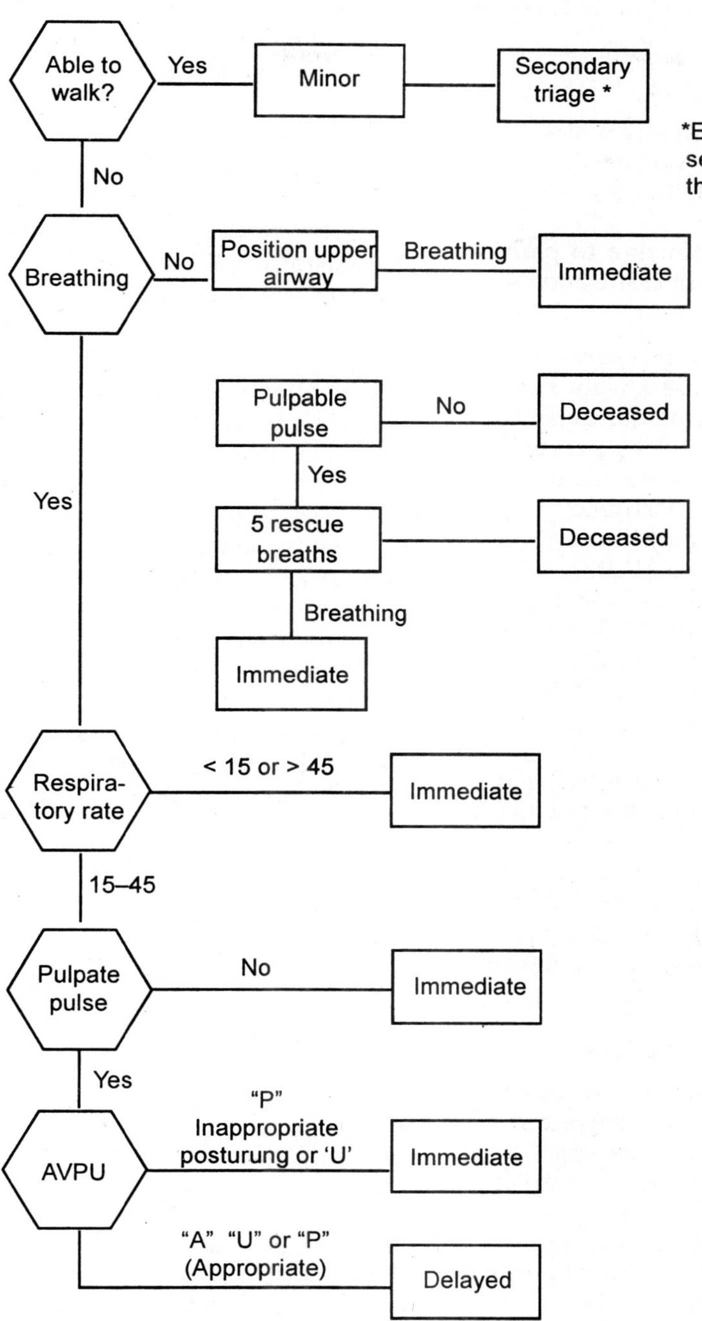

*Evaulate infants first in secondary triage using the entire JS algorithm

Fig. 46.3

- If no peripheral pulse is present (in the least injured limb), tag patient immediate and move on.

JumpSTART: Mental Status

- Use AVPU scale to assess mental status.
- If Alert, responsive to verbal, or appropriately responsive to pain, tag as delayed and move on.
- If inappropriately responsive to pain or unresponsive, tag as immediate and move on.

Modification for nonambulatory children

- Infants who normally can't walk yet.
- Children with developmental delay.
- Children with acute injuries preventing them from walking *before* the incident.
- Children with chronic disabilities.
- Evaluate using the JS algorithm.
- If any RED criteria, tag as RED.
- If patient satisfies YELLOW criteria:
  - YELLOW if significant external signs of injury are found (i.e., deep penetrating wounds, severe bleeding, severe burns, amputations, distended tender abdomen).
  - GREEN if no significant external injury.

Individuals with special health care needs may also be MCI victims!

Patients' limitations in ambulation and communication and differentiation between acute and chronic neurological conditions are the main challenges in the triage of children with special needs and disabilities.

Note for Black Category Victims

Unless clearly suffering from injuries incompatible with life, victims tagged in the BLACK category should be reassessed once critical interventions have been completed for RED and YELLOW patients.

- The physiology of adults and children differ; therefore different primary triage systems should be used.
- Use JumpSTART for infants through older children.
- Use START for young adults and older.
- Primary triage is just the first look at an MCI victim, similar to the primary/initial survey/assessment.

The Triage Sieve

The Triage Sieve can be used to quickly triage patients when at the scene of a multiple casualty incident and involves a rapid assessment as follows:

- Can the patient walk?
  - Yes: Priority 3 (Green – see above)
  - No.
- Is the patient breathing?
  - No, even after opening airway: Dead.
  - Yes, after opening airway: Priority 1 (Red).
  - Yes, without resuscitation.
- What is the respiratory rate?
  - Above 30/minute or less than 10/minute: Priority 1 (Red).
  - 10-30/minute.
- What is the pulse rate (or capillary refill time)?
  - Less than 40 or more than 120 (or capillary refill time greater than 2 seconds): Priority 1 (Red).
  - Between 40 and 120 (or capillary refill time less than 2 seconds): Priority 2 (Yellow).

Evaluation	*Cold or poor lighting*	*Triage category*
Walking		Priority 3 (delayed)
Not breathing with an open airway		Dead
Respiratory rate < 10 or > 29 breaths per minute		Priority 1 (immediate)
Capillary refill <= 2 seconds	Pulse <= 120 beats/minute	Priority 2 (urgent)
Capillary refill > 2 seconds	Pulse > 120 beats/	Priority 1 (immediate)

Comments and Performance

The sensitivity was low at 45%, with specificity about 88%. Counting respirations may be difficult in a fully clothed person and in poor lighting conditions.

Further Reading

Garner A, Lee A, *et al*. Comparative analysis of multiple-casualty incident triage algorithms. Ann Emergency Medicine. 2001; 38: 541-548.)

Modified sieve systems are available for use in children.

The Triage Sort

The triage sort it is one method used for triage at a casualty clearing station and is assessed as follows:

Physiological variable	*Value*	*Score*
Respiratory rate	10-29	4
	>29	3
	6-9	2
	1-5	1
	0	0
Systolic blood pressure	>90	4
	76-89	3
	50-75	2
	1-49	1
Glasgow coma scale	13-15	4
	9-12	3
	6-8	2
	4-5	1
	3	0

A total score of 1-10 indicates priority T1(P1), 11 indicates T2(P2), and 12 indicates T3(P3).

Trauma Scoring

Trauma scores are often audit and research tools used to study the outcomes of trauma and trauma care, rather than predicting the outcome for individual patients. Many different scoring systems have been developed, some are based on physiological scores (e.g., Glasgow Coma Scale) and other systems rely on anatomical description (e.g., Abbreviated Injury Score). There is however no universally accepted scoring system and each system has its own limitations.

1. Anatomical Scoring Systems

Abbreviated Injury Scale (AIS)

- Since its introduction as an anatomical scoring system in 1969, the AIS has been revised and updated many times. The AIS scale is similar to the Organ Injury Scales introduced by the Organ Injury Scaling Committee of the American Association for the Surgery of Trauma, however AIS is designed to reflect the impact of a particular organ injury on patient outcome.

Injury threat	*AIS score*
Minor	1
Moderate	2
Serious	3
Severe	4
Critical	5
Unsurvivable	6

Limitations

- The AIS scale does not provide a comprehensive measure of severity.
- The AIS scale does not represent a linear scale, i.e. the difference between AIS1 and AIS2 is not the same as the difference between AIS4 and AIS5.
- When used alone, the current AIS version is not useful for predicting patient outcomes or mortality; instead it forms the basis of the ISS and TRISS.

Injury Severity Score (ISS) and New Injury Severity Score (NISS)

- The ISS was introduced in 1974 as a method for describing patients with multiple injuries and evaluating emergency care. It has since been classed as the 'gold standard' of severity scoring.
- Each injury is initially assigned an AIS score and one of six body regions (head, face, chest, abdomen, extremities, external).
- The highest three AIS scores (only one

from each body region may be included) are squared and the ISS is the sum of these scores.

- Limitations:
  - Inaccurate AIS scores are carried forward.
  - Many different injury patterns can yield similar ISS scores.
  - It is not useful as a triage tool.
- Only considers one injury per body region and therefore may underestimate the severity in trauma victims with multiple injuries affecting one body part.
- The NISS is a modified version of the ISS developed in 1997. The NISS sums the severity score for the top three AIS injuries regardless of the body region, hence NISS scores greater than ISS values indicate multiple injuries in at least one body region.

Organ Injury Scale (OIS)

- This scale provides a classification of injury severity scores for individual organs.
- The OIS is based on injury description scaled by values from 1 to 5, representing the least to the most severe injury.
- The Organ Injury Scaling (O.I.S.) Committee of the American Association for the Surgery of Trauma (A.A.S.T.) developed the OIS in 1987; the scoring system has been updated and modified since that time.

2. Physiological Scoring Systems

Glasgow coma score and Glasgow paediatric coma score

- The Glasgow Coma Score (GCS) and Glasgow Paediatric Coma Score (PGCS) are simple and common method for quantifying the level of consciousness following traumatic brain injury.
- The scale is the sum of three parameters:
  - Best Eye Response.
  - Best Verbal Response.
  - Best Motor Response.
- Scales are based on values ranging between 3 (worst) to 15 (best) (See next page for table).

Revised Trauma Score

- Used as a triage tool in a pre-hospital setting.
- It is a common physiological scoring system based on the first data sets of 3 specific physiological parameters obtained from the patient.
- The three parameters are: the Glasgow Coma Scale (GCS), systemic blood pressure (SBP), and the respiratory rate (RR).

Limitations include the inability to accurately score patients who are intubated and mechanically ventilated.

The acute physiology and chronic health evaluation (APACHE):

- APACHE was first introduced in 1981. APACHE III is an updated version introduced in 1991.
- This evaluation system is used widely for the assessment of illness severity in intensive care units (ICUs).

Glasgow coma scale	*Systolic blood pressure*	*Respiratory rate*	*Value*
13-15	>89	10-29	4
9-12	76-89	>29	3
6-8	50-75	6-9	2
4-5	1-49	1-5	1
3	0	0	0

- RTS is equal to 0.9368 GCS plus 0.7326 systolic blood pressure plus 0.2908 respiratory rate.
- Range is 0-7.8408 and correlates with survival, e.g., a score of 4 indicates 40% mortality

Table II: Glasgow coma score or PGCS

	Infant < 1 yr	Child < 1-4 yr	Age 4-Adult
		Eye	
4	Open	Open	Open
3	To voice	To voice	To voice
2	To pain	To pain	To pain
1	No response	No response	No response
		Verbal	
5	Coos, babbles	Oriented, speaks	Oriented and alert
4	Irritable cry, consolable	Confused speech, disoriented, consolable	Disoriented
3	Cries persistently to pain	Inappropriate words inconsolable	Nonsensical speech
2	Moans to pain	Incomprehensible agitated	Moans, unintelligible
1	No response	No response	No response
		Motor	
6	Normal spontaneous movement	Normal spontaneous movement	Follows commands
5	Withdraws to touch	Localizes pain	Localizes pain
4	Withdraws to pain	Withdraws to pain	Withdraws to pain
3	Decorticate flexion	Decorticate flexion	Decorticate flexion
2	Decerebrate extension	Decerebrate extension	Decerebrate extension
1	No response	No response	No response

Interpretation of pupillary findings in head-injured patients

Pupil Size	*Light Response*	*Interpretation*
Unilaterally dilated	Sluggish or fixed	3rd nerve compression secondary to tentorial herniation
Bilaterally dilated	Sluggish or fixed	Inadequate brain perfusion Bilateral 3rd nerve palsy
Unilaterally dilated or equal	Cross-reactive (Marcus-Gunn)	Optic nerve injury
Bilaterally constricted	May be difficult to determine	Drugs (opiates) Metabolic encephalopathy Pontine lesion
Unilaterally constricted	Preserved	Injured sympathetic pathway, ego carotid sheath injury

3. Combination Scoring Systems

Trauma and Injury Severity Score (TRISS)

This score determines the probability of patient survival (Ps) from the combination of both anatomical and physiological (ISS and RTS, respectively) scores. A logarithmic regression equation is used:

- Ps = 1/ (1+e^{-b}), where b = bo + b1(RTS) + b2(ISS) +b3(AgeScore).

RTS and ISS are calculated as above and Age Score is either 0 if patient <55 years old or 1 if 55 and over. The coefficients b0 – b3 depend on the type of trauma (N.B. there is some variation in the published values for these). A TRISS calculator is available on the Trauma.org website.

Coefficient	*Blunt trauma or age <15 years*	*Penetrating trauma*
B0	-0.4499	-2.5355
B1	0.8085	0.9934
B2	-0.0835	-0.0651
b3	-1.7430	-1.1360

- Sort, Assess, Life Saving Interventions, Treatment and/or Transport (SALT).
- Secondary Assessment of Victim Endpoint (SAVE).
- Move, Assess, Sort, Send (MASS).
- Sacco Triage Method (STM).
- Multi-organ dysfunction score (MODS).
- Sequential organ failure score (SOFA).

Further Readings

1. Galler D; Critical Care Considerations in Trauma. eMedicine, January 2006.
2. Talmor D, Jones AE, Rubinson L, *et al;* Simple triage scoring system predicting death and the need for critical care resources for use during epidemics. Crit Care Med 2007 May;35(5):1251-6.

TRIAGE IN RADIATION HAZARD SITUATIONS

1. Contact radiation safety officer.
2. Assess External Contamination
   - Assess contamination pattern with radiation survey meter

Sequential Organ Failure Assessment (SOFA) Score*

Variable	*SOFA Score* 0	1	2	3	4
PaO2/FiO2 mmHg	> 400	301 – 400	201 – 300	101 – 200	≤100
Platelets, × 103/ìL or × 106/L	> 150	101 – 150	51 – 100	21 – 50	≤20
Bilirubin, mg/dL (μmol/L)	<1.2 (<20)	1.2-1.9 (20 – 32)	2.0-5.9 (33–100)	6.0-11.9 (101–203)	>12 (> 203)
Hypotension	None	MABP < 70 mmHg	Dop ≤5	Dop 6–15 or Epi < 0.1 orNorepi < 0.1	Dop >15 or Epi > 0.1 orNorepi > 0.1
Glasgow Coma Score	15	13–14	10-12	6-9	< 6
Creatinine, mg/dL (μmol/L)	< 1.2 (<106)	1.2-1.9 (106 – 168)	2.0-3.4 (169 - 300)	3.5-4.9 (301 – 433)	> 5 (> 434) or anuric

Note: Clinicians will determine the total SOFA score for each patient by summing the scores for each variable. Dopamine [Dop], epinephrine [Epi], norepinephrine [Norepi] doses in ug/kg/min. SI units are noted in parentheses ( ).

*Adapted from: Ferreira et al., 2001. Explanation of variables: PaO2/FiO2 indicates the level of oxygen in the patient's blood. Platelets are a critical component of blood clotting. Bilirubin is measured by a blood test and indicates liver function. Hypotension indicates low blood pressure; scores of 2, 3, and 4 indicate that blood pressure must be maintained by the use of powerful medications that require ICU monitoring, including dopamine, epinephrine, and norepinephrine. The Glasgow coma score is a standardized measure that indicates neurologic function; low score indicates poorer function. Creatinine is measured by a blood test and indicates kidney function.

- Evaluate for radioactive shrapnel.
- Document contamination pattern on a body diagram.
- Obtain nasal swabs for radioactivity assay if significant internal contamination suspected (survey meter shows head/neck contamination).

3. Decontaminate Whole Body
   - Decontaminate onsite or at other designated area.
   - Follow decontamination procedures.
   - Re-scan patient with radiation survey meter.
   - Repeat decontamination until radiation reading is < 2 times background radiation level.
   - Do not exceed 3 attempts.
   - Special issues for infants and children.
4. Evaluate if All Are True:
   - Decontamination successful (< 2 times background radiation).
   - Absent or minimal physical injury.
5. If All Are True:
   - Send home with follow-up instructions.
   - Register in event database.
6. Otherwise: Evaluate at Medical Facility.
   - Treat life- or limb-threatening injuries first.
   - Obtain sequential complete blood counts (CBCs) with differential to rule out whole-body exposure and acute radiation sickness (ARS).
   - Remove any remaining radioactive shrapnel and shield it safely.
7. Assess Internal Contamination
   - Scan patient with radiation survey meter (caveat).
   - Event responders or radiation safety officer will identify the isotope(s).
   - Swab body orifices (e.g., nostrils, ears, mouth, rectum) to help estimate body burden of isotope.
   - Collect 24-hr stool for isotope measurement (baseline and sequential after management).
   - Collect 24-hr urine for isotope measurement.
   - Label all specimens with time, date, and name.
   - Perform total body count if available; consider hospital nuclear medicine equipment.
8. Treat Internal Contamination of Specific Isotope
   - Decision to treat will depend on.
   - Level of internal contamination.
   - Size of radiation event.
   - Availability of resources/personnel.
   - Likelihood that patient will survive.
9. If No Recovery:
   - Management of the deceased.
   - Register data into event database.
10. For Patient Making a Recovery: Arrange for Continuing and Long-Term Follow-up.
    - Send home with follow-up instructions.
    - Register patient in long-term follow-up database.

NATO GUIDELINES

- *Red:* Airway obstruction, cardiorespiratory failure, significant external hemorrhage, shock, sucking chest wound, burns of face or neck.
- *Yellow:* Open thoracic wound, penetrating abdominal wound, severe eye injury, avascular limb, fractures, significant burns other than face, neck or perineum.
- *Green:* Minor lacerations, contusions, sprains, superficial burns, partial-thickness burns of < 20% BSA.
- *Black:* Head injury with GCS<8, burns >85% BSA, multisystem trauma, signs of impending death.

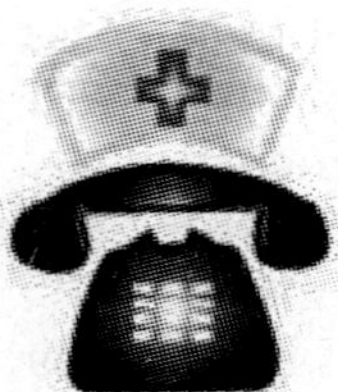

Fig. 46.4

TELEPHONE TRIAGE

Telephone triage is when a medical professional, usually a registered nurse, speaks by telephone to a patient and assesses the patient's symptoms or health concerns and offers advice. Telephonic programs are not a new methodology used to enhance health care advice to patients. The first recorded instance of assistance via telephone was recorded in 1879. By 1997, this had evolved to more than 500 nurse triage and advice systems serving 35 million Americans. Moreover, telephone advice nursing is the fastest growing nursing specialty. This growth has been exacerbated by a combination of concerns involving controlling unnecessary costs while providing quality services and maintaining customer satisfaction.This is done utilizing clinical protocols that help the nurse determine the severity of the patient's health issues and rank them according to urgency. Telephone triage nurses educate patients and guide them to appropriate care. Telephone triage services are offered by health care facilities, often for physician's offices to take calls from patients trying to contact the doctor. Known as nurse lines (NL), they provide guidance to callers regarding medical care. These are services provided by specially trained nurses to callers reporting a variety of medical complaints of varying severity. Nurses use decision support software to assist them in determining what advice to give the caller.

Overtriage and Undertriage

Effective triage requires balance not only between the demands on the system and the supply of resources but also between overtriage and undertriage. Overtriage and undertriage are related to the accuracy with which patients are triaged. Undertriage occurs when the severity of a patient's illness or injury is not appropriately recognized, which results in delayed treatment that places the patient at risk of dying. Particularly in day-to-day situations, undertriage is minimized through the use of protocols that tend to overtriage patients to higher levels of care than they require.

Such protocols are not foolproof, however, because overtriage has been shown to decrease overall survival rates among critically ill or injured victims. Overtriage may increase mortality by depleting resources, fatiguing staff, and impairing efficient flow of critically ill or injured patients through the system to definitive care. The accuracy of triage depends on both the reliability of the protocol in predicting patient outcomes and how the protocol is applied by the triage officers. Triage is a dynamic process that makes it more likely to correct inevitable instances of undertriage and overtriage.

Target levels for undertriage rates within a trauma system range from 0 to 5% of patients requiring Level I or Level II trauma-center care, depending on the criteria used to determine the undertriage rate (e.g., death and ISS) Target levels of overtriage vary (approximate range: 25%–50%). As field triage continues to evolve on the basis of new research findings, overtriage rates might be reduced while maintaining low undertriage rates.

IDEAL TRIAGE INSTRUMENT

Although a number of factors must be considered when selecting the most appropriate instrument to use during a MCI, one of the critical factors is the instrument's reliability and validity, which is the most critical characteristic of any instrument.The triage algorithms mentioned above and current research- Reliability means that the instrument is used to assess something in a reproducible way. Intra-rater reliability occurs when the instrument results in identical triage categories if the same evaluator rates the same patient twice (usually the two ratings are conducted within a short period of time at two different time points, at which the patient's condition is not expected to change). Inter-rater reliability occurs when the instrument also yields identical triage categories of the same patient from at least two different raters. None of the mass-casualty triage algorithms have been tested for intra or inter-rater reliability.

The construct validity of an instrument relates to its ability to assess what it is intended to assess. Although the validity of the secondary triage instruments has not been investigated, a few studies have examined the construct validity of the primary mass-casualty triage instruments. Garner *et al.* used trauma registry data from 1,144 adult trauma patients to retrospectively assign each one a triage level according to START, Triage Sieve and Care Flight Triage, and compared the ability of the use of the instruments to discriminate between patients with a critical injury (defined as a patient requiring a life-saving intervention).

The discriminant validity of Care Flight Triage and START was significantly better than Triage Sieve in this retrospective analysis. Sacco *et al.* compared the predictive validity of STM and START by estimating the use of the instruments to maximize the number of survivors using computer simulations that varied in terms of resources available and the number of patients that could be transported. The authors found that the use of the STM provided higher numbers of expected survivors than did the use of the START in all of the simulations, and that the difference between the results of using the two instruments increased as resources became more constrained.

Finally, Wallis and Carley prospectively evaluated the discriminant validity of Care Flight Triage, JumpSTART, START, and the PTT for triaging children aged d"12 years who were presented to a trauma unit within 12 hours of receiving an acute injury. From among 3,461 patients, the investigators evaluated the ability of the different triage algorithms to classify patients with serious injuries using different criteria such as the Injury Severity Score,the New Injury Severity Score (NISS), or requiring a life-saving intervention.The patterns were similar given the three criteria used. For example, when serious injury was defined as those with a NISS above 15, the sensitivity of placing them in the highest triage category (immediate) was calculated.

Care Flight Triage had the highest sensitivity for NISS above 15 for placing patients in the highest triage category at 31.5% (95% Confidence Interval (CI) 29%–34%),followed by PTT at 26.1% (95% CI 23%–29%), START at 22.3% (95% CI 16%–31%), and JumpSTART at 2.4% (1%–5%).20,21 Specificities were 99% for CareFlight, 98.9% for PTT, 97.8% for JumpSTART, and 77.3% for START.

Psychological Aspects of Triage

Psychological support services should be available both during and after the event because triage officers and their team members are likely to carry heavy emotional burdens stemming from the necessary decision making.

ETHICAL CONSIDERATIONS IN TRIAGE AND RESOURCE ALLOCATION

If faced with resource limitations, physicians will be forced to decide how best to distribute potentially life-saving care. Such decisions are complex and should be guided by an ethical framework. The use of a sound ethical framework not only aids in developing an appropriate triage protocol but also promotes effective application of the protocol. It is important for triage officers, healthcare workers, and the public to understand the ethical basis of triage decisions. Triage officers who do not understand the ethical basis of their decisions are likely to suffer a significant emotional Because the exclusion of some patients from critical care is implicit in tertiary triage decisions, the provision of palliative care and other alternatives must be fully integrated into the disaster response system. A few key ethical principles are: Bioethical concerns have historically played an important role in triage decisions, such as the allocation of iron lungs during the polioepidemics of the 1940s and of dialysis machines during the 1960s. As many health care systems in the developed world continue to plan for an expected influenza pandemic, bioethical issues regarding the triage of patients and the rationing of care continue to evolve. Similar issues may occur for paramedics in the field in the earliest stages of mass casualty incidents when large numbers of potentially serious or critical patients may be combined with extremely limited staffing and treatment resources.

There are a few common ways to distribute scarce resources: (1) first come, first served; (2) focusing resources where they will be the most effective in order to do the most good for the greatest number of people; and (3) directing the resources to those in greatest need.

Allocating scarce resources is an exercise in distributive justice. In medical triage, particularly if the goal is to do the most good for the most people or to direct resources to those in greatest need, one can look at either the medical or the social factors involved. Medical factors relate to how sick a person is. An individual's medical condition and outcome are the primary factors considered. Social factors pertain to such issues as a person's role in society (i.e. community leader, healthcare worker, criminal), a person's potential to contribute to society, and prior social injustices an individual may have faced. Although social issues seem important in lifeboat-style theoretical exercises, they are incredibly difficult if not impossible to judge at a bedside during an actual disaster. Because evaluation based on social factors is very subjective, medical triage typically focuses on the more objective medical factors.

A. *Principle of equal Chances: First Come, First Served:* The basic premise of the first-come, first-served approach is that all casualties deserve to be treated equally. The easiest way to give everyone an equal chance is to use a random allocation process, such as a lottery. Of course, a lottery would not be a useful tool in a disaster or pandemic because it is impossible to know in advance who is going to be injured or fall ill and require a medical resource. Thus, in a disaster or pandemic, first come, first served is the next best option, serving as somewhat of a cosmic random number generator. The primary strengths of this approach are that it is easy to apply and that at first glance it seems fair. However, closer examination reveals several fatal flaws. It has been well documented that the first patients to present to hospitals in a disaster are the walking wounded and minimally injured who can extricate and transport themselves. Many of those patients are suffering primarily from emotional stress. Giving priority to this group would rapidly consume resources before the truly injured ever arrived. Moreover, although vulnerable populations are more likely to be affected by a mass casualty incident, the people who are healthiest and wealthiest are often the best able to save themselves and seek help first. The calamities that accompanied Hurricane Katrina in 2005 are prime examples of this.

B. *Utilitarianism*: The greatest good for the greatest number: The utilitarian approach to triage focuses on the end result and aims to create the greatest good possible. Put another way, at the end of a disaster the available resources should have been used to help the most people to survive. This most commonly used guiding philosophy of medical triage dates back to the early 1900s. Its primary strength is that it holds out the hope that the greatest efficiency will be obtained from the resources available. This concept appeals strongly to medical personnel, especially in an era of outcome-driven, evidence-based medicine. However, the most significant shortcoming of this philosophy is that it necessitates an ability to predict the future. To achieve the goal of efficiency, healthcare workers must have some capacity to judge who is going to benefit from a resource, if applied.

C. *Egalitarianism*: Those Most in need Should receive. Under an egalitarian approach and the maximin principle the available critical care resources would be directed to the sickest patients. This approach, which is similar to how healthcare is practised on a daily basis, is morally comforting for many healthcare workers because it seems to minimize internal conflict by eliminating the need to make difficult decisions. It also fulfills the need to "do something" that many people feel when faced with someone who is suffering, especially in an emergency. However, the primary limitation of egalitarianism is that it will lead to a vast amount of resources being expended on many patients who will not survive. Further, the initial gratification of "doing something" for someone who is suffering may be short lived. As many seasoned ICU professionals report, the provision of care to a patient when the situation is futile produces significant moral distress. Unless a mechanism is included to limit critical care interventions, this approach could well lead to more harm than good. The World Medical Association states that it is unethical for physicians to waste resources by persisting to provide care in futile situations.

Overall, triage seeks to preserve and protect endangered lives. Because an overwhelmed system may deteriorate into a chaos in which no one will be helped, triage aims to provide a methodical approach to using the resources that are available to help the most people possible. Current triage approaches actually combine aspects of all 3 ethical theories by focusing care on patients who are in the greatest need but likely to survive and preserving the option to use first come, first served in cases where patients' needs and chances for recovery are equal. Further, many ethicists tend to look at the triage of critical care resources in isolation. Ultimately, the provision of critical care is only 1 small, albeit important, aspect of disaster response and must be viewed in the context of the overall government or societal response. Significant resources are also directed to disaster preparedness, mitigation, rescue and recovery.

DISASTER TRIAGE AND ALLOCATION OF SCARCE RESOURCES

The ability of a healthcare system to respond to a surge is determined by such factors as the resources available, the number of patients, the time period over which those patients arrive, and the need for specialized services.

Resource allocation strategies must take into account both supply and demand. When demand exceeds supply, scarcities will ensue and triage will be required to prioritize and ration resources.

Triage is a dynamic process requiring protocol adjustments to ensure that rationing (infringement on individual liberties) does not exceed the expected or experienced shortfall between demand and supply. Triage is commonly used throughout the healthcare system to set priorities for patient care. Only in rare disaster circumstances does it form the basis for rationing resources.

Disaster triage occurs at various points along the continuum of care and is classified accordingly as primary, secondary, or tertiary. Tertiary triage involves decisions related to allocating critical care resources. Standard tertiary triage protocols are lacking. Effective tertiary triage requires significant planning and an infrastructure that can support the process during a disaster. A strong ethical framework is necessary to guide the development and implementation of a triage protocol.

THE FUTURE

Triage in the future would be in the form of "Real-time" wave form analysis, heart rate variability R-wave amplitude, trend analysis, advanced/derived vital signs, pulse pressure, shock index and better monitors to support decisions.

47 Pre-Hospital Treatment

"When any calamity has been suffered, the first thing to be remembered is how much has been escaped."

—*Samuel Johnson*

SUCCESSFUL AIRWAY MANAGEMENT

This is a vital skill for first responders as it impacts patient outcome. This may have to be done in adverse environments, limited patient access and limited help from others. Patients may be intoxicated, have associated neck and head injuries and also a full stomach.

The fully conscious, talking patient is able to maintain his own airway and needs no further airway manipulation. However patients' status may deteriorate at any time, and ABC's must constantly be reassessed.

The following categories of patients require a definitively secured airway:

1. Apnoea.
2. Glasgow Coma Scale < 9 or sustained seizure activity.
3. Unstable mid-face trauma.
4. Airway injuries.
5. Large flail segment or respiratory failure.
6. High aspiration risk.
7. Inability to otherwise maintain an airway or oxygenation.

Indications for Airway Support

Inadequate ventilation, inability to protect the airway, upper airway obstruction, elevated ICP and hypoxia.

Requires 2-3 personnel minimum for:

Equipment preparation and check, perform Sellick' manouvre during intubation, provide suction, prepare drugs for premedication, sedation and muscle relaxation.

Delay in intubation can lead to aspiration, hypercarbia, hypoxia and rise in ICP and cervical spine injury.

Rapid sequence intubation: (7 P's)

- *Prepare*—Patient, medication and equipment—check suction, ETO, Ambu bag, oxygen, light, stylet.
- Preoxygenate (denitrogenation 3 to 5 min).
- Pretreat—sedation, amnesia.
- Protect in line traction of cervical spine-use collar, use forearm as stabilizing bridge, with elbows on chest and hands on occiput and zygoma during airway manipulations.
- Paralyze.
- Press: Sellick's manouver-cricoid pressure.
- Position: Check ETO in proper place.

Standby truphatek, McCoy laryngoscopes.

Jelly fish face masks give good seal despite facial hair and edentulous.

Fluid challenge 20 ml/kg in 10 min recommended if patient is hypotensive.

The urgency of airway intubation is the most important factor in planning which

Table 47.1: Indications for definitive airway

Need for airway protection	*Need for ventilation*
Unconscious	Apnea • Neuromuscular paralysis • Unconscious
Severe maxillofacial fractures	Inadequate respiratory effort • Tachypnea • Hypoxia • Hypercarbia • Cyanosis
Risk for aspiration • Bleeding • Vomiting	Severe closed head injury with need for hyperventilation
Risk for obstruction • Neck hematoma • Laryngeal, tracheal injury • Stridor	

technique of securing the airway is the safest and most appropriate. One must evaluate and assess the risk of further cord injury given head and neck movement, the degree of cooperation from the patient, anatomy and trauma to the airway and one's own expertise in each technique (Fig. 47.1).

Initially the airway should be cleared of debris, blood and secretions. It should be opened using the 'chin lift' or 'jaw thrust' manoeuvres. The 'sniffing the morning air' position for standard tracheal intubation flexes the lower cervical spine and extends the occiput on the atlas. However, the 'jaw thrust' and 'chin lift' both cause distraction of at least 5mm in a cadaver with C5/6 instability. This movement was unaffected by use of a rigid collar. Manual stabilization did however reduce movement.

Table 47.2: Approximate PaO_2 versus O_2 hemoglobin saturation levels

PaO_2 levels	*O_2 hemoglobin saturation levels*
90 mm Hg	100%
60 mm Hg	90%
30 mm Hg	60%
27 mm Hg	50%

An oral (Guedel) or nasopharyngeal airway may be necessary to maintain patency until a definitive airway is secured. Insertion of an airway produces minimal disturbance to the cervical spine. Bag and mask ventilation also produces a significant degree of movement at zones of instability.

Tracheal Tube

The safest method of securing a tracheal tube remains debatable. In general, the technique used should be the one the operator is most familiar with. The method is generally unimportant as long as the (potential) cervical spine injury is recognised and reasonable care taken (Flowchart. 47.1).

The ATLS recommends a nasotracheal tube in the spontaneously breathing patient, and orotracheal intubation in the apnoeic patient. MANUAL in-line axial stabilization must be maintained throughout. The hard collar may interfere with intubation efforts and the front part may be removed to facilitate intubation as long as manual stabilisation is in effect.

Blind nasal intubation is successful in 90% of patients but requires multiple attempts in up to 90% of these. Nasotracheal intubation

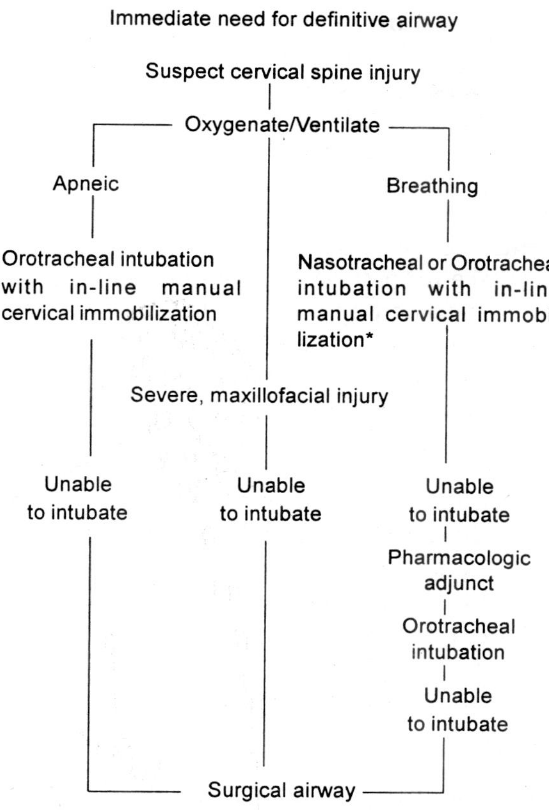

Flowchart 47.1: Airway algorithm

is (relatively) contraindicated in patients with potential base of skull fracture or unstable mid-face injuries. In addition, it may produce haemorrhage in the airway, making other airway manipulations difficult or impossible. Nasotracheal intubation in non-trauma patients is often accomplished by rotating or flexing the neck to align the tube correctly. This is not possible in the trauma patient and the procedure becomes more difficult. In the spontaneously breathing patient however, one can hear movement of air at the end of the tracheal tube and thus line the tube up with the trachea.

Orotracheal intubation is generally accepted as the more usual method for securing the airway in the trauma patient. It is the fastest and surest method of intubating the trachea using a modified rapid sequence induction technique with pre-oxygenation and cricoid pressure. Ten percent of these patients can have cervical spine injury but no neurological deterioration is likely following intubation.

Atlanto-occipital extension is necessary to bring the vocal cords within line-of-sight of the mouth. Thus patients with unstable C1 or C2 injuries might be at more risk from this

Table 47.3: Endotracheal tube size and position base on patient age

Age	*Internal diameter (mm)*	*External diameter (mm) Approximate, varying among manufacturers*	*French unit*	*Distance inserted from lips for tip placement in midtrachea (cm)n*
Premature	2.5	3.3	10	10
Full term newborn	3.0	4.0–4.2	12	11
1–6 months	3.5	4.7–4.8	14	11
6–12 months	4.0	5.3–5:6	16	12
2 years	4.5	6.0–6.3	18	13
4 years	5.0	6.7–7.0	20	14
6 years	5.5	7.3–7.6	22	15–16
8 years	6.0	8.0-8.2	24	16-17
10 years	6.5	8.7–9.3	26	17–18
12 years	7.0	9.3–10	28–30	18–20
14 years	7.0 (women)	9.3–10	28–30	20-24
14 years and older	8.0 (men)	10.7–11.3	32–34	

technique. Direct laryngoscopy has been shown to disturb the cervical spine both in anaesthetised volunteers and in cadavers. Manual axial in-line stabilisation reduces this movement by 60%. Quadriplegia following laryngoscopy without manual stabilization is a distinct possibility.

The use of induction agents and muscle relaxants to facilitate intubation are all safe and effective. If possible, patients requiring tracheal tube intubation should be anaesthetised unless very cooperative. In the obtunded head injured patient, anaesthesia is vital to prevent pressor responses to intubation increasing intracranial pressure. Carbon dioxide levels are also much better controlled in the anaesthetised patient.

The ideal induction agent probably does not exist, and once again it is down to operator experience. Propofol is not recommended for trauma because of the potential for hypotension (as with most IV agents) but has many advantages in these patients and is used in many centres. Its ability to provide total intravenous anaesthesia with good control over the depth of anaesthesia is also very valuable. Thiopentone (pentothal) requires making up to solution but otherwise is very effective and is the standard for rapid sequence induction. Etomidate has been reported to produce less cardiovascular depression than other intravenous induction agents, but this research was done on healthy individuals, and this is not the case for hypovolaemic patients. In addition, the potential adrenal and immunological suppression caused by even one bolus of etomidate puts a question mark on its use in these cases. Ketamine is a very under-used induction agent which maintains cardiovascular stability better than the other intravenous agents. As a non-competitive NMDA receptor antagonist it has neuroprotective effects. Its use is currently contraindicated in patients at risk from raised intracranial pressure as it has been shown to increase cerebral blood flow and so ICP in head injured patients. However, evidence is accumulating that this may not be the case, especially in hypotensive patients, and its effects on ICP may be modulated by agents such as propofol.

Awake intubation is also a feasible option and is favoured by some practitioners. It has been shown to be safe in the patient with cervical spine injury. It may be performed via the nasotracheal route, direct oral laryngoscopy or by fibreoptic technique.

Successful fibreoptic tracheal intubation requires a cooperative patient, a secretion and blood free airway, a pharynx unrestricted by oedema and adequate supraglottic and infraglottic anaesthesia. Such ideal conditions often do not exist, and local anaesthetic preparation of the airway is time consuming and might increase the risk of aspiration.

Failed Intubation

Failed or difficult intubation is always a problem. It is important not to waste time with repeated attempts at intubation while the patient is desaturating. Alternative methods of securing the airway should be instituted as soon as a problem is recognised.

Laryngeal Mask Airway (LMA)

The LMA is gaining wider support in the management of patients with cervical spine injury. As well as maintaining the airway, a tracheal tube (size 6 or less) may be placed, either blindly or via flexible fibreoptic laryngoscopy. The LMA does not, however, completely protect the airway from aspiration but can be inserted in lighter planes and better tolerated. Its use should probably be limited to maintenance of the airway after a failed attempt at intubation (Fig. 47.1).

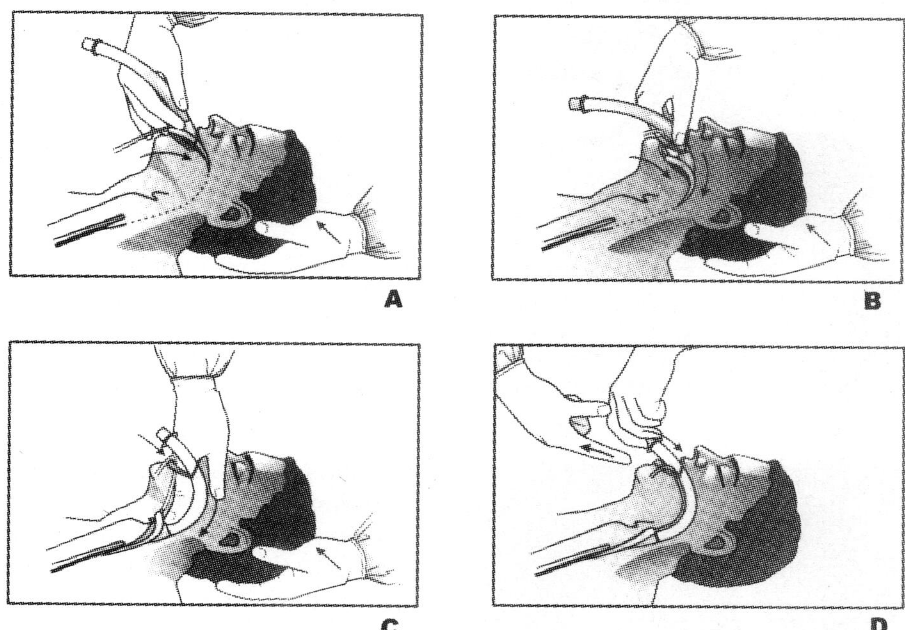

Fig. 47.1: Insertion of the LMA (A) The tip of the cuff is pressed upward against the hard palate by the index finger while the middle finger opens the mouth (B) The LMA is pressed backward in a smooth movement; note that the nondominant hand is used to extend the head (C) The LMA is advanced until a definite resistance is felt (D) Before the index finger is removed, the nondominant hand presses down on the LMA to prevent dislodgement during removal of the index finger; the cuff is subsequently inflated; an outward movement of the tube is often noted during this inflation

Combitube

The combitube is a double lumen tube inserted blindly into the oesophagus or trachea. The position of the tube is confirmed by the presence of breath sounds or capno-graphy. By inflating one of the two cuffs present, the lungs may then be ventilated. Problems arise after positioning with definitive securing of a tracheal tube, and again with protection of the airway from aspiration, although stomach suctioning is possible through the gastric port (Fig. 47.2 A & B).

Cricothyroidotomy

The need for a surgical airway should be recognised quickly and performed by an experienced person without delay. It may be used as a primary airway, with injuries to the pharynx for example, or after failure of orotracheal intubation. It may be a full surgical approach or via a percutaneous needle cricothyroidotomy with high flow oxygen. The potential for carbon dioxide retention with this technique must be remembered and the levels in arterial samples monitored. There are no studies regarding movement of the neck during cricothyroidotomy, ease of crico-thyroidotomy with neck immobilisation, or neurological deterioration following crico-thyroidotomy (Fig. 47.3).

Verification of Tracheal Tube Placement

It is vital that the position of the tube is confirmed to be in the trachea. Clinical

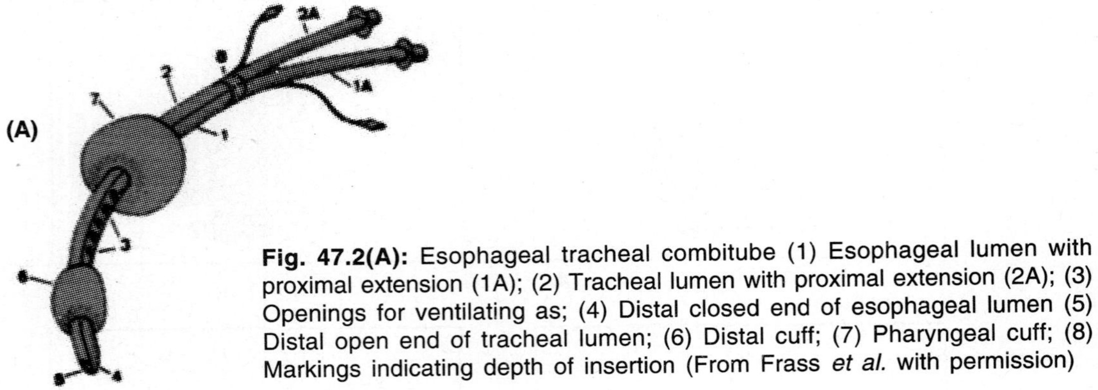

Fig. 47.2(A): Esophageal tracheal combitube (1) Esophageal lumen with proximal extension (1A); (2) Tracheal lumen with proximal extension (2A); (3) Openings for ventilating as; (4) Distal closed end of esophageal lumen (5) Distal open end of tracheal lumen; (6) Distal cuff; (7) Pharyngeal cuff; (8) Markings indicating depth of insertion (From Frass *et al.* with permission)

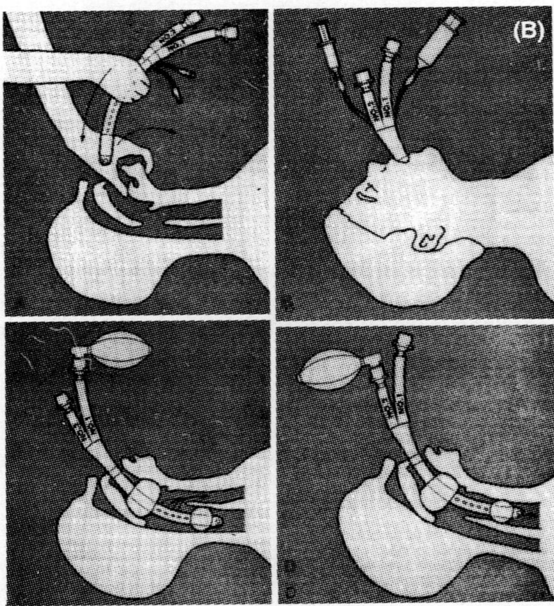

Fig. 47.2(B): Insertion of the combitude (A) The tongue and mandible are lifted with one hand and the combitube is inserted in the direction of the natural curvature of the pharynx with the other hand. The printed ring is aligned with the teeth. (B) The blue pharyngeal cuff is inflated with 100 mL of air while the white distal cuff Ls inflated with 15 mL. (C) Ventilation is begun through the longer blue tube as placement is usually in the esophagus. If ventilation is absent and the stomach is being insufflated, begin ventilation through the clear connecting tube

methods of verificationlike auscultation are notoriously unreliable, and patients with chest injuries increase the likelihood of mistakes in this area. Capnography is the gold standard in the operating room to assess tracheal tube position, and this should probably be transferred to the trauma area too.

Assessment of Victim

Level of consciousness is important as an awake patient can usually maintain his or her airway with an active cough reflex. If airway is obstructed and respiration noisy or laboured, oxygenation may be compromised. A central pulse cannot be felt if the blood pressure is below 50 mmHg and peripheral pulses are lost below 70 mmHg. A fast pulse rate and low blood pressure associated with cold skin (peripheral vasoconstriction), sweating and bluishness of tongue and nails warrants on-the-spot interventions by the first responder.

Head tilt, chin lift, jaw thrust and jaw lift with suctioning and insertion of airway and oxygenation may be life saving. Application of MAST is useful in shocked victims.

Intravenous line, fluid infusion and medications will be required for serious patients.

Direct pressure and splinting will be required to arrest bleeding.

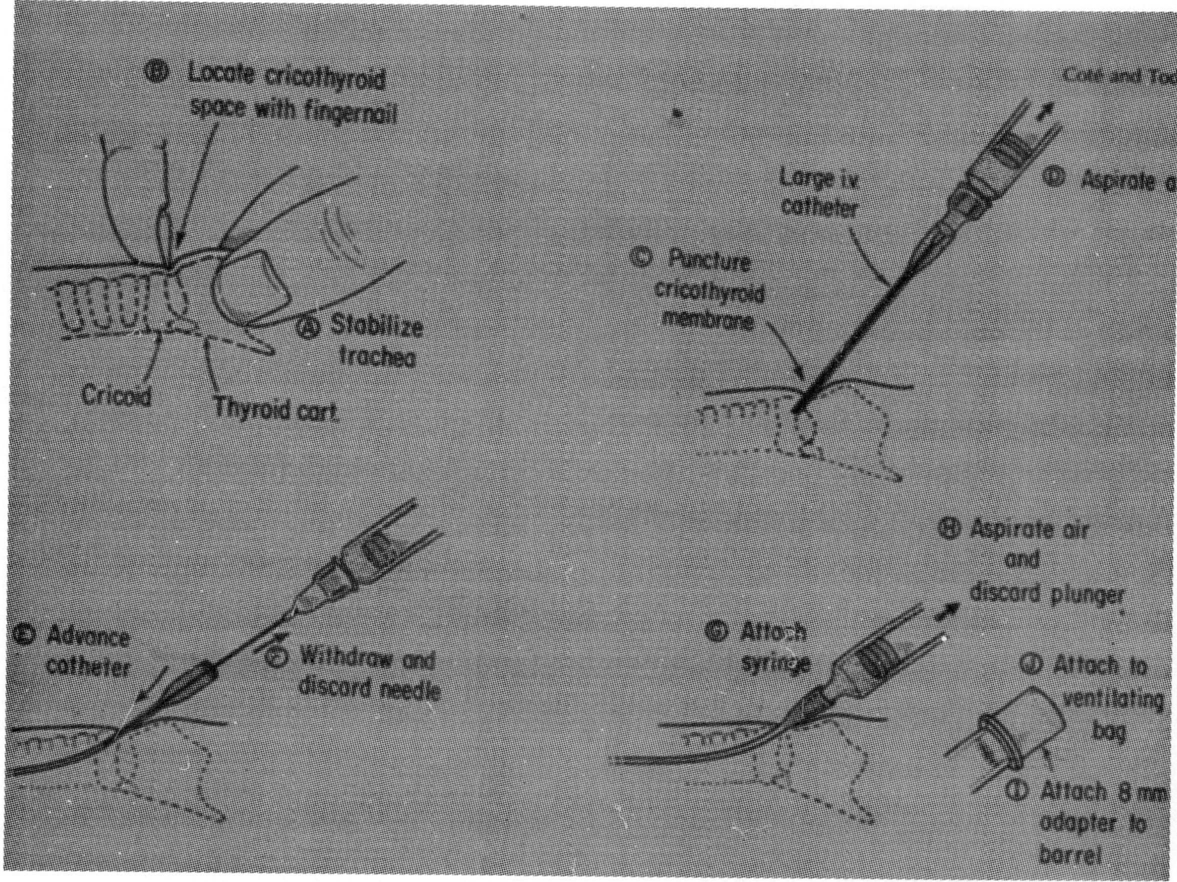

Fig. 47.3: Percutaneous cricothyroidotomy. Extend the head in the midline with a rolled towel on folded sheet transversely beneath the shoulders. Stabilize trachea (A). The cricothyroid membrane is located with the fingertip between the thyroid and cricoid cartilage (B). This space is so narrow (1 mm) that only a fingernail can palpate it in an infant. A large intravenous catheter (12-14 gauge) is inserted through the cricothyroid membrane (C) and air aspirated (D) The catheter is advanced into the trachea through the membrane (E) and the needle discarded (F); intraluminal position is reconfirmed by attaching a 3 ml syringe (G) and aspirating for air (H). The 3 ml syringe barrel without plunger is attached to the catheter. An 8 mm endotracheal tube adapter is attrahed to the syringe barrel (J). (Reprinted from stinsor TW III: A sample connector for treacheal ventilation. Anesthesiology 47;343, 1977. With permission). Connection are made to standard equipment (15 mm connections). As an alternative, a 3 mm airway adapter will fit any IV catheter

If breathing remains unsatisfactory, needle thoracostomy will be life saving in victims having tension pneumothorax.

Those with weakness of limbs may have a neck bone injury. They will require application of a cervical collar/immobilization device.

Victims in collapsed state will require artificial respiration and external cardiac compression.

Mechanical ventilation if required is usually done with an Ambu bag or the very versatile Siemens 90°C that can be powered by a car battery (Flowchart 47.2).

NEIGHBOURHOOD EMERGENCY TEAM (NET)

Despite the presumption that the public cannot participate actively in a disaster scenario, it is frequently observed that victims and bystanders perform a useful primary role. They often respond effectively and creatively by forming spontaneous groups that have roles, rules, leaders and a division of labour. This emergent collective behavior has amazed everyone as first responders and ordinary folks have rescued the majority of victims, well before arrival of the military, Red Cross or formal EMS providers. The locals tend to

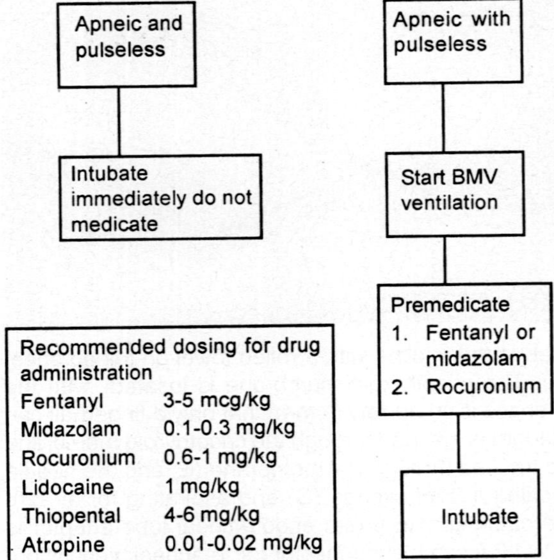

Flowchart 47.2: Protocol for airway management for (A) apneic patients and (B) those breathing spontaneously with or without associated head trauma. Insert contains current recommendations for appropriate medication doses

know the local language, culture and terrain better while the latter often arrive late due to multisite events like disruptions of communications, traffic routes etc. It becomes important therefore that the public be considered as partners in disaster situations and that is it is advantageous to decentralize response and work with local civic organizations, churches, RSS, schools, neighbourhoods and corporations that the locals trust and are familiar with in a chaotic situation. During Hurricane Andrew, a local AM disc jockey advised listeners to get into a bathtub and cover themselves with a mattress and saved more lives than anybody in the government! It is vital, therefore, to work with the public and not see them as some sort of adversial functionary. An informal training program can be instituted at grassroot levels to train lay public on vital aspects of disaster care and response. The NET program is one such and they have a continued awareness schedule aimed at educating lay public on the following aspects:

1. Disaster awareness: Personal, family and workplace preparedness.
2. Utility handling: Gas, water, electricity how and when to switch on or off, hazardous materials handling and aspects of fire fighting.
3. Disaster medicine: Recognition and treatment of life-threatening injuries, triage, secondary patient assessment, treatment of common injuries, set up of medical treatment area.
4. Public health considerations: Hygiene, pathogens, disinfection, search and rescue, patient extrication and transportation and disaster psychology.
5. Team management.

48 Basic Life Science

> "If we put the emphasis upon the right things, if we live the life that is worth while and then fail, we will survive all disasters, we will out-live all misfortune. We should be so well balanced and symmetrical, that nothing which could ever happen could."
>
> —*Orison Swett Marden*

INTRODUCTION

Cardiac arrest is the number one killer of modern times. Two out of every three deaths occur before the victims even reach a hospital. Survival of the event depends on a series of critical interventions. Even if one of these critical actions is neglected or delayed, survival is unlikely. The American Heart Association (AHA) uses the term chain of survival to describe this sequence. Communities with a strong chain have achieved survival rates as high as 30%. This is achieved by training lay public, first responders, ambulance personnel, paramedics, doctors and nurses to function as coordinated team to aggressively tackle cardiac arrest. Basic Life Support (BLS) is the phase of emergency cardiac and respiratory care that prevents circulatory insufficiency and supports ventilation of a victim of cardio respiratory arrest so that oxygenation and perfusion to the brain and vital organs is sustained until appropriate and definitive medical treatment is instituted. Also referred to as cardio pulmonary resuscitation (CPR), it is the most successful public health initiative in recent times. CPR is defined as the artificial delivery of oxygenated blood to systemic circulation at rates sufficient to preserve vital organ function until return of spontaneous circulation. The overall survival rate of such efforts averages 15%. The rate can be better if it is instituted within 4 minutes of the arrest and if advanced life support is initiated within 8 minutes. In situations of pure respiratory arrest, the survival rates are higher. Almost all neurologically intact survivors of out-of-hospital cardiac arrest emerge from a well defined group of victims whose cardiac arrest was witnessed and whose CPR was initiated within minutes, those who were in ventricular fibrillation and those for whom advanced life support care was rapidly provided. Evaluation of paramedic care has demonstrated that the single most effective intervention in the care of this group of victims was rapid defibrillation by paramedics or emergency medical technicians (EMTs). Automatic external defibrillators (AEDs) developed in the late 1970s enables first responders like fire fighters, emergency personnel, prehospital rescuers etc to effect defibrillation with consistent automated ECG interpretation, less performance variability, faster countershock delivery and less expense for both training skilled manpower and maintenance when compared to standard defibrillators.

BLS TECHNIQUE IN ADULTS

Shake the victims shoulders and shout Are you okay? If he or she responds go on to the next victim. If the victim is unresponsive but obviously breathing and there is no evidence of any major trauma, place the victim on the side with head end at a lower level, insert an airway if tolerated, and go on to the next victim. When the victim shows no response and is NOT breathing, call for help and place the victim on firm level ground. Perform a quick primary survey of the victim, assessing injuries, vital signs and injury mechanisms and establish a logical, sequential treatment priority with victim completely undressed. Ascertain airway patency first, inspecting for foreign bodies, facial and jaw fractures that may result in airway obstruction. Obtain patency of the airway by an initial chin lift-jaw thrust manouvre, taking great care to prevent excessive movement of the neck and avoiding hyperextension, hyperflexion or rotation movements for cervical spine protection. Always assume a cervical spine injury in a victim with mutlisystem trauma, altered consciousness or a blunt injury above the collarbone. Stabilize the victims head and apply a cervical collar or any other immobilization device. Place one hand on the victims forehead and the other hand behind his/her neck. Gently push down on the forehead and lift the neck to extend the neck. This places the airway passages in a favourable position for airflow. If the victim begins to breathe as assessed by looking for up and down rhythmic movements of the chest, listening with ears close to the victims nose for respiratory sounds and feeling the chest for movement, place the victim on his or her side. If not, give two slow expired air rescue breaths by mouth-to-mouth technique after ensuring a clear upper airway by finger sweeping victims mouth with a clean handkerchief, suctioning and insertion of an oropharyngeal or naso-pharyngeal airway. In a domestic accident, a vacuum cleaner can be used to improvise an effective and powerful suction, taking care not to exceed 1seconds at a time to prevent hypoxia. Ensure that the chest rises with each breath administered (Fig. 48. 1).

Check for pulse in the neck over the carotid arteries just adjacent to the voice box (Adams apple). If there is a pulse felt, continue rescue breathing until help arrives. If no pulsation is palpable, leave the airway, administer a sharp precordial thump and then give 3 chest compressions with a 25-3 kg force (upper torso weight) with both hands placed one on top of the other, the heels of both hands being kept parallel to one another over the lower central breastbone, with fingers pointed away from the resuscitators body and shoulders directly over the compressing hands. Compressions are given at a rate of one downward thrust per second with elbows held straight. Thrusts must be directed directly downwards with enough force to depress the sternum 1 to 2 inches (4 to 5 cm). Go back to the head end and give two more forceful rescue breaths, taking care not to inflate the victims stomach. If another person is available, get the other to give the chest compressions at a rate of above 100 per minute while you administer two rescue breaths during the pause at every 30th chest compression. This is not mandatory and mouth-to-mouth breathing can be continued uninterrupted through cardiac massage as this can actually be beneficial. External chest compression can produce systolic blood pressures of 100 mmHg and higher but diastolic pressures will be only 10-40mmHg. Sternal compressions alone produces minimal ventilation but it better than no intervention at all. Circulation of deoxygenated blood will not sustain cerebral viability. Survival from CPR is directly related to coronary perfusion pressure produced during chest compression and high impulse manual chest compression produces superior coronary perfusion pressures and aortic blood flow. This drill constitutes the ABC of Basic Life Support, an acronym for Airway, Breathing and Circulation. The cycle is continued until medics arrive to initiate advanced life support. Reassess the victim after four cycles of 30:2 CPR for presence of spontaneous breathing, palpable pulse, pupillary constriction and skin colour turning to pink from gray blue. Tearing at the eyes, some quasi-purposive movement to vigorous rubbing of knuckles over the victims mid sternal area, swallowing and cough efforts by the victim are all good indicators of recovery. AVPU is a simple acronym to assess the level of consciousness. A for alert patient, V for response to vocal stimuli, P for response only to painful stimuli and U for being totally unresponsive (Table 48.1 and Flowchart 48.1).

BLS IN CHILDREN

In neonates, cardiac massage is done with both thumbs over the lower sternum as the other four fingers encircle the chest behind. Under 1 year of age, head tilt-chin lift is as for adults, with rescue breathing given with the force of puffed up cheeks to inflate the lungs to avoid barotrauma. Chest compressions are done with just two to three fingers over the lower sternum at a minimal rate of 100/minute. Compression-ventilation ratio is kept at 30:2. If the infant is suspected to have choked, suspend it by the heels and administer firm blows to its back. In children ages 1-8 years, the heel of one hand is used for administering external cardiac compression while the rest of the drills are identical. Above 8 years of age, the two handed cardiac massage is acceptable (Fig. 48.1).

COUGH CPR

Cardiac arrest occurring before loss of consciousness can be tackled by the victim by forceful cough efforts within 1 to 15 seconds of the arrest. The increase in intrathoracic pressures that occurs with coughing generates adequate blood flow to the brain. This is particularly useful when the victim is already hooked to a cardiac monitor that is displaying gross slowing of heart rate.

Heimlich Manoeuvre or Manual Abdominal Thrusts

This procedure is useful to dislodge objects obstructing the lower airway. Four rapid upward thrusts are delivered by grabbing the victim from behind, with fist over the midline of the victim's upper abdomen. Four sharp back blows between the shoulder blades with a conscious victim sitting or standing and the unconscious victim lying on one side can also dislodge foreign materials in the airway. Infants and children are positioned face down over the forearm so that their head lower than the trunk while delivering the blows.

PRIMARY SURVEY RESUSCITATION PROTOCOLS

Look: Take 15 to 20 seconds to assess obvious injuries in a head to toe survey.

Listen: For air movement at victims mouth and nose. Elicit history from pre hospital personnel.

Ask: Patient to describe injuries, details of last meal, drugs and diseases, drug habituations/ addictions, drug allergies and blood group

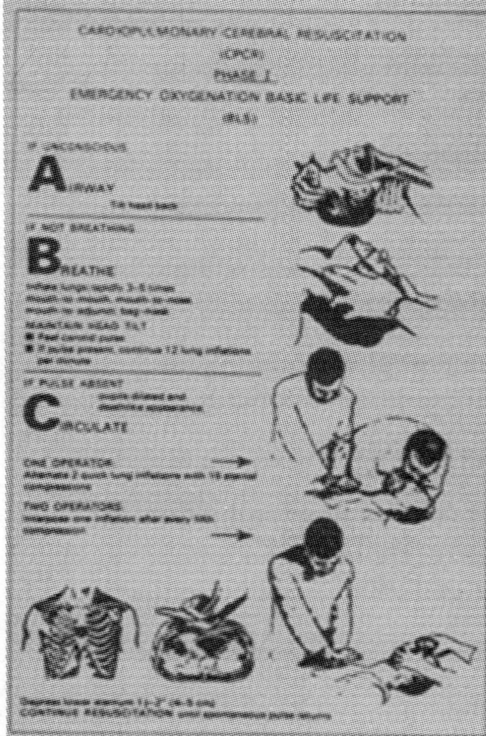

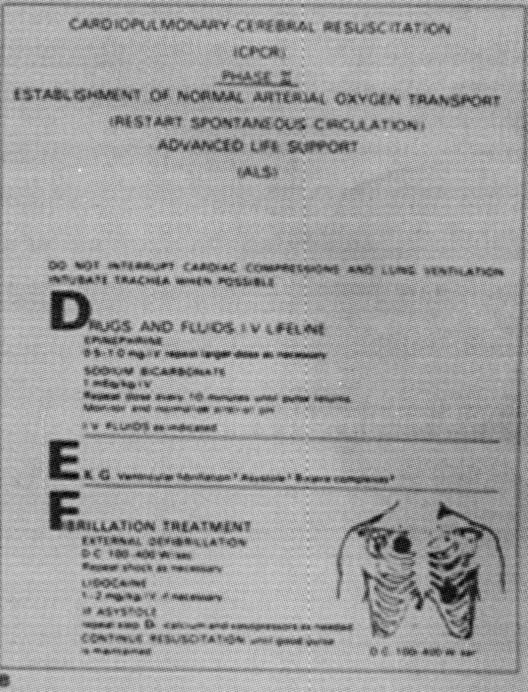

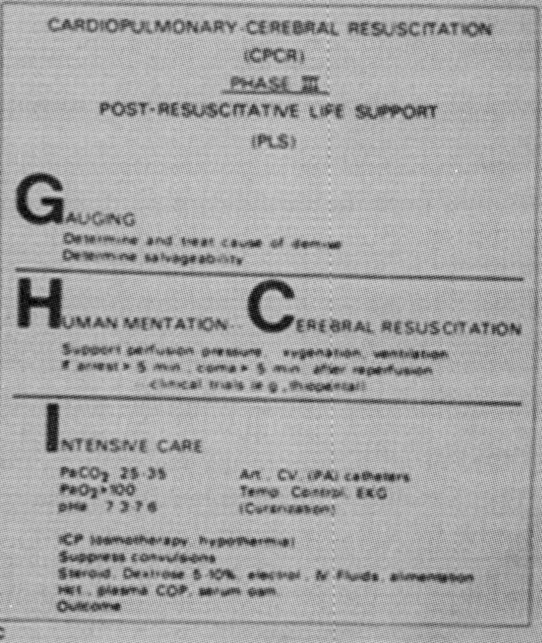

Fig. 48.1: (A) Basic life support: emergency oxygenation, a temporizing measure provided by a rescuer or rescuers. (B) Advanced life support; techniques to aid restoration of spontaneous oxygen delivery by the cardiac arrest victim (C) Post-resuscitative life support critical care therapies to support and maintain the resuscitated victim with particular emphasis on the cause of the cardiopulmonary arrest. Its treatment and prevention, and the post-CRR cardiopulmonary, neurologic, and renal status (Reproduced permission from Safar P Cardiopulmonary-cerebral resuscitation including emergency airway control in Schwartz GR, Safter P, Stone JH et al level: Principles and Practice of Emergency Medicine, p 177 Phladelphia, WB Saunders, 1978)

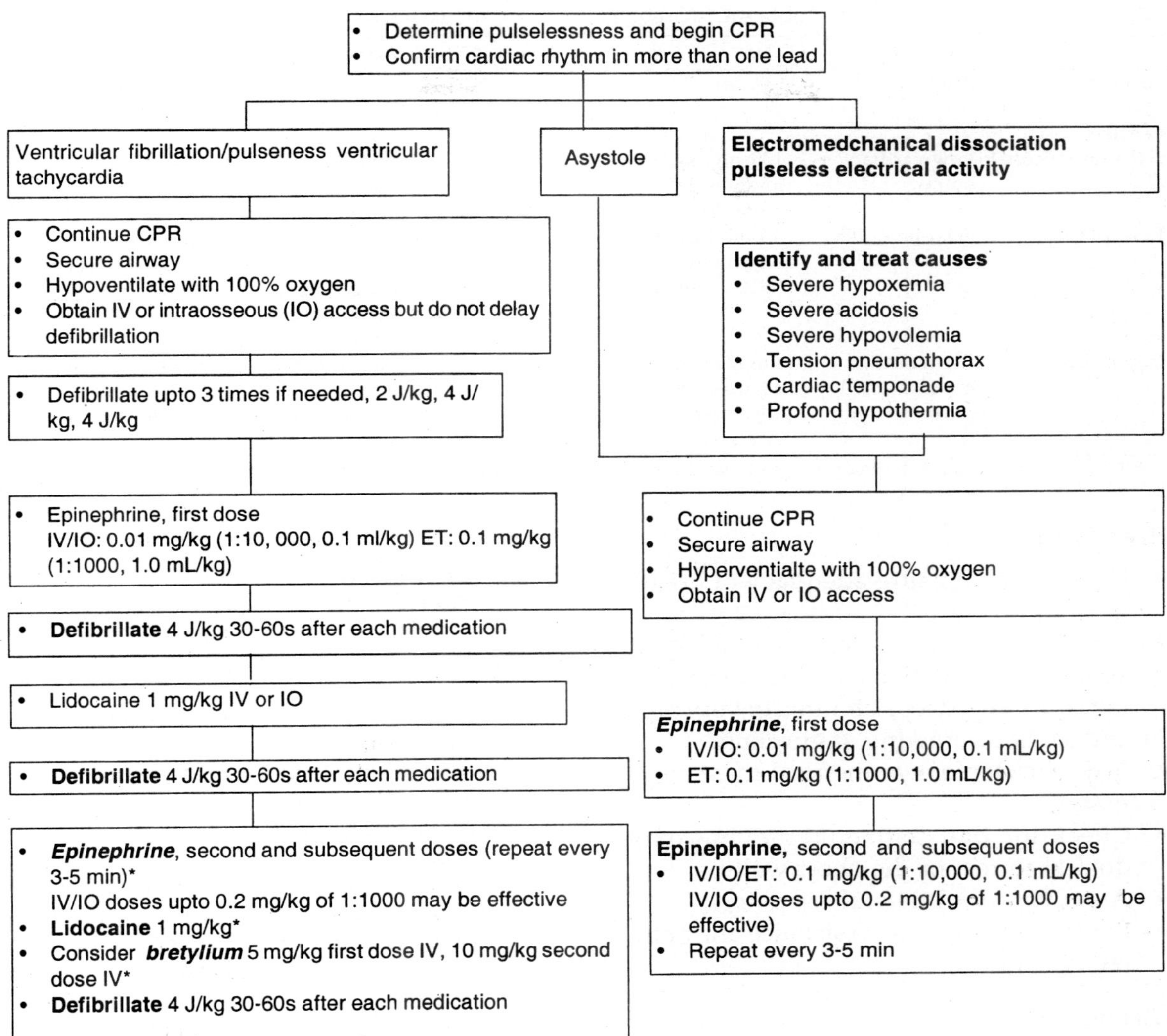

Flowchart 48.1: Asystole and pulseless arrest decision tree (Modified from Chaneides 246. Reproduced with permission. Copyright American Heart Association)

Feel: For air expired through patients nose and mouth.

ASCERTAIN THE ABCDES

Airway: Patent. Assure an open airway passage.

Look: For chest wall movements, retraction, nasal flaring, bluishness of nails, lips and tongue.

Listen: To breath sounds, stridor, stertorous or crowing respiration.

Feel: Air movement at the nares.

Table 48.1: Drugs used during resuscitation

Drug	*Indication*	*Dose*	*Route*	*Response*	*Complication*
Atropine	Bradycardia	0.03 mg/kg	IV	Increased	Marked tachycardia, heart rate diminished
cardiac					output
Calcium gluconate	Low cardiac output	100 mg/kg over 5-10 minutes (ECG monitoring		Improved cardiac arrhythmias	Bradycardia
Epinephrine	"Flat-line" ECG	0.1 ml/kg over 5-10 minutes (ECG monitoring)	IV	"Flat-line" ECG converted to some rhythmic response	Hypertension: ventricular fibrillation
Isoproteerenol	Bradycardia, hypotension, low cardiac output	4 mg/250 ml 5 percent dextrose in water, until heart rate increases	IV	Increased heart rate, improved cardiac output	Arrhythmias, low cardiac output if heart rate more than 180-220/min

* Doses give are in general starting doses and may have to be increased. Most drug tend to be more effective when pH > 7.15.

Breathing

- Obstruction. Ensure adequacy of breathing.
- Determine absence/presence of adequate spontaneous ventilation. Check if breathing is gasping, deep, laboured or very rapid and shallow, crowing or gurgling?
- Inspect chest for symmetrical chest movements.
- Check for flail segments moving paradoxical to rest of the chest wall.
- Auscultate for bilateral air entry.
- Provide mechanical assistance for ventilatory failure.

Circulation

- Adequate perfusion. Be sure heart is beating and any bleeding is controlled.
- Check blood pressure, peripheral pulsations, capillary refill at the nail bed. Is the skin cold and clammy or hot and dry, or are there goose pimples?
- Obtain ECG.
- Treat fibrillation with DC shock and asystole with effective cardiac massage.

Table 48.2: BLS summary for infants children

Manoeuvre	Infant < 1yr	Children 1-8 years
Airway	Head tilt-Chin lift	Head tilt-Chin lift
	(Unless there is suspicion of spinal injury)	
	Jaw thrust	Jaw thrust
Breathing		
Initial	Two breaths	Two breaths
	At 1-1.5 sec/ breath	At 1-1.5 sec/breath
Subsequent	2 breaths/min	2 breaths/min
Circulation		
Pulse check	Brachial/femoral	Carotid
Compression		
	Lower third sternum	Lower third sternum
	Compression with thumbs	Heel of one hand
Depth	Approx 1/2to 1 inch	Approx 1 to 1 1/ 2 inch
Rate		
	At least 100/min	100/min
Compression-	30:2,	30:2
Pause for ventilation	optional	
Foreign body obstruction		
	Back blows	Heimlich manoeuvre

- Grade shock by vital signs.
- Correct shock- blood samples for lab tests/ crossmatching, administer I/V fluids via two large bore cannulaes. Chose

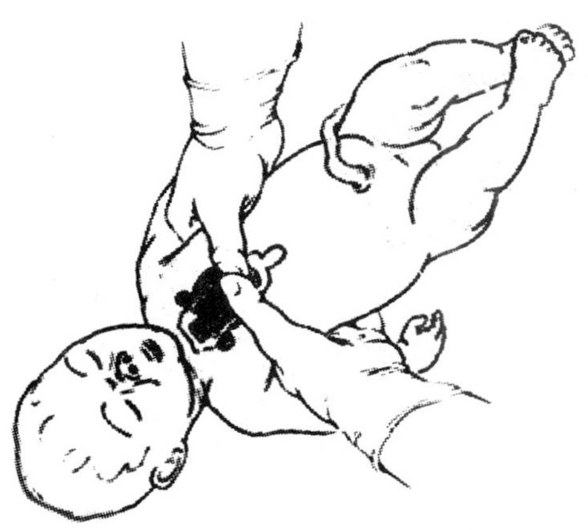

Fig. 48.2: Closed chest massage, for simplification, ventilation is not shown (From Gregory 85 with permission).

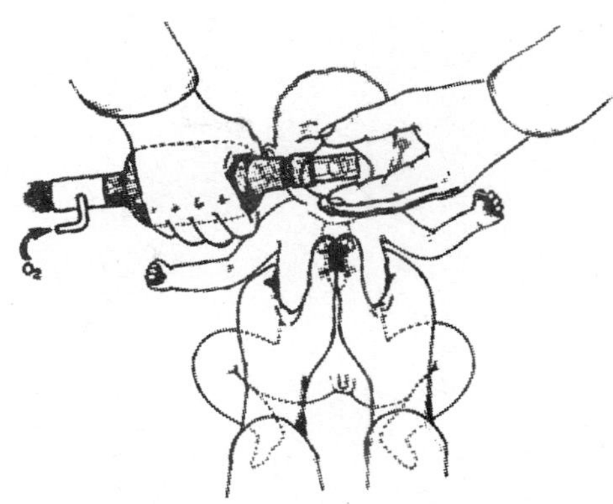

Fig. 48.3: Chest encircling method for cardiac compression of the neonate; recent guidelines recommend thumb pressure just below the nipple line (Reproduced with permission from Todres ID, Rogers MC: Method of external cardiac massage in the newborn infant J. Pediatr 86:781-782, 1975)

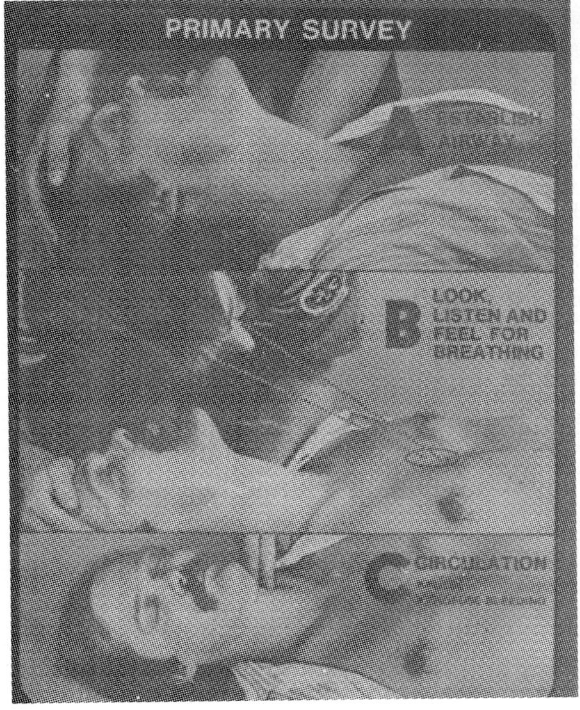

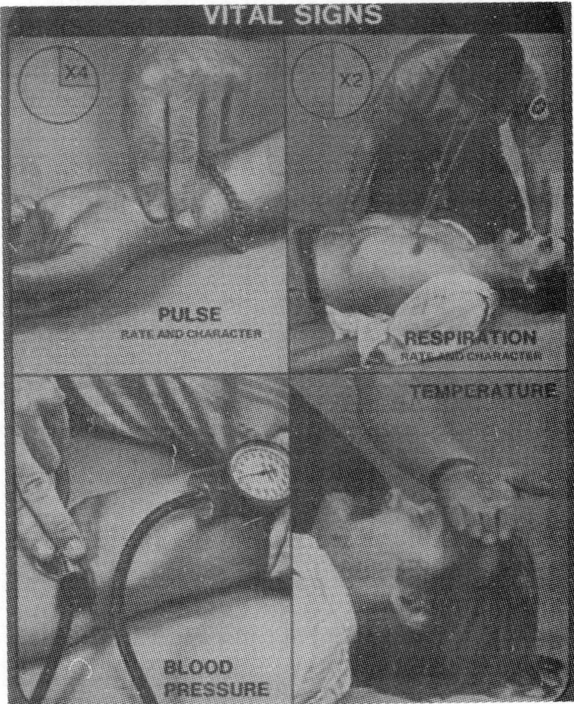

Fig. 48.4

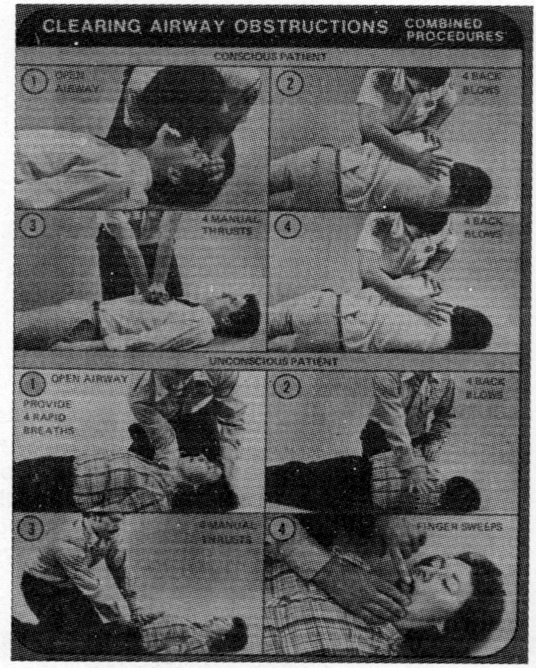

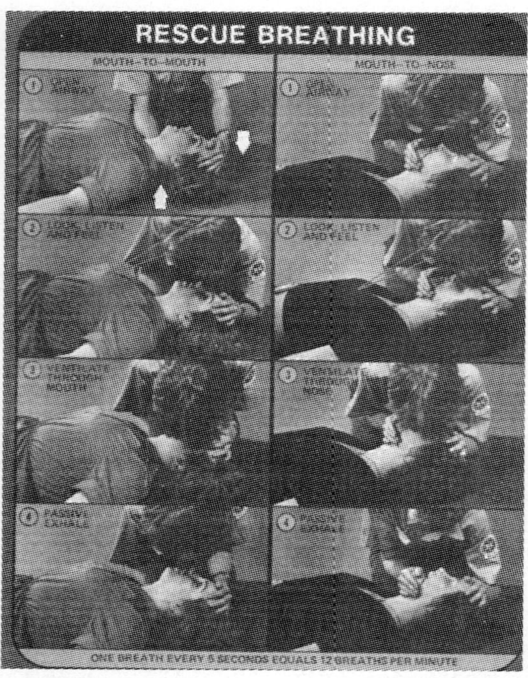

Fig. 48.5

Table 48.2: American Heart Association Basic Life Support Sequences for adults, children and infants

		Actions		
	Objectives	Adult (over 8 yrs.)	Child (1 to 8 yrs.)	Infant (under 1 yr.)
A. Airway	1. Assessment : Determine unresponsiveness	Tap or gently shake shoulder. Say, "Are you okay?"		Observe
	2. Get help	Call out "Help"		
	3. Position the victim	Turn on back as a unit, supporting head and neck if necessary. (4-10 seconds)		
	4. Open the airway	Head tilt/chin lift		
B. Breathing	5. Assessment: Determine Breathlessness	Maintain open airway. Place ear over mouth, observing chest Look, listen, feel for breathing (3-5 seconds)		
	6. Give 2 rescue breaths.	Maintain		

warm infusate of normal saline, Ringer lactate, polyethylstarch or polygeline.

Disability: Neurological injury.

Evaulate: Central function.

A alert

V response to vocal stimuli. Shout Are you Okay?

P -response to painful stimuli.

U -unresponsiveness.

- Evaluate pupil size in both eyes and response to light
- Determine motor function, test reflexes in all 4 limbs
- Assess Glasgow Coma Scale score

Expose patient for complete examination and then covering him or her with warm blankets to prevent hypothermia and infusing intravenous fluids warmed to 37-40°C.

Treat the problem as it is identified and do not wait for completion of primary survey for this.

BASIC LIFE SUPPORT ALGORITHM

Is the victim responsive? Yes you are not needed!

↓ No
↓
Call for help open victim's airway
(Head tilt-chin lift method)
Is the victim breathing? Yes keep airway patent and victim
(Look,listen feel) patient in left lateral position
↓ No
↓
Give 2 slow rescue breaths (Chest must rise)
Is there a pulse in the neck? Yes maintain rescue breathing
↓ No
↓
Leave the airway and give 3 chest compressions in 9-11 seconds then go back to airway and give 2 rescue breaths
In 2 rescuer bls, one keeps airway open and delivers rescue breaths while the other gives chest compressions 80-100 per minute, pausing after every 5th compression for other rescuer to give rescue breaths.

Table 48.4: Resuscitation protocols—primary survey

1. Look: 15-20-s overview for obvious injuries.
2. Listen to history from prehospital personnel.
3. Ask patient to describe injuries.
4. Ascertain the 'ABCDEs:
   A. Airway—patient?
      1. Look—chest wall movements, retraction, nasal flaring.
      2. Listen–breath sounds—stridor, stertorous respirations.
      3. Feel—air movement.
   B. Breathing—any obstruction? (may require intubation)
      1. Determine presence or absence adequate spontaneous ventilation.
      2. Inspect thoracic cage for symmetrical chest movement (open pneumothorax—sucking chest wound).
      3. Check for flail segments.
      4. Ausculate for bilateral air movement.
      5. Provide mechanical ventilatory assist for ventilatory failure.
   C. Circulation—adequate perfusion?
      1. Check peripheral pulses, capillary refill, arterial blood pressure.
      2. Obtain electrocardiogram.
      3. Grade shock by vital signs.
      4. Correct circulatory shock—start intravenous line and obtain blood sample for crossmatch and laboratory analysis.
   D. Disability—neurological injury?
      1. Evaluate central function:
         a. A—alert
         b. V—responds to vocal stimuli
         c. P—responds to painful stimuli
         d. U—unresponsive
      2. Evaluate pupil size and responsiveness to light.
      3. Determine motor function, reflexes in all four extremities.
      4. Use Glasgow coma scale.
   E. Expose patient for complete examination.
5. Remember: Treat problem when identified–do not wait for completion of primary survey.

Reprint by permission Stene JK, Grande CM, Bernhard WN, Barton CR 1991. Overview of preoperative anesthetic management of the trauma patient; thoracoabdominal and orthopedic injuries. In: Stene JK, Grande CM (eds) Trauma anaesthesia. Williams and Wilkins, Baltimore, pp 177-246.

THE COMPRESSION-VENTILATION RATIO IS KEPT AT 5:1 (AMERICAN HEART ASSOCIATION GUIDELINES)

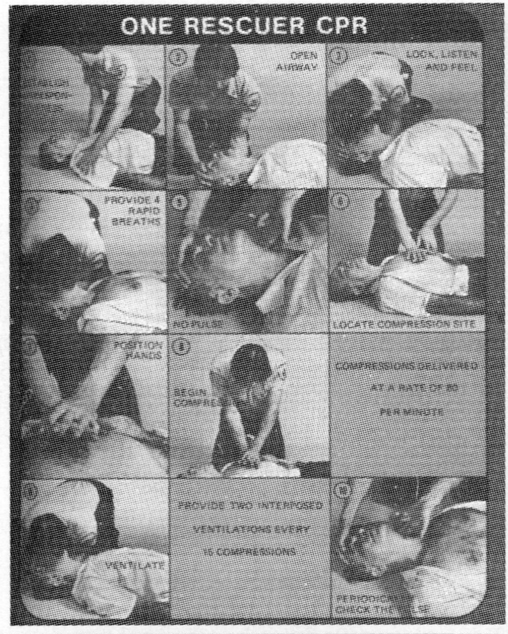

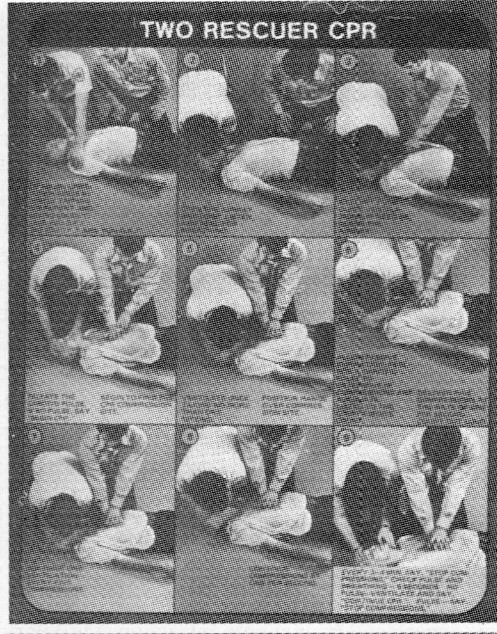

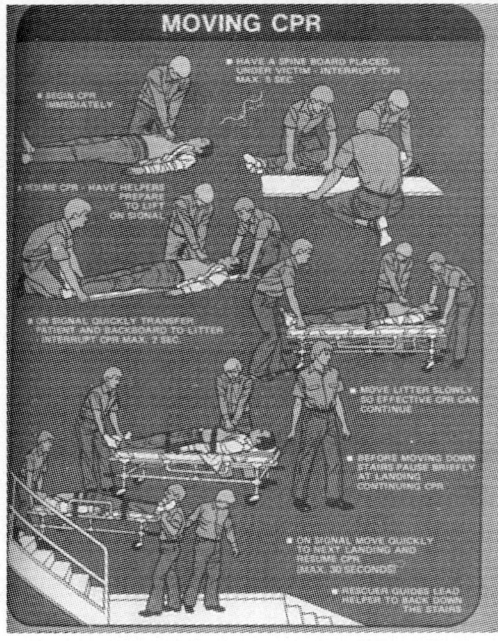

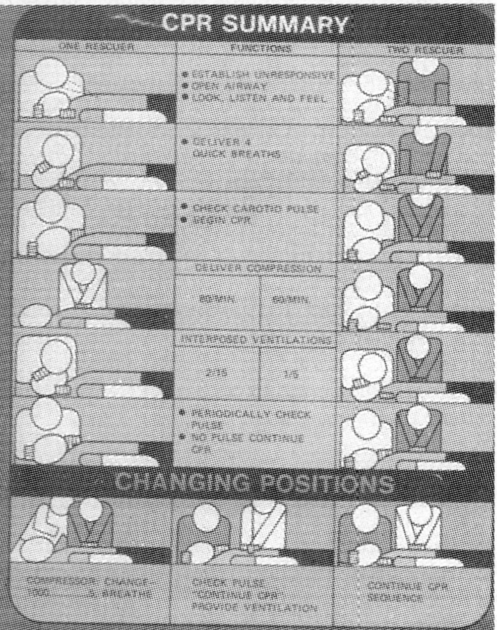

Fig. 48.6

Secondary survey

Item to assess	*Establishes identifies*	*Assess*	*Finding*	*Confirm by*
Level of consciousness	Severity of head Injury	GCS Score	≤8, severe head injury 9-12, moderate head injury 13-15, minor head injury	CT scan Repeat Without paralyzing agents
Pupils	Type of head injury Presence of eye injury	Size Shape Reactivity	Mass effect Diffuse axonal injury Ophthalmic injury	CT scan
Head	Scalp injury Skull injury	Inspect for lacerations and skull fractures Palpable defects	Scalp laceration Depressed skull fracture Basilar skull fracture	CT scan
Maxillofacial	Soft-tissue injury Bone injury Nerve injury Teeth/mouth injury	Visual deformity Malocclusion Palpation for crepitus	Facial fracture Soft-tissue injury bones	Facial bone X-ray CT scan of facial bones
Neck	Laryngeal injury C-spine injury Vascular injury Esophageal injury Neurologic deficit Pain, tenderness of c-spine	Visual inspection Palpation Auscultation	Laryngeal deformity Subq emphysema Hematoma Bruit Platysmal penetration	C-spine X-ray Angiography/ duplex exam Esophagoscopy Laryngoscopy
Thorax	Thoracic wall injury Subq emphysema Pneumo/hemothorax Bronchial injury Pulmonary contusion Thoracic aortic disruption	Visual inspection Palpation Auscultation	Bruising, deformity, or paradoxical motion Chest wall tenderness, crepitus Diminished breath sounds Muffled heart tones Mediastinal crepitus Severe back pain	Chest x-ray CT scan Angiography Bronchoscopy Tube thoracostomy Pericardiocentesis TE ultrasound
Abdomen/Flank	Abdominal wall injury Intraperitoneal injury Retroperitoneal injury	Visual inspection Palpation Auscultation Determine path of penetration	Abdominal wall pain/ tenderness Peritoneal irritation Visceral injury Retroperitoneal organ injury studies	DPL/ultrasound CT scan Celiotomy Contrast GI X-ray Angiography
Pelvis	GU tract injuries Pelvic fracture(s)	Palpate symphysis pubis for widening Palpate bony pelvis for tenderness Determine pelvic stability only once Inspect perineum Rectal/vaginal exam	GU tract injury (hematuria) Pelvic fracture Rectal, vaginal, perineal Injury	Pelvic X-ray GU contrast Studies Urethrogram Cyst gram IVP Contrast-enhanced CT
Spinal cord	Cranial injury Cord injury Peripheral nerve(s) injury	Motor response Pain response	Unilateral cranial mass effect Quadriplegia Paraplegia Nerve root injury	Plain spine X-rays MRI
Vertebral column	Column injury Vertebral instability Nerve injury	Verbal response to pain, lateralizing signs Palpate for tenderness Deformity	Fracture vsdislocation	Plain X-rays CT scan
Extremities	Soft-tissue injury Bony deformities Joint abnormalities Neurovascular deficits	Visual inspection Palpation	Swelling, bruising, pallor Malalignment Pain, tenderness, crepitus Absence/diminished pulses	Specific X-rays Doppler examination Compartment pressures

49 The MAST Suit

> "The pains felt by Asian countries are our own pains. Disaster in Asia is nothing but ours as well."
>
> —*Junichiro Koizumi*

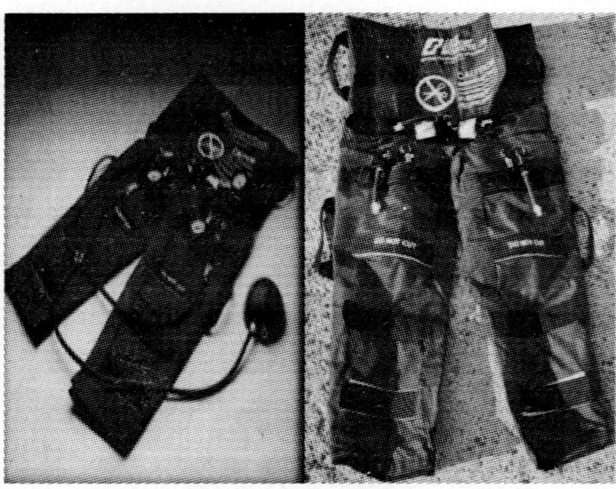

Fig. 49.1

INTRODUCTION

The MAST suit has become a regular component of the pre-hospitalization armamentarium. Various synonyms for the equipment are medical antishock trousers, military antishock trousers, antishock garment (PASG), G-suit, antishock air pants, external counterpressure device and pneumatic antishock garments. It consists of a pair of trousers with three inflatable bladders held in place by Velcro fasteners or zippers. It resembles a large blood pressure cuff tailored into a pair of pants. The suit consists of three components, two leg and an abdominal cuff portion, each of which can be inflated separately. The pants are incomplete in that the perineum is left uncovered. A foot pump with pressure gauges inflates the suit and pop off valves (set at 104 mmHg) to regulate generated pressures. Separate pediatric sized MAST suits are available.

HISTORY

Crile used an inflatable rubber suit to tackle postural hypotension in 1903 and later used it to tackle hemorrhagic shock. The air force later developed G suits to prevent ischemic blackouts and faints due to G forces during rapid ascent in flight. As pre-hospital care improved, the use of these suits in hypovolemic shock has been established. Their portability, easy application and minimal associated complications have made them popular.

Physiology

While it was thought that the beneficial effects of MAST suits were due to auto transfusion of 750 to 2000 ml blood from regions covered by the suits, later day research showed that this was to the tune of 4 ml/kg only. Further research has brought out the fact that these suits increased systemic peripheral vascular resistance (PVR) by direct mechanical compression and generalised pressor response by 48 to 50% to raise mean arterial pressure (MAP). It also promotes hemostasis in areas directly under the suit and stabilizes blood pressure.

Indications

The three general indications for MAST suit application are shock, stabilisation of fractures and hemostasis.

1. *Shock:* All types of shock states (except cardiogenic shock) can be treated where BP ranges between 80 to 100 mmHg, commonly associated with tachycardia and peripheral vasoconstriction. A wide spectrum of cases have been treated with MAST suits. Traumatic shock due to penetrating/ blunt injuries, non traumatic hemorrhagic shock due to ruptured ectopic/aneurysm, GI bleed and extracellular volume loss due to vomiting, diarrhea or polyuria, as well as loss of vascular volume into the extra cellular fluid in conditions like septic shock, anaphylaxis, drug overdosage/ poisoning have been treated. Low cardiac output states due to tamponade, tension pneumothorax have also been treated with MAST device along with specific measures required to resuscitate such patients. Where such facilities are not available in the pre-hospital phase, it is advised to apply MAST cautiously and without inflating the abdominal compartment.
2. *Fracture stabilization:* When inflated, the suit behaves like a pneumatic splint and stabilises lower limb and pelvic fractures.
3. *Haemostasis:* Where direct pressure cannot be applied over bleeding vessels, MAST suits have been successfully applied in ruptured abdominal aortic aneurysm, intractable bleeding after percutaneous renal biopsies, retroperitoneal hemorrhage, hemorrhage with multiple pelvic fractures and postoperative abdominal hemorrhage.

Contraindications

Pulmonary edema was considered a contraindication, under the belief that autotransfusion of 1-2 litres blood into the central circulation following MAST application would aggravate the situation. More recent evaluation has shown that MAST primarily increases afterload and only minimally enhances the preload. Nevertheless caution in such situations would be advisable and MAST cannot be categorized as an absolute contraindication. In cardiogenic shock MAST was considered a contraindication until a study by Wayne argued that differentiating a hypovolemic, hypervolemic and normovolemic state in cardiogenic shock would be difficult for prehospital EMTs and application of MAST could serve as a reversible fluid challenge, when those with hypovolemic state would benefit significantly. In the face of recent evidence that MAST increases afterload more than preload, MAST application would increase cardiac work and compromise coronary perfusion. It would be safer to avoid MAST in such a situation. Another possible contraindication is in postpartum patients in whom the placenta has not separated when inflation of the abdominal chamber could create negative pressure in the chest and cause air embolism through the uterine sinusoids.

There are five clinical situations in which the abdominal compartment of MAST should not be applied. Pregnancy, impaled foreign body of the abdominal wall, evisceration of abdominal contents, tension pneumothorax and cardiac tamponade.

Technique of MAST application

The recommended protocol for MAST application is as follows:

1. A quick examination of the abdomen, pelvis and legs, for once the suit is applied, these areas would be beyond scrutiny.
2. Empty all contents in trouser pockets of the patient before application of MAST to prevent puncture of the inflation chambers by sharp objects.
3. If possible, reduce all grossly angulated fractures.
4. Pad areas of bony prominence like the anterior superior iliac spines.
5. Place the patient on the open suit so that it extends from the ankles to the lower border of the lateral rib cage by either carefully sliding the suit under the patient or by logrolling the patient.
6. The suit is then applied by fastening the Velcro straps or zippers so that it fits snugly around the legs and abdomen.
7. The hose of the foot pump is then connected to the three compartments. Stopcocks are then opened and the leg compartment is inflated first and the abdominal compartment last.
8. Initial inflation pressures of 30-40 mmHg are reasonable if a pressure gauge attachment is available or else inflation is done till creates a firm palpable tension.
9. The patients blood pressure is checked frequently and inflation continued in a step-ladder manner so that systolic blood pressure reaches 90-100mmHg. Some suits have an incorporated pop off valve that releases air when pressures reach 104 mmHg.
10. Close all stopcocks and disconnect the foot pump tubings.
11. Monitor patients status and suit pressures frequently to detect leaks.

Optimal MAST Suit Pressures

The ideal pressure is the minimum pressure that yields the desired response. Lower pressures of 20 to 25 mmHg exceeds that of the venous capacitance vessels and increases CVP and blood pressure. Further increase in circumferential pressure may not increase blood pressure in a linear fashion. Experiments on healthy volunteers have shown an increase in MAP of 8 mmHg at 40 mmHg inflation pressures and 21 mmHg at inflation pressures of 100 mmHg. In acute settings, inflation pressures must be kept to those levels that yield stabilization of the patients vitals.

Environmental changes in altitude and temperature must be considered during MAST suit use. During air transport, air pressure drops with altitude and the air within the suit expands. Intra-suit pressures may triple as altitude changes from 2500 to 9500 feet. Suit pressure increases by 0.5 to 1.0 mmHg for each centigrade rise in ambient temperature and sufficient caution must be exercised in hot, arid conditions.

Decision to deflate must be considered based on patients underlying problem, volume status, cardiovascular stability and the need and availability of definitive surgical therapy. The suit must not be deflated prematurely to allow personnel to examine underlying areas. Intravenous fluid therapy must ensure stable blood pressures before deflation. Induction of anesthesia should be a slow, careful procedure to avoid precipitous fall of blood pressures as the abdominal section of the MAST suit is deflated first. A small amount of air is released, keeping a check on the systemic blood pressure (SBP). If there is a fall, further intravenous fluids are infused until BP is restored. When BP is stable, air is released in small increments followed by decompression of the leg compartments in a similar, stepwise fashion.

POTENTIAL COMPLICATIONS WITH MAST

Compartment Syndrome

This can occur if application of the suit is for prolonged periods at high inflation pressures. The incidence is however very rare and the risk factors for development of this complication must always be kept in mind and careful observation kept up throughout the period of its use.

Changes in Pulmonary Function

This was observed with the original prototype G-suits which had a single-piece construction extending upto the xiphoid process. Present day suits have separate leg and abdominal compartments and the latter extends only till the lateral rib margin. This has no material effect on the respiratory function and there have been no significant changes in the ABG seen, except in those with co existent head injuries. Studies on normal healthy normovolemic, supine volunteers has shown no significant change in the forced expiratory volume, lung volumes or in the arterial blood gases (ABG).There have been no changes in the vital capacity at inflation pressures of 0 to 60 mmHg and only a 5% decrease at pressure of 100 mmHg.

Intracranial Pressure Changes

Experimental studies in dogs have not shown any significant changes in ICP despite increased MAP. In cases of hemorrhagic shock, the MAST suit does not increase ICP and is actually more likely to improve cerebral perfusion.

Alterations of Renal Function with MAST

No significant change in renal blood flow was seen with tagged iodine in patients exposed from 4 to 24 hours of 15 mmHg counterpressure with MAST. There is a report of renal failure after MAST in 1 of 37 patients. Wayne and MacDonald's retrospective study found 8 out of 821 patients to have developed renal failure following MAST (an overall incidence of 0.97%), a prevalent rate comparable with that of other studies on hypotensive patients. The prevalence rate is very low and there exists no cause-effect relationship between the application of MAST and renal dysfunction.

Acidosis

MAST may aggravate metabolic acidosis by compromising blood supply to areas under the inflated garment. Ransom and McSwain observed severe metabolic acidosis in dogs at the end of 3 hours of inflation and further deterioration after deflation when systolic blood pressures were 80mmHg and counterpressures greater than 100mmHg. In human studies however, ABG values after 2 hours inflation showed an average pH of 7.36 before deflation and 7.31 following deflation in 505 out of 821 patients studied. There were no cases where the acidosis could not be primarily controlled by ventilation, perfusion and use of sodium bicarbonate. Washout of accumulated lactic acid from leg compartments after MAST is not a serious or common problem.

Future Use

Both animal and human studies suggest that MAST augments CPR with significant improvement in mean arterial, systolic and diastolic pressures and a two-fold increase in carotid blood flow over controls. In a study of 8 human subjects in cardiac arrest, ECC showed an average increase of 15mmHg in systolic BP with MAST. MAST has been proved to be of value in cases of refractory pre-hospitalisation cardiac arrest. In patients with pulseless idioventricular rhythm and ventricular fibrillation, a statistically significant improved outcome is reported when MAST was applied. MAST application helps maintain aortic diastolic and coronary perfusion pressures by increasing PVR and aids resuscitation. Inflation of the abdominal compartment must be done with care as this could cause liver lacerations during CPR.

CONCLUSION

The use of MAST suit has become common place and it is a practical and useful device if properly applied and removed. A number of potential complications exist but are infrequent and should not preclude its application.

50 Hospital Major Accident Planning Procedures and Documentation

> "When it is dark enough, you can see the stars."
>
> —*Charles Beard*

INTRODUCTION

A disaster or major incident plan involves techniques and procedures to provide prompt and efficient care during a disaster situation, provided by personnel who have specially trained for such an event. Disaster plans are worked out for every possible contingency that may occur within a given community allowing for agencies, personnel and support services to work together in the best possible manner. It must answer each aspect of disaster management.

AIM

To enable every member of the hospital staff to work on familiar tasks in a familiar environment with familiar material so that every casualty is guaranteed maximal therapy.

QUESTIONS TO BE ADDRESSED IN A HOSPITAL DISASTER PLAN

- Who is in authority for the overall plan?
- Who controls each aspect of the management protocols?
- How is communication to be set up and regulated?
- How is transportation to be set up and regulated?
- What needs to be done?
- Where specific procedures should be done?
- Who is needed for a particular job or procedure?
- What are the support services required, their location and contact numbers?
- Which are additional sources of help?

Every major hospital must be prepared to deal with an incident of disaster proportions at any time. In the USA, all accredited hospitals are required by law to draw up a detailed written disaster plan and institute two simulated drills each year. Disaster planning has to be dynamic, as every fresh experience teaches new lessons and raises previously unconsidered problems. Disasters can occur any time, in any place and in any weather. It is a time honored estimate that two incidents of disaster magnitude can be expected to occur each year.

Disaster planning in common with disaster management requires multidisciplinary team-work. However, the ultimate responsibility for planning must be borne by one person. The head of the Accident and Emergency depart-ment is best suited for this

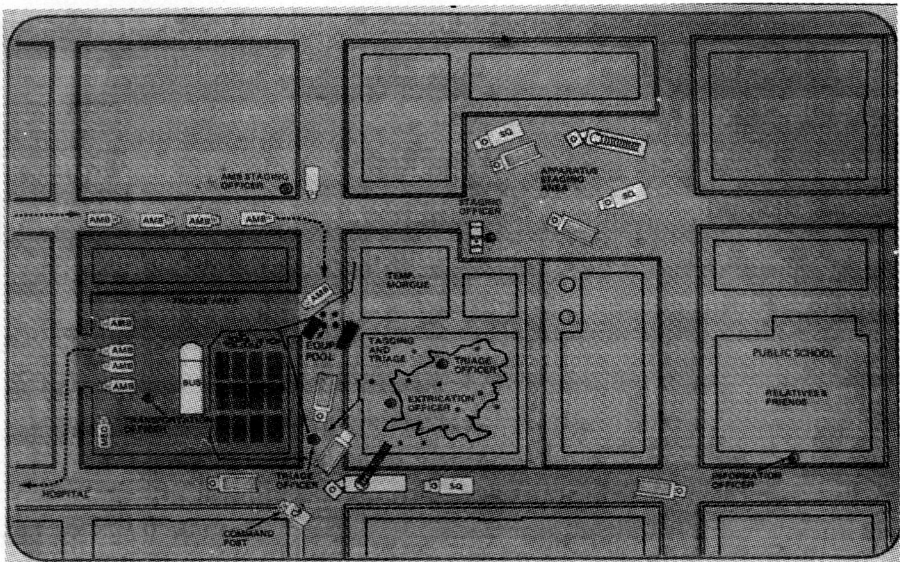

Fig. 50.1: The disaster scene

onus. Good planning must ensure good functioning on a routine basis and must be reviewed periodically by all the major disciplines involved. It must be accepted that disasters result in a compromise in the optimal management of casualties, and the greater the disaster, the greater the compromise (Fig. 50.1).

THE HOSPITAL PLAN

The general principles for dealing with any major disaster must have the following attributes:

Simplicity: It should be capable of taking immediate effect.

Flexibility: It must allow for very considerable variations in the type of disaster.

Adaptibility: To the silent hours at nights and weekends when the available staff would be considerably less than during the normal working day.

Be Non-specific: Individual names must not be included but only their appointments, specially the posts represented in the hospital at all times.

Be Routine: It should follow normal hospital procedure as far as possible because few people can be expected to act or think clearly in the confusion, noise, horror and tragedy of a disaster situation.

The plan must not be voluminous or else few of those issued with the manual would care to read it. And fewer still remember anything about it. The plan must present the essentials to include the general alert code, general principles of conduct and a brief synopsis of the total hospital plan. It must have a section devoted to the responsibilities and requirements of individuals/ departments, some principles of medicare, and specific problems peculiar to disaster management. These sections must be concise and best expressed as lists/tables and algorithms. All medical staff and all key personnel are required to read the plan on appointment and sign a declaration that they have done so.

ACTION CARDS

All personnel are then issued with an Action Card specific to the individuals appointment, with instructions regarding his or her action post and responsibilities in a disaster situation as well as to whom he or she is responsible to. A list of essential telephone numbers is displayed on the back of this card. The card must be carried on person at all times. A specific watch and station bill is placed in all departmental notice boards tabulating the action posts of the personnel for quick reference during exigencies.

INITIAL ALERT

On receipt of information regarding the occurrence of a disaster at the main switchboard of the hospital, details regarding the type, place and time of the accident must be ascertained including the identity of the person giving the information. All neighbouring hospitals must then be alerted, preferably by a hot line established specifically for such an event. A simple code such as Major Emergency- Red Alert with other colour codes to indicate early warning/standby/exercise can be evolved. The switchboard operator must announce over the public address system, thrice at 5 second intervals – *"Attention please! This is a mass casualty red alert. All doctors and hospital personnel notify your departments and report to your assigned stations."* The duty operator must then call up or page the designated staff listed in the hospital emergency/disaster plan without any delay. All those on duty are not to be relieved at the end of their shift and all leave should stand cancelled. All off-duty staff are summoned to hospital and clear sign posting of triage and emergency service areas must be undertaken (Fig. 50.2).

COMMAND STRUCTURE

Disaster management requires leadership and decisiveness. The hospital disaster plan is executed by an apex team comprising of the medical controller/duty senior registrar, senior nursing staff/matron and the hospital administrator sharing a common base and working closely together. The role of the medical controller is to mobilize, co ordinate and communicate and NOT be embroiled in the clinical care of individual casualties. Available medical staff report to him or her

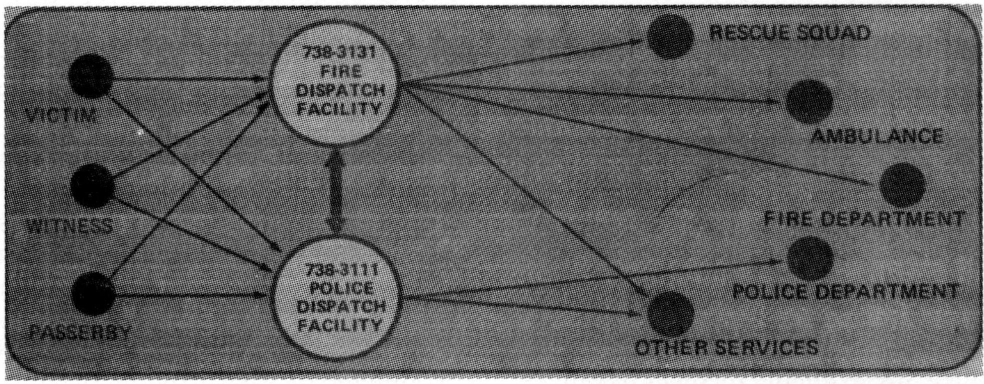

Fig. 50.2: Many communities are served by separate dispatching facilities. Direct telephone and radio links between the centers help reduce the problems caused by misdirected calls

and are assigned to various hospital areas based on their seniority, experience and skills, especially ensuring that the most experienced are involved in the treatment of the most seriously injured patients. The senior nursing staff is responsible for identifying the nursing needs and allocating extra nursing staff to certain essential areas. These are preferably those already familiar with such areas of work to handle work stresses. The hospital administrator is responsible for the many and varied non-clinical aspects of hospital response like information services, liaison cell, documentation, store inventory and ensuring the availability of sufficient ancillary staff like housekeeping and catering. There must be only one entrance for all casualties whether ambulant or stretcher-borne, and a separate egress point for efficient triage and documentation.

The anesthesiologist is particularly suited to play a prominent role in all stages of management of a seriously injured patient. They are skilled at advanced airway management, peripheral and central venous accessing, analgesia protocols, clinical pharma-cology and training of ambulance and EMT personnel. Anesthesiologists are now increasingly being involved in the vital pre-hospital care of trauma victims. In France the anesthesiologist is in overall charge of each ambulance of the SAMU (Service d'Aide Medical Urgents) services. In West Germany, the majority of ambulance and helicopter physicians are anesthesiologists. From the available medical staff, the medical controller must select four of the more experienced to perform the following duties:

THE TRIAGE OFFICER

In the first few hours after a sudden influx of casualties, the available medical resources may be overwhelmed. The triage procedure aims to ease this pressure by identifying the critically injured and sick that should have priority over the less seriously affected and those beyond the hope of recovery, thus precluding unnecessary loss of life. Triage is a French word that means sorting. The German equivalent is Sichtung while Warsaw Pact countries prefer to use the word Einstufung to mean categorization of the wounded according to the urgency of their treatment and transport. Triage determines severity of injury, injury to specific parts of the body and the special circumstances surrounding the mechanism of injury. It identifies special populations like extremes of age, presence of co morbid medical conditions and directs the casualties to the most appropriate regional facility. The triage officer is preferably a surgical registrar assigned to assess the casualties as they arrive in the emergency department and assess their priority for medical attention. This is a skilled and vital task and the triage officer is not required to become involved with the actual treatment of these victims. He or she is most effective when extending his normal role in a busy surgical OPD rather than having someone else learning a new task in that slot. He must be a senior professional capable of diagnosing quickly with the simplest means, capable of quick decisions for suitable and appropriate interventions, and courageous enough to assume responsibility and withstand criticism for errors of judgement. He must be calm amidst the turbulence of fast unfolding events, able to exert authority and arrive at the right decisions under extreme pressure. Orthopedic and anesthesiology consultants must also conduct triage in their respective departments within the hospital after the initial triage by the triage officer. He would be the first member of the hospital staff encountered by each arriving casualty. Triage is a continuous process and the only thing worse than triage is no triage. Without this vital sorting process there would be chaos, frustrating disorder and vastly darker prospects of recovery of the victims of a disaster.

TRIAGE PRIORITIES

These are essentially of four priorities:

1. The highest priority is Priority One (P-1) for those critically injured requiring urgent resuscitation and urgent surgery e.g. those with respiratory arrest, airway obstruction, severe breathing difficulties, cardiac arrest, uncontrolled severe bleeding, severe head injuries, open chest wounds, open abdominal wounds, severe shock, burns more than 50% BSA or smoke inhalation syndrome, unconsciousness due to any cause, severe medical problems including acute myocardial infarction, stroke, poisoning, heatstroke, hypothermia etc.P-1 tags are colour coded in red.
2. Second Priority or Priority Two (P-2) are allotted yellow colored tags. They are less critically injured and require admission for interventions (not immediate) and observation, but not in need of resuscitation e.g. spinal injuries, moderate bleeding, burns, multiple fractures, head injuries without loss of consciousness.
3. Lowest Priority or Priority Three (P-3) are allotted green colored tags. No life or limb threatening injuries identified and they require some treatment and investigations and probably return home shortly thereafter e.g. minor bleeding, minor fractures and soft tissue injuries, minor burns.
4. Priority Four (P-4) are those with obviously mortal wounds, the dying and dead for whom all interventions would have no consequence on outcome. Approximately 2% of the injured would be in this category. Tag color is black (Flow Chart 50.1).

The Triage Officer is responsible to fill out the appropriate colour coded triage tags to ensure that those in need of priority treatment do in fact receive it. In most disaster situations, P-3 patients outnumber P 1and2 and tend to reach the hospital first. A large open area within the hospital preferably of 9 square metres size with few fixed furniture, adequate storage spaces, good lighting and separate entrance and exits must be identified and designated as the triage area. It should preferably be located near the emergency departments and provided with adequate seating arrangements, stretchers, blankets and refreshments. Two treatment areas may be established designated as RED AREA for P-1 2 victims and GREEN AREA for P-3 cases. The desired equipment in this facility would be a large, high quality OR light with two peripheral satellite lights for multiple, simultaneous procedures, an OR table capable of plain radiography and fluoroscopy, four suction connections, eight electrical outlets, a rapid infusion device, a blood salvage device, a multipurpose anesthesia machine capable of high minute ventilation upto 300 l/min, multichannel monitor, a large X-ray viewing box, electrocautery, trauma trays including rib spreader, sternal retractor, vascular clamps , chest drains, water seal drains, and also theatre staff gowns and linen. The activities in the triage area would include airway management, resuscitation, control of haemorrhage, insertion of chest drains, central vein cannulations, mobilization of major fractures, wound dressings, analgesia and sedation. The conduct of essential investigations like blood grouping and cross matching and minimal and very essential X-Rays are also performed here. Patients condition does not always remain stable, hence triage is a continuous process and needs to be periodically reviewed and updated. Patients must be rapidly dealt with and shifted to wards and the theatres to prevent cluttering and chaos. Priority 3 cases can be administered first aid and asked to

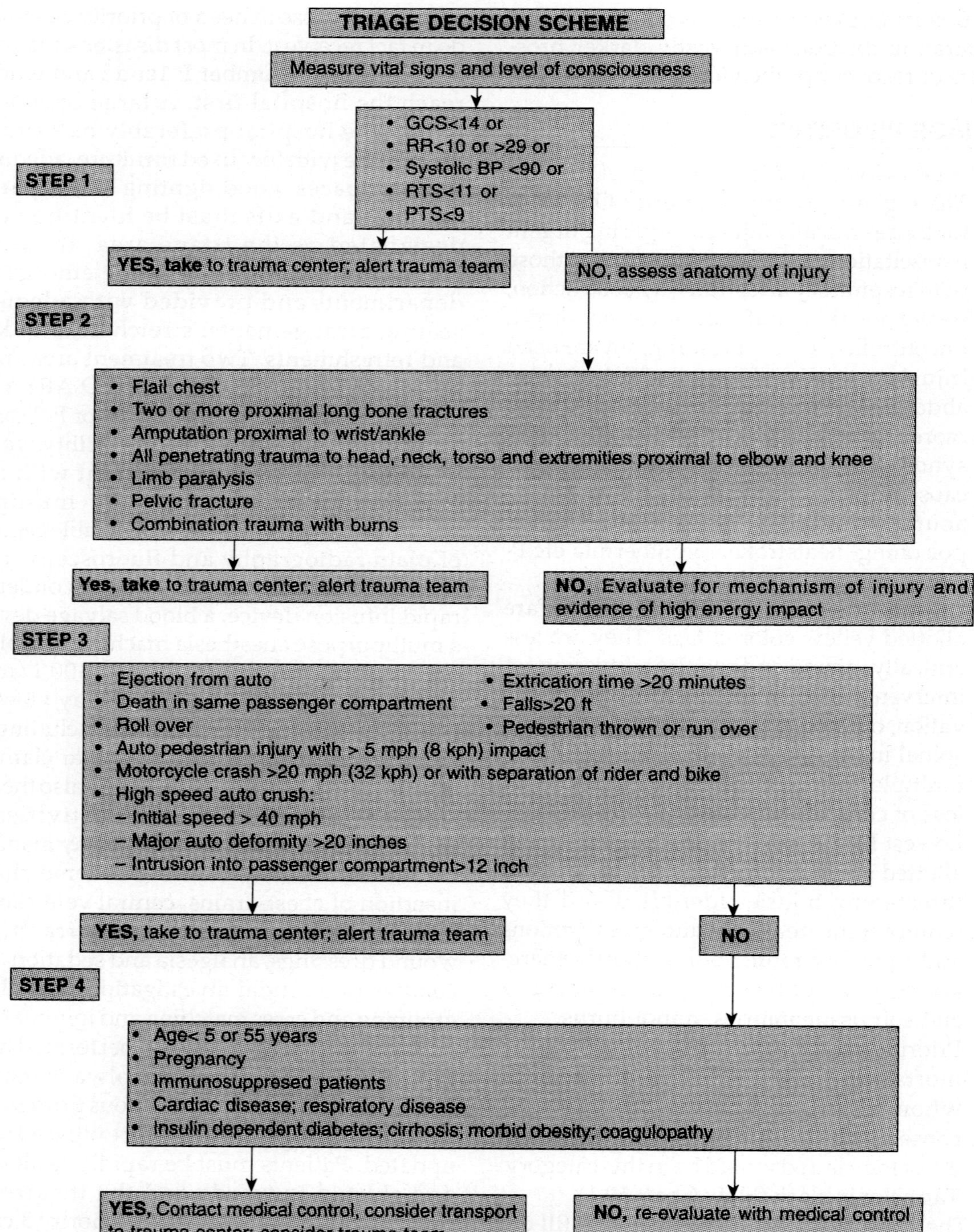

Flowchart 50.1

consult their own G.P.'s or return the following day to avoid congestion in the A & E and triage areas. Some can be diverted to nearby smaller hospitals. A supply of large labeled polyethylene bags must be stocked in the triage area to deposit personal property and clothing of all admitted casualties. Their sorting and listing is done later on. In the event of casualties contaminated by radioactivity or chemicals, all clothing items and personal effects are removed and deposited in the bags. This ensures removal of 90% of surface contamination.

Reception of such contaminated victims is limited to a large dirty area where a plentiful supply of soap and running water is available for the initial decontamination scrub. Special protective clothing for hospital staff must be made available in this area and the standard theatre attire is usually quite sufficient. Monitoring of levels of radioactivity using dosimeters will be required here. These casualties would require isolation and management on the lines of immuno compromised patients with strict barrier and reverse barrier nursing implementation. It would be useful to have a nourishment room/ pantry of about 7 metres square in the vicinity of the triage area for serving hot and cold beverages (Fig. 50.3).

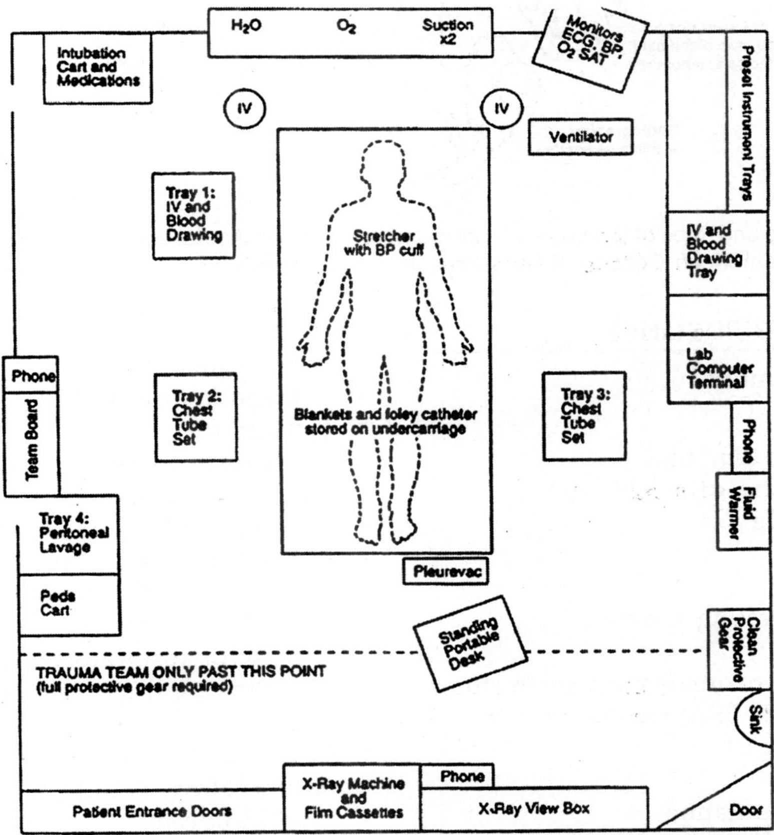

Fig. 50.3: Layout of the trauma resuscitation area. (From committee on trauma, American College of Surgeons. Resoruces for the optimal care of the injured patient. Chicago: American College of Surgeons, 1993 with permission

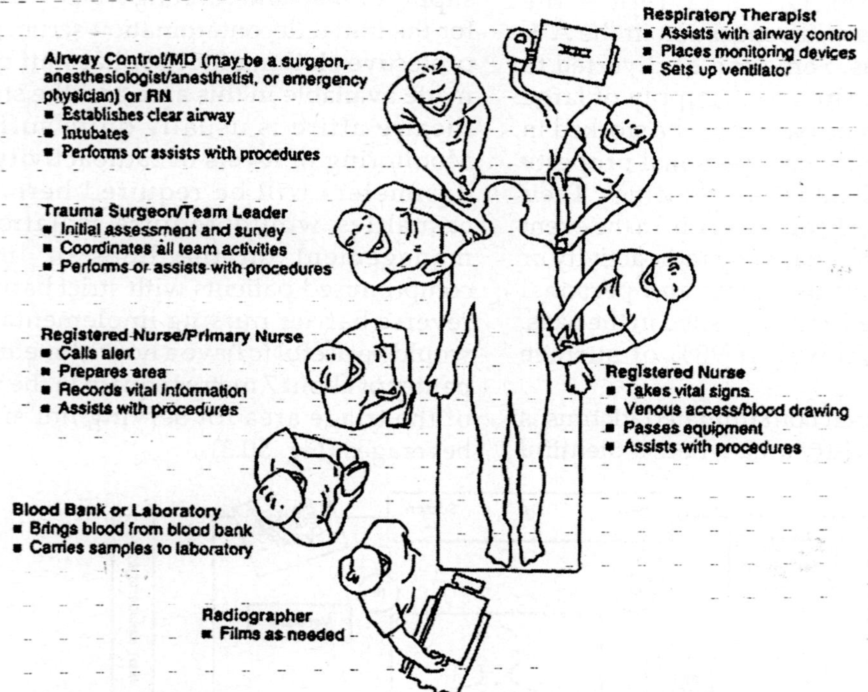

Fig. 50.4: Positions and roles of the trauma team members (From Resources for the optimal care of the injured patient. Chicago: American College of Surgeons, 1993 with permission).

FIELD TRIAGE GUIDELINES

Patient Assessment

- Physiologic.
- Pulse <60 or >100/ min.
- Respiratory rate <1or >29/min.
- SBP <90mmHg.
- GCS <14.
- Anatomic.
- Serious penetrating injuries.
- Flail chest.
- Two or more proximal long bone fractures.
- Burns on >15% BSA, face or airway.
- Pelvic fractures.
- Paralysis.
- Extremity amputation.
- Mechanism of injury.
- Ejection from vehicle.
- Death of victim in the same passenger compartment.
- Extrication time >20/min.
- Fall >15 ft.
- Roll-over accident.
- High-speed crash.
- Auto versus pedestrian >5 mph.
- Motorcycle crash >2 mph.
- Pre or Comorbid conditions.
- Age <5 or >55 years.
- Cardiac or respiratory disease.
- Diabetes mellitus (especially if using insulin).
- Cirrhosis or liver disease.
- Active cancer/malignancy.
- Morbid obesity.
- History of bleeding disorder or anti-coagulant therapy.

5. Other Issues

- Potential for decline in patient condition
- Availability of resources Personnel and level of training, Equipment and supplies, Transport vehicles (ground versus air), Turnaround time for vehicles, Local facilities and bed availability (Adult and pediatric trauma centres, Burn centres, Special care centres, Presence of ongoing hazards).

SIMPLE TRIAGE AND RAPID TREATMENT SYSTEM (START)

This is based solely on clinical presentation. Patients are categorized as immediate or delayed priority, based on evaluation of three parameters – ventilation, perfusion and mental status. An abnormality with any one parameter places the victim in the immediate transport category.

TRIAGE TAGS

Triage tags are most effectively used in systems that use the tags routinely for large and small multivictim accidents. Problems that can occur with triage tags include separation of the tag from the victim, contamination of tag by blood or body fluids or limited space for documentation. Code Red indicates critically injured patients with major injuries to the head, chest and abdomen requiring immediate surgery or specialty care. Code Yellow indicates less critically injured, who require surgical or specialty care, but not immediately. Code Green indicates no identifiable life or limb-threatening injury Code Black connotes patients who are dead or those with mortal injuries that preclude survival.

Limitations of Triage

Perfect triage is difficult to achieve. Overtriage of up to 50% may be necessary to achieve an undertriage rate of 10%. Overtriage can burden existing resources with patients sustaining non critical injuries and also prevents patients with serious injuries receiving appropriate care. Undertriage occurs when the field team underestimates the severity of a patients injuries and can cause delays in treatment, transfer of patients with serious injuries or transport of patients with serious injuries to hospitals lacking the appropriate resources.

LIST OF EQUIPMENTS IN THE TRIAGE AREA

- Drip stands.
- Oxygen.
- CVP lines and modules.
- Mobile operating lamp.
- Sphygmomanometer and stethoscope.
- Torch and scissors.
- Oxygen and delivery system.
- Powerful Suction Unit/portable V-Vac suction unit and suction catheters.
- 15 and 5 amp plug banks/extension boxes.
- Opthalmoscope and auriscope.
- Chest drains and underwater seal drainage system.
- Foleys catheter and sterile collection systems.
- Laryngoscope(adult and child).
- Laryngeal mask airways.
- Endotracheal tubes and tracheostomy tubes.
- Ambu bag- adult pediatric with silicone face masks.
- I/V cannulaes.
- Ryles and feeding tubes.
- Dressing, cutdown and tracheostomy drums.
- Marking pen and triage tags.
- Tape measure.
- Cardiac monitor.
- Pulse oximeter.

- I/V fluids, hexastarch and haemacel.
- Blood.
- Portable X-ray machine.
- Ventilator.
- Emergency drugs crash cart.
- Portable ultrasound.
- ITU bed with side railings and variable positioning.
- Patient warming system.
- Assorteds plints.
- Stiffneck extrication collars sizes A to F.
- Headbed cervical immobilization device.
- Bins.
- Large plastic bags for personal effects.
- Body bags.

Further Reading

Emergency Medicine. Medical Corps International, 1987, 1, p:10- 13).

THE CLINICAL CONTROLLER (A and E)

The duty anaesthesiology registrar is best suited for this job during the initial phase and could be replaced by the surgical consultant later on. He or she has the immediate responsibility of supervising the resuscitation and management of patients who are critically ill and transferring them to the ward, once their condition has been stabilized.

THE CLINICAL CONTROLLER (WARD)

The doctor accompanying the first casualty to the ward is designated as the clinical controller of the ward. He performs an independent triage there and draws up the operation list in consultation with the theatre controller. Once the initial rush of casualties has subsided, it should be possible for the roles of triage officer and clinical controller (A andE) to be undertaken by the same person. The duty consultant surgeon then becomes free to become the clinical controller of the ward.

THE THEATRE CONTROLLER

This is usually the duty consultant anesthesiologist. His or her responsibility is to ensure that sufficient number of theatres and anesthesiologists are available and to liase with the clinical controller (Ward) and A and E.

Apart from those designated within the hospital, it may become necessary to depute a site medical officer and a mobile medical team to the scene of the disaster as soon as possible.

THE SITE MEDICAL OFFICER

He has the difficult task of co-ordinating all the medical and first aid services at the disaster site, maintaining liaison with other rescue services and transmitting accurate information including requests for drugs and equipment to the parent hospital. He is not a member of the mobile medical team and is to keep away from personal involvement in medical/surgical treatment of casualties. He or she must perform triage on site in a relatively safe area, ensuring that all patients pass through him and are funneled through the triage area, however minor or major their injuries, so that no patient reaches a hospital unheralded. He or she must not make forays into the actual disaster area or get involved in extrication/disentanglement as the risks of falling masonry, radiation, toxic fumes, electrocution and explosions are still present. Hazard control must be first ensured by firefighters and law enforcement personnel and the area declared safe before attempting triage and patient care activities. Ambulance facilities must be reserved for those with chances of responding to treatment and not infructiously utilised for P-4 category patients. The site MO must be a competent generalist with skills in resuscitation. A staging area must be set up for incoming ambulances so that they do not directly go to the triage area and add to the congestion there. All ambulance drivers must stay with their vehicles. A second triage area can be set up to determine the order of transportation for treated patients. Details of procedures conducted and drugs administered must be documented and securely attached to each patient. Marker pens can be used to log the drug code and time of administration on the patients forehead to prevent duplication and dangers of overdosage, especially in respect to narcotic drugs. The site medical officer must ascertain from the command post before deciding which ambulance goes to which hospital. Avoid positioning too many doctors here as this may lead to duplication of treatment and a delay in evacuating the injured.

Transfer to Definitive Care

Definitive care, whether it is support and monitoring in an ICU or surgical intervention, requires the presence and active involvement of the intensivists and the surgical team. If neither are unavailable at a local hospital, it is better that a disaster victim is evacuated to a facility that has the resources and capabilities to care for the patient. It is no longer considered proper to transfer a trauma victim to the closest hospital, but rather, to the closest appropriate hospital. It is vital to do no further harm, and care of a trauma victim must improve with each step from the site of the incident, and it is mandatory that the level of care never declines from one stage to another. Patient outcome depends directly on the time between injury to that of properly delivered definitive care. Pre hospital communication must be such that hospitals without full time, in-house emergency doctors are identified to avoid inter hospital transfers and delays and also to ensure that victims with injuries requiring super specialist care are evacuated directly to hospitals capable of handling such cases.

When hospitals reach their maximum capacity, the command post must be notified. A special area may have to be set up to receive relatives and friends of disaster victims and care taken to pass on only reliable information to them. A temporary morgue may be set up out of sight and properly guarded at all times. A refrigerated container van is a useful alternative. Video taping of the disaster site, disentanglement and extrication procedures of the victims and all hazard containment activities is recommended for forensic, legal, audit and educational purposes. The LOTAS project (Level One Trauma Anesthesia Simulation) utilises video analysis of actual trauma patient management to produce realistic computer simulation for teaching trauma anesthesia and resuscitation. This method allows for intellectual, psychomotor and decision-making skills with regard to trauma-management without risk to patient safety.

THE MOBILE MEDICAL TEAM

This team is useful when casualties are trapped or when the hospital is some distance away from the actual site of the disaster. The composition of this group and the stores and equipment to be carried needs to be planned carefully depending on the nature of the disaster. The unit must be fully self-sufficient and capable of operating independently for 6-8 days at a stretch. The team must work in close collaboration, often in extremely difficult conditions without opportunity for much breaks or relaxation. They should be able to cope with their own fears and stresses and be able to keep their emotions in check at all times. They are given work schedules containing regular rest periods whenever possible. Someone in authority must keep a constant watch for signs of emotional distress and fatigue. Personnel must be encouraged to sleep and eat whenever they can and encouraged to talk and interact with their colleagues. They must take particular care to avoid the use of gallows humour as a safety valve for dealing with stress. What may seem a harmless joke, can upset fellow workers and bother them long after the disaster is over.

MORTUARY ARRANGEMENTS

In the event of a major disaster, it may be necessary to set up an emergency mortuary within the hospital or outside. Refrigerated containers have been used for this purpose. It is imperative however that all available information, personal clothing and belongings accompany the body to facilitate identification of the victims. Some coding system must be evolved to avoid mix ups.

ADMINISTRATIVE PROBLEMS

(A) Communications

An efficient hospital response relies heavily on effective communication and the relay of minute-by-minute, accurate feedback of information. The hospital requires incoming, internal and outgoing lines, independent of the main switchboard that would invariably be swamped by calls from outside. A radio line is required between the site medical officer and the controller (A and E). The hospital internal communication network may be supplemented with a small number of runners familiar with the hospital layout and drawn from clerical staff or medical students/trainee staff. For outgoing calls, existing public telephones and additional emergency lines may be requested from the P and T authorities. Radio communications must be kept as brief as possible, making sure that the text of a message is vetted for clarity, using the correct terminology and accuracy before going on air. Avoid slang, lay terms and incomplete sentences and also avoid interrupting someone else on the channel and use codes only if they are an acknowledged part of the system. Oral communications must be in a calm, steady, professional manner using a neutral tone. Do not shout or whisper, and pitch must be deliberately raised if announcers voice is gruff. Check walkie-talkie batteries, do not interrupt any ongoing transmissions and wait for 1-2 seconds after pressing transmit button before speaking to avoid the first few words being lost in static. To initiate, always say the receivers call sign and then your own, ending with over to indicate the receiver should reply or over and out to end transmission. For Example "Charlie Two from Mike One, message over. Charlie Two, go ahead, over. Mike One, casualty estimate two zero zero, out."

Ensure that the transmit button is released after speaking to permit others to transmit on that frequency. VHF radios have a longer range than UHF. Use the NATO phonetic alphabet to spell long or difficult words. Roger or OK means that you have understood. 406 MHz transmitters are preferred as they have global coverage, digital signals and first alert capability.

Mass Casualty Communication Procedure

The term mass casualty is used when an incident requires three or more ambulances to transport victims.

a. Assign medical channel to C-Med
b. Notify all hospitals in vicinity of number and extent of casualties expected request for additional medical resources. Establish hotline with all of them.
c. Detail one communications person to the triage officer.
d. Establish two way communication with all ambulances being dispatched with C Med and Triage Officer.
e. Ambulance drivers to call up C Med on leaving disaster scene with details of casualties.

f. Hospital C Med to direct ambulance to other hospitals to prevent overload or offer better tertiary/specialized care.

The communications plan must be based on user requirements and must be planned by a specialist based on 8 R's. It must be appropriate and designed for the situation in which it is expected to operate.

1. Required: Based on user requirement.
2. Reasonable cost.
3. Robust-yet light and portable.
4. Reliable: avoid network overload.
5. Really easy: To use without/with minimum technical support.
6. Resource constrained: operation from multiple power csources, weather proof.
7. Routine: must be in use regularly to see if they work in critical situations.
8. Reviewed: Regarding capabilities and costs.

Telemedicine in Disasters

Disaster management utilizes diverse technologies to accomplish a complex set of tasks. Telemedicine or clinical care at a distance enabled by telecommunication-based digital information exchange has been utilized to improve future disaster medicine outcomes since the mid-1980s. Emergency care providers must plan effectively to utilize disaster specific telemedicine to provide quality health care and disaster aid to persons whose access is otherwise restricted by geography or environment. Transmission modalities include direct hard-wired connections over standard phone lines or specialized data lines like coaxial and fibreoptic cables. These cannot support mobile operations and cannot be extended at short notice to reach remote locations economically. Wireless transmission, on the other hand, utilizes the entire frequency spectrum from 10 KHz to several Gigahertz, is independent of local telephone and electric infrastructures, and also effective over long distances using infra red, radio, television, microwave and the internet. Satellite-based linkages are more versatile but they rely on land based radio towers, base stations and repeaters and are very expensive. Recent developments like geostationary satellites embedded with more powerful transceivers and low earth orbit (LEO) non-geostationary satellites have permitted smaller, hand-held earthbound terminals. Telemedicine capabilities include video teleconferencing using real-time voice and video for remote consultations, transmission of high-resolution still digital color/black and white images of radiographic films, CT scans, ultrasound, ECG and other medical images and also to access medical records, laboratory data and track patient evacuations. The technology is particularly useful where all land based forms of communication are disrupted as it offers immediate, effective, reliable and personalized communication for disaster responders, regardless of the severity and magnitude of the surrounding damage. The Global Health Network (GHNet) and the Global Health Disaster Network (GHDNet) provide online medical expertise with lists of organizations involved in disaster relief worldwide and also a disaster database to all, irrespective of country or status. UN's Relief Web supports humanitarian relief efforts and disseminates information on prevention, preparedness and response during disasters with a 24 hours access and user language preference.

(B) Documentation

Adequate documentation is often the most difficult aspect of the internal organization and one that the medical staff tends to dangerously ignore. All documentation must be done with speed, safety and accuracy, preferably using familiar documents. A senior receptionist or nursing staff working by the side of the triage officer must perform the initial documentation at the reception area. Each patient is allotted a number and his or her name is entered. Among the injured there may be many who are unconscious, too serious to yield personal information, children separated from their parents, foreigners unfamiliar with the local language, and those stunned or deafened by the explosions or just too shocked to speak for a while. The admission/attendance code number allotted would then be the only identification at this stage and the same is marked on the hospital bracelet issued to each patient. A folder with the number and name, if elicited, must accompany the patient, containing normal admission documents, investigations, consent forms, envelopes for patients personal effects and clothing together with a check list, all using the same alpha numerical identification system. Lists of admitted patients must be made in triplicate so that a copy can be made available to the police and relatives. In the diagnosis column, the triage priority can be stamped. For clinical assessment a single folded form would suffice with minimum writing and formatted in such a manner that clinical findings and treatment can be ticked off on the chart itself.

(C) Forensic Identification

A police documentation team must be created to identify and note the details of the injured and the dead and notify the next of kin. In the absence of a positive identification, descriptive details are made. All foreign bodies removed from the person of the victims are placed in labeled, sealed containers.

(D) Crowd Control

Pre-designated assembly points must be located to handle the relatives, press and voluntary workers. The medico-social worker is best suited to man this area and provision for adequate refreshments must be provided here. Chaplains and priests may also play a useful role at these points. Potential blood donors must be received graciously and directed to the blood bank. Regarding the press and media, denying access to information may result in publication of inaccurate facts. One hospital spokesperson must be designated to supply information, supervise photography and arrange interviews.

(E) Rehearsals/Drills

A disaster plan can only be tested by a real or simulated event. Drills can be conducted without the presence of casualties and conducted on the lines of a fire-exercise. Mobilization of hospital staff, designation of entry and exit points, establishing communication lines and triage areas as well as aspects of documentation must be effectively rehearsed at least twice a year. This must be concluded with a debrief session/hot wash up to bring out lacunaes in the existing protocols and system.

51 Details for Hospitals Preparedness During Mass Casualties

> "If we put the emphasis upon the right things, if we live the life that is worth while and then fail, we will survive all disasters, we will out-live all misfortune. We should be so well balanced and symmetrical, that nothing which could ever happen could."
>
> —*Orison Swett Marden*

EXECUTIVE SUMMARY

Disasters and incidents with hundreds, thousands, or tens of thousands of casualties are not generally addressed in hospital disaster plans. Nevertheless, they may occur, and recent terrorist actions around the globe suggest that it would be prudent for hospitals to improve their preparedness for a mass casualty incident so as to serve effectively, if a mass casualty incident arose in any community.

Mass casualty preparedness is very different from Y2K because of its uncertainty. No one knows when an incident will occur, where it will occur, or what will be its cause. Of course, most hospital leaders hope their communities never experience a mass casualty incident. It must also be remembered that resources for mass casualty preparedness have to compete with other initiatives hospitals are being encouraged, or required, to adopt at the present time.

Preparedness needs to be grouped into four broad categories:

A. Community-wide preparedness;
B. Staffing;
C. Communications and
D. Public policy.

A. Community-Wide Preparedness

By definition, mass casualty incidents overwhelm the resources of individual hospitals. Equally important, a mass casualty incident is likely to impose a sustained demand for health services rather than the short, intense peak customary with many smaller scale disasters. This adds a new dimension and many new issues to the preparedness planning for hospitals.

Hospitals, because of their emergency services and 24 hours a day operation, will be seen by the public as a vital resource for diagnosis, treatment, and follow up for both physical and psychological care.

Hospital preparedness for disasters has focused historically on a narrow range of potential incidents. To increase their preparedness for mass casualties, hospitals have to expand their focus to include both internal and community-level planning.

Traditional planning has not included the scenario in which the hospital is the victim of a disaster and may not be able to continue to provide care. Hospita.l planners should consider the possibility that a hospital might need to evacuate, quarantine, or divert incoming patients.

There are limited data on hospital emergency capabilities. In multi-hospital communities and regions there is a need to develop a real time database, including an unduplicated count of potential staff.

B. Staffing

Preparedness would benefit from development of a community-wide concept of reserve staff identifying physicians, nurses and hospital workers who are (1) retired, (2) have changed careers to work outside of healthcare services, or (3) now work in areas other than direct patient care (e.g., risk management, utilization review).While developing the list of candidates for a community-wide reserve staff will require limited resources, the reserve staff concept will only be viable if adequate funds are available to regularly train and update the reserves so that they can immediately step into roles in the hospital which allow regular hospital staff to focus on incident casualties.

Hospital preparedness can be increased if medical practitioners from allied specialities and alternative medicine fields could be inducted or co-opted.

Hospital preparedness can be increased if temporary privileges can be given to trained medical workers in emergency or disaster situations and if hospitals in a community regularly share lists of the medical staffs.

C. Communications

Everyday communications systems used in the community are likely to be overwhelmed in a mass casualty incident. Backup and redundant systems need to be developed, tested and drilled.

A single community spokesperson for the mass casualty incident needs to be identified in advance, press and media briefings need to be regularly scheduled away from the hospital(s) but with supporting medical expertise.

Community-wide systems for locating patients need to be planned with a single point of contact.

D. Public Policy

In the present financial environment, where each payer wishes to pay only for the immediate costs of its patients, there is a need for a means to pay for the planning, education, standby supplies, and training costs of preparedness.

Safe harbor provisions may be needed so that a hospital assigned a role of caring for unexposed patients can divert contaminated victims, even in an emergency, to maintain its status as a clean facility.

A new governmental approach is needed which expresses its commitment to assist hospitals in disaster recovery. The government needs to provide necessary catastrophic financial relief to assist hospitals in caring for disaster victims and in disaster recovery. This funding should recognize economic loss during disasters and establish the central governmental cost sharing role besides that provided by the state.

Finally, hospital preparedness can be increased more rapidly if standardized but scalable national resources for staff training, building design, and facilities operations are developed and widely disseminated.

Implemented together, these recommendations would increase hospital preparedness for mass casualty incidents.

Preface

Hospitals have multiple missions like patient care, clinical education, clinical research, and community service.

Two of these missions come together when a community prepares for and faces an emergency or disaster patient care and community service.

The hospitals patient care role begins with and follows the disaster. The hospitals community service role begins long before the disaster as the hospital develops, tests, and implements its disaster plan. The objective is to prepare the hospital through the development of emergency response systems, staff training, and purchase of equipment and materials so that it can continue caring for its present patients, protect its own staff, and respond to the needs presented by the disaster.

A hospitals disaster plan usually addresses both internal emergencies, such as loss of electric power or potable water, and external disasters. Some of the external disasters are the results of events in nature. For some natural disasters like hurricanes and floods, hospitals are likely to receive advance warning and be able to activate their disaster plan before the event. For other natural disasters, such as earthquakes, there is no advance warning. Many man-made disasters, or emergencies, also provide no advance warning. These include chemical plant explosions, industrial accidents, building collapses, and major transportation accidents.

Terrorist acts can result in deaths and a significant number of injuries. There exists a potential for biological terrorism with the agents of anthrax, smallpox, Ebola, plague or other infections.

Most disasters have been characterized by heavy property damage and a large number of deaths or injuries requiring attention. Natural or man-made disasters could realistically result in hundreds or thousands of casualties. Some terrorists appear to desire a high casualty count to provoke public anxiety and undermine social order.

Incidents with hundreds, thousands, or tens of thousands of victims are not generally addressed in hospital disaster plans. For that reason, the financial support of the National Calamity Fund may be inevitable to tackle the volume presented.

Strategies about mass casualty preparedness for hospitals must involve emergency medical technicians, epidemiologists, members of the community, town planners, fire brigade, Red Cross, home guards, military, civil defence, administrators, industrialists, school principals and more.

Background and Framework

Most hospital leaders hope their community never experiences a mass casualty incident. This makes it much more difficult for hospitals to allocate the staff time and financial resources necessary to establish a preparedness plan for a mass casualty event. Most hospitals would prefer to use their limited resources to address the needs of today's patients rather than the potential, hopefully unlikely, mass casualty preparedness needs.

Developing recommendations and strategies for mass casualty preparedness requires addressing a careful balance. In the ideal world, every hospital would be fully prepared to address every contingency. In the real world, however, resources committed to one purpose are often unavailable for another, although some contingencies can benefit from the planning for others.

Recommendations and strategies for mass casualty preparedness have to address a broad range of institutions. To appreciate the challenge of recommendations on preparedness, the group must review the background characteristics of the hospitals in the community as they will vary considerably in size and ownership. Initiatives to encourage mass casualty preparedness must accommodate this diversity.

Resources for mass casualty preparedness have to compete with other initiatives hospitals are being encouraged to adopt at the present time. These include, in no particular order:

- Billing system accuracy and compliance.
- Safer handling of sharps and implementation of a needle-less system.
- Limitations on medical device reuse.
- Medical error reduction.
- Medication error reduction.
- Privacy and security of personal medical information.
- Filtering of blood products.
- New requirements for restraint and seclusion.
- Ergonomic standards for employees.
- Reduce solid wastes, especially of heavy metals.
- Heightened productivity to be financially autonomous.
- Uniform billing procedures and processes for all payers.

Each of these initiatives addresses a public need. Unfortunately, they compete with each other and with mass casualty preparedness for hospital attention, funds and personnel.

Existing Preparedness Requirements

The hospital must have an emergency preparedness system for managing the consequences of power failures, natural disasters or other emergencies that disrupt the hospital's ability to provide care.

a. Standard hospitals providing full-time emergency services. If the hospital provides emergency services on a 24-hour-per-day, 7-day per week basis, the hospital meets the following requirements at all times.
   The hospital has sufficient numbers of personnel, including doctors of medicine other practitioners and registered nurses, to meet patient needs for emergency care.
   The services are appropriate to patient needs.
   The emergency services provided are integrated with other departments of the hospital.
b. Standard Hospitals providing part-time emergency services. If the hospital provides emergency services, but not on a 24-hour per day, 7-day per week basis, the hospital meets the following requirements:
   - The hospital has fewer than 10 beds and is located in a rural area
   - The hospital establishes regular hours and days when the emergency services are available, and actually has services available at all of those times.
   - The hospital notifies local emergency services personnel, law enforcement agencies, physician offices, and other health facilities of when it does and does not offer emergency services, and provides those it has notified with at least 5 calender days' advance notice of any changes in its emergency services schedule.
   - The hospital posts its days and hours of operation of emergency services in a conspicuous place where the public most commonly is informed of the hospital's location.
   - The hospital does not offer emergency services.
c. Standard hospitals not providing emergency services. If the hospital does not provide emergency services, the hospitals must provide for appraisal of emergencies, initial treatment, and referral when appropriate.

Spectrum of the Mass Casualty Plan

A. Emergency preparedness management plan.
B. Security management plan.
C. Hazardous materials and waste management plan and
D. Emergency preparedness drills

A. The Emergency Preparedness Management Plan

It requires hospitals to address the following:

- Specific procedures in response to a variety of disasters or emergencies.
- Role in community-wide plan.
- Role of external authorities.
- Space, supplies, security.
- Radioactive or chemical isolation decontamination.
- Notifying and assigning personnel.
- Evacuation and alternative care site.
- Managing patients.
- Backup for utilities and communication.
- Orientation and education.
- Performance monitoring.
- Annual evaluation.

B. The Hospital's Security Management Plan.

In this component of its plan, hospitals must address:

- Access to/egress from sensitive areas.
- Vehicular access to urgent care areas.
- Security incident or failure.
- Civil disturbance, media.
- Control of human and vehicle traffic.

C. The Hospital's Hazardous Materials Plan

Including incidents such as chemical accidents or industrial explosions must address:

- Applicable laws and regulations.
- Handling and disposing of wastes.
- Space and equipment.
- Emergency procedures for exposures.
- Personal protective equipment.

D. Emergency Preparedness Drills

All major hospitals are required to conduct two emergency preparedness drills every year. These simulations are designed to provide training exercises as well as to identify unanticipated shortcomings of the current plan so that revisions may eliminate weaknesses. The hospital is responsible for determining the particular disaster scenarios, but one drill must involve an influx of patients beyond those presently being treated by the hospital. The second drill may involve either an internal or an external disaster when the hospital must:

- Clearly identify who is in charge of what and when they are in charge.
- Establish a command structure.
- Manage the logistics of critical supplies.
- **Assure that Emergency Management includes management of:**
  - Patient scheduling, services, information, transportation.
  - Ensure security.
  - Have consideration for staff family support.
  - Maintain interaction with family members.
  - Have good liaison with news and electronic media.
- **Have critical processes when an alternative care site is necessary:**
  - Have patient packaging (medications, admissions, medical records) and tracking, inter-facility communication, transportation of patients, staff, equipment.
  - Make available essential utilities (electricity, water, fire protection, fuel sources, medical gas, vacuum)
  - Have back-up systems for internal and external communications.

Disasters are seen as something that overwhelms, at least temporarily, the capacity of a hospital. An industrial explosion or airplane crash may result in a patient load that does overwhelm a single hospital or even a small number of hospitals. Thus, drills based on these incidents are appropriate.

If the disaster is a mass casualty event, such as a major earthquake or biological terrorism, the patient load may overwhelm all of the hospitals, the offices of physicians, and the general resources of the community. A disaster plan limited to an individual facility is inadequate. A single facility's plan may address part of the spectrum of disasters appropriately, but its weakness is that it may ignore larger scale incidents. Therefore, hospital preparedness should expand from planning within the context of a single hospital organization to planning by the hospital to become part of a community-wide initiative to address mass casualties. This would necessitate participation in community-wide preparedness drills.

All hospitals should include responding to the basic elements of mass casualty incidents in their preparedness plan. In a disaster, especially one for mass casualties, the hospital may receive more patients than it can handle. Or, if the incident results from chemical or biological exposure, the community may need to protect itself by designating some hospitals as open to victims and others as open only to patients who have not been exposed to the chemical or biological contaminants.

A hospital may deny access to patients when it is in diversionary status because it does not have the staff or facilities to accept any additional emergency patients at that time. However, if the ambulance disregards the hospitals instructions and brings the individual on to hospital grounds, the individual has come to the hospital and the hospital cannot deny the individual access to hospital services.

Individuals coming to the emergency department must be provided a medical screening examination beyond initial triaging. Triage is not equivalent to a medical screening examination. Triage merely determines the order in which patients will be seen, not the presence or absence of an emergency medical condition.

A hospital, regardless of size or patient mix, must provide screening and stabilizing treatment within the scope of its abilities as needed, to the individuals with emergency medical conditions who come to the hospital for examination and treatment.

Thus, if mass casualty patients present themselves physically at the hospital or on hospital property, the hospital has a legal obligation to provide at least a medical screening examination.

Framework for Forum Discussions

Mass casualty incidents, by definition, overwhelm the resources of individual hospitals. They may overwhelm the resources of a community's entire health care system. Therefore, mass casualty incidents should be seen as community-wide concerns likely to require a broad array of community resources to supplement the health care system. Local government will assuredly be involved, including both the public health department and the public safety systems of police and fire departments. Other community resources are likely to also be called upon. This may include schools, churches, public transportation, news media, telephone and communication systems, voluntary organizations (e.g., Red Cross and the Armed Forces), restaurants and food suppliers.

Because of their emergency services and 24 hour a day operation, hospitals will be seen by the public as a vital resource for diagnosis, treatment, and follow up for both physical and psychological care.

While some mass casualty incidents may follow the pattern of an intense, short-time peak of activity, others (e.g., bioterrorism incidents) will present the community and health system with rapidly increasing demands that plateau and have to be addressed for days or weeks.

The local community is the primary resource for initially responding to the incident and providing subsequent clinical care. To assemble and transport resources to the site of the incident, state and central governments will need time. They may supplement local resources across time, but no community should plan on its state government or the government as either the initial or primary clinical resource in a mass casualty incident.

Mass casualty incidents that result from infectious causes are different from all other types of incidents for many reasons, including the onset of the incident may remain unknown for several days before symptoms appear, even when symptoms appear, they may be distributed throughout the community's health system and not be recognized immediately by any one provider or practitioner. Once identified, the initial symptoms are likely to mirror those of the flu or the common cold so that the health system will have to care for both those infected and the worried well, having gone undetected for several days or a week, some infectious agents may already be in their second wave before the first wave of casualties is identified, Public confidence in government officials and health care authorities may be undermined by the initial uncertainty about the cause of and treatment for the outbreak, health care authorities and hospitals may want to restrict those infected to a limited number of hospitals but the public may seek care from a wide range of practitioners and institutions, and health care workers may be reluctant to place themselves or family members at increased risk by reporting to work.

Hospitals lack a toolkit of best practices in facility design, engineering operations, and facilities management systems which they can use to identify best practices for planning and implementation. While no single set of tools will be appropriate for all hospitals because of their variation in size, clinical programs, and patient community, a toolbox of scalable options with their estimated costs could facilitate more rapid development of hospital preparedness. Central government support for development and dissemination of the toolkit would be valuable because it would minimize duplication and provide most consistency across the nation.

There is a need to develop a widely understood and widely used classification system for mass casualty incidents so that communities can communicate their needs internally and with outside resources.

Recommendations on Community-wide Preparedness

Disasters in communities come in all shapes and sizes. Some impact a small number of people, place intense demands on the health system for a short period and conclude. Others may involve large number of casualties but reach a plateau only after a latent period, placing heavy continuing demands on the health system. Bioterrorism incidents, by their very definition, are much closer to the second.

Hospitals have a long history of preparing for and responding to short, intense disasters. Numerous examples of one of more hospitals responding to a plane crash, a train wreck, a flood, or an earthquake provide evidence that hospitals had appropriate plans in place, staff understood how to implement the plan, and the plan was sufficiently flexible to respond to the specifics of the incident.

Mass casualty incidents will overwhelm any single organization. Mass casualty incidents require the hospital to operate on three planes simultaneously it must respond as:

- An organization in its own right.
- As part of the community's health care system; and
- As one component in a community-wide effort that extends far beyond the health system.

Hospitals must adopt a community-wide perspective and leadership role in planning and preparing for a mass casualty incident. This leadership role does not mean that the hospital needs to necessarily take primary responsibility for the community planning, just that hospitals work with other community leaders to effect an integrated community-wide plan. This broad perspective needs to begin with trustee development and education. Hospital trustees need to understand that their role involves both fiduciary responsibility for the institution and establishing linkages with the broader community

Within the hospitals, there exists a need to broaden the scale and scope of their disaster plans to link with and involve the community.

Suggested linkages include:

Communities need to develop horizontal and vertical relationships between the organizations, governmental and private, that will be called upon to work together in a mass casualty incident. Hospital participation in these functions is essential. While each community leader is primarily responsible for his or her organization, it is essential that senior representatives from each organization know each other personally, have developed working relationship with each other, and understand the roles that are planned for each organization. In the midst of responding to a mass casualty incident, there is no time to develop the infrastructure or trust and awareness necessary for the community to respond as a whole.

Establish an open and ongoing relationship with the local health department and its leadership. While some mass casualty incidents may be easily identified and defined, biological incidents in particular require a community-wide surveillance and control effort to assemble apparently isolated incidents into a recognizable pattern that identifies the gravity of the challenge and institutes appropriate public health interventions, e.g., immunizations and prophylactic antibiotics.

. Develop periodic meetings with police and fire officials whose staff will be first responders to some mass casualty incidents and may be required by the hospital to enforce crowd control as the number of casualties increases. These meetings should be used to create a shared understanding of the different cultures between health care, public safety, and law enforcement organizations. They also should provide the opportunity to build the personal trust necessary for mutual action in the developing and potentially chaotic stages of a mass casualty incident.

Develop and test daily a community-wide communications network. Recent disasters have demonstrated that different organizations may use different media and/or different frequencies in their communications. Unable to communicate with one another, precious time can be lost at the start of a mass casualty incident.

Because of the broad scope of the incident, communications overload throughout the community is possible. Backup and redundant systems should be identified in advance to help assure communications. This should include an agreed-upon and tested courier service in case voice communications fail or are overloaded.

Within the health care community, hospitals have an opportunity to use their existing emergency medical system (EMS), trauma coordination, and neonatal care relationships as a framework on which to build expanded relationships for mass casualty preparedness. The existing programs provide a framework for communications linkages, joint and complementary funding, and data collection and sharing.

Communities and regions need to create and/or link existing data reporting systems to provide a community-wide assessment of health needs and resources. Mass casualty incidents will increase demands simultaneously on all of the community's health resources. There will not be adequate time or unused personnel to survey hospitals, community health centers, multi-specialty clinics, nursing homes, and public facilities to inventory capabilities after the incident starts. Data systems which have a common architecture to integrate streaming data from institutional operations will provide the best means of matching community needs to available resources.

Community-wide mass casualty drills should supplement the individual hospital and small casualty community drills generally in use today. At the state and national levels, steps can be undertaken to facilitate the community and regional preparedness essential for mass casualty incidents.

Biological incidents will be the most difficult for the community to understand and effectively coordinate its response. Valuable time is lost if public health officials are unable to rapidly identify and communicate the threat represented by what appears to be a series of unrelated illnesses. The central government should continue to provide support for epidemiological programs which allow hospitals to submit rapidly information on atypical patients so that community-wide patterns can be identified as soon as possible.

The traditional separation between the medical care community (e.g., hospitals, physicians, and nursing homes) and the public health community needs to be bridged in preparation for mass casualty incidents. Mass casualties will provide more work than any organization itself can address. Coordination is the key, and the historic separation is a genuine disadvantage.

Special funding for the development and testing of mass casualty preparedness plans and drills are essential. To obtain the greatest benefit for the community, the funds should be provided to a community-wide organization which is required to involve the community's political leadership, public safety services, public health services, hospitals, and community health centers.

Hospital associations, alliances, and systems can facilitate mass casualty preparedness of their members by establishing linkages with the public health community, identifying and communicating best practices, identifying and sharing lessons learned from disasters and emergencies of all sizes, and facilitating more uniform data definitions and reporting systems for institutional capacity.

Recommendations on Staffing

As previously stated, mass casualty incidents are likely to overwhelm the capacity of individual hospitals and, perhaps, all of the hospitals in the community. Traditionally, hospital capacity has been described in terms of the availability of beds. Having unoccupied beds to use for casualties remains important the availability of adequate numbers of trained staff is a better indicator of the capacity of the health system to respond to mass casualty incidents.

Numbers of Staff

In hospital disaster plans, staff augmentation is regularly addressed in a variety of ways, including extending hours of present staff and calling in supplemental staff. If all of the disaster plans in a community are collected, they appear to provide for a substantial augmentation of staff. This includes medical staff, nursing staff, technicians and technologists, and support services staff. However, it is common for each hospitals disaster plan to be prepared individually. Thus, there is a real potential for double counting of potential staff. That is, two (or more) hospitals may envision using the same resources for staff augmentation. In a mass casualty incident where the full human resources of the community are stressed, attendees recommend that hospitals improve their preparedness by working together to develop an unduplicated estimate of the number and sources of additional staff.

A number of very basic steps can expand hospital staffing for mass casualty incidents:

Development of a community-wide concept of reserve staff identifying physicians, nurses and hospital workers who are (1) retired, (2) have changed careers to work outside of healthcare services, or (3) now work in areas other than direct patient care (e.g., risk management, utilization review).While developing the list of candidates for a community-wide reserve staff will require limited resources, the reserve staff concept will only be viable if adequate funds are available to regularly train and update the reserves so that they can immediately step into roles in the hospital which allow regular hospital staff to focus on incident casualties and develop protocols for where and how to use such staff efficiently and safely.

It may be possible to expand the reserve staff concept to include medical, nursing, and allied health students training in programs affiliated with the hospital(s). Attendees recognize that this potential is untested and may not be feasible if the students actually reduce available staff time because of their needs for supervision.

Under defined emergency conditions, medical personnel from allied and alternative specialties can be co-opted.

In a mass casualty incident, physicians may be unable to reach the hospital where they usually admit patients. Hospital preparedness can be increased if medical staff lists are drawn up and circulated on a regular basis to allow for flexibility in their employment in other hospitals in such situations.

In the initial hours of a mass casualty incident, first responders (i.e., EMS, police, and fire personnel) may be fully occupied in the on-scene care and potential decontamination of casualties. However, as the duration of the incident progresses, first responders may be potential sources to help augment hospital staff. Attendees were unaware of communities which have developed and tested this concept. There needs to be an effort to identify communities who have tested, by design or default, this approach. If actual experience can not be identified, funding to explore the concept in communities of various sizes is needed.

In many disaster drills, the incident places a short-term but intense demand upon the hospital. As a result, the clinical personnel experience a substantial increase in demands, but the support staff (e.g., food service workers, housekeepers) may have only a limited change in demands. In a mass casualty incident, the demand for both care and support services may be more sustained. Hospital preparedness will be facilitated by providing for augmentation of both clinical and non-clinical, support staff.

Some biological incidents are different because of their risk of infecting hospital staff. Biological terrorism will pose additional challenges of both uncertainty and fear. Reactions to unknown infectious agents can perhaps best be gauged by the reaction of health workers to AIDS/HIV in the early 80s, when some workers were reluctant to care for infected patients. Attendees recognize that staff concerns can be reduced through appropriate education and the use of universal precautions until the nature of the disease agent is understood. However, hospital preparedness plans need to include contingency plans in case medical professionals, and or volunteers do not show up.

Communities have a long history of helping hospitals in times of crisis. A frequent demonstration of this community support is the willingness of individuals with four-wheel drive vehicles to provide transportation assistance to hospital patients and staff during snowstorms or inclement weather. The potential for untrained volunteers to assist with a mass casualty incident is very limited and the hospital staff will be under enormous demands and stress. There will be only limited time to identify, train on site, and supervise volunteers. In some cases, volunteers may add to the problems of staff identification and crowd control.

Staff Training

In mass casualty incidents, there is unlikely to be time to conduct intensive staff training between identification of the incident and its onset. Weather related natural disasters like floods and hurricanes may provide little lead time for training, but most of the available time will be consumed by implementing the disaster plan. Staff will need to arrange care for members of their families and for pets.

Mass casualty incidents require a prompt response and implementation of both the institutional and community-wide disaster plans. A more prompt response will be forthcoming from the full range of staff if education on potential incidents and their expected risks and consequences are taught to all hospital staff prior to the onset of any incident.

While many hospitals rely on information resources originally developed by the military services for addressing chemical and biological exposure, some of the information and supplies assumed in a combat situation are not representative of civilian hospital environments. Standardized materials oriented to training hospital personnel need to be developed and made widely available. Such materials would facilitate training, allow for a more standardized body of information across the hospital field, reduce the loss of expertise that accompanies employee turnover, and be cost efficient. State and Central governmental grants are seen as the only realistic source for developing the necessary training resources. Upon development, central agencies should work with medical, nursing, and hospital associations to make the availability of the materials widely known through newsletters, member advisories, and association web pages.

Hospital preparedness for mass casualty incidents will be increased if hospitals engage in regular, ongoing in service training programs and in readiness drills. But, the resources required for this training are expensive. Training materials must be developed, trainers must be trained, staff must be released from other obligations, and supplies must be consumed. No payer for hospital services includes in their payments funds for the staff education necessary for hospital preparedness. The costs of hospital preparedness can be reduced in a number of ways:

a. A standardized curriculum and set of training materials for mass casualty preparedness must be drawn up. Access to these materials and subsidies for their purchase should be made available to all hospitals. The subsidies may result from central or state grants, from grants from national or community foundations, or from local charities, such as the Red Cross.
b. Historically, training has relied upon printed materials and training films. While both remain relevant, training materials using videotapes, CDs, and web-based technologies should be explored to provide more cost-effective and readily revised resources.

Staff Support

Faced with the demands of a mass casualty incident, physicians and hospital staff will be called upon to provide extraordinary service to their communities. Pressure and stress will be high. Casualties will be numerous and may include friends and neighbors. To allow staff to function at their highest potential, the following recommendations are made:

A. Facing long hours of work and the likelihood of limited communications, hospital staff do not need the distraction of worrying and arranging for the needs of family members. In some communities, the network of an extended family or established group of friends may provide coverage during the incident. In many communities, however, population mobility, nuclear family structures, and single parent families may mean that many staff member do not have existing arrangements to care for their families. Mass casualty preparedness will be facilitated if hospitals work with community resources, school systems, places of worship, and employers to include in their disaster plan pre-arranged supervision, shelter, and feeding for the families of those working in the hospital. These pre-arranged community support systems can be activated using public service announcements on radio and television stations.

B. Arrangements for the care of the pets of hospital workers can be just as necessary and often more complex. The congregate living arrangements that are possible for family members do not work well for pets. This may provide an opportunity for the veterinary medicine community to contribute to improving hospital preparedness. For example, hospital staff could provide a registry of pets which could be shared with both veterinarians and veterinary assistants for feeding and care if staff are confined to the hospital for extended periods.

C. Those who have studied or experienced mass casualty incidents have reported the enormous stress and pressure faced by health workers. Effective response by these workers to the crisis requires that they have the necessary supportive services for themselves. These include access to vaccines, infection control advice, adequate rest and relief, and mental health counseling. In a sustained, mass casualty incident, the inclusion of these resources in the disaster plan will assist staff in meeting the other demands the plan places on them.

D. At the onset of the mass casualty incident, there is likely to be confusion and conflicting information about the incident. This lack of certainty may distract hospital workers wishing to understand the risks they personally face in caring for incident victims. The use of universal precautions and a system for sharing information with staff prior to any incident are likely to facilitate implementation of the disaster plan.

E. Crowd control will be essential in a mass casualty incident. There will be the sick and injured, relatives searching for each other, the worried well, and the curious. To facilitate access to the hospital by physicians, hospital workers, and any reserve staff component, preparedness plans must include photo identification cards issued or authorized by the hospital. Prior to any incident, public safety officials must have information on the characteristics of authentic identification cards for each facility in the community. For reserve staff and pre-designated volunteers, identification cards can be coded with number and/or letter systems so that public safety officials can readily identify those authorized to cross any crowd control perimeter.

Recommendations on Communications

Mass casualty incidents may be sudden, such as explosion, or gradual, such as a biological infection. In both cases, the scale of the incident will create a demand for public information. In most cases, at least some of the information will not be readily available while the incident develops.

We live in a mass media and multi-media culture. Every news and information source will seek access to the latest and most up-to-date information. Absent clear and credible information, speculation may reign and increase the stress and pressure of the incident, especially on the hospital and its staff.

Planned and structured arrangements for communication throughout the incident and during its response are critical components of hospital and community preparedness. The following recommendations and insights are made:

1. *External communications:* A mass casualty event will become a Tower of Babel if every organization in the community attempts to establish its own media briefings. Unaware of what others are saying and despite the best of intentions, the use of different words and phrases will confuse the public and undermine the trust essential to the orderly chaos of a well-managed disaster. All organizations involved in the community preparedness plan for mass casualties, including hospitals, need to agree in advance on who will serve as the single, regional spokesperson. If a government official is designated as the spokesperson, health experts must be provided to assist the official with responses to medical questions.

A community-wide spokesperson system will minimize disruption of hospitals if the press events are conducted away from health care facilities and using regularly scheduled and pre-announced media briefing times.

All organizations participating in the community preparedness plan will facilitate communications and reduce disruption of their own staff, if the plan for a pre-arranged community spokesperson also clearly identifies what others are not to say. While each organization responding to community need will want to tell its story, a pre-existing agreement that the focus will be on a single point of communication will minimize disruptions while still allowing each organization to tell its story after the incident has concluded.

Hospitals often have established relationships with the local health reporters. In a mass casualty incident, the health reporter may not be the prime media contact. The government reporter, or crime reporter in the case of terrorism, may have the lead on the incident. The community spokesperson needs to be known and trusted by this reporter prior to any incident. Health experts who will be used to complement the spokesperson also should be known in advance to the reporter(s).

The present language being used by some to describe mass casualty incidents is unnecessarily inflammatory. When addressing potential incidents caused by terrorists, some have used the terms weapons of mass destruction or weapons of mass effect to characterize the incident. Both of these terms have heavy emotional and psychological overtones which are apt to increase community anxiety and fear in the face of any incident. Attendees encourage the use of more neutral words in communications.

2. *Internal communications:* Hospitals need an ongoing, open channel of communications with emergency response teams who may have first awareness of the incident. In a mass casualty incident, this channel of communications can not be limited to a set of dyads where the EMS unit has to use a different channel or means of contact with each organization. A community-wide network using the same channel is necessary. The network should be tested daily, with the test rotating across the various hospital and EMS shifts. Redundant backup capability must be built into the preparedness plan in case the usual means of communications are ineffective. The backup capability also requires regular testing.

The arrival of casualties will be accompanied by calls from family and friends seeking to learn where the person is and their condition. These well-meaning calls can rapidly overload the hospitals telephone system and isolate the hospital. Community-wide mass casualty preparedness plans will improve the responsiveness of health organizations if they include a single, community site for obtaining patient locator information. In many communities, the Red Cross is equipped and experienced in serving as this third-party, off-site source of information.

A mass casualty incident overloads the resources of the hospital(s) if not the whole community. Staff morale and effectiveness will be facilitated by developing clear information systems that use both telecommunications and a position-to-position cascade in the event that telecommunications are unavailable or overloaded. Such a cascade should be designated in terms of position, not person. The combination of hospital turnover, the multiple shifts of hospitals, and the reassignment of personnel during the incident have been found to undermine systems where the cascade specified names rather than positions.

The use of cellular phones, pagers, and the internet is increasing and must be fully utilized in a disaster situation. The ham radio operators can be called upon to bridge disruptions in communication lines.

A post-event critique and evaluation of the communications plan must be made.

Recommendations on Public Policy

Mass casualty incidents are community-wide incidents. They are not confined to individual hospitals. They involve hospitals, employers, transportation systems, food and medical suppliers, schools, and more co ordination and response to large-scale disasters is a legitimate responsibility of the government and is unlikely to be borne by any other entity. Moreover, the governmental responsibility rests first and primarily on local government. The local community is where the event occurs. Local government provides the first responder to explosions, chemical contamination, and natural disasters. Local governments manage the roads and public transportation systems, the school systems, and often the drinking water.

State and central governments will be involved if the incident is large enough. But, state and central governments will not lead. They are often outside the immediate area, lack the critical mass of immediate clinical resources, and will be unable to be present immediately.

There are actions in public policy that state and central governments can take to help communities and hospitals develop and implement preparedness plans. The following needs to be kept in mind.

The hospital has a dual role, one as a community social institution and the other as health care business ventures. Hospitals need to educate policy makers about the role of hospitals in mass casualty disasters. Hospitals are the last link in the community's response to a mass casualty incident. They are the most comprehensive community health resource. They are open 24 hours a day, 7 days a week, 365 days a year. People turn to the hospitals emergency department when they do not know where else to turn. Hospitals will receive the most seriously injured and ill casualties. Authorities need to acknowledge this role and its implications for preparedness plans.

Mass casualty incidents and disasters are community events. While hospitals expect to be paid for the health services provided to the injured, there is no stream of funding for the costs of developing preparedness plans, training staff, purchasing standby equipment, and conducting disaster drills. Government(s) need to develop a fund for hospital preparedness, especially mass casualty preparedness. This may involve a special assessment and budgetary allocation from industries that pose special risks of nuclear, chemical, or infectious contamination. General revenue support is also likely to be needed if the health care system is going to be adequately prepared to meet the contingencies of mass casualty incidents.

The National Calamity Fund must provide necessary catastrophe financial relief to assist hospitals in caring for disaster victims and in disaster recovery. This funding should recognize economic loss and establish the central government, perhaps with a cost-sharing role with the states.

CONCLUSIONS

Community Wide Preparedness

By definition, mass casualty incidents overwhelm the resources of individual hospitals. Equally important, a mass casualty incident is likely to impose a sustained demand for health services rather than the short, intense peak customary with many smaller scale disasters. This adds a new dimension and many new issues to preparedness planning for hospitals.

Hospitals, because of their emergency services and 24 hours a day operation, will be seen by the public as a vital resource for diagnosis, treatment and follow up for both physical and psychological care.

Hospital preparedness for disasters has focused historically on a narrow range of potential incidents. To increase their preparedness for mass casualties, hospitals have to expand their focus to include both internal and community-level planning.

Traditional planning has not included the scenario in which the hospital is the victim of a disaster and may not be able to continue to provide care. Hospital planners should consider the possibility that a hospital might need to evacuate, quarantine, or divert incoming patients.

Staffing

Preparedness will be enhanced by development of a community-wide concept of reserve staff identifying physicians, nurses and hospital workers who are (1) retired, (2) have changed careers to work outside of healthcare services, or (3) now work in areas other than direct patient care (e.g., risk management, utilization review).While developing the list of candidates for a community-wide reserve staff will require limited resources, the reserve staff concept will only be viable if adequate funds are available to regularly train and update the reserves so that they can immediately step into roles in the hospital which allow regular hospital staff to focus on incident casualties.

Communications

Everyday communications systems used in the community are likely to be overwhelmed in a mass casualty incident. Backup and redundant systems need to be developed, tested and drilled.

A single community spokesperson for the mass casualty incident needs to be identified in advance, press and media briefings need to be regularly scheduled away from the hospital(s) but with supporting medical expertise.

Community-wide systems for locating patients need to be planned with a single point of contact.

Public Policy

There is no financial framework for funding hospital preparedness and mass casualty costs. In the present financial environment, where each payer wished to pay only for the immediate costs of its patients, there is a need for a means to pay for the planning, education, standby supply, and training costs of preparedness.

The Central Government needs to provide necessary catastrophic financial relief to assist hospitals in caring for disaster victims and in disaster recovery. This funding should recognize economic loss and establish the federal government, perhaps with a cost sharing role with the states.

Finally, hospital preparedness can be increased more rapidly if standardized but scalable national resources for staff training, building design, and facilities operations are developed and widely disseminated.

Emergency Preparedness Management Plan

A management plan addresses emergency preparedness.

The emergency preparedness management plan describes how the organization will establish and maintain a program to ensure effective response to disasters or emergencies affecting the environment of care. The plan provides processes for the following:-

a. Implementing specific procedures in response to a variety of disasters.
b. Defining and, when appropriate, integrating the organization's role with community-wide emergency preparedness efforts.
c. Notifying external authorities of emergencies.
d. Notifying personnel when emergency response measures are initiated.
e. Assigning available personnel in emergencies to cover all necessary staff positions.
f. Managing space, supplies, and security.
g. Evacuating the facility when the environment cannot support adequate patient care and treatment.
h. Establishing an alternative care site when the environment cannot support adequate patient care; and
i. Managing patients during emergencies, including scheduling, modification, or discontinuation of services, control of patient information, and patient transportation.

The plan identifies

i. An alternative source of essential utilities.
ii. A backup communication system in the event of failure during disasters and emergencies.
iii. Facilities for radioactive or chemical isolation and decontamination.
iv. Alternate roles and responsibilities of personnel during emergencies; and an orientation and education program for

personnel who participate in implementing the emergency preparedness plan.

The plan establishes

1. Specific roles and responsibilities during emergencies.
2. The information and skills required to perform duties during emergencies.
3. The backup communication system used during disasters and emergencies.
4. How supplies and equipment are obtained during disasters or emergencies.
5. Emergency preparedness knowledge and skills for staff.
6. The level of staff participation in emergency preparedness management.
7. Monitoring and inspection activities.
8. Emergency and incident reporting procedures that specify when and to whom reports are communicated.
9. Inspection, preventive maintenance, and testing of applicable equipment.
10. Use of space.
11. Replenishment of supplies and management of staff.

Security Management Plan

Management plan addresses security. A security management plan describes how the organization will establish and maintain a security management program to protect staff, patients, and visitors from harm. The plan provides processes for:

a. Designation of personnel responsible for developing, implementing, and monitoring the security management plan.
b. Addressing security issues concerning patients, visitors, personnel, and property.
c. Reporting and investigating all security incidents involving patients, visitors, personnel, or property.
d. Providing identification, as appropriate, for all patients, visitors and staff.
e. Controlling access to and egress from sensitive areas, as determined by the organization; and
f. Providing vehicular access to urgent care areas.

In addition, the plan establishes:

1. Processes for minimizing security risks for personnel in security sensitive areas
2. Emergency procedures followed during security incidents.
3. Processes for reporting security incidents involving patients, visitors, personnel and property.
4. Performance improvement standards that address staff security management knowledge and skill.
5. The level of staff participation in security management activities.
6. Monitoring and inspection activities.
7. Emergency and incident reporting procedures that specify when and to whom reports are communicated.
8. Inspection, preventive maintenance, and testing of security equipment.

It also includes emergency security procedures that address:

1. Actions to be taken in the event of a security incident or failure.
2. Handling of civil disturbances.
3. Handling of situations involving VIPs or the media; and
4. Provision of additional staff to control human and vehicle traffic in and around the environment of care during disasters.

Hazardous Materials and Waste Management Plan

A hazardous materials and waste management plan describes how the organization will establish and maintain a program to safely control hazardous materials and waste. The plan provides processes for:

a. Selecting, handling, storing, using, and disposing of hazardous materials and waste from receipt or generation through use or final disposal.
b. Establishing written criteria consistent with applicable law and regulation, to identify, evaluate, and inventory hazardous materials and waste used or generated.
c. Managing chemical waste, chemotherapeutic waste, radioactive waste, and regulated medical or infectious waste, including sharps.
d. Monitoring and disposing of hazardous gases and vapors.
e. Providing adequate and appropriate space and equipment for safe handling and storage of hazardous materials and waste and reporting and investigating all hazardous materials or waste spills, exposures, and other incidents.

In addition, the plan establishes an orientation and education program for personnel who manage or have contact with hazardous materials and waste that addresses:

i. Precautions for selecting, handling, storing, using, and disposing of hazardous materials and waste.
ii. Emergency procedures for hazardous material and waste spills or exposure.
iii. Health hazards of mishandling hazardous materials; and
iv. Orientation and education about reporting procedures for hazardous materials and waste incidents, including spills or exposures for appropriate personnel.

Performance improvement standards that address one or more of the following:

1. Staff knowledge and skills necessary for their role in managing hazardous materials and waste.
2. The expected level of staff participation in materials and waste management activities.
3. Monitoring, inspection, and corrective action.
4. Routine procedures for emergency and incident reporting that specify when and to whom reports are communicated.
5. Inspection, preventive maintenance, and testing of applicable equipment.
6. Emergency procedures that describe in detail the specific precautions, procedures, and protective equipment used during hazardous material and waste spills or exposures.
7. An annual evaluation of the hazardous materials and waste-management plan's objectives, scope, performance, and effectiveness.

Emergency Preparedness Drills

Drills are regularly conducted to test emergency preparedness.

The emergency preparedness plan is executed twice a year, either in response to an emergency or in planned drills. Organizations that offer emergency services or designated disaster receiving stations must perform at least one exercise yearly, that includes an influx of volunteer or simulated patients. Exercises are conducted at least four months apart and no more than eight months apart.

Suggested Issues for Hospital Mass Casualty Preparedness

The potential issues and priorities for mass casualty preparedness are:

a. Ensuring an adequate supply of food and water for staff, patient, and families at a time when normal supply patterns may be interrupted.
b. Management of a large number of fatalities, including awareness of and respect for religious customs.
c. Coordination of volunteers.
d. Adequate, advanced staff education, including identification of who needs training, who provides training and who pays for training. Training must include

recognition of the spectrum of causal agents and their respective treatments.

e. Setting priorities for high yield and low yield activities.
f. Coordination of regional resources to assure that hospitals are not double counting the same contingency suppliers.
g. Coordination of media relations. This will require coordination with others who will speak to the media and also the education of media representatives before any event occurs.
h. Open and reliable communication across the community to enable monitoring of the big picture.
i. Need for a plan to maintain a connection with the local community.
j. Communication across agencies, organizations, and communities.
k. Establishing logistics, especially with respect to patient and equipment transportation.
l. A staff augmentation plan, especially for a prolonged crisis.
m. Stockpiling and inventory of supplies so that they are readily available.
n. Mental health interventions during the incident and follow-up until recovery.
o. Advanced, ethical guidelines and policies for triage of patients, supplies, and drugs. In the military, the triage concept is focused on making decisions to facilitate completing the mission. In the civilian community, triage has traditionally meant treating the most injured first. In a mass casualty incident, it may be necessary to use a triage approach more similar to the military's definition that the traditional civilian one. Moreover, depending upon the duration and pattern of the incident, the definition of triage may change over time.
p. A biological incident may initially manifest itself with vague symptoms. There must be a balance between early identification of incidents and undermining public confidence with false positives.
q. Need to establish an inventory of successful practices. Hospital associations could inventory members. There is less legal resistance if inventory is of factual information rather than judgmental information.
r. Integration of support staff from non-traditional sources. Nurses who work in physician offices can be used to supplement hospital staff. Also technicians and technologists in private clinical laboratories can be relocated to the hospital laboratory.
s. Isolation of air handling systems so that airborne contaminants are not spread throughout the hospital or vented into the community.
t. Clear policies in the community and at the hospital as to who is in charge. The list must include redundancy to provide coverage for vacation, business and personal travel, and other contingencies. Recognition that a mass casualty event depends primarily on a local response.
u. Clear roles and coordination of the response triad of fire, police, and medical services.
v. The development of large, geographically dispersed health systems has moved hospital governance and management outside of local communities. This makes it more difficult to obtain approval for disaster planning. The constraints include that of:
    i. Space and facilities for handling a large volume of patient.
    ii. Identification of educational resources on the awareness of the several mass casualty threats.
    iii. The weak relationship between many hospitals and health departments.

iv. The weak relationship between many hospitals and community health centers.
v. The need for hospital leaders to look beyond their institution in order to develop and appropriate plan and allocation of resources. This may necessitate some guidelines that provide safe harbors for collaborative actions across facilities in a community.
vi. Communications with media, especially when information is incomplete on cause or response. Clear agreements on who will coordinate? Avoidance of the media's divide and conquer tactic. Community-wide agreement not to speculate when facts remain unknown.
vii. Outbreak control.
viii. A plan for a backup strategy when hospitals are at capacity.
ix. Coping with and addressing ethnic and religious customs for diets, death, and burial.
x. Funding for mass casualty preparedness, especially in financially vulnerable hospitals.
xi. Need a preparedness plan template for mass casualty plan to download and customize.
xii. Fatalities resulting from the incident may be seen as evidence by the law enforcement community. This will result in religious and family conflicts.
xiii. Conflict in culture between health care organizations, law enforcement, and media organizations. Health care is based on the premise of open communications with the assumption of honest, if incomplete, information. Law enforcement organizations often question every source and consider every action suspicious. The media seeks to probe and question. In this triangle of cultures, each party questions the behaviors of the other two.
xiv. The public sees terrorism as an act of war but doesn't want their health insurer to deny claims under a war exclusion provision.
xv. Management of fear, prejudice, and hatred among providers.
xvi. Need for real-time data to inform public and maintain their trust.
xvii. Temporary or bridge funding to make emergency purchases, especially when alternative vendors must be used.
xviii. Plan for tapping into wider network of professionals beyond the local community.
xix. Sustaining competence in disaster skills. Hospital employee turnover in many communities ranges from 16-20% annually. What is the feasibility of rapid re-education of new staff?
xx. Database for community and regional capacity of facilities, staff, supplies, local experts, etc.
xxi. Protecting the safety of staff. How do they get into facilities? Who gets past crowd control?
xxii. A national pharmaceutical stockpile. What is the hospital role in distribution? Are there standing priorities determined in advance of any incident? How does a community recognize and define the at risk population? What will be the health rules for allocations of the stockpile versus the politics?
xxiii. What are the best strategies for information management of medical records, patient tracking, confidentiality, and cyberterrorism?
xxiv. What if the hospital is site of event?
xxv. Cellular phone systems often have built-in but unknown priorities for access in overload situations. Will the hospital and health providers be given

priority during a mass casualty incident?

xxvi. Plans for auxiliary treatment facilities.

Other important considerations would be:

a. An inventory of laboratory preparedness which may be used during a mass casualty incident.
b. Wide communication of the effectiveness of biological prophylaxis.
c. Vehicles for transportation. Need equipment and directions for out-of-town personnel who arrive to supplement local resources.
d. Facility protection from contamination and crowds.
e. Effective regional mutual aid across communities for supplies, equipment, and staff privileges.
f. Methods to locate next of kin.
g. Decontamination facilities.
h. Toolbox of options and costs so that every hospital and community does not have to reinvent the wheel.
i. Political policy to get plans implemented.
j. Addressing denial (i.e., it won't happen here!) throughout the community.
k. An inventory of non-health private industry that could support health care providers during an incident.
l. The identification of quarantine facilities available for use during a biological incident.
m. A contingency plan for an incident with no effective treatment.

52 Education in Emergency and Disaster Medicine

"Quem in ipsa re trepidare noleuris, ante rem exerceas Seneca"
(If you want someone not to tremble when in danger, train him before danger comes)

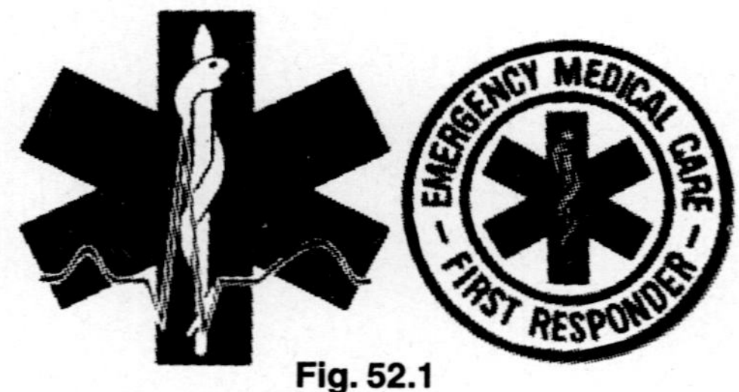

Fig. 52.1

INTRODUCTION

The key to preparedness is training and the scope of training has broadened considerably from focusing on top-level managers to first responders the local health workers and the community. Their education must be on aspects of mass casualty management, refugee camps and elementary sanitation procedures to ensure safe water and food for victims. Training in triage to enable them sort victims into categories for care and transport based on the severity of their injuries is a vital aspect. This provides for quick and organized response to disasters. Medical schools allow little time in their curricula for the teaching of resuscitation procedures and pre hospital care of trauma victims. Even in a strife-riddled country like Israel, 75% of surveyed graduates had finished internship without a single endotracheal intubation, cardiac massage, central vein cannulation, insertion of a chest drain or application of anti-shock trousers. Nearly 15% of them had performed these procedures only once. A committed program needs to be evolved for skill-oriented training of these vital procedures. A step-by-step supervised training protocol using video films and mannequins, followed by actual hands-on performance of these procedures is required. Computer simulation can effectively teach triage in mass casualty situations. Check list skill cards must be used to keep a tab on the procedures actually performed by each student followed by a strict evaluation procedure, brooking no compromise. Paramedics and non-medics also need to be indoctrinated in resuscitation methods for first-responder medical aid. The chain of survival must be clearly impressed on them, i.e., Early access, Early CPR and Early ACLS. Resusci Anne, injector dummies/mannequins etc from the house of Laerdal can be used as simulators and the tasks covered should include casualty evaluation, triage, pressure dressing methods for wounds, first aid for burns, CPR techniques, resuscitation, spine stabilization methods and splint applications.

Training must incorporate 61 protocols, 28 procedures and cover the use of 18 emergency drugs, inclusive of intravenous fluid administration. Level 1 training is a 5 week on-entry training for probationers in first aid, basic life support, adjunctive care (to include insertion of oropharyngeal airway, use of suction equipment and oxygen powered resuscitators), triage skills, disentanglement and evacuation skills, recording of vital signs, patient assessment and history taking. Level 2 is for certification as a paramedic and provides higher level training in all ambulance skills. Level 3 teaches advanced life support and qualifies for a registered nurse certification. The last includes application of medical anti-shock trousers (MAST), intravenous cannulation, endotracheal intubation, intravenous fluid therapy, drug therapy, interpretation of cardiac dysrrhythmias and their treatment, synchronized cardioversion and insertion of a chest tube to decompress tension pneumothorax. The curriculum requires 76 hours of full time tuition and supervision.

In the U.K., the Intercollegiate Board for Training in Intensive Care Medicine (IBTICM) has recommended a staged process of struct-ured training in critical care medicine from the undergraduate to the post graduate level. An initial 3 months basic training for all senior house officers in a recognised ICU, followed by a 12 months intermediate training and then another 12 months advanced training in intensive care medicine before certification.

In the USA, the emergency and critical care medicine (ECCM) system targets development of ambulance services, prehospital emergency care, national standards for ambulance design and equipment, training of basic emergency medical technicians, advanced paramedic training and mobile intensive care, categorization of hospitals based on the infra structure available and training and certification of intensivists and emergency physicians. Under the helm of Dr Peter Safar, it was recognized that the ECCM system was only as strong as its weakest component and that the earlier modern life support was instituted, the greater the chances for a victim's recovery and savings in hospitalization costs. First year medical students are offered a 30 hour elective course in emergency medical care to prepare them for the state EMT 1 examination and American Heart Associations basic rescuers test in CPR. Second year students have to qualify in the ABCs of CPR and execute manikin drills to perfection. Third year students receive an obligatory 3 weeks clerkship in anesthesiology and critical care medicine so that they are competent to swiftly treat respiratory, circulatory and cerebral failure. Student performances and skill acquisition are tested and graded at the end of this attachment. Fourth year students are offered a variety of six-week electives in operating rooms, mobile ICU-type ambulances, emergency departments. One to three months rotation is mandatory for residents. To qualify as Critical Care Medicine fellows, candidates must have completed a three year residency and then qualify in a two year program in Level 1 ICUs. The EENET (FEMA's Emergency Education Network) provides a distance learning system while the Asian Institute of Management at Manila offers short term and long courses on various aspects of disaster management. The Advanced Disaster Management Simulator (ADMS) and the U.S. Army Simulation and Instructional Command (STRICOM) have evolved complete training protocols on all aspects of disaster management in a virtual setting. In India, the Indian Institute of Ecology and Environment, New Delhi, offers 2 years PG diploma in disaster mitigation.

SYLLABUS

The International Society for Disaster Medicine has recommended the following syllabus for training in disaster medicine:

- Advanced Life Support (ALS).
- Triage.
- Mass casualty treatment at site and in hospital.
- Initial management of burns and smoke inhalation.
- Specific disaster problems e.g. NBC.
- Psychological aspects of disasters.
- Health aspects of displaced populations.
- Definition, classification and scoring of disasters.
- Disaster epidemiology risks and prevention.
- Disaster relief organizations.
- Disaster management—field, transportation and hospital.
- Evacuation of large populations.
- Command, coordination and communication.
- Legislative aspects.
- Media Relations.
- Theoretical and practical exercises.

Skills determined essential in the emergency medicine training programs are as following:

Primary procedures:

- Endotracheal intubation.
- Coniotomy.
- Intercostal tube insertion.
- External internal cardiac massage.
- Central vein cannulation.
- Venous cut down.
- Control of bleeding.

Second procedures:

- Application of MAST.
- Initial management of wounds.
- Fracture splinting.
- Management of spinal injuries.
- Nasogastric tube insertion.
- Bladder catheterization.
- Intravenous medications.

Instruction in emergency medicine and the initial management of mass trauma casualties must be formally included in the curriculum of medical schools during the clinical years, as an integral part of the surgical clerkship. Particular emphasis must be placed on pre-hospital care and full use of training aids like video tapes, slides, posters, mannequins, computers and animal laboratory must be made. Evaluation of skills through an examination covering all theoretical and practical aspects of emergency medicine and initial management of trauma casualties is essential. Pass mark scores must be 60% and above.

Suggested Body of Knowledge

- Emergency resuscitation.
- Pre-hospital emergency care.
- Field management of life-threatening emergencies.
- Communications by radio and telemetry (telemedicine).
- Mobile ICU design and equipment.
- Monitoring (invasive and non invasive).
- Mechanical ventilation and respiratory therapy(insertion of chest tubes, ventilator settings, intubation, bronchoscopy, tracheostomy, ABG interpretation, chest physiotherapy).
- Circulatory support (arrhythmia recognition and treatment, defibrillation, cardioversion, pacing, treatment of shock states, assisted circulation techniques, pre and after load management).
- CNS management (coma evaluation, EEG interpretation, ICP monitoring, cerebral resuscitation, management of spinal cord injuries, brain death evaluation and certification).

- Renal support (electrolyte, fluid therapy, acid base balance, peritoneal and hemodialysis).
- Management of metabolic and endocrine derangements.
- Tube and parenteral nutrition.
- Infection control.
- Aspects of anesthesia, biomedical engineering, humanities and social sciences.
- Pediatrics–considerations of perinatology, infancy and childhood.
- OBGY–Fetal well being assessment and conduct of normal deliveries.

The reputed Advanced Trauma Life Support Course or ATLS Program for doctors aims to provide participants with a safe, reliable method for immediate management of the injured victim, with emphasis on competent initial assessment and management of the trauma patient. It provides essential information and skills to identify and treat life-threatening as well as potentially life-threatening injuries. On completion, every participant is expected to:

- Undertake primary and secondary patient assessment
- Establish management priorities in a trauma situation.
- Initiate primary and secondary management for the emergency care of acute, life-threatening emergencies.
- Establish a patent airway and initiate artificial ventilation.
- Treat shock states.
- Perform venous cutdowns.
- Accomplish pleural decompression by chest tube insertion.
- Undertake emergency pericardiocentesis.
- Identify thoracic injuries from X-rays.
- Perform peritoneal lavage, ultrasound and CT evaluation of acute abdomen.
- Head and neck trauma assessment and neuro scoring with Glasgow Coma Scale.
- Identify intracranial lesions by CT scan.
- Identify spinal injuries by imaging techniques.
- Assess and manage neurotrauma and musculoskeletal problems.

The Pre Hospital Trauma Life Support (PHTLS) course is a parallel scaled-down version of the ATLS course conducted for emergency medical technicians, paramedics and nurses.

DART RESCUE CERTIFICATION (DART)

The Disaster Assistance and Rescue Team (DART) Certification Requirements (Per Year):

- Rescue systems – 5 hours of heavy rescue and basics of rope rescue.
- First responder drills – 4 hours including work with hazardous chemicals.
- Operation of Respirators and Self Contained Breathing Apparatus – 8 hours.
- CPR and Basic Life Support – 8 hours.
- Emergency Medical Treatment – 48 hours.
- Confined Spaces Rescue – 4 hours.
- Incident Command System – 16 hours.
- Fire fighting – max 13 hours.

THE WHITE HELMETS COMMISSION

The White Helmets Commission is a humanitarian aid and peacekeeping agency based on an initiative launched by Argentina in 1993, and adopted by the United Nations General Assembly in 1994 and the Organization of American States in 1998. It has more than 4,000 trained volunteers and has participated in missions in numerous countries of the Americas and other continents.

TRAUMA MOULAGE

A moulage is a practice scenario hosted by Trauma.Org, where you have a patient to assess and manage appropriately. These moulages were the first on the internet and more are planned for the future. The moulages require Netscape Navigator 2.0+, Internet Explorer 3.01+ or another internet browser that supports frames and must be Javascript is enabled. Though they work in most screen modes, they are optimised for 800 x 600 with font size set to small.

In the first moulage on the Internet you are designated as an emergency room doctor and must assess and adequately treat an injured patient. You will have an assistant to help you, but they can be of variable help, as in real life. Remember to apply the basic principles of trauma resuscitation to avoid going wrong.

Prehospital Care

Having finished with the last patient, you will be required to head up to the helipad to escape from the ER for a while. Things never go as planned however and 5 minutes later you will be on a motorway 15 miles away. This is a prehospital scenario, but the principles of trauma management still hold, perhaps more so. You will have an experienced paramedic to help you, and all the kit you might need.

Cervical Spine Clearance

Suddenly and inexplicably you are transferred to the spinal service, where you have to assess and evaluate six patients with potential cervical spine injuries.

Paediatric Moulage

Transferred back to the ER after generating too much work for the hospital's lawyers on the spinal service, you will be required to manage a child injured in a motor vehicle accident. The child's parameters and response to your treatment will change with each run through, and you'll get a full appraisal of your performance at the end of the moulage (Fig. 52.2).

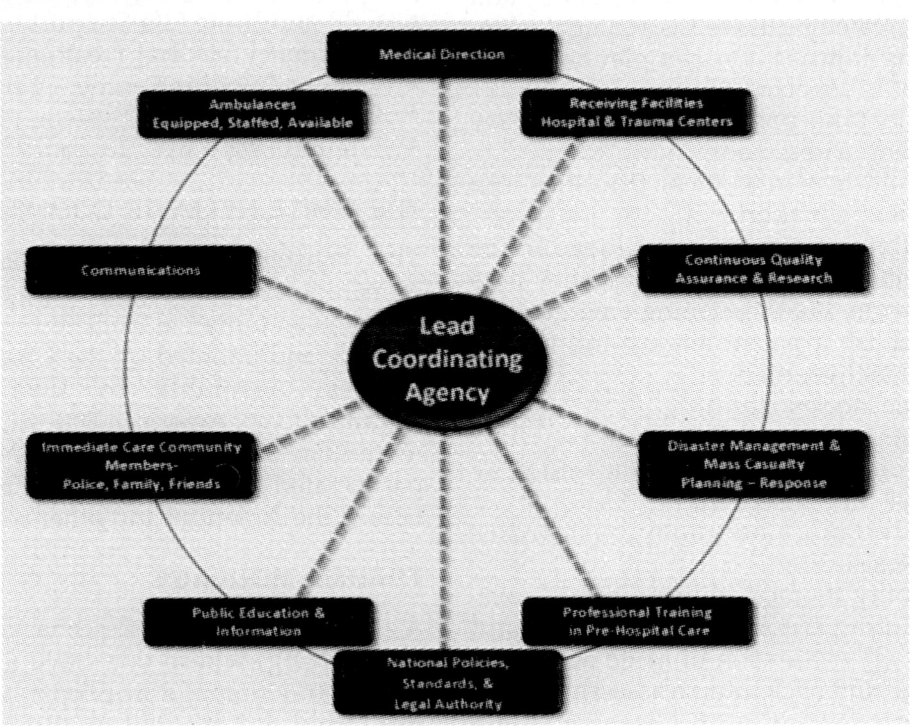

Fig. 52.2

Neurotrauma Moulage

The Neurotrauma Moulage demonstrates the principles behind the care of the head injured patient. Using a mathematical model to approximate brain neurophysiology it is able to simulate a wide range of conditions that affect brain injury management, both in the emergency room and intensive care unit.

Trauma Team Leader Decision Scenarios

Multiple short scenarios where you, as team leader, will be required to tread the path of the enlightened trauma doctor.

REFERENCES

1. Disaster Medicine-Towards Unifying Teaching and Training in Tomorrows Europe. Bernd DomresMedical Corps International 1991;2:32.
2. Undergraduate education in emergency medicine and initial management of trauma casualties in Israel.Joseph M. Klausner and Ron R. Rozin. Military Medicine 1987, Vol 152, No.9, p458-460.
3. Critical Care Organization and Education. Anesthesiology, Aug 1977, Vol 47, No 2.
4. Organization and Physician Education in Critical Care Medicine. Peter Safar and Ake Grenvik 1977, Vol 47, p-82-95.
5. American Association of Critical Care Nurses Recommended course content for use in development of crticial care nursing curricula. Heart Lung. J Crit Care 1972,1:317-323.
6. Public Health Reports, 2001 Supplement 2, Vol 116. Understanding Public Response to Disasters, p 71-73.
7. ATLS Student Course Material, American College of Surgeons, Committee on Trauma 1997).

53 Major Vehicular Accidents

> "Road traffic injuries are a major but neglected public health challenge that requires concerted efforts for effective and sustainable prevention. Of all the systems with which people have to deal every day, road traffic systems are the most complex and the most dangerous. Worldwide, an estimated 1.2 million people are killed in road crashes each year and as many as 50 million are injured. Projections indicate that these figures will increase by about 65% over the next 20 years unless there is new commitment to prevention. Nevertheless, the tragedy behind these figures attracts less mass media attention than other, less frequent types of tragedy."
>
> —*WHO*

INTRODUCTION

Trauma remains among the top-ten causes of death with 1 in 10 deaths resulting from injury. It commonly affects young adults. Disability-adjusted life years (DALY) is an indicator of the burden of injury, with 1 DALY equivalent to 1 lost year of healthy, productive life. Using this methodology, 16% to 20% of the world's burden of disease can be attributed to trauma. The main injury-related causes of DALY are road traffic accidents, falls, interpersonal violence and self inflicted injuries. 50% of deaths take place at the scene of injury or within minutes of the event.

Every year nearly 1.3 million people die in road accidents worldwide. By 2030, the figure is expected to touch 2.4 million. Road accidents are the 9th leading cause of death from all causes and is slated to climb to the 5th leading cause, surpassing even AIDS and Tuberculosis. Pedestrians, cyclists and motorcyclists are the most common victims. Traffic accident is also the leading cause of death in the age group 10-24 years. In addition, nearly 20-50 million people are involved globally in non fatal accidents every year. Nearly 90% of all road mishaps occur in poor and developing countries which account for 48% of the world's total vehicles on road. Causes being poorly designed roadways, inadequate enforcement of traffic rules, poor vehicular maintenance,alcoholism, overburdened health care infrastructure and a non efficent emergency medical response system. The financial implications of road accidents approaches $518 million annually. In India, road mishaps account for nearly 33.6% of all accidental deaths with most numbers occuring in the states of Tamil Nadu, Maharashtra, Karnataka, Kerala and Andhra Pradesh.

In an accident situation, the first rule must be to prevent further injury. This is done by defending the scene- by switching on hazard lights, deploying warning triangles, radio and highway alerts to prevent further pile-ups at the site.

COLLISION INJURIES

Injuries sustained in motor vehicle accidents are produced by a rapid decrease in velocity over a short distance – also termed as deceleration injuries. Severity of the injury depends on the energy transferred during deceleration.

Collisions

Three separate collisions can occur:

1. The primary collision when the vehicle impacts another object.
2. Secondary collision(s), when the victim inside impacts the internal parts of the vehicle.
3. The collision shearing forces that cause differential movement of fixed versus static parts.

Such injuries are inversely related to the size and weight of the vehicle and injury patterns vary based on front seat versus back seat occupants, use of restraints, and air bags that minimize secondary collisions and prevent ejections. Restraining devices are effective only if they worn correctly, while improperly applied devices can cause unusual injuries. But injury risk is always greater in unrest-rained victims. Lap belts alone decrease mortality by 50%, but they increase the risk of abdominal injuries, especially small bowel rupture and lumbar spine fractures. The three-point restraint coupled with airbag decreases mortality even further, especially in front end collisions and prevents ejection, when contact of the victims head with the car frame is prevented. Extremity injuries are however, not prevented and they are of no use in side impact collisions. The shoulder belt alone is inadvisable and back seat passengers can easily slide out from under the belt in a collision. The air bag allows for a gentler deceleration than the three-point restraints resulting in fewer rib and thoracic injuries and preventing head contact with the steering wheel or car frame. The proportion and severity of lower extremity injuries are more frequent when compared to torso and head injuries. The air bag does not prevent injuries to those who are out of position, facing backwards, leaning against the steering wheel or leaning into the passenger compartment at the moment of impact. Chance of major injury increases 300-500% when occupant is ejected, with chance of spinal injury being 1 in 13.

DIRECTION OF IMPACT

Frontal Impact

These are the commonest (64%) direction of impact in most accidents. Facial and chest injuries are most frequent and lower limb injuries are three times more than in lateral impacts and overall mortality rate is lower. Often victims are not belted and intoxicated. Facial injuries are common, caused by shattering of windscreen, impact over the steering wheel and internal rear view mirror (Fig. 53.1 and 53.2).

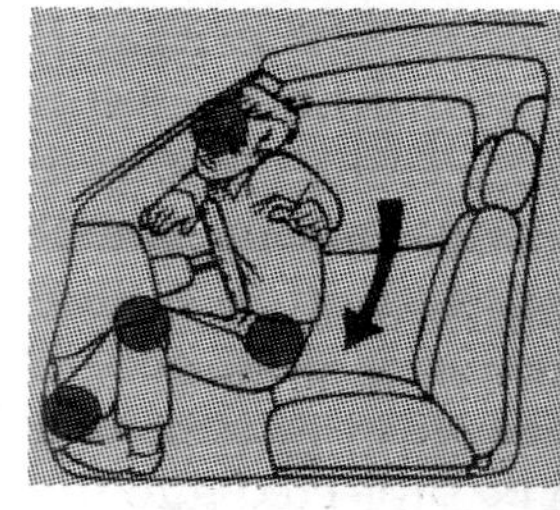

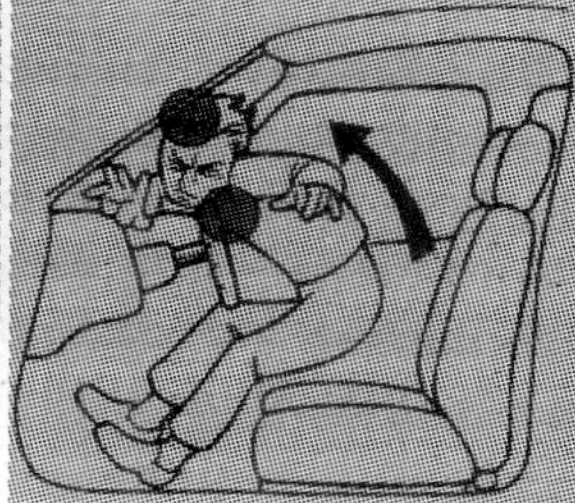

Fig. 53.1: Patterns of injury for unbelted driver in head on collison (A) Down-and-under mechanism. (B) Up-and-over mechanism. Note that the patient will exhibit characteristic cluster of injuries, including head and neck, chest, abdomen, and lower extremity fracture, depending on bow the body strikes the steering wheel (From Parr and Crande)

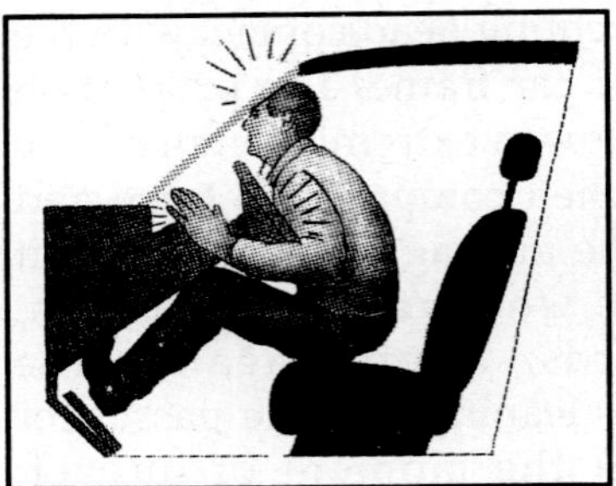

Fig. 53.2a: Frontal impact, unrestrained driver

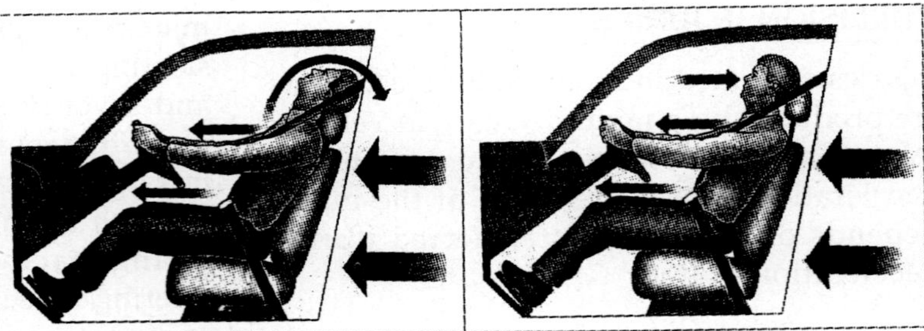

Fig. 53.2b: Rear impact, improper and proper headrest use

Rear End Impact

Only 8% of rear impacts produce serious injuries with cervical sprains and whiplash injuries being commoner.

Rollover Collisions

Force vectors can vary and kinetic energy is often dissipated over a long distance, which results in less injuries to passengers if they are belted. Roof collapse can produce severe head injuries and compression fractures of the spine from axial loads are common. Unrestrained occupants can be ejected or suffer severe crush injuries.

Lateral Crashes

The mortality rates are twice that of frontal collisions as impact is more direct with little space or metal to cushion forces. Thoracic and abdominal injuries are commoner and unrestrained drivers can be projected into the passenger compartment.

Pedestrian-Automobile impact

They account for 20% of all traffic injuries and 13% of traffic-related deaths, usually in children or older persons. 35% are musculoskeletal (low tibial and pelvic) and 27% intracranial injuries (Waddle's triad of lower limb fracture, truncal and craniofacial injury). Children are usually run over and sustain degloving injuries (Fig 53.3).

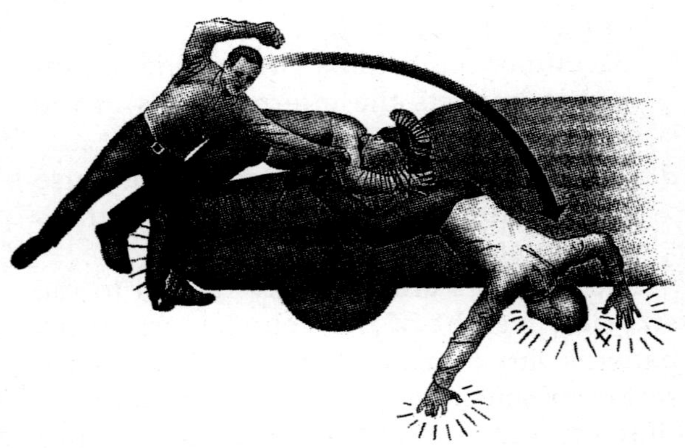

Fig. 53.3: Adult pedestrian injury triad

Motor Cycle Crashes

Victims tend to absorb all impact and kinetic energy with high risk of limb, pelvic and head injuries. The last account for 75% of motorcycle accident deaths. Risk decreases by 50% if helmets are worn. The helmet is designed to reduce the force to the head by changing the kinetic injury of impact to the work of deformation of the padding and distribute the force over as large an area as is possible, reducing the energy delivered to the head by translation. Unhelmeted motorcycle crash patients suffer more severe brain injuries, consume more resources, and have the worst payor mix. Society bears a large financial burden for these uninsured unhelmeted patients. There is a survival advantage for helmeted patients. All states should have universal motorcycle helmet laws that are aggressively enforced.

Fall Injuries

Nature of injuries depends on elevation, surface struck and position on impact. Mortality is 50% for falls from 25 to 30 feet and associated with multiple injuries, frequently fractures of the thoracolumbar spine, cervical region and limbs (Table 53.1).

Assaults

Usually seen among young men, injuries depend on weapon used, victims position and intensity of attack. 72% have injuries to head and face, 10% defensive wounds of upper and lower extremities.

GAINING ACCESS TO ACCIDENT VICTIMS

Gaining access to patients can be a major problem at times and can be even more challenging than the care to be rendered to the victim. Locked gates, doors, windows etc may stand in the way. Training in gaining access is required for EMTs and they must have the necessary minimum tools in the ambulance itself. Waiting for a rescue squad or a fire brigade can result in fatal delays. If the EMT or member of the medical team

Table 53.1: Mechanisms of injury and related suspected injury patterns

Mechanisms of injury	*Suspected injury patterns*
Frontal Impact • Bent steering wheel • Knee imprint, dashboard • Bull's-eye fracture, windscreen	• Cervical spine fracture • Anterior flail chest • Myocardial contusion • Pneumothorax • Traumatic aortic disruption • Fractured spleen or liver • Posterior fracture/dislocation of hip, knee
Side Impact • Automobile	• Contralateral neck sprain • Cervical spine fracture • Lateral flail chest • Pneumothorax • Traumatic aortic disruption • Diaphragmatic rupture • Fractured spleen/liver, kidney depending on side of impact • Fractured pelvis or acetabulum
Rear Impact • Automobile collision	• Cervical spine injury • Soft-tissue injury to the neck
Ejection, vehicle	• Ejection from the vehicle precludes meaningful prediction of injury patterns, but places patient at greater risk from virtually all injury mechanisms' • Mortality significantly increased
Motor vehicle-pedestrian	• Head injury • Traumatic aortic disruption • Abdominal visceral injuries • Fractured lower extremities/pelvis

reaches the site first, they must radio to the police for help and commence their efforts to gain access. There is no sense in trying to gain access by yourself, only to fail and then waste time trying to get help. The first priority for a rescuer is his or her own safety and to do only what they are trained to do. Motivation must not be allowed to overcome common sense.

DISENTANGLEMENT PROCEDURES IN VEHICULAR ACCIDENTS

Definition

The procedure of disentanglement is one of altering or removing wreckage to allow for a pathway or access, so that proper care can be rendered and the victim released for evacuation to the nearest hospital for further attention.

The Process

During the process, the victim has to be protected from further harm and full communication kept up, where possible, to keep the victim posted of the developments and allay his or her anxiety. Though patient assessment and care are the primary duties of an Emergency Medical Technician (EMT), there will be times when access to a victim is not possible by wreckage and entrapment, precluding adequate access to provide first aid or to evacuate the victim from mangled superstructures. The process of disentanglement would then be the sole option to solve this problem. Specially trained personnel from the rescue squad, fire brigade or home guard usually conduct this procedure. But sometimes, when even basic life support cannot be rendered to such victims, and the victims condition is deteriorating, the EMT and bystanders may have to begin the process themselves, while simultaneously calling for assistance from such trained personnel. Gaining access to a victim may be nothing more than getting a jammed door open or a complex procedure requiring removal of the entire top of a vehicle.

Disentanglement procedures can provide both the rescuers and the victim to hazards from broken glass, sharp metal edges or to flammable materials like leaking gasoline. While rescuers are required to wear adequate body protection, helmets, eyeshades, gloves etc, the victim must be also protected. Blankets, clothing, dressing materials must be available and adequate ventilation ensured under these heavy drapes. A volunteer must always be standby with a fire extinguisher. Extrication time must be as brief as possible as victims can become exsanguinated from even scalp lacerations and fracture sites by delays.

The Principles of Extrication

- Stabilize the vehicle where it lies movement can exacerbate injury.
- Make the vehicle safe - switch off ignition, immobilize the battery, swill away inflammable substances like fuel.
- Identify the patients that need immediate extrication to save life or limb.
- Read the wreckage to relate vehicle damage to potential injuries major chassis distortion = major injuries, deformed steering wheel = chest injury etc.
- Try opening the doors first, before removing the windscreen or the roof !
- Remove the wreckage from the casualty, not the casualty from the wreckage.
- Do not try to extricate victims through small apertures and access ways.
- Stabilize the victim on site before shifting into an ambulance.

MAKING A PATHWAY THROUGH THE WRECKAGE

The objectives of this procedure are twofold. The first allows rescuers with tools and appliances to reach the victim and, secondly, it establishes a route by which the victim can be evacuated once he or she is disentangled.
A Posts: Vertical support from the sides of the windshield.
B Posts: Vertical support located between the front and rear doors.
C Posts: Vertical support located behind the rear door: **C posts**.

Raising a Crushed Roof

Where the roof is crushed, the occupants inside will be encased in the wreckage and access to them would require prying a door open or raising a corner of the crushed roof. To extricate victims without causing additional harm, it may sometimes be required to remove the entire top of the vehicle. It would be necessary to identify a space between the body and the roofline and then wedge the toe and footplates of a bumper jack or a screw jack and raise the roof. If not, it would be necessary to cut directly behind the A-posts and fold back the roof. Shoring block placements may be required under the wedge or spreader each time it is fully opened and closed. Once the top is raised as far as possible, it may permit space to force the doors open. If the victims within have spinal injuries or extremity fractures, it may be impossible to immobilize them effectively prior to their extrication. Hence, removing the entire top of the vehicle is always a better alternative than displacing a seat to gain good access to victims. It is also a faster method and takes 10 to 15 minutes to execute. A hacksaw can be used to cut through the roof pillars. If several hacksaws are available, this can be accomplished even faster. Two blades can be in the saw and positioned to allow for cutting in both directions of the sawing stroke. Spare blades must be available to replace broken ones. In some cases, cutting oil may have to be applied to ease friction. Once the forward and middle pillars (A and B posts) are cut, the roof can be folded back, just ahead of the rear pillar or C-post. Before this can be done, the windshield must be removed or broken and, once the glass has been removed, the roof can be cut and folded. Use a pry or a flat bladed screwdriver, plastic and chrome trim around the posts must be trimmed and all rubber gaskets and sealant scrapped off. Chrome trim is cut off and may take more time. The A-post and the B-post on the same side are cut, holding the hacksaw firmly, and making smooth even cuts while exerting a steady downward force. Rushing it or using excessive force will cause blades to break and must be avoided. As cutting progresses, an assistant supports the roof on the same side. The same procedure is repeated on the other side. Lastly, a right-angled cut is made in the roof just ahead of the C posts with the hacksaw. An assistant stands at the rear, with his one foot placed approximately where the roof will fold, dimpling the metal while others fold back the roof back like that of a convertible. The severed pillars with sharp jagged edges are then covered with duct tape or rags or short sections of used fire hose. The use of air-operated chisels lends speed and efficiency to top-removal operations. The chisel tips sometimes get bound if the correct chisel bit is not selected for the job.

Cutting Through the Roof

Stabilize the vehicle before attempting rescue with chocks, spare tires, ropes or jacks. Try opening the doors or unlock the door through a half-open window. A half-conscious victim can be persuaded to unlock or open the door. If all these attempts fail, tools will be required to gain access without causing aggravation of the victims condition. After stabilizing the vehicle, an air operated cutting chisel is used to drill into a lower corner of the roof, about 6 inches from the windshield edge. The chisel is driven up one side, across the top and down the other side in one uninterrupted sweep and the resulting flap pulled down. The roof supports are then cut and the headliner ripped away, pulling out any rod struts that support the headliner. Ideal operating pressures for the air chisel is 100 to 125 psi. In the absence of this tool, an axe and sledgehammer is used to open the roof, using full personal protection. Here too the approach is made with the leading edge 6 inches away from the windshield edge and 6 inches from the rain gutter. One person holds the axe firmly against this point while the other strikes with the sledgehammer repeatedly till the axe blade crunches through the metal.

The axe is then turned till its blade is parallel to the roof and then steered with subsequent blows to make three cuts, one down the right side, one across the top and the third down the left side, leaving a smooth edge for the flap to be pulled down for safe extrication of the trapped victim. Spectators and other rescuers must keep well away during this exercise as fragments can break away and fly considerable distance. Duct tape or split old rubber hose/tyre tubing lengths must be applied over all sharp edges when removing victims. In dire emergencies, roof openings have been done with flat blade screwdrivers and short handled hammers but this is time consuming and exhausting.

Cutting Through the Floor

When a vehicle has come to rest on its top with the roof crushed flat against the body, access to trapped victims will have to be through the floor. After stabilizing the vehicle, the rear foot well is located and the

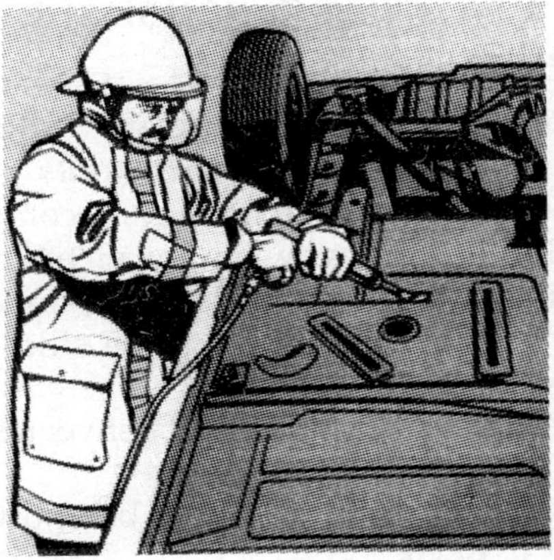

Fig. 53.4: Access can be gained through the floor of an overturned vehicle

rubber drain plug pulled out. Gentle probing is done through this opening to ensure no victims are jammed onto that portion being cut away. As described above, three cuts are then made and a flap pulled away. The floor carpet is then removed or cut with scissors so that the EMT can crawl in, head first while being supported by two persons. He then uses his hands to move body parts of trapped victims sufficiently until he can be fully lowered in (Fig. 53.4).

Widening Door Openings

Seldom do doors open to full 90º to the body of the vehicle and it is often impossible to evacuate a patient on the floor of the vehicle when the seat must also be pulled back at the same time. Most doors can be ripped off from its hinges by the combined efforts of three rescuers. Otherwise chock blocks are put ahead of the front wheel and behind the rear wheel on the same side where a door is to be removed. Have one rescuer push the door with two others pulling it. Most doors will open beyond their usual limit after one or two efforts. Wait for any rocking motion of the vehicle to stop before attempting again, otherwise one of the wheels may ride over the wheel chocks. Where tools are available, a combination of a hand winch and two chains can be used to open a jammed door.

Seat belts quick-release buckles will usually work well even after an accident. Otherwise the belt can be snipped off using scissors or cutters.

Displacing the Steering Column

It is wise to first make sure that plastic coverings around the steering column and plastic parts of the dashboard are not cracked or splintered. The steering wheel must be removed first and then the steering column is displaced upwards by manual force or use of power tools like a jack handle or hydraulic jack and ram tool. A hand winch and chain cam also be used for this purpose to displace the steering column from outside the vehicle after removing the windshield.

Displacing Floor Pedals

Brake and clutch pedals may sometimes hold a victims foot firmly against the floor of a wrecked vehicle in head-on collisions. A length of rope with a loop at one end is slipped over the pedal to be removed. The other end is tied to the doorframe on the same side. Pulling the door open sharply will displace the pedal.

Displacing the Dash

Combined use of a small pry and a hand winch usually suffices for this task.

Displacing Seats

A hand winch and a chain set would be required for this. The winch is positioned on the rear trunk deck, running the rear winch cable or chain through the rear window opening and snapping the hook over the ring of the short chain that has been wrapped around the lower seat. Shore blocks are placed under the chain where it may snag. The winch handle is then operated while another depresses the seat adjustment mechanism till it is freed. The spring component of the seat adjustment mechanism may have to be cut as soon as it becomes visible so that it does not break loose. A hydraulic jack can also be used by placing the foot of the ram against the doorframe and the wedge of V-bloc end of the unit against the seat support. The seat is then forced upward with a wedge or spreader. An air-operated chisel if available can be used to cut the seat supports or the bolts from underneath, one side at a time.

VEHICLE FIRES

- 1 out of 5 fires involves motor vehicles.
- 1 out of 8 fire deaths results from motor vehicle fires.
- 600 people are killed and 1,200 firefighters are injured a year from motor vehicle fires.

Fires in motor vehicles can produce toxic gases. Automobiles, trucks, and other motor vehicles are made of many synthetic materials that emit harmful, if not deadly gases when they burn. A main by-product of fires is carbon monoxide, an odorless colorless and tasteless gas that causes death in high concentration. Fire can cause fatal or debilitating burn injuries. A vehicle fire can generate heat upwards of 1,500 degrees F. Keep in mind that water boils at 212 degrees F, and that most foods are cooked at temperatures of less than 500 degrees F. Flames from burning vehicles can often shoot out distances of 10 feet or more.

Parts of the vehicle can burst because of heat, shooting debris great distances. Bumper and hatchback door struts, two-piece tire rims, magnesium wheels, drive shafts, grease seals, axle, and engine parts, all can become lethal shrapnel. Although relatively rare, gas tanks of motor vehicles can rupture and spray flammable fuel, posing a clear potential for serious injury. In even more extraordinary instances, gas tanks have been known to explode. Hazardous materials, such as battery acid, can cause injury even without burning.

Vehicle fires are so dangerous that firefighters wear full protective fire resistant equipment and self-contained breathing apparatus to keep themselves safe. They have the ability to quickly put out vehicle fires with large amounts of water or other extinguishing agents.

Avoid standing directly in front of the blazing vehicle and ensure that the wind is at your back. Do not try to throw the hood open as this may induce a flare up. Spray fire extinguisher under hood opening, grill, window or wheel-well using the extinguishing agent no more than necessary. Try to direct force of extinguisher to sweep flames away from the passenger compartment. The NEGATIVE battery cable must always be snipped off as cutting the positive cable could generate a hot spark and ignite spilled fuel. Fuel tank caps can be removed to minimize the explosion caused by heated, sealed fuel tanks.

HELMET REMOVAL

Accident victims wearing helmets must have it removed with the neck held in a neutral position, using a two-person procedure, with one providing in-line manual immobilization from below while the other expands the helmet laterally and removes it from above. Helmets can also be removed using a cast-cutter while stabilizing the head and neck to minimize cervical spine motion where cervical spine injury is suspected. Detailed technique is as follows:

- One person stabilizes the victims head and neck by placing one hand on either side of the helmet with his or her fingers on the patient's lower jaw to prevent slippage if the strap is loose.
- The second person loosens or cuts the helmet straps at the D-rings.
- The second person then places one hand over the angle of the lower jaw, with his or her thumb on one side and the fingers on the other. The rescuers other hand is placed under the head at the occipital region and applies pressure. This transfers the responsibility of in-line immobilization to the second person.
- The first rescuer then removes the visor and expands the helmet on the sides to clear the ears, and carefully removes the helmet. If the helmet provides full facial coverage, the helmet must be tilted backwards and raised over the victim's nose, ensuring that the second rescuer maintains continuous in-line immobilization from below to prevent the victims head from tilting.
- After helmet removal, inline manual immobilization is re established from above and a cervical immobilization

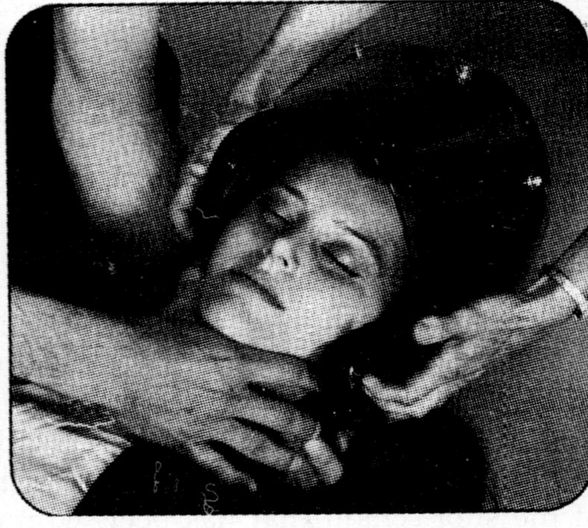

Fig. 53.5: Maintaining traction when removing helmets

device applied before shifting and transporting the victim.

- If helmet removal causes pain or tingling of nerves or if x-rays show evidence of c-spine injury, the head and neck are stabilized and a cast cutter used to divide the helmet in the coronal plane at the level of the ears. The outer FRP layer is removed and the inner Styrofoam cut and removed from front and back, maintaining neutral alignment of the head and neck (Fig. 53.5).

IMPROVING MOTOR VEHICLE SAFETY

Safety Features in Motor Vehicles

The terms "active" and "passive" are used in several seemingly-conflicting ways in the context of automobile safety. "Active safety" is often used to refer to crash avoidance and "passive safety" to crashworthiness. However, the terms may also be applied to the vehicle occupant's involvement in the function of the safety device or system. Under such nomenclature, **active** safety devices and systems are those which the vehicle occupant must *act* to make functional, as for example by fastening a seat belt. **Passive** safety devices and systems are those(such as air bags) which operate without any input or action from the vehicle occupant. Terminological conflict can arise from the fact that passive safety devices and systems—those requiring no input or action by the vehicle occupant—can themselves operate in an active manner. An example is active head restraints, which move to a position optimal for preventing neck injury when a collision is imminent.

SEAT BELTS

In the event of a crash, seat belts are designed to keep the passengers inside the vehicle. They also reduce the risk that of collision with the steering wheel, dashboard, or windshield. New seat belt designs have the following additional features that improve seat belt performance (Fig. 53.6):

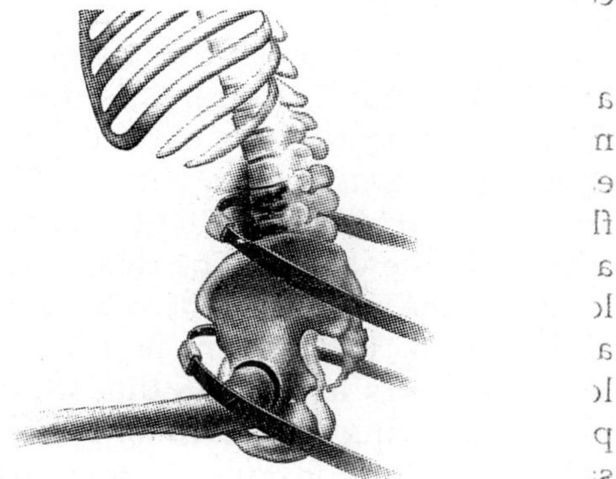

Fig. 53.6: Proper versus improper lap belt application

Adjustable upper belts: An adjustable upper belt lets the passenger change the position of the shoulder strap to accommodate a person's size. This feature may encourage passengers to wear their belts, since it increases shoulder belt comfort.

Seat belt pretensioner: Pretensioners retract the seat belt to remove excess slack, almost instantly, in a crash. However, one still needs to adjust one's seat belt so that it fits as snugly as possible, since pretensioners are not powerful enough to pull one back into one's seat in the event of an impact.

Energy management features: Energy management features allow seat belts to "give" or yield during a severe crash to prevent forces on the shoulder belt from concentrating too much energy on the passenger's chest. These features include "load limiters" built into the shoulder belt retractor and/or "tear stitching" in the webbing that causes the seat belt to extend gradually.

Rear center seat lap/shoulder belts: Some manufacturers provide a rear center lap/ shoulder belt. This added feature is especially beneficial to older children and children in booster seats who are often seated in the rear center position.

LATCH: An acronym for "Lower Anchors and Tethers for CHildren", is designed to make proper installation of child safety seats easier. Child safety seats with LATCH have flexible or rigid anchors that attach to rigid anchors in the vehicle. The rigid anchors are located at the junction of the vehicle seat back and bottom. The system features built-in lower anchors and top-tether attachment points allowing LATCH-compatible child safety seats to be installed without using the vehicle's safety-belt system. The LATCH system helps child-seat installation by reducing incompatibilities that safety-belt installation may present (Table 53.2).

Air Bags

Depending on the speed at impact and the stiffness of the object struck, front air bags inflate to prevent occupants from hitting the dashboard, steering wheel, and windshield. Side air bags reduce the risk that occupants will hit the door or objects that crash through it. Although air bags provide life-saving benefits for the vast majority of people, there are situations in which air bag deployment can have adverse effects, such as when occupants are unbelted. Front air bags do not eliminate the need for seat belts and are not designed to offer protection in rollovers, rear, or side impacts. In fact, maximum air bag effectiveness depends upon seat belts, which help keep the passenger in place should a collision occur. One can significantly reduce the risk of injury from an air bag by buckling one's seat belt and keeping about 10 inches or more between one's breastbone and the air bag. Children can be killed or seriously

Table 53.2: Truncal and cervical injuries from restraint devices

Restraining device	*Injury*
Lap Seat Belt	
Compression	Tear or avulsion of mesentery Rupture of small bowel or colon Thrombosis of iliac artery or abdominal aorta
Hyperflexion	Chance fracture of lumbar vertebrae
Shoulder Harness	
Submarining	Intimal tear or thrombosis in innominate, carotid, subclavian, or vertebral arteries Fracture or dislocation of c-spine
Compression	Intimal tear or thrombosis in subclavian artery Kib fractures Pulmonary contusion Rupture of upper abdominal viscera
Air Bag	
Contact	Corneal abrasions, keratitis Abrasions of face, neck, chest
Contact/deceleration	Cardiac rupture
Flexion (unrestrained)	C-spine or thoracic spine fracture
Hyperextension (unrestrained)	C-spine fracture

injured by an air bag, so one should always put children age 12 and under in the rear seat. One should never use a rear-facing child seat in the front seat of a vehicle equipped with a front passenger air bag unless the air bag is off.

Head Injury Protection

Head injury protection consists of foam or other energy absorbing material under the trim of the vehicle interior and is likely to be invisible to vehicle occupants. Some vehicles have head air bags. While all head air bags are designed to deploy in side impacts, some are also designed to deploy during rollovers. Both types of air bags are designed to help protect occupants from injuries caused when their head strikes the upper interior of a vehicle.

Head Restraints

Head restraints are extensions of the vehicle's seats that limit head movement during a rear-impact crash, thus, reducing the probability of neck injury. Head restraints meeting specific size and strength requirements are required in front seats, but not in rear seats. While one must adjust most head restraints manually, some adjust automatically with changes in seat position or dynamically in a crash. In general, dynamic head restraints provide the best protection.

Antilock Brake System

An antilock brake system (ABS) prevents a vehicle's wheels from locking during "panic" braking, which allows the driver to maintain greater steering control—a key factor in avoiding a collision. However, an ABS does not guarantee one's ability to avoid a crash. Furthermore, one still may lose control when driving at excessive speeds or when using extreme steering maneuvers. Learning to use the ABS correctly will provide one with the greatest benefit from the system. All passenger cars equipped with ABS have four-wheel ABS. Sport utility vehicles, trucks, and vans equipped with ABS can have either four-wheel or two-wheel ABS. Four-wheel ABS monitor and control all the wheels of the vehicle, while two-wheel ABS only monitor and control the rear wheels of a vehicle. Some ABS's also include brake assist, which senses emergency braking by detecting the speed or force at which the driver presses the brake pedal and boosts the power as needed. Under certain conditions, brake assist may reach the braking force needed to activate the ABS more quickly and easily compared with vehicles without brake assist, and can potentially reduce overall stopping distance by eliminating the delay caused by not braking hard enough or soon enough.

Traction Control

Traction control systems improve vehicle stability by controlling the amount the drive wheels can slip when one apply excess power. The system automatically adjusts the engine power output and, in some systems, applies braking force to selected wheels during acceleration. Traction control is mainly found in vehicles with four-wheel antilock brake systems.

All-Wheel Drive

All-wheel drive distributes power to both front and rear wheels to maximize traction. Unless combined with traction control, all-wheel drive systems do not prevent the drive wheels from slipping when you apply excess power during acceleration.

Electronic Stability Control

Electronic stability control (which is offered under various trade names) is designed to assist drivers in maintaining control of their vehicles during extreme steering maneuvers. Electronic stability control senses when a vehicle is starting to spin out (oversteer) or plow out (understeer), and it automatically applies the brake to a single wheel. It is intended to reduce the occurrence of crashes in which vehicles veer off the road and strike curbs, soft shoulders, guard rails and other objects that initiate rollovers. However, it can't keep a vehicle on the road if its speed is simply too great for the curve and the available traction.

Weight

Crash data show that heavy vehicles offer more protection than light vehicles with the same safety equipment, particularly in two-vehicle crashes.

Crash Avoidance

Crash avoidance systems and devices help the driver—and, increasingly, help the vehicle itself—to avoid a collision. This category includes:

- The vehicle's headlamps, reflectors, and other lights and signals.
- The vehicle's mirrors.
- The vehicle's brakes, steering and suspension systems.

Driver Assistance

A subset of crash avoidance is *driver assistance* systems, which help the driver to detect ordinarily-hidden obstacles and to control the vehicle. Driver assistance systems include:

- Infrared night vision systems to increase seeing distance beyond headlamp range.
- Adaptive highbeam assist which automatically and continuously adapts the headlamp range to the distance of vehicles ahead or which are oncoming.
- Adaptive headlamps swivels headlamps around corners.
- Automatic high beams which automatically adapts the headlamp range to the distance of vehicles ahead or which are oncoming.
- Reverse back up sensors, which alert drivers to difficult-to-see objects in their path when reversing.
- Back up camera.
- Adaptive cruise control which maintains a safe distance from the vehicle in front.
- Lane departure warning systems to alert the driver of an unintended departure from the intended lane of travel.
- Tyre pressure monitoring systems or deflation detection systems.
- Traction control systems which restore traction if driven wheels begin to spin.
- Electronic stability control, which intervenes to avert an impending loss of control.
- Anti lock brakinng systems.
- Electronic brakeforce distribution systems.
- Emergency brake assist systems.
- Cornering brake control systems.
- Precrash system.
- Automated parking system.
- Crashworthiness systems and devices prevent or reduce the severity of injuries when a crash is imminent or actually happening. Much research is carried out using anthropomorphic crash test dummies. Laminated windshields remain in one piece when impacted, preventing penetration of unbelted occupants' heads and maintaining a minimal but adequate transparency for control of the car immediately following a collision. Tempered glass side and rear windows break into granules with minimally sharp edges, rather than splintering into jagged fragments as ordinary glass does. Crumple zones absorb and dissipate the energy of a collision, displacing and diverting it away from the passenger

compartment and reducing the impact force on the vehicle occupants. Side impact protection beams, collapsible steering columns reduce the risk and severity of driver impalement on the column in a frontal crash. Padding of the instrument panel and other interior parts of the vehicle likely to be struck by the occupants during a crash.

Pedestrian protection systems. A minimum/maximum hood (bonnet) height and ban on fitting *"bull bars" in SUVs.*

Post-Crash Survivability

Post-crash survivability devices and systems help minimise the chances that vehicle occupants who survive a crash will be injured or killed by secondary effects of the collision, such as fire. Examples include technical standards for vehicle fuel system integrity and fire resistance and retardation of vehicle interior materials. Advanced automatic collision notification systems will alert authorities automatically after an accident has occurred.

54 Basic Principles of Accessing and Moving Patients in Disaster Situations

> "The period of greatest gain in knowledge and experience is the most difficult period in one's life."
>
> —*Dalai Lama*

ACCESSING VICTIMS

Gaining access to patients can be a major problem at times and can be even more challenging than the care to be rendered to the victim. Locked gates, doors, windows etc may stand in the way. Training in gaining access is required for EMTs and they must have the necessary minimum tools in the ambulance itself. Waiting for a rescue squad or a fire brigade can result in fatal delays. If the EMT or member of the medical team reaches the site first, they must radio to the police for help and commence their efforts to gain access. There is no sense in trying to gain access by yourself, only to fail and then waste time trying to get help. The first priority for a rescuer is his or her own safety and to do only what they are trained to do. Motivation must not be allowed to overcome common sense.

Patients Trapped in Buildings

The hazards one may have to face are fire and structural give-outs, confrontation with pets and guard dogs, tackling locked doors and windows and exiting from heights. Burning buildings must never be entered alone and without the proper gear. A well fitting helmet with headlight, canvas/asbestos gloves, boots, breathing apparatus and a fireman's axe are standard gear for such an exercise. The breathing apparatus is a self-contained demand regulator apparatus. Fire in a confined space generates a large amount of heat and flammable gases that are deficient in oxygen. The heated gases rise and, when air is admitted into the room, it explodes to create a backdraft that can throw one off his feet. Excess of gray yellow smoke is suggestive of possible backdraft conditions and those areas must be avoided and vented at the highest point to allow potentially explosive gases to escape without igniting. Never swing open doors. Feel the top of the door with bare hands and, if it is hot, there is probably a blaze on the other side. Opening a door suddenly can result in a blast of lung-searing heat. If it feels just warm, open the door carefully keeping the foot braced at the bottom to prevent the door slamming open. Enter and exit a smoke filled room by crawling on all fours to keep below the heated and toxic gases. If the top of the door feels hot, use wet towels and mattresses to seal all cracks and crevices around the door and plug all openings through which smoke may enter the room such as a/c vents, exhaust fan vents and open all windows to let in fresh air. If the smoke is too thick and billowing, use blankets and strong sheets to stem exit of smoke from the room and stick your head out from beneath the drapes to breathe in fresh air. Phone for help and hang out brightly coloured and highly visible sheets and materials outside the windows to attract attention. NEVER PANIC. On the prevention side and keeping in mind that fire is responsible for the third largest number of accidental deaths and injuries, there is sufficient evidence to endorse and merit installation of smoke detectors and rapid response automatic water sprinklers in all new residential and non residential buildings.

Structural Hazards

One must be alert for weak spots in the ceilings and floors in any building. Always keep a powerful flashlight when entering a building for a rescue. Unstable piles of broken concrete slabs, columns, structural materials, furniture will have to be cut and lifted carefully to avoid endangering those buried under rubble. Sophisticated sound detectors are used to discern noises from buried survivors and helps experts to burrow a way to rescue them by digging access tunnels. Long improvised tubing may be required to supply oxygen to such victims from an external source. A plentiful supply of jacks would be required to prevent a cave-in. Sniffer dogs can also be pressed into service to detect trapped survivors. Do not try to save trapped animals and pets. Animal-control experts, if available, are best suited for this. In case of locked doors, see if another gate is open or if a duplicate or master key can be obtained. Remember to both push and pull the door and look around to see if its key is stashed in a niche or on the top of the doorway. Sometimes a neighbor may have the key. Wear a face shield, helmet, gloves and protective coat before trying to force through locked doors. A long- handled bolt cutter may be used to cut padlocks and chain-links. A hacksaw can be tried as an alternative. Plate glass doors are very tough and an improper blow with a pry-axe can cause it to bounce back onto your face. Every forcible entry generates flying particles and adequate personal protection must always be ensured. Use a sharp awl or the pike of an axe to strike as close to the frame as possible in a lower corner. Be wary of all loose wiring as they may be energized. Mobile cranes, earth moving machines, caterpillars, and excavators would be required to rescue buried victims and it would be wise to have an inventory of places and organizations with such equipment so that they could be mobilized in short time to the scene of a calamity.

Cave Ins (Trench Rescue)

Persons or children can be trapped in landslides, dirt pile, grain or sludge and speed is vital in reaching a trapped victim as dirt covers their mouth and nose and also packs around the chest to prevent its movements. The fire department and rescue squads are alerted and hand tools used to dig in at sites pointed out by witnesses if any. Digging must be done carefully to prevent further shift of material that may endanger the life of the rescuers themselves. Once located, the victim is freed upto the waist as resuscitation is pointless till the chest is freed. The mouth and nares are cleaned and sucked out and oxygen is administered and digging continued to free him totally. DO NOT PULL THE PATIENT FREE as he or she may have neck or spinal injuries as well. If the patient is hypothermic, swaddle him in blankets or Bair Hugger type warming envelope or just immerse one forearm in a tub of water at 40°C for gradual warming.

LIST OF TOOLS RECOMMENDED FOR RESCUE OPERATIONS

Over 600 tools and appliances could be used in a rescue operation. Keeping in mind their weight, size, cost and the requirement of an external power supply for some, the following list of tools are considered essential:

- A 12 inch adjustable wrench.
- A 12 inch screwdriver.
- A hacksaw with many spare blades.
- A vise-grip pliers.
- A 5 pound hammer.
- A flat headed fire-axe.
- A long handled sledge hammer.
- A pry axe.
- A 51 inch pinch point bar.
- A bolt cutter.
- Shoring blocks.
- A pointed shovel.
- Double action tin snips.
- Assorted Manila ropes.
- A hand winch of 2 tonne capability.
- Aluminized blankets.
- Manually powered hydraulic tools.
- A heavy duty knife.

SPECIAL CACHE OF EQUIPMENT

- Hydraulic and electric jack hammers.
- Hydraulic concrete cutting saws.
- Hydroelectric reinforcement bar cutters (rebar).
- Gas powered circular saws.
- Hydraulic spreaders, cutters and rams (a.k.a. Jaws of Life).
- High pressure pneumatic airbags.
- Gas and electric powered concrete core drills.
- Electric concrete breakers, chippers and roto hammers.
- Oxyacetylene torch kits.
- Gas powered electrical generators.
- Woodworking tools (Hand and electric powered).
- Stokes litters, backboards, Miller boards, KEDS, SKEDS.
- Trauma kits, cervical immobilization collars, oxygen and medical gear.
- Pry bars, sledge hammers and roller pipes.
- Ladders.
- Trash/dewatering pumps.
- Light stands and arc lights.
- Lumbar piles.
- SCUBA and bottle charging apparatus.
- Search cameras, infrared abled videocams.
- Atmosphere analysers.
- Rapid response trailer or mobile command post with onboard 7 kw generator, computer with wireless broadband internet access, interactive videoconferencing and telemedicine facilities, fax machine, printer, cellphone, base station radio, television camera and workstation for staff.
- Boats/Gemini with outboard motor.
- Wet suits, dry suits, exposure suits.

SUMMARY

Disentanglement involves altering and removing wreckage so that appropriate care can be rendered to the patient and facilitate their evacuation to the nearest hospital facility. Personal safety of the rescuers is of prime concern. As far as the victim is concerned, adequacy of ventilation, stabilization of the spine, arrest of bleeding and pain relief would be the major areas of concern.

MOVING AND EVACUATING DISASTER VICTIMS

Emergency moves of patients from the scene of a disaster would have to be done before full assessment of his or condition can be done and before basic life support, wound dressing or splinting of fractures can be made. This may be especially necessary where the scene is hazardous for both the victim and the rescuer or when the victims condition is rapidly on the decline. The types of moves may be:

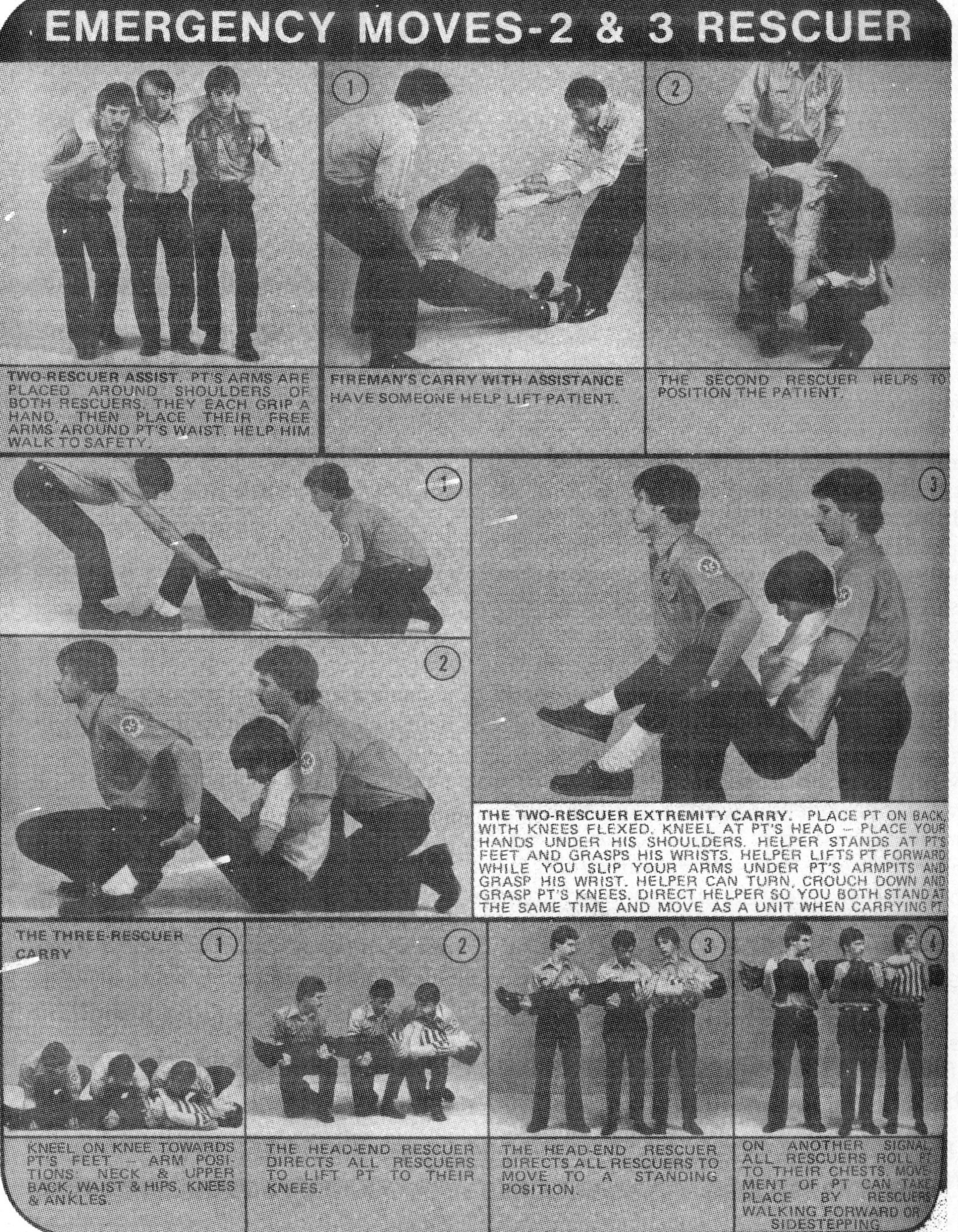
EMERGENCY MOVES-2 & 3 RESCUER
TWO-RESCUER ASSIST. PT'S ARMS ARE PLACED AROUND SHOULDERS OF BOTH RESCUERS. THEY EACH GRIP A HAND, THEN PLACE THEIR FREE ARMS AROUND PT'S WAIST. HELP HIM WALK TO SAFETY.
1
FIREMAN'S CARRY WITH ASSISTANCE
HAVE SOMEONE HELP LIFT PATIENT.
2
THE SECOND RESCUER HELPS TO POSITION THE PATIENT.
1
2
3
THE TWO-RESCUER EXTREMITY CARRY. PLACE PT ON BACK WITH KNEES FLEXED. KNEEL AT PT'S HEAD — PLACE YOUR HANDS UNDER HIS SHOULDERS. HELPER STANDS AT PT'S FEET AND GRASPS HIS WRISTS. HELPER LIFTS PT FORWARD WHILE YOU SLIP YOUR ARMS UNDER PT'S ARMPITS AND GRASP HIS WRIST. HELPER CAN TURN, CROUCH DOWN AND GRASP PT'S KNEES. DIRECT HELPER SO YOU BOTH STAND AT THE SAME TIME AND MOVE AS A UNIT WHEN CARRYING PT.
THE THREE-RESCUER CARRY
1
KNEEL ON KNEE TOWARDS PT'S FEET — ARM POSITIONS: NECK & UPPER BACK, WAIST & HIPS, KNEES & ANKLES.
2
THE HEAD-END RESCUER DIRECTS ALL RESCUERS TO LIFT PT TO THEIR KNEES.
3
THE HEAD-END RESCUER DIRECTS ALL RESCUERS TO MOVE TO A STANDING POSITION.
4
ON ANOTHER SIGNAL ALL RESCUERS ROLL PT TO THEIR CHESTS. MOVEMENT OF PT CAN TAKE PLACE BY RESCUERS WALKING FORWARD OR SIDESTEPPING.

Fig. 54.1

- *One Rescuer Moves:* One rescuer assist type where the victim can walk with assistance, piggyback carriage where victim is conscious and has no extremity injuries, cradle carriage, fireman's lift or one rescuer drag.
- *Two Rescuer Moves:* Here too, the two rescuer assist, extremity carriage and fireman's carriage may be employed.
- *Three Rescuer Moves:* Three-rescuer carriage of conscious or unconscious victims with no extremity injuries.

Transferring a Victim

Early day stretchers were rectangular boards of wood fitted with handles and covered with straw. They were provided with a two wheeled undercarriage to lend better mobility. Heavy and cumbersome, they certainly did not provide any comfort for the patient being transported on them. It was only during the beginning of the 20th century that improvements in stretcher design were attempted. The Army stretcher 12 was introduced into the German Armed Forces in 1912. Made of organic textile fabric fastened to the sides of wooden bars that allowed it to be folded and stowed. The British armed forces used wooden bars with nailed canvas, protruding handles and wrought iron feet. Later the handles were made of aluminium tubing. The Army Stretcher 38 used by the German army in 1920s had oval tubes, a central hinge, a blockable transverse hinge and detractable handles. The whole device was covered with canvas that was fastened to the spars by eyelets and cords. Later, the canvas was clamped with sectional plates. In 1957, canvas was replaced with water proof polyethylene fabric that was disinfectable and porous.

THE PRINCIPLES OF PATIENT TRANSPORTATION

1. First select a proper patient-carrying device.
2. Then package the patient for transfer,
3. Move the victim to the ambulance.
4. And lastly load the victim onto the ambulance.

The Commonly Used Patient Carrying Devices or Stretchers

In principle, a stretcher must have the following characteristics:

A. Subject the patient to as little strain as possible.
B. Fulfill hygienic requirements for thorough disinfection.
C. Be appropriate to the local climate.
D. Be big enough, lightweight, water and dirt resistant.
E. Have arrestable and collapsible or detractable handles.
F. Be foldable for easy stowing.
G. Have neutral oscillation behavior.
H. Be simple to handle.
I. Have arrestable transverse hinges when taut.
J. Have stable feet at the spars and have quick fitting, arrestable wheel supports and mountings.
K. Incorporate tilting design for quick head low positioning.
L. Have dimensions 1900 mm length, 600 mm width and max 8.5 kg weight.
M. Also serve as a treatment table with infusion bar for holding infusions.

Varieties of Stretchers

Wheeled ambulance stretchers: These can be multi level devices with adjustable headrest and provision for Trendelenberg (head-low) positioning. The victim is secured securely and then either wheeled or carried for evacuation.

Portable stretchers: Made of foldable light steel U-frames and a canvas or nylon fabric hammock.

Collapsible stretchers: With two rear leg wheels, useful for transferring victims down stairs or narrow spaces.

Spine boards: Designed to immobilize spinal injury victims.

Scoop style orthopedic stretchers: Designed to pick up seriously injured victims with a minimum of body movement.

Basket stretchers: These are wire and plastic devices used to move victims from heights by ladder, rope or helicopter over debris and obstacles with four point suspension bridles, patient security straps and adjustable footrest.

Pole stretchers: Consisting of two wooden poles and a canvas harness.

The Neil Robertson stretcher: A bamboo and canvas framework stretcher useful for shifting victims down stairways, hatches on board ships and also for winching to helicopters or by jackstay to another ship while underway. It has restraining torso and head straps leaving the victims hands free.

The multi purpose Nor Hosp Stretchers: These are army stretchers with telescopic handles based on NATO standards. They have great flexibility and can also function as a stackable bed for transport of patients in transports of all types, serve as a shelter when outdoors and as a treatment table with or without wheels with a detachable intravenous stand. Also suited for the field is the rescue and military foldable stretchers, mobile model 48, model 60 (length=1140mm width=670 mm, height = 785 mm, weighing17 kg with case of dimensions 1080x350x120 mm weighing 11 kg, with stand and 2 inflated tyre wheels. This is compatibile with most ambulances/rescue vehicles. Manufacturers are Hans Stollenwerk and Cie, W Germany (Fig. 54.2).

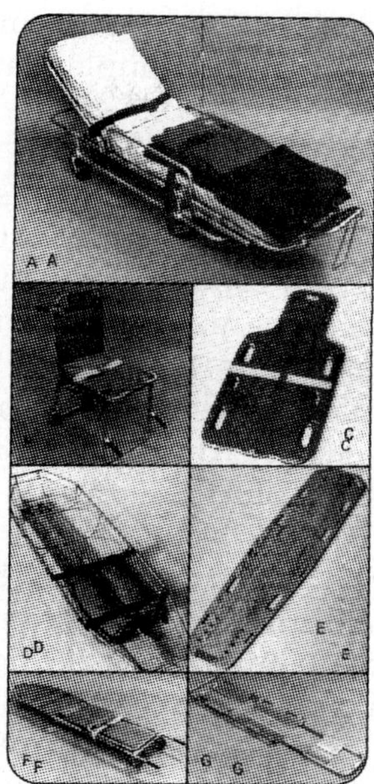

Fig. 54.2: Patient carying devices (A) Wheeled (B) Folding stair chair (C) Short spine board (D) Basket (E) Long spine board (F) Folding (G) Scoop

Further Reading

Stretchers – Yesterday and Today. Ingka E Reimann. Medical Corps International, 1986;4:14-19.

PACKAGING/SECURING A VICTIM

This involves a sequence of operations to ready the victim for a move without aggravating his or her condition. Wound dressing and fracture immobilization must be completed and impaled objects must be stabilized. The patient is swathed in a bed sheet and blanket and secured to the victim-carrying device. Metalline rescue and carrying blankets are sterile sheets 140 x 205 cm in size when opened and ideal for short-range transportation of injured patients and prevention of heat losses as well as being non adherent to wounds due to their porous and aluminized finish. Textile bands enable snug binding of victims especially those with thermal injuries. Lohmann GmbH Co of FDR manufactures this. Drapes must not hang loose and a plastic sheet may be needed during wet weather. For thermal injuries, Water-Jel dressings available from full blanket size 244cm x 183 cm down to 5cm x 15 cm size confers wound protection by preventing further contamination, stabilizes skin temperature, prevents hypothermia and eases pain in one fast and simple manner.

Patients With Spinal Injuries

Injury to the spine must be considered whenever there are serious injuries to other parts of the body. A complete patient assessment is vital to recognize such a problem, especially where there have been sudden deceleration trauma, e.g., being thrown against the dashboard etc. The dorsal spine and the sacral spine are usually unaffected due to attachments of to the ribs and pelvis respectively. The cervical and lumbar vertebrae are without such supports and vulnerable to whiplash accidents and while lifting heavy weights. In the whiplash type of injury, the neck quickly whips back and forth far in excess of the normal range of motion, e.g., during car collisions, striking an object dead-on. The spine can also be injured during falls from heights, sports accidents, diving-board mishaps and during contact sports.

The spine should be protected at all times during the management of the multiply injured patient. The ideal position is with the whole spine immobilised in a neutral position on a firm surface. This may be achieved manually or with a combination of semi-rigid cervical collar, side head supports and strapping. Strapping should be applied to the shoulders and pelvis as well as the head to prevent the neck becoming the centre of rotation of the body. Manual spinal protection should be instituted immediately. The application of definitive immobilisation devices should not take precedence over life-saving procedures. If the neck is not in the neutral position, an attempt should be made to achieve alignment. If the patient is awake and co-operative, they should actively move their neck into line. If unconscious or unable to co-operate this is done passively. If there is any pain, neurological deterioration or resistance to movement the procedure should be abandoned and the neck splinted in the current position. Long spine (rescue) boards are valuable primarily for extrication from vehicles. Repeated transfers to and from the board may compromise spinal protection and induce a significant amount of spinal movement. Patients may also be transferred on a scoop stretcher and/or vacuum mattress. There is little place for the short spine board or spinal extrication devices in the prehospital environment (Fig. 54.3).

Indicators of Spinal Injury

Pain, tenderness, deformity over the spinal column area, impaired breathing, numbness, tingling or loss of sensation or motor power in limbs, involuntary/ loss of bowel/bladder function and priapism (Fig. 54.4).

First aid protocols for suspected cases of spinal injury

Manual traction for head and neck in the axial plane by applying a rigid-type of cervical collar of appropriate size such that the front width of the collar fits snugly between the point of the chin and the chest at the jugular notch (Figs. 54.5 and 54.6).

Immobilization using short spine boards or Kendrick extrication devices for sitting patients. The board is slipped behind the victim with its smooth side towards the patient and properly centred while employing a modified log-roll to ensure neutral alignment of the entire spine. Four rescuers are needed for this manouver. One applies gentle manual inline immobilization of the victims head and neck and applies a semi-rigid cervical collar. The other places the victims arms alongside the torso with palms facing inwards and the victims legs straight in neutral alignment with ankles bound by a cravat. The third person holds the victim at the shoulder and wrist, while another grasps the victims

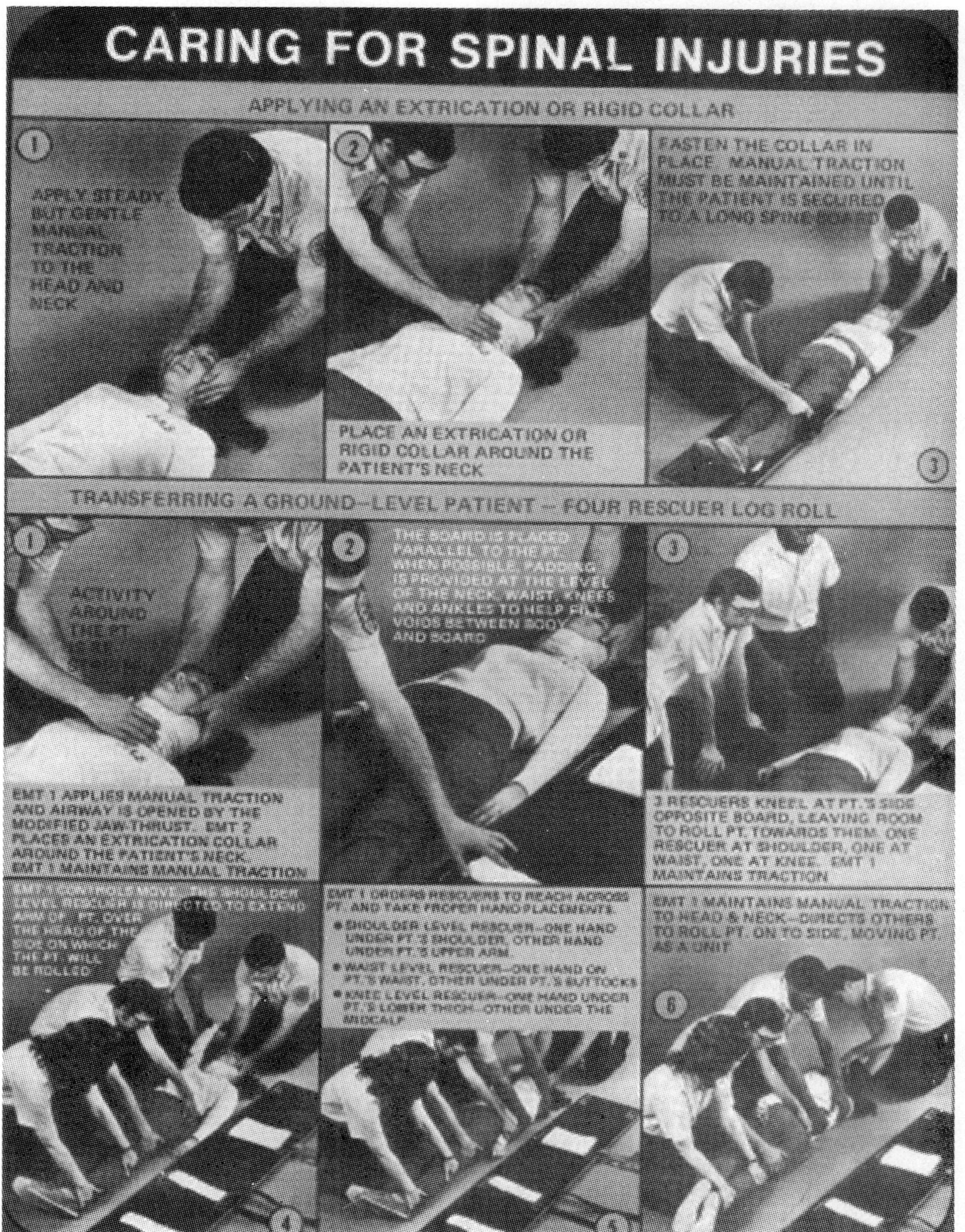
CARING FOR SPINAL INJURIES
APPLYING AN EXTRICATION OR RIGID COLLAR
1
APPLY STEADY BUT GENTLE MANUAL TRACTION TO THE HEAD AND NECK
2
PLACE AN EXTRICATION OR RIGID COLLAR AROUND THE PATIENT'S NECK
FASTEN THE COLLAR IN PLACE. MANUAL TRACTION MUST BE MAINTAINED UNTIL THE PATIENT IS SECURED TO A LONG SPINE BOARD
3
TRANSFERRING A GROUND–LEVEL PATIENT – FOUR RESCUER LOG ROLL
1
ACTIVITY AROUND THE PT.
EMT 1 APPLIES MANUAL TRACTION AND AIRWAY IS OPENED BY THE MODIFIED JAW-THRUST. EMT 2 PLACES AN EXTRICATION COLLAR AROUND THE PATIENT'S NECK. EMT 1 MAINTAINS MANUAL TRACTION
2
THE BOARD IS PLACED PARALLEL TO THE PT. WHEN POSSIBLE. PADDING IS PROVIDED AT THE LEVEL OF THE NECK, WAIST, KNEES AND ANKLES TO HELP FILL VOIDS BETWEEN BODY AND BOARD
3
3 RESCUERS KNEEL AT PT.'S SIDE OPPOSITE BOARD, LEAVING ROOM TO ROLL PT. TOWARDS THEM. ONE RESCUER AT SHOULDER, ONE AT WAIST, ONE AT KNEE. EMT 1 MAINTAINS TRACTION
EMT 1 CONTROLS MOVE. THE SHOULDER LEVEL RESCUER IS DIRECTED TO EXTEND ARM OF PT. OVER THE HEAD OF THE SIDE ON WHICH THE PT. WILL BE ROLLED
4
EMT 1 ORDERS RESCUERS TO REACH ACROSS PT. AND TAKE PROPER HAND PLACEMENTS
• SHOULDER LEVEL RESCUER—ONE HAND UNDER PT.'S SHOULDER, OTHER HAND UNDER PT.'S UPPER ARM
• WAIST LEVEL RESCUER—ONE HAND ON PT.'S WAIST, OTHER UNDER PT.'S BUTTOCKS
• KNEE LEVEL RESCUER—ONE HAND UNDER PT.'S LOWER THIGH—OTHER UNDER THE MIDCALF
5
EMT 1 MAINTAINS MANUAL TRACTION TO HEAD & NECK—DIRECTS OTHERS TO ROLL PT. ON TO SIDE, MOVING PT. AS A UNIT
6

Fig. 54.3a

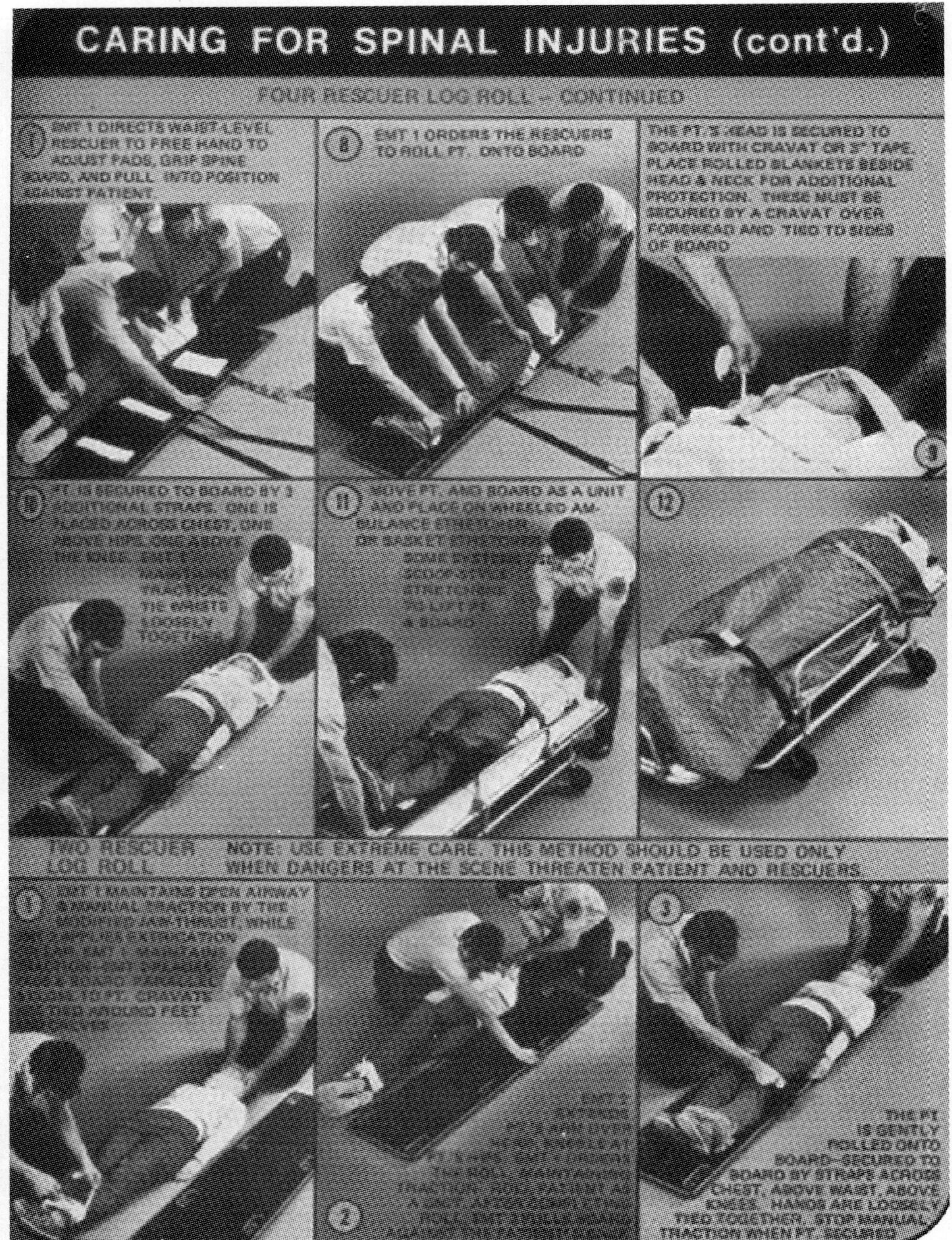
CARING FOR SPINAL INJURIES (cont'd.)
FOUR RESCUER LOG ROLL – CONTINUED
EMT 1 DIRECTS WAIST-LEVEL RESCUER TO FREE HAND TO ADJUST PADS, GRIP SPINE BOARD, AND PULL INTO POSITION AGAINST PATIENT.
8
EMT 1 ORDERS THE RESCUERS TO ROLL PT. ONTO BOARD
THE PT.'S HEAD IS SECURED TO BOARD WITH CRAVAT OR 3" TAPE. PLACE ROLLED BLANKETS BESIDE HEAD & NECK FOR ADDITIONAL PROTECTION. THESE MUST BE SECURED BY A CRAVAT OVER FOREHEAD AND TIED TO SIDES OF BOARD
PT. IS SECURED TO BOARD BY 3 ADDITIONAL STRAPS. ONE IS PLACED ACROSS CHEST, ONE ABOVE HIPS, ONE ABOVE THE KNEE.
11
MOVE PT. AND BOARD AS A UNIT AND PLACE ON WHEELED AM-
12
TWO RESCUER LOG ROLL
NOTE: USE EXTREME CARE. THIS METHOD SHOULD BE USED ONLY WHEN DANGERS AT THE SCENE THREATEN PATIENT AND RESCUERS.
EMT 1 MAINTAINS OPEN AIRWAY & MANUAL TRACTION BY THE MODIFIED JAW-THRUST, WHILE
THE PT IS GENTLY ROLLED ONTO BOARD—SECURED TO BOARD BY STRAPS ACROSS CHEST, ABOVE WAIST, ABOVE KNEES. HANDS ARE LOOSELY TIED TOGETHER. STOP MANUAL TRACTION WHEN PT. SECURED

Fig. 54.3b

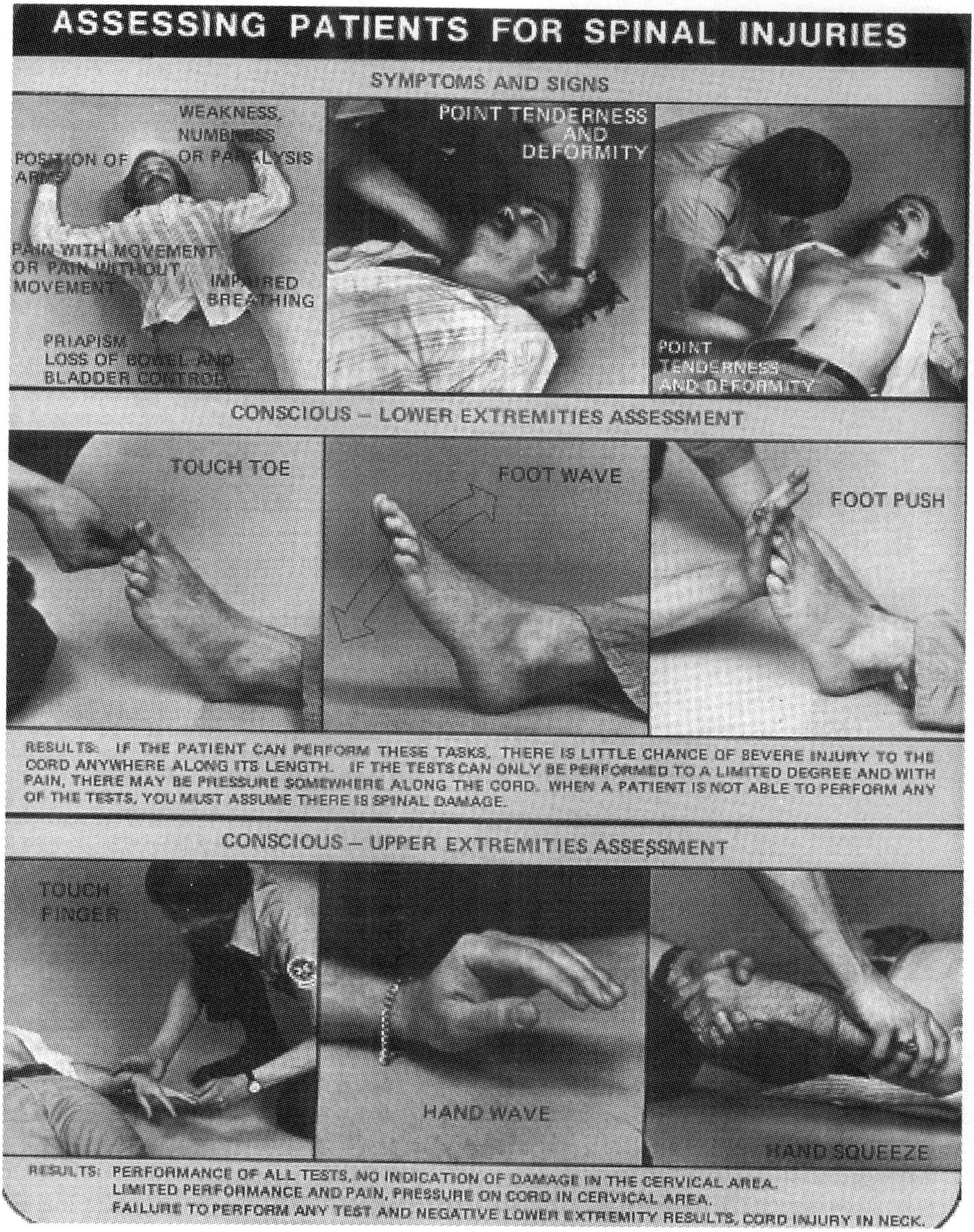

ASSESSING PATIENTS FOR SPINAL INJURIES

SYMPTOMS AND SIGNS

WEAKNESS, NUMBNESS OR PARALYSIS

POSITION OF ARMS

PAIN WITH MOVEMENT OR PAIN WITHOUT MOVEMENT

IMPAIRED BREATHING

PRIAPISM LOSS OF BOWEL AND BLADDER CONTROL

POINT TENDERNESS AND DEFORMITY

POINT TENDERNESS AND DEFORMITY

CONSCIOUS – LOWER EXTREMITIES ASSESSMENT

TOUCH TOE

FOOT WAVE

FOOT PUSH

RESULTS: IF THE PATIENT CAN PERFORM THESE TASKS, THERE IS LITTLE CHANCE OF SEVERE INJURY TO THE CORD ANYWHERE ALONG ITS LENGTH. IF THE TESTS CAN ONLY BE PERFORMED TO A LIMITED DEGREE AND WITH PAIN, THERE MAY BE PRESSURE SOMEWHERE ALONG THE CORD. WHEN A PATIENT IS NOT ABLE TO PERFORM ANY OF THE TESTS, YOU MUST ASSUME THERE IS SPINAL DAMAGE.

CONSCIOUS – UPPER EXTREMITIES ASSESSMENT

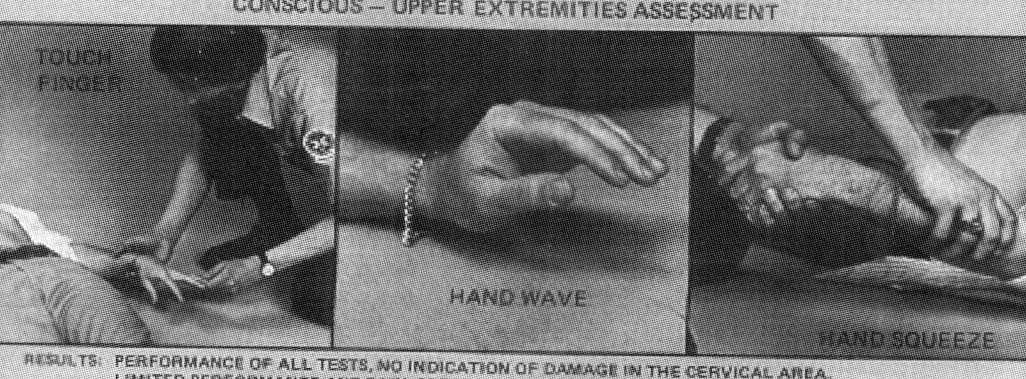

RESULTS: PERFORMANCE OF ALL TESTS, NO INDICATION OF DAMAGE IN THE CERVICAL AREA.
LIMITED PERFORMANCE AND PAIN, PRESSURE ON CORD IN CERVICAL AREA.
FAILURE TO PERFORM ANY TEST AND NEGATIVE LOWER EXTREMITY RESULTS, CORD INJURY IN NECK.

Fig. 54.4

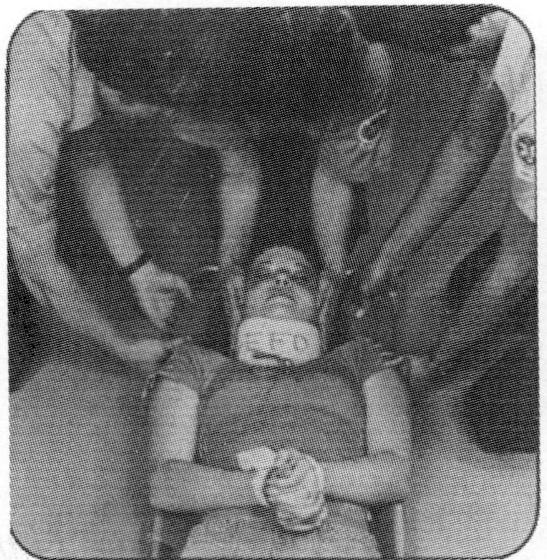

Fig. 54.5: The vinyl head support is properly positioned

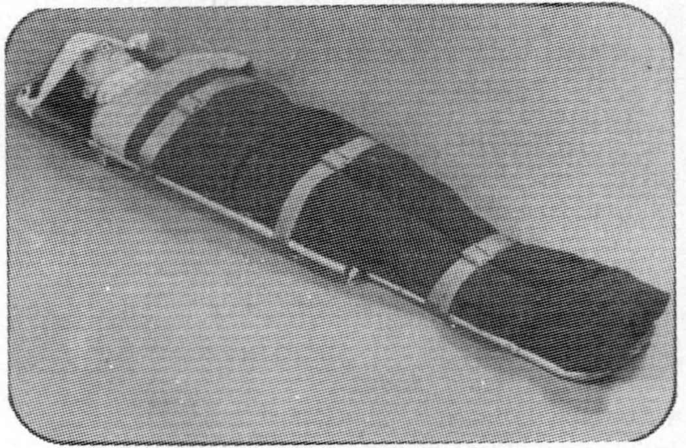

Fig. 54.6: A patient properly positioned, covered and secured on a scoop-style stretcher

hips beyond his wrist with one hand and the cravat binding the ankles with the other and then gently log-rolls the victim while the spine board is slipped underneath. The straps are then applied with adequate padding to ensure patient comfort and total immobilization. If the victim is retained on a spine board for more than 2 hours, good padding must be ensured over the occiput, scapulae, sacrum and heels to prevent pressure sores. Three inch cravats can be used to secure the lower head and neck. Removal of the victim from the spine board must be done by a similar pre planned drill, taking care to avoid rotation, flexion, extension, lateral bending and shearing-type movements of the back in any direction. No part of the victims body must be allowed to sag during transfer (Fig. 54.7).

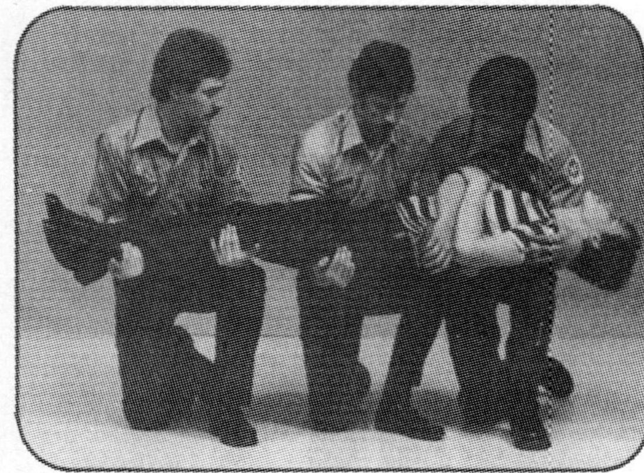

Fig. 54.7: The EMTs raise the patient to their knees so that he can be placed in the stretcher

For those wearing helmets, two rescuers are needed to remove the device. One to maintain manual traction in the axial plane with either hand on the side of the lower jaw while the other removes the chin strap and maintains traction by counter pressure applied with the hands placed under the chin and occipital process.

For lying patients, long spinal boards are used.

A newer immobilization device, the Dispos-O-Bag is a lightweight foam-filled sandbag made of puncture-resistant sealed-seam envelope and suitable for head and neck stabilization. No single method can consistently place the spine in neutral position or prevent all motion in the axial spine. Cervical Collars (c-collars) encircle the cervical spine and soft tissues of the neck, effecting snug fit between the tip of the chin and the suprasternal notch of the anterior chest, occiput and the suprascapular region of the back. These collars limit movement of the head in the coronal and transverse planes, minimizing lateral and rotary motion. They do not, immobilize in the sagittal plane (flexion-extension motion) For this reason, a rigid cervical collar alone is inadequate for effective spinal immobilization and must used with CID (Cervical Immobilization Device)and spine board (short or long). Soft neck collars are ineffective at limiting motion of the head in all planes and must not be used for spinal immobilization. CIDs are made of plastic, cardboard or foam. They act to pad the lateral aspects the head and limit both lateral and rotary motion, fixing the patient head and c-collar to a rigid spine board by restraining straps. CIDs can be fashioned from blanket rolls, blocks, or sand bags placed alongside the head and fixed to the spine board by 2 to 3 inch silk tapes placed over the forehead and chin.

Too much traction will cause distraction of the cervical spine and aggravate spinal cord injury.

Intubation, if indicated, is best done by the oral route, avoiding flexion of the neck and using in-line immobilization and newer laryngoscopes like

GUIDELINES FOR SCREENING PATIENTS WITH SUSPECTED

C-SPINE INJURY

1. **The presence of paraplegia or quadriplegia is presumptive evidence of spinal instability.**
2. **Patients who are awake, alert, sober, neurologically normal, and have no neck pain; and have no other painful distracting injury:** These patients are extremely unlikely to have an acute c-spine fracture/subluxation. With the patient. in a supine position, remove the c-collar and palpate the spine. If there is no significant tenderness, ask the patient to voluntarily move his or her neck from side to side. If there is no pain, have the patient voluntarily flex and extend his or her neck. Again, if there is no pain, c-spine films are not mandatory.
3. **Patients who are awake and alert, are neurologically normal, but do have neck pain:** The burden of proof is on the doctor to exclude a spinal injury. All such patients should undergo lateral, AP, and open-mouth X-rays of the c-spine. If these films are normal, remove the c-collar. Under the care of a knowled-geable doctor, ask the patient to voluntarily flex his or her neck and obtain a lateral flexion X-ray. If the film shows no subluxation, the patient's c-spine can be cleared and the c-collar kept off. However, if any of these films are suspicious or unclear, replace the collar and obtain a CT scan of the levels in question.
4. **Patients who are comatose, have an altered level of consciousness, or are too young to describe their symptoms:** All such patients should at least have a lateral and AP c-spine X-ray. Whenever possible, an open-mouth view also should be obtained. If the entire c-spine can be visualized and is found to be normal, the collar can be removed after appropriate evaluation by a neurosurgeon or orthopedic surgeon.
5. **When in doubt, leave the collar on:** A cervical CT scan can be obtained somewhat later when the patient's other acute problems have been managed.
6. **Consult:** The neurosurgery or orthopedic service should be consulted in all cases where a spine injury is detected of suspected.

7. **Backboards:** Patients who have neurologic deficits (quadriplegia or paraplegia) should be evaluated quickly and taken off the backboard as soon as possible. A paralyzed patient who is allowed to lie on a hard board for more than 2 hours is at high risk for developing serious decubiti.
8. **Never force the neck:** Under no circumstances should a patient's neck be forced into flexion or extension. When performed voluntarily by the patient, these maneuvers are generally safe.
9. **Emergency situations:** In certain instances, the presence of an intracranial. hematoma or other emergency may require the patient to be rushed to the operating room before a complete work-up of the spine can be completed. In such instances the c-collar should be left on and the patient moved carefully as though a spinal fracture were present. The surgical team should then take particular care to protect the neck as much as possible during the operation. The anesthesiologist should be informed of the status of the work-up.
10. **Assess the c-spine film for** (a) bony deformity, (b) fracture of the vertebral body or processes, (c) loss of alignment of the posterior aspect of the vertebral bodies (anterior extent of the vertebral canal), (d):l increased distances between the spinous processes at one level, (e) narrowing of the vertebral canal, and (f) increased prevertebral soft-tissue space (>5 mm Opposite C-3).

Inj methylprednisolone 30mg/kg I/V over 45 minutes within the first 15 minutes following injury (and not later than 8 hours after the injury) can improve neurologic outcome. This is followed by the same drug in a dose of 5.4 mg/kg/h I/V over the next 23 hours by infusion. Inj Methylene blue is also an exciting new development.

Table 54.1: Spine X-ray suggestions

Abnormal findings	*Diagnoses to consider*
Any c-spine bony abnormality	Cord compromise
C-spine injury	Airway compromise
Facial fracture	C-spine injury
Upper rib fracture	C-spine injury Upper thoracic spine injury Great vessel injury Brachioplexus injury
Clavicular fracture	C-spine injury Upper thoracic spine injury Great vessel injury Brachioplexus injury
Head injury	C-spine injury Upper thoracic spine injury.
Lower thoracic spine fracture	Pancreatic injury

Crush Syndrome

Crush syndrome was first described by Bywater in the British Medical Journal in 1941 after the London Blitz. Also known as traumatic rhabdomyolysis or *Bywaters' syndrome,* it is a serious condition characterized by shock and renal failure following a crushing injury to skeletal muscle. Incidence is 2-5% in victims trapped under fallen masonry or rubble. Crush syndrome is a reperfusion injury that appears after the release of the crushing pressure. The mechanism is believed to be the release into the bloodstream of muscle breakdown products – notably myoglobin, potassium, phosphorus, CPK-MM and urate that are the products of the breakdown of skeletal muscle damaged under ischemic conditions. There is increased permeability of the cell membrane and to the release of potassium, enzymes, and myoglobin from within cells. If a significant amount of skeletal muscle is damaged (>100 g), excess myoglobin is filtered by the kidneys and can cause renal tubular obstruction and acute renal failure as myoglobin is nephrotoxic. Ischemic renal dysfunction secondary to hypotension due to sequestration of water in the injured muscle cells results in diminished renal perfusion reflected as raised urea, creatinine and oliguria in victims. Metabolic acidosis due to release of cellular phosphate and sulphate from the injured muscle cells is compounded by hypoxia due to asphyxiation. Hypocalcemia can also occur. Disseminated intravascular coagulopathy is a usually terminal event.

Presentation

Clinical features can include:

Obvious muscle injury with pain, swelling, bruising and tenderness, tea-coloured urine may be an early sign, nausea, vomiting, confusion and agitation, profound hypovolaemic shock, there may be loss of sensation and muscle power in the affected body part and the limb/body part may be pulseless.

Blood Tests

These should include: Urea and electrolytes, including potassium, creatinine, calcium (there may be hypocalcaemia), phosphate, creatine kinase (rhabdomyolysis has been defined as total creatine kinase levels 5-10 times above normal in a patient with typical symptoms and/or risk factors), uric acid (may be raised), full blood count and clotting studies (to look for evidence of DIC), liver function tests (may show hepatic dysfunction), arterial blood gas studies and correction of base deficit if any.

Other Investigations

- Urine dipsticks for myoglobin (but this is only positive in 50% of cases of rhabdomyolysis so a negative dipstick does not exclude it).
- ECG may show changes secondary to hyperkalaemia.
- The usual assessment for trauma, including X-rays should be performed.
- Assessment of compartment pressures may be needed if compartment syndrome is a concern (focal muscle tenderness and firm muscle compartment).

Treatment

- The patient must be assessed in keeping with the usual criteria for assessing a severely injured person.
- Assessment of Airway, Breathing and Circulation should be carried out initially.
- Attention should be given to life-threatening injuries. Give Inj Tetglob 250-500 IU and a broad spectrum antibiotic early.
- Early, vigorous hydration helps preserve renal function.
- Venous access should be obtained as early as possible, ideally before the trapped limb is freed and decompressed.
- Because of the very high risk of acute renal failure, a catheter should be inserted at an early stage and urine output monitored.
- Because of the need to maintain fluid balance, a CVP line is usually required.
- A high index of suspicion is necessary at the time of extrication and a saline infusion of 1000-1500 ml/h should be initiated to ensure a urine output of 300ml/h. If the urine remains tea-colored forced mannitol-alkaline diuresis up to 8 litres/day should be maintained keeping urine pH greater than 6.5 as alkalinization with sodium bicarbonate increases the urine solubility of acid hematin and aids in its excretion. This must be continued until myoglobin is no longer detected in the urine. Mannitol also is an effective scavenger of oxygen free radicals and may help reduce the reperfusion component of injury. Once the

patient reaches hospital, 5% dextrose should be alternated with normal saline to reduce the potential sodium load. Creatine kinase levels peak within 24 hours and should then decrease by 30-40% per day. Serial measurements will be needed. If levels continue to elevate, consider ongoing muscle injury or compartment syndrome. Haemodialysis may be needed in some cases and DIC will need treatment with fresh frozen plasma, cryoprecipitate and platelets.

Compartment Syndrome

Defined as increased pressure within a confined space that leads to micro-vascular compromise and ultimately to cell death as a result of oxygen starvation. It can occur after a crush injury because of the uptake of fluid into muscle cells contained within a tight compartment. Once compartment pressure exceeds capillary perfusion pressure (about 30 mmHg), the tissue inside the compartment becomes ischaemic, with disastrous consequences, including paralysis, loss of limb or life itself.

Causes

- Trauma—hematoma, animal/insect bites, crush injury.
- Edema related—frostbite, burns, overuse injuries.
- Cooagulopathies—genetic, iatrogenic or acquired.
- Other causes—external compression (MAST, tight bandaging).

Signs and Symptoms—The 5 P's

Pain: This is most common and consistent sign; described as out of proportion to normal clinical condition. The pain is usually diffuse and intense, exacerbated by movement, touch, pressure or stretch.

Paresthesias (or anesthesia): numbness or complete loss of feeling below compartment area with distal radiation.

Passive stretch: severe pain when muscles in the affected compartment are stretched.

Pressure: Palpable tenseness in affected compartment (very tight to feel, sometimes warm).

Pulselessness: Least reliable and often seen only in late stages as microvasculature is affected. The major vessels are not affected initially.

Management

- Do not try to cool area with ice as it exacerbates the existing vasoconstriction.
- Do not elevate the limb but keep in a position of comfort.
- Splint for comfort and protect only when necessary (during transportation).
- Transport to appropriate medical facility.

Administer Inj Fentanyl 1 mcg/kg I/V as it provides pain relief comparable to Morphine without causing vasodilation.

Surgical

- Fasciotomy is useful in reducing muscle damage from compartment syndrome. It should be done early. Field fasciotomy may be performed; cut through tissue and fascia, tweeze muscle fibers apart, don't cut muscles.
- It may be necessary to amputate crushed limbs. Amputation at an early stage may prevent crush syndrome and gangrene. This can be done as an emergency on site under ketamine anesthesia after suitable premedication and with oxygen supplementation.

Complications

- Hyperkalaemia and infection are the commonest causes of death. Hyperkalaemia can lead to dysrrhythmias and cardiac arrest. Infection is a major cause of death in disaster zones.

- Acute renal failure can occur.
- Disseminated intravascular coagulation can occur when tissue damage is extensive.
- Creatine kinase levels peak within 24 hours and should then decrease by 30-40% per day. Serial measurements will be needed. If levels continue to elevate, consider ongoing muscle injury or compartment syndrome.

Prognosis

- Adequate fluid support improves prognosis.
- The earthquake in Marmara, Northern Turkey in 1999 has been well documented when the mortality rate for crush syndrome was estimated at 15.2%.
- Time duration under the rubble did not seem to have an adverse effect on outcome but this may have been due to survivors being less severely injured. It has been recommended that recovery of survivors should continue for at least 5 days.
- Anyone who has been buried under rubble for a length of time may have other injuries like chest compression and spinal injuries.
- Tissue damage followed by irreversible tissue death usually occurs within 4-12 hours depending on compartmental pressure; permanent disabilities can develop from undiagnosed compartment syndrome.

Prevention

- In any major disaster, adequate triage must carried out to identify those in need of urgent attention. This may have a marked effect on morbidity and mortality.
- Adequate rehydration reduces the risk of acute renal failure in crush syndrome.
- Amputation at an early stage may prevent mortality from crush syndrome.

Further Reading

1. Malinoski DJ, Slater MS, Mullins RJ; Crush injury and rhabdomyolysis.; *Crit Care Clin.* 2004 Jan;20(1):171-92.
2. Craig S; Rhabdomyolysis. eMedicine, August 2008.
3. Knochel JP; Mechanisms of rhabdomyolysis. Curr Opin Rheumatol 1993 Nov;5(6):725-31.
4. Sauret JM, Marinides G, Wang GK; Rhabdomyolysis. Am Fam Physician. 2002 Mar 1;65(5):907-12.
5. Wheelers' Textbook of Orthopaedics; Reperfusion Injury/Crush Injury.
6. Atef-Zafarmand A, Fadem S; Disaster nephrology: Medical perspective. *Adv Ren Replace Ther.* 2003 Apr 10(2):104-16.
7. Kazancioglu R, Cagatay A, Calangu S, et al; The characteristics of infections in crush syndrome.; *Clin Microbiol Infect.* 2002 Apr;8(4):202-6.
8. Sever MS, Erek E, Vanholder R, *et al.*, Lessons learned from the catastrophic Marmara earthquake: factors influencing the final outcome of renal victims.; *Clin Nephrol.* 2004 Jun;61(6):413-21.
9. Sever MS, Erek E, Vanholder R, *et al.*, Lessons learned from the Marmara disaster: Time period under the rubble.; *Crit Care Med.* 2002 Nov; 30(11):2443-9.
10. Bulut M, Fedakar R, Akkose S, *et al.*, Medical experience of a university hospital in Turkey after the 1999 Marmara earthquake.; *Emerg Med J* 2005 Jul 22(7):494-8.

CONCLUSION

Good pre hospital trauma care (PHTC) can prevent fatalities and limit or halt the cascade of events that may otherwise prove disastrous. Immediate care of wounds and hemostasis, immobilization of fractures, ensuring ade-quate airway, oxygenation and blood pressure at the site of an accident will improve outcome. PHTC must be simple, sustainable, practical, efficient and flexible. It is essentially a 3 tiered system. The first tier targets the first responders – the lay public, taxi drivers, firefighters, police personnel etc and teaches them basic first aid so that they can recognize an emergency, call for help and provide basic medical treatment and ensure safe rescue and transport of victims. They must be able to transport victims to the nearest hospital capable of definitive care which need not be the closest hospital or medical facility.The second tier teaches basic life support i.e. rescue, stabilization and treatment of the injured victims. The third tier teaches advan-ced life support to medical personnel. The PHTC system must be integrated into the existing health care, public health and transportation infrastructure. It cannot function in isolation and must be competent enough to attend to all emergencies including pediatric, adult and OBGY acute medical and surgical problems. It must have a universal, toll free, easy-to-remember telephonic access.

Keeping things moving in the right direction is one of the biggest challenges in the care of the critically ill victim. The chain of critical care must never be broken. From the field to the hospital, medical care must be continuum, if the therapeutic gains initiated by first responders are to be maintained. Behind even very small improvements in a severely ill patient, there is often a whole-hearted effort based on patience, knowledge, experience, untiring observation supported by high technology equipments. The transport of Priority 2 and 3 victims can easily upset the clinical condition dramatically during critical minutes. Hours of dedicated work can be wasted and, at best, be reconstructed with great effort. Transportation is often the weakest link in the chain of evacuation and every interruption carries a serious risk for the victim. With the right method, there is no patient who cannot be transported or evacuated. One must balance the risk of transportation against the benefits and ascertain that the patient is in a reasonably stable condition before any move. Flexibility and a patient-oriented attitude are vital to such efforts. Transportation adds stresses like pain due to movement and vibration, noise, heat or cold and mental stress. Monitoring must never be discontinued. Speed in transport can be decisive and all equipment must be lightweight and easy to handle. The sensitive transport phase is never the right situation to start therapeutic experiments. The rule here is 'noli me tangere' – translated to mean 'don't touch my patient' during transport. It is better to switch off audio alarms during transportation as these can create disturbing noises and add to the victim's stress. A well performing team is everything in emergency situations and competent staff must be assigned to transporting the critically ill.

55 Presence of Attenders/ Relatives During Trauma Resuscitation

THE ARGUMENTS AGAINST

Sensory Disturbance

Trauma resuscitations can be visually disturbing, even to the most experienced clinical staff. At an olfactory level, burns, blood and other secretions can result in unpleasant, upsetting smells in the trauma room. Similarly, one would imagine that patients who are crying out due to pain, hypoxic confusion or anxiety would cause an auditory disturbance for the relatives.

Confidentiality

If the patient is unconscious, it is not possible to gain their consent for witnessed resuscitation. Consequently, patient confidentiality may be broken if the patient's wishes are not known. Not only would the relatives see everything happening to the patient, they may hear information of an intensely personal nature. At a professional level, nursing and medical governing bodies suggest that no one, not even a loved one or relative is entitled to information which the patient does not want them to have.

Complaints/Litigation

Staff may fear that during a witnessed resuscitation, an observed action or remark may offend relatives, leading to a complaint. Fear of allowing observation of medical procedures may increase the risk of litigation against the hospital or the practitioner.

Staff Response

Nursing, medical and paramedical staff use a variety of methods to deal with the stress of trauma resuscitations. Some bleak situations may be peppered with a small degree of humour, which can help to keep the team functioning under stress. The presence of a relative may inhibit this coping mechanism, thereby affecting team perfor-mance. Doctors and medical personnel may want to be detached about what is going on around, and even making occasional light-hearted comments.

Relatives Emotional Response

This is often cited as an argument against witnessed resuscitation. Emergency room staff interviewed about this suggested that panic by relatives disrupts medical efforts. There is a fear that uncontrollable relative grief can disrupt the team.

Clinical Performance

With a relative present, there is a pressure for the trauma team to perform well. This may be inhibited by a reluctance to discuss the patients condition in front of the relative and unable to voice an opinion about the patients deteriorating condition. In addition, decision making may be delayed and the resuscitation may be kept going longer than usual. Furthermore, many procedures learned by doctors and nurses have to be done first time in vivo during a trauma call as there is a commitment to train junior colleagues. A senior doctor talking a more junior doctor through a chest drain insertion or a junior nurse taking blood from her first trauma patient may not be viewed positively by a grief stricken relative.

THE ARGUMENTS FOR

Respecting the Relatives (and Possibly the Patients) Wishes

It is presumed that patients are resuscitated to save their lives and return them to their family and friends. The wishes of close relatives should be respected. Most professionals would prefer relatives not to be present but near and dear would be keen to be present and just hold the victim's hand to offer a token comfort.

Seeing

By allowing relatives to see what is happening to their loved one, even for a short period of time, may help to dispel terrible imagery or anxiety. Relatives can then see that everything possible is being done for their loved one(s).

Media Influences

Whilst it would be naïve to imagine that a medical docu-drama or soap could completely prepare a relative for trauma resuscitation, the public may be more informed than we think. The media obsession with this type of programme does graphically bring to the living room the close up workings of an emergency room as never before.

Staff Attitudes

Some emergency personnel are accepting and comfortable with witnessed resuscitation. Results from a study into medical and nursing staff attitudes showed that the more senior and experienced the member of staff (in both resuscitation and caring for upset relatives), the more likely it was for them to agree with allowing relatives into the emergency room. The emergency room staff have developed guidelines and a support structure for these interactions with some success as evidenced by the following:

- No evidence of relatives interfering.
- Some incidence of hysteria where relatives were led away from the resuscitation.
- Witnessed trauma resuscitation is now practiced.
- Children are allowed to be present.
- An excellent support system is available for relatives.
- Staff regard patients as part of a community, not merely a clinical challenge.

In a study into whether relatives wished to be present during resuscitation and also if there were any adverse psychological side effects, the hospital staff made the following observations:

- No relatives commented on any technical procedures – problems (including a difficult intubation).
- All relatives felt that it had been beneficial to be present.
- Trends towards lower degrees of intrusive imagery, post traumatic stress disorder, and grief related symptoms.
- Staff viewed the patient as a valued family member.

There was little evidence to support the exclusion of relatives who wished to be present during resuscitation.

In summary, this complex and controversial issue has many implications. It is an area that needs more research. Considerations of staff availability, support personnel, training costs and relative follow up all need to be addressed. Language and cultural barriers can be problematic when discussing this sensitive issue with relatives. However, one recommendation that can be made *is to treat each trauma case individually, considering the patient's and relatives' wishes.*

Further Reading

1. Fullbrook S, 'Medico legal insights, legal implications of relatives witnessing resuscitation' British Journal of Theatre Nursing 7, 1998;10:33-35.
2. United Kingdom Central Council, 'Code of Professional Conduct for the Nurse, Midwife and Health Visitor' 3rd Ed. London, June 1992.
3. Schilling R 'No room for spectators' (letter) BMJ 309 406,1994.
4. Redley B, Hood K, 'Staff attitudes towards family presence during resuscitation' Accident and Emergency Nursing 1996;4:145-151.
5. Hanson C, Strawser D, 'Family presence during cardio-pulmonary resuscitation: Foote Hospital ED nine year perspective' Journal of Emergency Nursing 1992;18:104-106.
6. Adams S, Whitlock M, Bloomfield P, Baskett P, 'Should relatives be allowed to watch resuscitation?' BMJ 1994;308:1687-1689.
7. Martin J, 'Rethinking traditional thoughts' Journal of Emergency Nursing 1991;17:67-68.
8. Mitchell M, Lynch M, 'Should relatives be allowed in the resuscitation room?' Journal of Accident and Emergency Medicine 1997;14:366-369.
9. Robinson SM, Mackenzie-oss S, *et al.*, 'Psychological effect of witnessed resuscitation on bereaved relatives' The Lancet 1998;352:614-617.
10. Small G and Pryse B, 'Witnessed resuscitation and bereavement services' 3M A and E Focus 3M Health Care 1999;10:19-21.

56 Oil Rig Disaster

INTRODUCTION

Drilling or digging for oil has occurred in one way or another for hundreds of years. The Chinese, for instance, invented a bamboo rig to obtain oil and gas for lighting and cooking. But only in the last 40 years has humankind been able to efficiently extract petroleum from beneath the seas – an achievement to rank with this century's mightiest technological triumphs.

Nearly 90 per cent of our petroleum wealth is found offshore. The search is difficult, extremely expensive, and often fruitless—but critical to a nation's economic future. Locating an oil and gas "trap"—as it is known—and extracting the oil and gas is difficult enough on land. But offshore, in deep and often stormy waters, it becomes an awesome undertaking.

Potential traps are identified by analysing seismic survey data but whether they contain oil or gas won't be known until a drill bit penetrates the structure. Directing the drill bit to a precise location—perhaps several kilometres away—requires sophisticated computer technology. A navigation device installed above the drill bit feeds back information which enables the exact position of the well to be measured and monitored. A steerable motor within the drill pipe can be remotely controlled to adjust the direction of the drill.

Four Drilling Rig Types

In the early days of offshore drilling, explorers simply fitted a derrick to a barge and towed it to their site. Today, four types of offshore rigs are used to drill wildcat or exploration wells.

- *Submersibles:* These are rarely used. They can be floated to shallow water locations then ballasted to sit on the seabed.
- *Jackups:* Usually towed to a location. Their legs are then lowered to the seabed and the hull is jacked-up clear of the sea surface. Used in waters to about 160 metres deep.
- *Drill ship:* These look like ordinary ships but have a derrick on top which drills through a hole in the hull. Drill ships are either anchored or positioned with computer-controlled propellers along the hull which continually correct the ships drift. Often used to drill "wildcat" wells in deep waters.
- *Semi submersible:* Mobile structures, some with their own locomotion. Their superstructures are supported by columns sitting on hulls or pontoons which are ballasted below the water surface. They provide excellent stability in rough, deep seas.

Production Platforms

Once oil or gas is discovered, the drilling rig is generally replaced by a production platform, assembled at the site using a barge equipped with heavy lift cranes. Platforms vary in size, shape and type depending on the size of the field, the water depth and the distance from shore. For medium to large fields, fixed production platforms are commonly used. These are made of steel and fixed to the seabed with steel piles. These platforms house all the processing equipment and accommodate up to 80 workers who typically work a 12 hours day, one week on and one week off. There are also concrete structures which are big enough to store oil. Gravity holds them on the seabed. The world's biggest platforms are bigger than a football field and rise above the water as high as a 25 storey office tower. They are home to nearly 500 workers.

If the field is in shallow water and near land or another platform, small remotely controlled monopod platforms may be used. Another system is a floating structure, either anchored or tethered, called a Floating Production Storage Offloading (FPSO) vessel.

Another platform type, suitable for deep water production, is the Tension Leg platform, built of steel or concrete and anchored to the sea floor with vertical "tendons".

Drilling For Oil

The first stage of drilling is called "spudding" and drilling starts when the drill bit is lowered into the seabed. The bit can be of two types: - a roller cone or rock bit which usually has three cones armed with steel or tungsten carbide : teeth:; or buttons; or—a diamond bit, imbedded with small industrial diamonds. The drill bit is attached to drill pipe (or a drill string) and rotated by a turntable on the platform floor. As the hole deepens, extra lengths of drill pipe are attached. A length of drill pipe is 30 feet long, or 9.1 metres (oil workers use the old imperial measurement system). The drill bit ranges in diameter from 36 inches or approximately 91.4 centimetres (used at the start of the hole) to eight and a half inches (approximately 21.5 centimetres). Drilling may take weeks or months before the targeted location is reached. The major potential environmental effects from offshore drilling result from the discharge of wastes, including drilling fluids, drill cuttings and "produced formation water" (PFW).

Drilling Fluid

Drilling fluid is pumped down the drill pipe and into the hole at high velocity through nozzles in the drill bit. The fluid is usually a mixture of water, clay, a weighting material (usually barite), and various chemicals. The drilling fluid serves several purposes. It raises the drill cutting to the surface for disposal; it provides the "weight" to keep the underground pressures in check; it keeps the hold stable by caking the wall with a thin layer of clay; and it cleans and cools the bit. The fluid is recycled through a circulation system where equipment mounted on the drilling rig separates out the drill cuttings and allows the clean fluid to be pumped back down the hole. Most have been drilled using water-based drilling fluids, not oil-based. The ISRC is of the opinion that drilling waste discharges have only minor effects on water quality and pelagic ecosystems and that acute toxic effects of drilling fluids on marine organisms are only found at very high concentrations within a few tens of metres from the point of discharge and only for short times after discharge. As the plume of drilling fluid and cuttings falls to the seabed, it disperses, with 90 percent of it settling within 100 metres of the platform. Soluble waste concentrations will have fallen by a factor of 10,000 within 100 metres and suspended sediment concentrations by a factor of at least 50,000.

Drill Cuttings

As the well is drilled, the "cuttings", consisting of crushed rock and clay, are brought to the surface by the drilling fluid and discharged overboard.

Produced Formation Water

Where you find oil, you often also find water. As oil is drawn from a reservoir, it is necessary to separate the water and return it to the ocean. This is what is known as "produced formation water" (PFW). Great emphasis is placed on ensuring that the water returned to the ocean is as free as possible from oil and chemicals. Strict regulations apply on how much petro-leum hydrocarbon is contained in PFW. The regulatory limit is 30 mg/litre average. Mechanical separation devices and chemical treatments are used to separate oil and water efficiently.

Directional Drilling

Drilling an oil well may not be a case of going straight down. Directional drilling has been developed where drill bits are steered laterally over a distance of up to several kilometres towards the petroleum reservoir. One production platform is often used to drill a number of wells, in a variety of directions and inclinations. To steer the drill bit, a downhole motor may be used. It is turned by pumping the drilling mud through it.

Completing the Well

When the well has been drilled to its target depth, production casing is set and cemented.Tubing is lowered into the hole together with "packers" which seal the space between the tubing and the casing. Finally, at the end of the well, the casing is perforated at predetermined depths by small explosive charges detonated remotely. The small holes in the casing allow the oil or gas under its natural pressure to flow to the surface.

A Dry Well

If the drilled hole is considered to be "dry" or not worth developing, the decision is made to "plug and abandon" it. This involves setting several cement plugs in the well.

Formation Kick

A kick can be the result of improper mud density control, an unexpected overpressured (shallow) gas pocket, or may be a result of the loss of drilling fluids to a formation called a *thief zone*. If the well is a development well (and not a wildcat), these thief zones should already be known to the driller and the proper loss control materials would have been used. However, unexpected fluid losses can occur if a formation is fractured somewhere in the open-hole section, causing rapid loss of hydrostatic pressure and possibly allowing flow of formation fluids into the well bore. Shallow overpressured gas pockets are generally unpredictable and usually cause the more violent kicks because of rapid gas expansion almost immediately.

The primary means of detecting a kick is a relative change in the circulation rate back up to the surface into the mud pits. The drilling crew or mud engineer keeps track of the level in the mud pits, and an increase in this level would indicate that a higher pressure zone has been encountered at the bit. Conversely, a drop in this level would indicate lost circulation to a formation (which might allow influx of formation fluids from other zones if the hydrostatic head at depth is reduced from less than a full column of mud). The rate of mud returns also can be closely monitored to match the rate that it is being pumped down the drill pipe. If the rate of returns is slower than expected, it means that a certain amount of the mud is being lost to a thief zone, but this is not necessarily yet a kick (and may never become one). In the case of a higher pressure zone, an increase in mud returns would be noticed as the formation influx pushes the drilling mud toward the surface at a higher rate.

The first response to detecting a kick would be to isolate the well bore from the surface by activating the BOPs and closing in the well. Then the drilling crew would attempt to circulate in a heavier *kill fluid* to increase the hydrostatic pressure (sometimes with the assistance of a well control company). In the process, the influx fluids will be slowly circulated out in a controlled manner, taking care not to allow any gas to accelerate up the wellbore too quickly by controlling casing pressure with chokes on a predetermined schedule. In a simple kill, once the kill-weight mud has reached the bit, the casing pressure is manipulated to keep drill pipe pressure constant (assuming a constant pumping rate); this will ensure holding a constant adequate bottom hole pressure. The casing pressure will gradually increase as the contaminant slug approaches the surface if the influx is gas, which will be expanding as it moves up the annulus and overall pressure at its depth is gradually decreasing. This effect will be minor if the influx fluid is mainly salt water. And with an oil-based drilling fluid it can be masked in the early stages of controlling a kick because gas influx may dissolve into the oil under pressure at depth, only to come out of solution and expand rather rapidly as the influx nears the surface. Once all the contaminant has been circulated out, the casing pressure should have reached zero.

Sometimes, however, companies drill underbalanced for better, faster penetration rates and thus they "drill for kicks" as it is economically sounder to take time to kill a kick than to drill overbalanced (which causes slower penetration rates). Under these circumstances, always with qualified personnel on the rig, calling in a "well control" specialist may not be necessary.

A Blowout

When all the controls described above fail, a blowout occurs. A blowout is the uncontrolled release of formation fluid from a well, typically for petroleum production, after pressure control systems have failed.

Blowouts are dangerous since they can eject the drill string out of the well, and the force of the escaping fluid can be strong enough to damage the drilling rig. Blowouts often ignite due to the presence of an ignition source, from sparks from rocks being ejected along with flammable fluids, or simply from heat generated by friction. (Rarely the flowing gas will contain poisonous hydrogen sulfide and the oil operator might decide to ignite the stream to convert this to less hazardous substances.) A well control company will then need to extinguish the well fire and/or cap the well, and replace the casing head and hangars.

Sometimes, blowouts can be so forceful that they cannot be directly brought under control from the surface, particularly if there is so much energy in the flowing zone that it does not deplete significantly over the course of a blowout. In such cases, other wells (called relief wells) may be drilled to intersect the well or pocket, in order to allow kill-weight fluids to be introduced at depth. (Contrary to what might be inferred from the term, such wells generally are not used to help relieve pressure using multiple outlets from the blowout zone.)

An "underground blowout" is a special situation where fluids from high pressure zones flow uncontrolled to lower pressure zones within the open-hole portion of the well bore. Usually they come up the well bore to shallower formations (typically near the last casing shoe) that have been fractured from the overall effect of hydrostatic mud head plus casing pressure imposed at the time of the initial kick. Underground blowouts can be very difficult to bring under control although there is no outward flow at the drill site itself. However, if left unchecked, in time the fluids may find their way to the surface elsewhere in the vicinity (possibly "cratering" the rig), or may pressurize other zones, leading to problems when drilling subsequent wells.

Cause of Blowouts

A blowout is caused when a combination of well control systems fail – primarily drilling mud hydrostatics and blow-out preventers (BOPs) – and formation pore pressure is greater than the well bore pressure at depth. When such an incident occurs, formation fluids begin to flow into the well bore and up the annulus and/or inside the drill pipe, and is commonly called a kick. If the well is not shut in (common term for the closing of the blow-out preventer valves), a kick can quickly escalate into a blowout when the formation fluids reach the surface, especially when the fluid is a gas which rapidly expands as it flows up the well bore, further decreasing the effective weight of the fluid, and accelerates to near the speed of sound. The flash point of gasoline is -43°C (-45°F), and considered highly flammable and its explosive range ranges from 1.3 to 6.0% vapor in air. Methane has a relatively high spontaneous ignition temperature of 537 deg. C (999 °F) and explosive range is 5 to 15%. This makes re-ignition of a methane fuel fire after extinguishment difficult. In practice, low-flash-point, low-spontaneous-ignition-temperature gas condensate blowouts present the greatest blowout ignition hazard. Crude oil is a highly volatile, explosive cocktail which is lighter than water and burns twice as hot as coal.

The gas and other hydrocarbons commonly ignite during a blow-out, creating explosions and vigorous fires which are difficult to extinguish. The pressure-feed fire of a blowout will totally destroy the surrounding steel structure in minutes. Derricks may collapse in less than 30 minutes after blowout ignition. The core temperature in a crude oil blowout can measure 1,677°C (3,051 °F) with a radiant heat temperature of 510°C (950 °F) at ground level. This can melt and fuse surrounding sand and stones. Common radiant heat exposure limits are:

- 0.5 KW/m^2: Maximum working level for unprotected personnel.
- 10.0 KW/m^2: Maximum working level with protective equipment.
- 15.0 KW/m^2: Maximum working level for equipment.

Steel loses most of its strength at 500 deg. C and melts at 1,500 deg. C . Blowouts can cause significant damage to drilling rigs, injuries or fatalities to rig personnel, and significant damage to the environment if hydrocarbons are spilled. Prior to the development of blow-out preventers, blowouts were common during drilling operations, and were referred to as gushers.

Preventing "Blow-Outs"

Sophisticated and reliable blowout prevention systems (BOP) are used in every production well to minimise the possibility of a blowout – where uncontrolled fluids flow from a well.

The weight of the drilling fluid acts as the first line of well control by keeping underground pressures in check. If an influx of pressurised oil or gas does occur during drilling, well control is maintained through the rig's blowout prevention system (BOP). This is a set of hydraulically operated valves and other closure devices (rams) which seal off the well, and route the well bore fluids to specialised pressure controlling equipment.

A blowout preventer (BOP) is a large valve that can seal off at the surface wellhead, a well being drilled or worked over. During drilling or well interventions, the valve may be closed if overpressure from an underground zone causes formation fluids such as oil or natural gas to enter the well bore and threaten the rig. By closing this valve (usually operated remotely via hydraulic actuators), the drilling crew can prevent explosive pressure release, thus regaining control of the downhole pressure. Once this is accomplished, often the drilling mud density within the hole can be increased until adequate fluid pressure is being placed on the influx zone, and the BOP can be opened for operations to resume. The invention and use of BOPs were instrumental in the end of oil gushers, which were dangerous and costly. BOPs come in a variety of styles, sizes and pressure ratings, and usually several individual units comprise a BOP Stack. Blind rams are designed to close an open well bore. Pipe rams seal around tubular components in the well (drill pipe, casing, tubing, wire line or coiled tubing). Shear-seal BOPs are fitted with hardened steel shearing surfaces that can actually cut through drill pipe and tool strings, if all other barriers fail. Since BOPs are important for the safety of the crew, as well as the drilling rig and the well bore itself, BOPs are regularly inspected, tested and refurbished. Tests vary from daily test of functions of critical wells to monthly or less frequent testing of wells with low likelihood of control problems. Any of these BOPs may be installed underwater, normally with two hydraulic actuators.

Types of BOPs

BOPs come in two types, ram and annular.

A ram BOP utilizes two horizontally opposed hydraulic rams that either close around the drill string, shear through the drill string and then seal, or close off a wellbore when no drill pipe or tubing is in it. The ram BOP was invented by James Smither Abercrombie and Harry S. Cameron in 1922, and was brought to market in 1924.

An annular BOP, also known as a spherical BOP, utilizes a hemispherical piece of rubber reinforced with steel. Unlike a ram BOP which closes with a sharp horizontal motion, an annular BOP closes around the drill string in a smooth simultaneous upward and inward motion. The geometry of this movement reduces internal stresses and friction between the BOP body and the sealing element, resulting in a longer field life with less maintenance. The annular design also allows a much lower operating pressure, reducing the number of hydraulic accumulators necessary and thereby reducing cost and complexity of the operation. It was invented by Granville Sloan Knox in 1946; a U.S. patent for it was awarded in 1952.

Both types are usually used together in oil well BOP stacks.

Trained personnel operating this highly reliable equipment minimise the possibility of a "blowout", or an uncontrolled flow of fluids from a well.

Fire at the Wellhead

Fire requires fuel, heat and oxygen to burn (the fire triangle principle). In fighting a fire at a wellhead (the portion of the well at and just above the ground's surface), sufficient water application by sprinkler heads and deluge nozzles and/or using offshore marine vessels delivering 10,000 gallons per minute allows water to reach even large platforms. Special air-transportable fire pumps deliver 4,000 gpm at 250-psi head via 4 inch aluminium pipes. Two of these pumps are used on a typical large fire on a land or inland barge rig to greatly reduce heat impact on surrounding structures. Truck-mounted pumps can provide 1,500 to 3,000 gpm, water works to extinguish blowout fires by various means:

- It cools fire below spontaneous ignition temperature by absorbing heat as it is flashed to steam.
- Water flashed to steam displaces oxygen and smothers fire.
- Powerful water streams displace fuel from fire.

Foam and dry chemicals have a limited role in oil well firefighting. Foam consists of water, foam concentrate and air. It is used on liquid hydrocarbon fires to smother the fuel surface (excludes oxygen), suppress vapor emissions (explosive vapor release is restricted), generate steam (removes heat and displaces oxygen), cool surface (heat absorption) and reflect radiant heat. Use on blowouts is restricted to gas condensate fires and oil wells where lateral flow has led to a large fire-surface area. 3M Lightwater ATC is commonly used with the William's Hydro Foam nozzle. This self-proportioning nozzle, when used with the ATC foam, allows foam to be thrown farther and can handle up to 6,000 gpm, but the 2,000-bpm nozzle is most used on oil well fires.

Dry chemical extinguishers work like water, but principally act as a smothering agent. Common compounds used are sodium bicarbonate, Purple K (potassium bicarbonate base) and Monnex (highest efficiency rating). Use is generally on methane well fires where explosives cannot be used and water supply is inadequate. The main problem is that these systems are "one shot" devices that can not be topped up or refilled during application. The largest systems commonly available have 68 kg of powder in storage. The William's Hydro-Chem nozzle allows one nozzle to start water cool down, add foam to knock out the liquid fire, and finally inject dry chemical to knock down the remaining gas fire. Main water use in blowout fire fighting is not to extinguish the fire, but to allow men and equipment to work near the fire. Early firefighters' efforts on burning blowouts involve removal of debris and working to get the fire burning vertically. Wells capped while burning may require more water than conventional extinguish-and-cap efforts.

Commonly available explosives such as 80% nitroglycerin grade dynamite are still used in oil well firefighting. It is believed that M. M. Kinley invented the presently used method, which was employed by experienced firefighters in the 1920s. Typically high explosives such as dynamite are used to consume all the local atmospheric oxygen and 'snuff' the flame first. Doing so removes the 'heat' but the 'fuel' (the natural gas or oil) is still present, often a huge 'fountain' of oil surrounds the work area, showering fuel upon the working crew. Depending on fire size and prior experience, up to 500 lb of explosive may be used. Typically, a smaller lube oil drum is used and packed with explosive. This drum is detonated using detonating cord run through the athey wagon boom. The cord is electrically detonated at the front of the athey wagon, some 60 to 70 ft away from the explosive drum. Heat insulating, silicon based cloth and water spray are used to protect the explosives from the fire. There is little risk of premature explosion as hot spots would only lead to non-detonation, and the explosives would burn up in the fire. This is, interestingly, the lowest cost fire fighting technique.

CAPPING

After snuffing, the wellhead must be 'capped' to stop the flow of fuel. During this time, the fuel and oxygen required to create another inferno is present in copious amounts. At this perilous stage, one small spark (perhaps from a steel or iron tool striking a stone) or other heat source might reignite the fuel.

To prevent reignition, brass or bronze tools, which do not strike sparks, or paraffin coated tools are used during the capping process. Meticulous care is used to avoid heat and sparks, or any other ignition source. The explosive re-ignition of a wellhead may take the form of an extremely powerful explosion, possibly even worse than the original 'blowout'.

Due to recent advances in technology as well as environmental concerns, many wells today are capped while they burn.

57 Coronal Mass Ejection

A coronal mass ejection (CME) (Also called the 'Hand of God") is an ejection of material from the solar corona, usually observed with a white-light coronagraph. It has a three part structure consisting of a cavity of low electron density, a dense core (the prominence, which appears as a bright region on coronagraph images) embedded in this cavity, and a bright leading edge. CME speeds range from about 20 km/s to 3,200 km/s with an average speed of 489 km/s. The average mass based on coronagraph images is 1.6×10^{15} g. Fast CMEs, ;those traveling faster than the ambient solar wind, take 3-5 days to reach earth and are responsible for triggering large, non-recurrent geomagnetic storms when they encounter the earth's magnetosphere. The average solar cycle lasts for eleven years and the frequency of ejections depends on the phase of the solar cycle: from about one every other day near solar minimum to 5–6 per day near solar maximum. The ejected material is a plasma consisting primarily of electrons and protons (in addition to small quantities of heavier elements such as helium, oxygen and iron), plus the entraining coronal magnetic field. Magnetic reconnection is the name given to the rearrangement of magnetic lines of force when two oppositely directed magnetic fields are brought together. This rearrangement is accompanied with a sudden release of energy stored in the original oppositely directed fields and is responsible for solar flares and CMEs.

When the ejection reaches the Earth as an ICME (Interplanetary CME), it may disrupt the Earth's magnetosphere, compressing it on the day side and extending the night-side magnetic tail. When the magnetosphere reconnects on the nightside, it creates trillions of watts of power which is directed back toward the Earth's upper atmosphere. This process can cause particularly strong aurora also known as the Northern Lights, or aurora borealis (in the Northern Hemisphere), and the Southern Lights, or aurora australis (in the Southern Hemisphere). CME events, along with solar flares, can disrupt radio transmissions, cause power outages (blackouts), and cause damage to satellites and electrical transmission lines. The runaway current would knock out and melt hundreds of key transformers within minutes. No power grids, no satellites, no computers and no mobiles phones will work. Ground-to-air, ship-to-shore, shortwave broadcast, and amateur radio (mostly the bands below 30 MHz) will be disrupted. Solar protons with energies greater than 30 MeV are particularly hazar-dous and can cause chromosomal damage.

A disaster that would begin on the surface of the sun and could end with tragedy on earth. The planet would be thrown into chaos as the technology that has become crucial to every day living suddenly gets taken away. There will be no power for heat, cooling or refrigeration until the electric grids are repaired. Hospitals may not be able to provide modern healthcare, and a lack of water and food will result in spreading disease. Pharmaceutical companies without electricity may not be able to produce the necessary medicines to meet the demand.

Suggested Action Before a CME

Build an underground shelter and have a ready supply of food and water Using the shelf life display as a guideline, maintain a three to five day supply of the following food groups for each family member:

1. Canned stew, spaghetti, corned beef hash, soup, beans, tuna, sardines, meats, fruits and vegetables like potatoes, baked beans, tomato puree, mushrooms.
2. Drinks such as canned juices, soda, coffee, tea, bouillon and cocoa.
3. Crackers and spreads for crackers such as peanut butter, canned meat and cheese.
4. Salt, pepper, ketchup and mustard.
5. Hard candies, raisins, canned nuts, instant puddings, honey, dried fruit, seeds, granola bars, etc.
6. Dried and/or evaporated milk, condensed milk.
7. Ready to eat cereals, rice stored in airtight containers.
8. Oatmeal cookies or crackers.
9. Salad oil.
10. Mineral water.
11. Install a high-quality surge protector with the highest possible rating on all AC power cords. Install coax surge protectors (available from most ham radio suppliers) within 6 feet of the radio equipment to be protected. Install a grounding antenna switch and keep the antennas grounded when not in use. Install good earthing—2 or more standard electrical grounding rods connected with #6 solid copper wire that is buried.
12. Stock hand held radios with short antennas (less than 14") as grid connected electronics would be more vulnerable, and stuff with long antennas worse still. Batteries and other emergency/cooking supplies would be advised as well.
13. Install basement shelters in your house. These have the following advantages.
    - They permit entry and exit without having to leave your home.
    - One can overpressure the entire basement as this allows you to store items out there and retrieve them without worrying about what you are breathing. You need to put an overpressure valve between your safe room and the basement.
    - With electricity, water, and sewer in your basement and also an NBC air filter, you will be assured of continuing your overpressure for many hours after a power outage.
    - You can easily incorporate a blast door into the side of your shelter in order to avoid lowering supplies, people, and pets down through a blast hatch and down a ladder.
    - Any radioactive fallout on your roof is about 10 feet from the roof of your shelter and less harmful.
    - Shelters can also serve as a vault for valuables, a panic room in case of a home invasion robbery, a communications center, and a food storage area.

58 Pediatric Trauma and Resuscitation

INTRODUCTION

Everyday, around the world, the lives of the more 2000 familes are torn apart by the loss of a child to unintentional injury that could have been prevented. Such losses impacts entire communities and such tragedies can change lives irrevocably. All children have a right to a safe environment and protection from injury and violence. But injuries are a major killer of children and responsible for nearly 950,000 deaths each year i.e. nearly 100 children dying needlessly every hour of every day!Trauma, especially road traffic injuries are the leading cause of mortality in children between the ages of 15 to 19 and the second leading cause in those aged 5-14 years, with more children succumbing to injuries and their sequelae than all other childhood diseases combined. Tens of millions of children require hospital care for non fatal injuries, many left with some form of disability, often with lifelong consequence. Of these, 95% of all injury deaths occur in low and middle income countries. Blunt trauma, mostly head injuries as the result of falls and motor vehicle collisions, accounts for nearly 90% of pediatric injuries while 10% of trauma victims have penetrating injuries. Long-term disability in pediatric trauma victims is estimated to be more than three times the mortality rate and is primarily the result of brain injury. As in adults, boys are more frequently injured than girls by a factor of 2:1, with the exception of burn injuries. Children with multi system injuries can deteriorate rapidly and develop serious complications. Such victims are best transferred early to a facility capable of managing the child with such problems.

Effective management in the first 20 minutes after injury can do much to reduce morbidity and mortality in children with trauma. The most common cause of preventable death in this group is errors in management of ventilation and circulation and failure to detect cryptic injuries. Early participation of senior staff familiar with surgical, anesthetic and medical management of children is vital. Because of their smaller size, multisystem injuries are commoner and combined thoracic and abdominal injuries due to blunt trauma are much more frequently seen than penetrating injuries. Less body fat, elastic connective tissue and close proximity of organ systems makes for greater energy transmission on impact. Appreciable internal injuries can occur in this age group without overlying bony fractures. Associated head injuries are also more common and an initial baseline Glasgow Coma Scale score and a pediatric verbal score for children below 4 years of age must be assessed in all cases

Table 58.1: Pediatric glasgow coma scale for infants and young children

Eye opening	*Pts*	*Best verbal response*	*Pts*	*Best motor response*	*Pts*
Spontaneous	4	Coos, babbles	5	Normal spontaneous movements	6
To speech	3	Irritable, cries	4	Withdraws to touch	5
To pain	2	Cries to pain	3	Withdraws to pain	4
None	1	Moans to pain	2	Abnormal flexion	3
None	1	Abnormal extension	2	None	1

(Table 58.1). Scores less than 08 merits prompt resuscitation including tracheal intubation. CT scan is indicated for all children with altered mental status or loss of consciousness with GCS of 14-15, for all children with GCS less than 13, or post traumatic incidence of repeated seizures or vomiting, children with bulging fontanelle or suture diastasis. NO ROLE EXISTS FOR SKULL X-RAY FILMS. Scalp lacerations can cause significant blood loss in children and must be examined carefully for underlying skull fractures. Remember that fontanelles and sutures are open in children below 18 months of age. Most skull fractures occur in the parietal bone and there is a 10 fold increased risk of intracranial hematomas when there is an associated skull fracture. Also, 60% of children with head injuries have concomitant intra-abdominal injuries. As regards spinal injuries, 85% of cervical spine fractures in children below 8 years occurs between C1 and C3, while in those above 10 years of age, pattern is similar to adults at C4-7.

Hypothermia due to exposure occurs rapidly in children because of their high body surface area to weight ratio, thin skin and lack of subcutaneous tissue. Clothes may have to be removed to facilitate initial examination and performing practical clinical procedures. Hence, monitoring of the core temperature in all children is a vital component of their initial assessment. Raising the ambient ambient temperature where feasible or swaddling the child in blankets, plastic sheets or aluminium foil are alternatives to prevent heat loss. Fall in body temperature would otherwise cause a rise in oxygen consumption with peripheral vasoconstriction and lactic acidosis.

Causes of Childhood Trauma

A number of physical characteristics make children vulnerable to injuries. They lack the knowledge, skills and levels of concentration needed to manage the road environment, no matter how calm the road conditions. Their physical and mental ability mismatch results in compromised balancing ability and reasoning. Their small size increases their risk in a road environment as they are less visible than adults, and when hit, are more likely to suffer a head or neck injury. Again due to their smaller size, children also have difficulty in seeing over vehicles, judging the speed of oncoming vehicles and the distance of an approaching vehicle. Concepts of speed and distance are not mastered until 5-7 years of age. Infants skin burns deeper, quicker and at lower temperatures than that of adults. Boys, especially those aged 9 to 14 years, exhibit higher activity levels, risk taking and impulsive behaviour and are more likely to be unrestrained by their parents and roam further and often alone. Those living in underdeveloped nations are more likely to be exposed to hazardous environments, lack of space and facilities for safe play, cramped, unsafe living conditions with unprotected windows, open roofs and stairs without handrails. Where traffic volume exceeds 150000 motor vehicles per day, where there are no safe and efficient public transport system, where traffic and speed is unregulated, where there is lack of playgrounds and lack of separation between road users and housing, schools and commercial outlets, children are at an increased risk of sustaining injuries. Methods to slow down traffic to below 30 km/h, separate lanes for cyclists and enforcement of helmet usage, use of child passenger restraints systems can all bring down injury related deaths and disabilities.

Age-wise Etiologies

- *Age 0-1 years:* Choking/Suffocation, burns, drowning, falls.
- *Age 1-4 years:* Road Traffic Accidents (as occupants of vehicles) burns, drowning, falls.
- *Age 5-14 years:* Road Traffic Accidents (as occupants or pedestrians), bicycle accidents, burns, drowning.

MANAGEMENT

The assessment of children with multiple injuries should follow the same protocols outlined for adults and the basic principles of resuscitation must be effected immediately without waiting for full evaluation. The airway in children has specific anatomical differences when compared to adults as following:

- Large head relative to body size.
- Small oral cavity with relatively large tongue.
- Large angle of the jaw, 140° in infants Vs 120° in adults.
- A more U (omega)shaped epiglottis compared to the adult (Fig. 58.1).
- A more cephalad larynx with anterior and inferior inclination. The glottis being at C3 level in infants against C5-6 in adults.
- The cricoid forms the narrowest part of the larynx and an endotracheal tube passing the glottis can be held up at this level (Fig. 58.2).
- The trachea is short (newborn 4-5 cm and at 18 months age 7-8 cm) and main stem bronchi emerge at equal angles against the more vertical right bronchus in adults.
- Infants under 6 months of age are obligatory nose breathers.

After airway assessment, supplemental oxygen must be given to all children with trauma, as their oxygen consumption is higher, their functional residual capacity lower, closing volume higher and physiological shunting greater. These factors are further exacerbated by injuries. Children tolerate nasal prongs better than masks but, for infants under 6 months of age, facemask is a better choice to avoid nasal obstruction. If there is any injury above the clavicle, it may be assumed that there is co existing cervical spinal injury also and an appropriate immobilization device-collar type or improvised sandbags and tape-positioned. The airway is then cleared and, if gag reflex is present, insertion of an artificial airway must be avoided as it may precipitate choking, laryngospasm or vomiting. If gag reflex is absent, an airway of appropriate size is inserted and IPPV with 100% oxygen commenced using gentle pressures not exceeding 20 cm H_2O for fear of distending the stomach and causing splinting of diaphragm and the added risk of silent

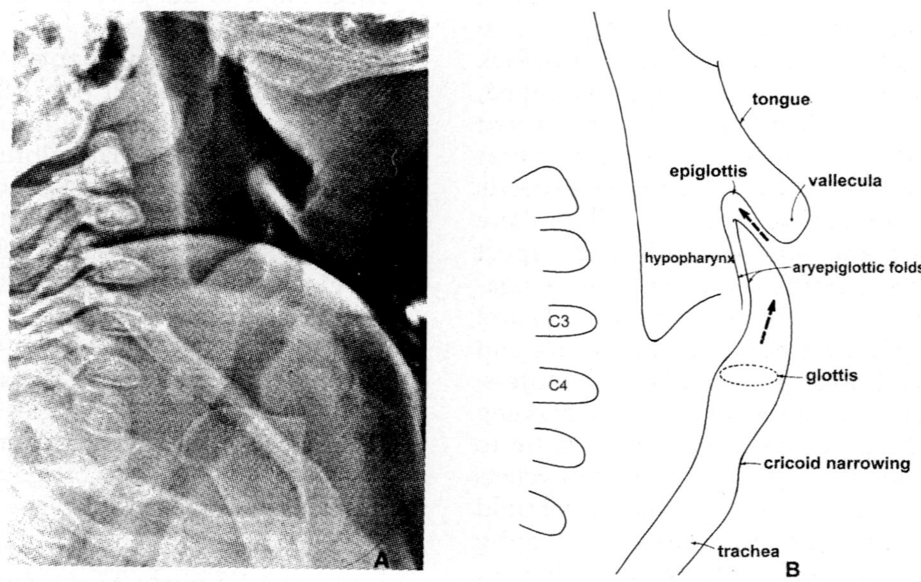

Fig. 58.1: Lateral neck xerogram (A) and schematic (B) of the infant larynx. Note the short, angled epiglottis and the narrow cricoid cartilage

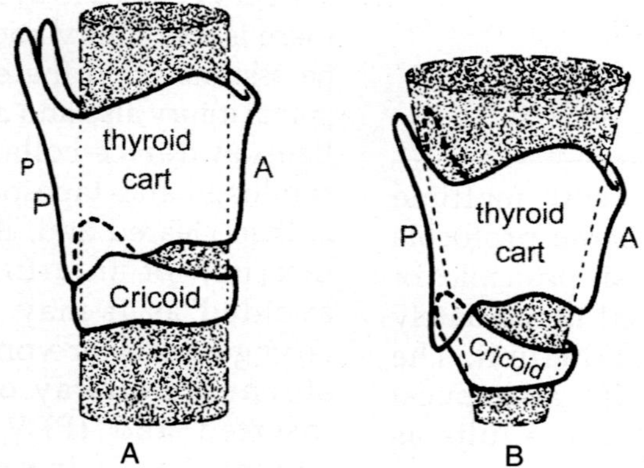

Fig. 58.2: Configuration of the adult (A) in the infant larynx (B). Note cylinder shape of adult larynx, infant larynx is funnel shaped due to narrow undeveloped cricoid cartilage

regurgitation. Oral or nasotracheal intubation must be attempted ONLY AFTER hypoxia has been overcome with mask, airway and Ambu bag compressions. For children less than 1 year age, a straight blade laryngoscope is used and a tube selected of the size of the nostril or the victims little finger. Plain tubes are selected for all children below the age of puberty and passed 2-5 cm below vocal cord (depending on the age) and the chest auscultated at the infra-axillary region to exclude accidental endobronchial intubation and then double fixed firmly to avoid migration (Table 58.2). A minimal leak of gas around the tube as the lungs are inflated is both acceptable and desirable. Rate of inflation is based on normograms for age. Cyanosis should disappear and pulse oximeter saturation must be above 90% at this stage. If, at any stage, ventilation is unsuccessful, a needle cricothyrotomy with a 14 swg intravenous cannula is performed. Tracheostomy must be resorted to only in hospitals. A stressed child swallows air and acute gastric dilatation is common in children and mask ventilation may compound the problem further. This can precipitate regurgitation, aspiration and vomiting, besides splinting the diaphragm, compressing the inferior vena cava and reducing venous return. A nasogastric tube must be passed in all children unless there is epistaxis and signs to suggest injury to the cribriform plate, when the oral route is unavoidable. Instill nasal decongestant into the nares and lubricate the nasogastric tube liberally to permit its smooth, atraumatic passage. Check correct positioning by dipping the proximal end under water to check for emerging stream of air bubbles if the tube has found its way into the trachea. If this is absent, inject 5 ml of air into the proximal port and auscultate over the epigastrium to confirm correct placement in the stomach. Always

Table 58.2: Equipment guidelines according to age and weight

	Age 50th Percentile weight					
Equipment	*Premie (1-2.5 kg)*	*Neonate (2.5-4.0 kg)*	*6 months (7.0 kg)*	*1-2 years (10-12 kg)*	*5 years (15-18 kg)*	*8-10 years (24-30 kg)*
Airway—oral (00)	Infant (0)	Infant/small (1)	Small (2)	Small (3)	Medium/large (4/5)	
Breathing						
Self-inflating bag	Infant	Infant	Child	Child	Child	Child/adult
O2 ventilation	Premature	Newborn	Infant/child	Child	Child	Small/adult
Endotracheal tube	2.5-3.0 (uncuffed)	3.0-3.5 (uncuffed)	3.5-4.0 (uncuffed)	4.0-4.5 (uncuffed)	5.0-5.5 (uncuffed)	5.5-6.5 (cuffed)
Laryngoscope blade	0 (straight)	1 (straight)	1 (straight)	1-2 (straight)	2 (straight or curved)	2-3 (straight 0 or curved)
Suction/stylet (F)	6-8/6	8/6	8-10/6	10/6	14/14	14/14
Circulation						
BP cuff	Newborn	Newborn	Infant	Child	Child	Child/adult
Venous access						
Angiocath	22-24	22-24	22-24	22-22	18-20	18-20
Butterfly needle	25	23-25	23-25	23	20-23	18-21
Intracath	–	–	19	19	18	14
Arm board	6″	6″	6″-8″	8″	8″-15″	16″
Orogastric tube (F)	5	5-8	8	10	10-12	14-18
Chest tube (F)	10-14	12-18	14-20	14-24	20-32	28-36

From Chamedies L (ed): TB of Pediatric Advanced Life Support. Reproduced with permission of the American Heart Association, Dallas, 1988).

aspirate tube to inspect gastric contents. If blood is mixed in gastric juice, administer an injectable dose of an H2 antagonist and instill iced saline mixed with a non-particulate antacid into the NGT.

Always ensure that oxygen saturation is above 95%, $PaCO_2$ between 32 and 35 mmHg. Chest tube insertion for pneumothorax in children is best done via the second interspace along the midaxillary line, as midclavicular line insertion can injure the pulmonary artery.

CIRCULATORY ACCESS AND FLUID THERAPY

Blood volume is estimated at 80 ml/kg. Suspect hypovolemia if heart rate is more than 10% of value calculated for age or blood pressure is less than 5th percentile of calculated value. Hemorrhage is controlled by direct pressure. Because of increased physiological reserve in children, changes in vital signs occur late despite blood loss. Early diagnosis of shock is based on appearance of skin, temperature of extremities, capillary refill time and sensorium (Table 58.3).

A child's normal blood pressure is systolic calculated by the formula {70 mmHg + (2 x age in years)}, and fluid therapy must be initiated BEFORE there are abnormalities in the vital signs (Table 58.4). Children can maintain their blood pressure until almost 45% blood volume has been lost. Stroke volume is relatively fixed in infants and young children and depends on venous return. They respond to hypovolemia by increase in heart rate and maintain blood pressure. When the pressures actually start to drop, blood loss is usually quite severe and venous access in hypovolemic children becomes very difficult and usually requires a cutdown (Fig. 58.3 and Table 58.5).

An interim intraosseus infusion is a useful

Table 58.3: Relationship of skin color, capillary refill time, pulse volume, and extremity temperature to hypovolemia

Amount of volume depletion (%)	*Skin color*	*Capillary refill time (seconds)*	*Posterior tibial pulse volume*	*Skin temperature*
None	Pink	<2	++++	Warm
5	Pale	3-4	++	Cold from midcalf and midforearm out
10	Gray	4-5	0	Cold midthigh and upper arm
15	Mottled	>5	0	Entire extremity cold

Symbols ++++ full; ++, moderately full; 0, markedly diminished or absent.

Table 58.4: Age-specific vital signs

Age (years)	*Weight (kg)*	*Pulse (per mlin)*	*Systolic blood pressure (mmHg)*	*Respiratory rate*	*Tidal volume (mL)*
Newborn	3	160	70	60	240
1	9	130	85	40	700
3	15	120	89	30	1,200
6	24	110	94	25	2,000
10	35	90	100	20	2,800
Adults	75	70	120	15-20	5,000

(From the Child Hospital of Pittsburgh, Benedum Pediatric Trauma Program, Pediatric Field

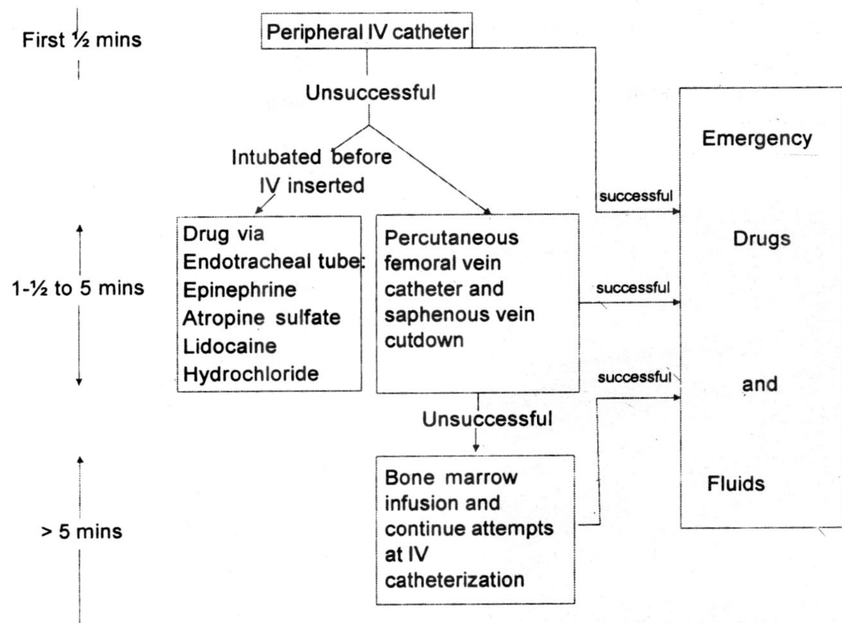

Fig. 58.3: Protocol for emergency intravenous (IV) access during pediatric resuscitation (From Kanter *et al.* with permission)

Table 58.5: Resuscitation medications, by weight and age, for infants and children 0-12 years

Age	*50th percentile weight (kg)*	*Epinephrine*		*Atropine*		*Bicarboante**	
		mg	*mg+*	*mg*	*mg+*	*mEq*	*mg+*
Newborn	3.0	0.03	0.3	0.1	1.0	3.0	6.0
1 month	4.0	0.04	0.4	0.1	1.0	4.0	8.0
3 months	5.5	0.055	0.55	0.11	1.1	5.5	11.0
5 months	7.0	0.07	0.7	0.14	1.4	7.0	7.0
1 year	10.0	0.10	1.0	0.20	2.0	10.0	10.0
2 years	12.0	0.12	1.2	0.24	2.4	12.0	12.0
3 years	14.0	0.14	1.4	0.28	2.8	14.0	14.0
4 years	16.0	0.16	1.6	0.32	3.2	16.0	16.0
5 years	18.0	0.18	1.8	0.36	3.6	18.0	18.0
6 years	20.0	0.20	2.0	0.40	4.0	20.0	20.0
7 years	22.0	0.22	2.2	0.44	4.4	22.0	22:0
8 years	25.0	0.25	2.5	0.50	5.0	25.0	25.0
9 years	28.0	0.28	2.8	0.56	5.6	28.0	28.0
10 years	34.0	0.34	3.4	0.68	6.8	34.0	34.0

The use of bicarbonate in cardiac arrest is controversial (see text), Good ventilation must be established before bicarboante is used

+Volume (ml) is based on the follwoing concentrations:

Epinephrine: 1:10,000 (0.1 mg+ml^{-1})
Atropine: 0.1 mg/ml^{-1}
Bicarbonate: $\leq$3 months = 4.2% solution (0.5 mEq ml^{-1})
>3 months = 8.2% solution (1 mEq ml^{-1})

From Chamedies L (ed): TB of Pediatric Advanced Life Support. Reproduced with permission of the American Heart Association, Dailas, 1988)

alternative in such situations. Sites chosen are the anterior tibial plateau 1 cm inferior and medial to the tibial tuberosity or the inferior one third of the femur 3 cm above the lateral condyle (Fig. 58.4).

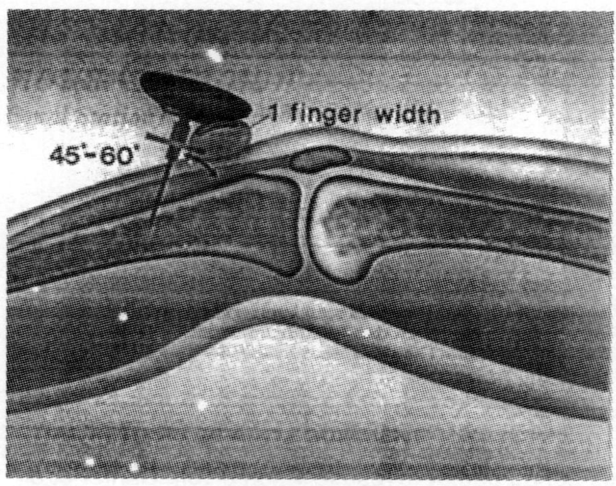

Fig. 58.4: Intraosseous puncture

Use a 18-20 gauge cannula for children to 1 year of age and 13 to 16 gauge needle for those above 1 year of age, inserted perpendicular to the bone and confirming correct positioning by marrow aspiration. Injection of 5-6 ml of saline expels clots and there should be no evidence of any local swelling. Crystalloids, colloids and drugs can be administered through this route as they are absorbed by the rich network of venous sinusoids of the medullary cavity that drain via the venous canal, nutrient and emissary veins into the systemic circulation. Any fracture in the same leg or pelvic fractures are contraindications to i/o line and osteomyelitis is a potential complication if infusions are continued beyond 4 hours by this route. Epiphyseal plate damage can be avoided by inserting the needle away from the joint space. Whatever route of access is chosen, blood samples must be taken for grouping, cross matching, full blood count, urea and electrolyte estimation. Basic life support measures must be continued throughout. Infusate should be a bolus of 20 ml/kg of Ringer Lactate or normal saline that can be repeated up to three times. If there is no improvement 10ml/kg of packed cell transfusion can be given. Alternatively, a colloid (Haemacel, hexastarch or albumin) warmed to body temperature and administered at a rate of 20 ml/kg over 20 minutes initially. Dextrose containing fluids are not recommended during the initial resuscitation period because of hyperglycemia from elevated catecholamine response to traumatic stress. A return towards hemodynamic normalcy is indicated by slowing of the heart rate to less than 130/min, increased pulse pressure to more than 20 mmHg, return of normal skin color, increased warmth of extremities, improving GCS score, systolic pressures above 80 mmHg and urine output of 1-2 ml/kg (Table 58.6).

Table 58.6

GCS	*Systolic blood pressure*	*Pulse*	*Resp rate*	*Score*
14-15	Normal	Normal	Normal	3
10-13	Mild-mod hypotension	tachy-cardia	Tachy-pnea	2
4-9	Severe hypo-tension	Brady-cardia	Hypo-venti-lation	1
3	0	0		
0 or intubated				

Pediatric Trauma Scoring

The pediatric trauma score is an index to predict outcome and based on anatomic and physiologic parameters and injuries sustained. Values are assigned to six components and a combined score of <8 is associated with poor outcome (Table 58.7).

Age Specific Pediatric Trauma Score (ASPTS)

Current pediatric trauma scores are not age specific. The ASPTS incorporates age-specific values for systolic blood pressure, pulse and respiratory rate in addition to the Glasgow Coma Scale. Values are assigned from to 3 for each parameter (Table 58.8).

CHILDREN AND DISASTERS

The unique characteristics of children make them more vulnerable in infectious, natural or man-made disasters. While all children have these vulnerabilities, children with special health care needs may also have specific conditions which can place them at even greater risk.

The vulnerabilities of children to natural or man-made disasters and in infectious situations are:

- Because their skin is thinner and they have a larger surface-to-mass ratio than adults, children are more vulnerable to agents that act on the skin.
- Children are particularly vulnerable to aerosolized biological or chemical agents because their respiratory rate is faster and they inhale relatively larger doses of the substance than an adult would in the same period of time. Also, because the breathing zone of children is closer to the ground, children are more vulnerable to agents like sarin and chlorine because these agents are heavier than air and accumulate close to the ground.

Table 58.7: Pediatric trauma scale

Component	*+2*	*+1*	*-1*
Airway	Normal	Maintainable	Unmaintainable
CNS	Awake	Obtunded	Comatose
Weight	>20 kg	10-2 kg	<1 kg
Systolic BP	>90 mmHg	50-9 mmHg	<5 mmHg
Open wounds	None	Minor	Major/Penetrating
Fractures	None	Closed	Open/Multiple

Table 58.8

GCS score	*SBP*	*Pulse*	*Resp rate*
14-15	Normal 3	Normal	Normal
10-13	Mild-Moderate 2	Tachycardia	Tachypnea
4-9	Severe hypotension 1	Bradycardia	Hypoventilation
3	0	0	
0 or intubated	0		

ASPTS is the sum total of coded values for all 4 variables.

- Children have less fluid reserve than adults and can become dehydrated faster, so they are more vulnerable to the effects of agents that produce vomiting and/or diarrhea.
- Infants, toddlers, and young children do not have the motor skills to escape from the area of a chemical, biological or other terrorist incident.
- Children lack cognitive decision-making skills that would help them to figure out how to flee danger or to follow directions from others.
- Children have smaller circulating blood volumes than adults so if treatment is not immediate, relatively small amounts of blood/fluid loss can lead to irreversible shock or death.
- Because children are more sensitive to changes in body temperature, have a faster metabolism, and less blood and fluid reserves, a child's condition can shift from stable to life-threatening very rapidly.

Mass Casualties Involving Children

Children are likely to be among the victims in most mass casualty events and, because of their anatomy and physiology, have a higher likelihood of morbidity or mortality. Recent history has proven that children may also be targets of terrorism. For these reasons, every hospital should anticipate having pediatric victims appear on their doorstep in the event of disaster and must start planning to address the issue of treating pediatric patients.

A frequently recommended first responder triage system specifically for children, named JumpSTART, derived by Romig in 2002, is based on an adult triage system called START (Simple Triage and Rapid Treatment). This pediatric triage system places an emphasis on assessing and opening up the airway, along with providing rescue breaths and pulse checks; recognizing the unique physiology of children in whom respiratory failure, rather than cardiac failure, causes death.

However, JumpSTART is a triage system designed to be used primarily in the pre-hospital setting to determine priority for transport. Hospital-based disaster triage encompasses more complex issues and must reflect the hospitals resources, space allocation, anticipation of numbers of incoming victims, and repeated reassessment of the patients. Additionally, hospital-based triage becomes even more complex if decontamination is required prior to entry into the hospital.

The core of this new triage system is the application of the clinical, history and physical assessment skills that are used in an emergency department triage on a day-to-day basis by experienced nurses and clinicians. However, the new triage structures the allocation of treatment/care and staffing to provide "the greatest good for the greatest number."

One priority for hospital based triage is to maximize care of the critically injured by preventing over-triage, which is defined as an overflow of minimally injured/sick and already treated into the critical care areas or emergency department. Quickly establishing treatment and evaluation areas for these minimally injured away from critical areas in the emergency department needs to be addressed.

Another priority of hospital based triage is triage accuracy. This depends largely on the experience of the clinical staff performing triage. It is acknowledged that clinicians not used to evaluating acutely ill children generally over-triage into more severe categories, thus potentially misallocating resources.

Pediatric experience is known to result in more accurate triage of infants and children. Pediatric patients may be sicker following a disaster because of their unique physiology and their appearance may be deceiving. Therefore, the triage officers triaging pediatric patients ideally should be pediatrics experienced.

Visual assessment of a patient's immediate status is done daily in every emergency department by experienced nurses and physicians who quickly decide who needs emergency treatment and who can go through a longer registration and routine triage. The visual assessment described here uses this same technique for rapid mass casualty sorting. The assessment done prior to decontamination would be done by staff in decontamination gear, making it difficult to physically assess patients or to have much more meaningful communication with them.

Reassessment in triage:

- Level 1 = Continuous
- Level 2 = Every 15 min
- Level 3 = Every 60 min
- Level 4 = Every 60 to 90 min
- Level 5 = Every 2 hours

The visual assessment described here is based on the Pediatric Visual Assessment Triangle: Respiration, Circulation, Appearance. The core element of primary triage is dependent upon identifying abnormal elements of these three areas. Once an abnormal criterion is identified, the patients are immediately sent to the RED Resuscitation Area, where the patient will receive immediate care.

Pediatric visual assessment triangle

First impression	
Appearance	*Breathing*
Body position	Visible movement
Muscle tone	Work of breathing
Mental status	(normal/increased)
Circulation	
Color	

Important Points to Remember

- Although the ABC mnemonic tool is very helpful in remembering the key elements of pediatric visual assessment, the order of assessment should be B, C, A (Breathing, then Circulation, then Appearance).
- With infants and young children, form a visual impression before you approach to begin the hands-on assessment process.
- Abruptly approaching a young child who is already distressed can increase the child's agitation, potentially exacerbating the child's clinical condition.
- Maintain a calm, reassuring manner whenever you assess a very young patient.
- To assess younger children, have a parent hold the child or allow the child to sit on a parent's lap if possible.
- Encourage the parent to participate in the examination.
- Take age-related factors into account throughout the assessment.
- Allowing infants to suck on a pacifier or gloved finger can calm them.
- If at any point during the first impression you identify a significant clinical problem, immediately discontinue your visual assessment, approach the child, and begin the hands-on initial assessment.
- Do not delay lifesaving interventions to initiate monitoring.
- Fever may make infants and children irritable or somnolent, which can affect the assessment.

Pediatric Airway Considerations

- More anterior than adult (less head tilt to open the airway).
- Smaller diameter of airway than an adult (easily blocked by secretions or blood).
- Large tongue in relation to jaw size (likely to cause obstructions when child is unconscious).

- Infants prefer to breathe through the nose (nasal obstructions can cause respiratory distress).
- In children, respiratory arrest is the primary cause of cardiac arrest.
- The critical window between onset of apnea and onset of cardiac arrest in children is very short—no more than a minute or two.
- A child's airway is narrower at all levels than an adult's. The child's anatomy results in higher airflow resistance, so when further narrowed by edema or secretions, the child experiences greatly increased resistance to airflow (Fig. 58.5).
- Avoid actions that could agitate or frighten a child who is in respiratory distress.
- *Tone:* Is there vigorous movement with good muscle tone, or is the child limp? Interactivity Is the child alert and attentive to surroundings, or apathetic?
- Will the child reach for a toy?

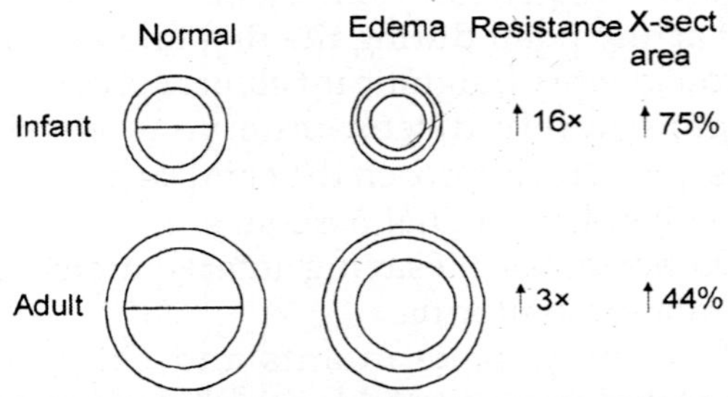

Fig. 58.5: Relative effects of airway edema in the infant and adult. The normal infant and adult airways are presented on the left, edematous airways (1 mm circumferential) on the right. Note that resistance to flow is inversely proportional to radius of the lumen to the fourth power for laminar flow, and the radius of the lumen to the fifth power for turbulent flow. The net result in the infant is a 75% reduction in cross-sectional area, and 16-fold increase in resistance, as compared to a 44 percent reduction in cross-sectional area and a 3-fold increase in resistance in the adult

- Does the child respond to people, objects, and sounds?
- *Consolability:* Does comforting the child alleviate agitation and crying?
- *Look/Gaze:* Do the child's eyes follow your movement, or is there a vacant gaze?
- *Speech/Cry:* Are vocalizations strong, or are they weak, muffled, or hoarse?
- Valuate work of breathing and breath sounds Is the child able to speak or cry vigorously? Ask the parent to lift the child's shirt. Look for signs of airway obstruction. Observe movement of the chest or abdomen.
- Inspiratory retractions in the suprasternal, supraclavicular, intercostal, or subcostal areas.
- Inspiratory nasal flaring.
- Head bobbing.
- Listen for stridor, grunting, gurgling.
- Count the respiratory rate for a 30-second period.
- Assess the respiratory depth and pattern.
- Evaluate central color at the lips, tongue, and oral mucosa.
- Inspect for chest trauma.
- Auscultate chest by placing stethoscope below each axilla in turn and compare breath sounds right and left lung fields to see if equal /Decreased breath sounds/ Wheezing/Crackles. Listen for sounds that indicate airway obstruction or excessive secretions. Stridor: A high or low pitched sound that occurs when the child breathes in, stridor indicates partial obstruction of the upper airway. Foreign body? Swelling (from disease, poison, etc)?
- *Optional:* Initiate pulse oximetry (this may be time consuming and is not needed for triage process during disasters).
- Note skin color at the lips and tongue, the palms, or the soles of the feet; abnormal skin color (pallor, mottling, or cyanosis) indicates an urgent condition.

Pediatric Circulation Considerations

- Palpate the central pulse. Recommended sites:
  - Newborn: Base of umbilical cord.
  - Infants and young children: carotid artery.
- If central pulse present, evaluate strength; weak pulse can indicate decompensated shock.
- Count rate for 30 seconds, double this figure for rate per minute.
- If child is uncooperative, count rate by ausculating with stethoscope over left side of chest between sternum and nipple.
- Compare peripheral and central pulses; they should be similar; weak or irregular peripheral pulses indicate either poor peripheral perfusion or exposure to cold ambient temperatures; hot skin may indicate fever, infection, or hyperthermia caused by very warm ambient temperatures (check body temperature, see below).
- Check capillary refill time; delayed capillary refill (more than 3 seconds) may indicate poor perfusion or exposure to cool ambient temperatures.
- Unlike adults, blood pressure is not a reliable indicator of poor perfusion in children and should not be determining factor used to decide if the child has hypoperfusion. Blood pressure can be measured in children over three, particularly when the condition is non-urgent and there is no need to expedite transport.
- Begin circulation assessment by detecting and stopping active bleeding. Use direct pressure, elevation and, when necessary, the proximal pressure point. Remember that seemingly small blood losses can be significant as a child has a much smaller blood volume than an adult.

Pediatric Mental Assessment Considerations

- *Level of Consciousness:* All well children will constantly interact with their environment. Proceed with initial assessment when child is markedly irritable, agitated, reduce responsiveness.
- *Interaction with Parent:* A child will respond to his/her name called. Proceed with initial assessment when the child is markedly slow or absent response, inconsolable crying, or failure to recognize a parent.
- *Response to Others:* A child will recognize your presence. Proceed with initial assessment when there is no response to your presence.
- *Muscle Tone and Body Position:* A child will assume a comfortable position. An infant will have his extremities in a flexed position. There will be equal movement with their limbs. Proceed with initial assessment when there is hypotonia, rigidity, or inability to sit.

Characteristics Unique to Each Age Group

- Infants (0 to 18 months)
  - Ambulation begins at approximately 1 year.
  - Easily consolable by caregiver, e.g., smile and coo with parent.
  - Appropriate reaction to the others–stranger anxiety, associated with crying is normal.
- Toddlers (18 months to 3 years)
  - *Normal:* Explores the environment, i.e., looking, walking around.
  - *Talking appropriate for development:* Simple words and short sentences.
- Preschool (3 years to 6 years)
  - *Talking:* More prominent and longer sentences; ability for others to understand.

- School aged (7 years to 12 years)
  - *Able to verbalize their needs:* However, the child may regress to earlier stage of development.

Prevention

Injuries can be prevented or controlled. Safety strategies include broad approaches to encourage a culture of safety and strong political commitment. Legislations in the form of specific standards and regulations for a wide range of goods and services such as childcare products, use of fire retardant material for children's bedclothes,building construction especially related to window guards, stair gates and guard rails and isolation of water hazards, child resistant packaging of drugs and poisons, product modification, environmental modification (lanes for cycles and 2 wheelers), development and promotion of safety devices like helmets, smoke detectors, child seats in 4 wheelers and also education and improved pre hospital care can reduce the burden of childhood death and disability from injury.

Further Reading

1. Pediatric Trauma Primary survey and resuscitation I . Lloyd-Thomas, AR. BMJ, 11 Aug 1990, Vol 301, 334-336.
2. Pediatric Trauma Primary Survey and resuscitation II. BMJ, 18-25 Aug 1990, Vol 301, 380-382.
3. Pediatric Trauma. Schiedler, MG, Lynch, JM and Ford,HR. The Trauma Manual, 2nd Edn, Lippincott Williams Wilkins, 2002, Chapter 47, 446-460.
4. ATLS Student Course Manual, 1997.
5. The Trauma Manual, 2nd Edn.,Lippincott Williams Wilkins, 2002, Chapter 47,Pediatric trauma.
6. World Report on Child Injury Prevention,2008. WHO and UNICEF/NMH/VIP08.01.

59 Trauma During Pregnancy

"Save the mother, save the fetus."

INTRODUCTION

It is estimated that accidental injury complicates 6 to 7% of all pregnancies, creating a unique situation in which immediate, multidisciplinary intensive therapy, sometimes invasive and aggressive, may have to be carried out simultaneously on behalf of two patients. Correct management, although difficult and demanding, will, in successful cases, result in over 100 years of combined potential life expectancy for both mother and child. A pregnant woman is naturally accident-prone. Her changing physical dimensions affects her maneuverability as well as her reaction to approaching dangers, and occurs more frequently in the third trimester than at any other time during the female adulthood. The enlarged blood volume which may be about 40% at term, predisposes to both hypovolemia and hypoxia which, in turn affects uteroplacental blood flow, and secondarily the fetal well being. The uterine vascular bed is a low resistance system that is completely dependent upon maternal arterial blood pressure to maintain uterine blood flow. Though incapable of further vasodilatation, vasoconstriction can occur in response to sympathetic stimulation.

Types of Accidental Maternal Injuries

- Blunt abdominal trauma (mainly motor vehicle accidents).
- Penetrating abdominal trauma.
- Electrical injuries.
- Burns.
- Attempted suicide.
- Blunt abdominal injury.

Motor vehicle injuries account for 50% of maternal trauma. Damage to the pregnant passenger is in direct relationship to the damage sustained by the automobile. Severe life-threatening injuries are usually multiple. Internal injuries are usually accompanied by intraperitoneal bleeding and hypovolemic shock. Victims with multiple injuries will usually suffer fetal loss through placental abruption or maternal shock. Maternal death is most often caused by head injury. Pelvic injuries occur frequently, mostly at the anterior half of the pelvic ring, usually the horizontal pubic rami. Pelvic fractures are highly correlated with concealed retroperitoneal hemorrhage, shock, uterine rupture, injuries to the urinary bladder, urethra and abruption.

Fetal loss is always proportional to severity of maternal injury. The most common cause of fetal death is death of the mother. The second most common cause of fetal death is placental abruption.

There is a lower mortality rate for a pregnant driver than for the other front or rear seat passengers, probably due to lesser risk of ejection. Ejection from the vehicle substantially increases the risk for the pregnant passenger. Abruption, when it occurs, is usually of a concealed variety and vaginal bleeding is less frequently seen. Delayed placental abruption is often seen following automobile accidents 5 to 6 days following trauma Premature labour is usual in third trimester injuries. Use of a seat belt restraint, preferably the three anchorage point lap-shoulder seat belts offers added protection to a pregnant woman passenger, increasing survival rates from 50 to 92%. Seat belts with shoulder harness distribute deceleration forces more evenly and prevent forward flexion shear forces. The lap belt restraint alone can produce uterine compression by flexion forces over it, and could intensify rather than reduce fetal and maternal injury.

Trauma caused by accidents is a common and important complication of pregnancy, involving 5-20% of pregnancies. Recent studies demonstrate that trauma is more likely to cause maternal death than any other medical complication of pregnancy. Direct and indirect obstetric factors caused maternal deaths in 31.5% of 95 cases. Trauma caused maternal deaths in 46.5% of the 95 cases, and, of these traumatic death cases, 34% were due to accidents, 57% to homicide, and 9% to suicide. The following describes the percentage of traumatic maternal deaths caused by each mechanism of injury.

- Gunshot wounds 23%.
- Motor vehicle accidents 21%.
- Stab wounds 14%.
- Strangulation 14%.
- Blunt head injury 9%.
- Burns 7%.
- Falls 4%.
- Toxic exposure 4%.
- Drowning 2%.
- Iatrogenic injury 2%.

Trauma has become the most frequent cause of maternal death in advanced countries. Although maternal mortality due to other causes such as infection, hemorrhage, hypertension, and thromboembolism, has declined over the years, the number of maternal deaths due to penetrating trauma, suicide, homicide and motor vehicle accidents has risen steadily. Accidental injuries occur in 6 to 7% of all pregnant patients. Penetrating trauma accounts for as many as 36% of maternal deaths. In the case of gunshot wounds to the pregnant abdomen, overall maternal mortality is low (3.9%). Fetal mortality, on the other hand, is high, ranging between 40 and 70%.

Although the initial assessment and management priorities for resuscitation of the injured pregnant patient are the same as those for other traumatized patients, the specific anatomic and physiologic changes that occur during pregnancy may alter the response to injury and hence necessitate a modified approach to the resuscitation process. The main principle guiding therapy must be that resuscitating the mother will resuscitate the fetus.

The approach to treating trauma is different in patients who are pregnant than in patients who are not pregnant. Unless the treating physician is aware of maternal physiologic adaptation to pregnancy, misdiagnosis and suboptimal treatment may ensue. On the other hand, a wide variety of obstetrical pathologies can obscure, confuse, and delay the diagnosis of intra-abdominal injury. A central focus is balancing the health and well-being of the fetus against the mother's need for surgery. When a surgical intervention is chosen, the effect of surgery on the fetus and the pregnancy often is very difficult to discern from the effects caused by the pathologic process (e.g., trauma) that created the need for surgery. A demonstrable increase in risk to the fetus occurs from surgery alone, and the risk appears to be greatest in the first and third trimesters. The concern for the fetus adds to complexity of diagnosis and management of trauma during pregnancy.

An understanding of normal maternal-fetal physiology is critical in the diagnosis, surgical management, and postoperative care of pregnant women who require major surgery or who have been injured. Normal clinical and laboratory findings in pregnant women would be suggestive of pathology in women who are not pregnant. The differentiation between normal physiology and pathology in these groups of women saves them from exposure to needless, and sometimes dangerous, diagnostic testing (Table 59.1).

Table 59.1: Changes in laboratory values during pregnancy

Value	*Non-pregnant*	*Pregnant*
Chloride (mEq/L)	100-106	90-105
Bicarbonate (mEq/L)	24-30	17-22
PCO_2 (mm Hg)	35-50	25-30
PO_2 (mm Hg)	98-100	101-104
Base excess (mEq/L)	0.7	3-4
Arterial pH	7.38	7.40-7.45
BUN (mg/dL)	10	4-12
Creatinine (mg/dL)	0.6	0.4-0.9
Creatinine clearance (mL/min)		3.5 2.0-3.7
Osmolality (mOsm/kg)	275	275-285
Alkaline phosphatase (mU/mL)		13 25-80
SGOT† (mU/mL)	10	10-40
Total protein (g/dL)	6.0	5.5-7.5
Albumin (g/dL)	3.5	3.0-4.5
Total cholesterol (mg/dL)	120	250
Triglycerides (mg/dL)	45-150	230
Hematocrit (%)	37-48	32-42
Hemoglobin (g/dL)	12-16	10-14
Leukocytes (cells/mm^3)	4300-10,800	5000-15,000
Lymphocytes (%)	38-46	15-40
Fibrinogen	250-400	600
Platelets	150,000-350,000	130,000-350,000
Iron saturation (%)	30-40	14-30
Ferritin (ng/mL)	35	10-12
Erythrocyte sedimentation rate (mm/h)	<20	30-90

* Partial pressure of oxygen

† Serum glutamic-oxaloacetic transaminase

PHYSIOLOGICAL CHANGES IN PREGNANCY

Intravascular Volume

The rapidly growing uteroplacental-fetal unit places a marked pressure on oxygen delivery. These demands are met by increasing oxygen carrying capacity (ie, blood volume), cardiac output, and minute ventilation. Total blood volume increases by 35-40%, and this increase in blood volume can help predict the normal adaptations in most organ systems. Plasma volume is the first component to respond to the new hormonal milieu of pregnancy. Plasma volume increases progressively from 5-7 weeks' gestation to a maximum volume of about 5000 mL at 32 weeks' gestation, an increase of 45% (about 1400 mL). This increase in plasma volume is more rapid than the increase in red cell mass. Red cell mass increases by about 350 mL by term, an increment of 25%. The greatest discrepancy between the increasing red cell mass and the increasing plasma volume occurs at 27-33 weeks' gestation; the hematocrit decreases during this period. A hematocrit less than 30% or a hemoglobin less than 10 g/dL is diagnostic of anemia.

Erythrocyte 2,3-diphosphoglycerate concentration increases during pregnancy, thus lowering the affinity of maternal hemoglobin for oxygen. This facilitates the dissociation of oxygen from hemoglobin as the blood passes through the intervillous space in the placenta. This process enhances the delivery of oxygen to the growing fetus. Pregnancy-induced decreases in colloid osmotic pressure (COP) place the gravid woman at greater risk of pulmonary edema. Colloid osmotic pressure describes the ability of large molecules (e.g., proteins) to retain fluid in the intravascular (or interstitial) space. Their large size prevents their transfer across the semipermeable endothelial membrane and sets up an osmotic gradient.

Non pregnant ambulatory patients have a mean COP value of 25 (± 2.5 standard deviation [SD]) mm Hg. In pregnancy, COP declines to about 22.5 (± 0.5 SD) mm Hg at term. After delivery (nadir at 6 h), COP drops to 15 (± 2 SD) mm Hg. The pulmonary capillary wedge pressure (PCWP) is a proxy for left ventricular cardiac function. When the COP-to-PCWP gradient is less than 4 mm Hg, a substantial risk for pulmonary edema exists. Preeclampsia reduces COP to 18 mm Hg antepartum and 14 mm Hg postpartum. The drop in COP in preeclampsia corresponds to the decrease in serum albumin that is associated with preeclampsia. The large transfusion (i.e., 2-3 mL/1 mL blood loss) of crystalloid solutions in association with trauma or burns results in earlier onset of pulmonary edema in pregnant women and immediately postpartum.

The loss of circulating blood volume and hemorrhage are major physiologic challenges associated with trauma. The typical pregnant woman is young and healthy and can adapt to the challenge more easily than older women with chronic diseases such as ischemic heart disease, diabetes, or chronic hypertension. In healthy individuals with normal oxygen carrying capacity, the traditional signs of hemorrhage and adaptation do not become evident at rest until 15-20% (i.e., 1200 mL) of total blood volume is lost. Pregnant women who are older (i.e., >35 y) or who have underlying medical disease may manifest symptoms with less significant blood loss. Because pregnancy is associated with an increase in blood volume, the actual amount of blood loss that results in clinical signs of response is greater in pregnant women than in non-pregnant women.

Once 20-25% (i.e., 1200-1500 mL) of blood volume is lost, systemic adaptation through sympathetic stimulation becomes apparent along with mild tachycardia (ie, 95-105 beats per min and peripheral vasoconstriction manifested as cold, pale extremities). Any decreases in blood pressure are mild, and mean arterial pressure (MAP) drops 10-15% (i.e., MAP is 70-75 mm Hg). Moderate hemorrhage, 25-35% (i.e., 1500-2000 mL) of blood volume, is associated with increasing evidence of sympathetic stimulation and the onset of tissue hypoxia, tachycardia (i.e, 105-120 beats per min), MAP drop of 25-30% (i.e, MAP is 50-60 mm Hg), restlessness, and oliguria (i.e, <0.5 mL/kg of actual weight). With severe hemorrhage (i.e, >30% or >2000 mL loss of blood volume), hemorrhagic shock is manifest along with significant tissue hypoxia, tachycardia (i.e, >120 beats per min), hypotension (i.e, MAP <50 mm Hg), altered consciousness, and anuria.

Fetal tolerance of maternal hemorrhage depends on the degree of maternal sympathetic response, the oxygen carrying capacity of the maternal blood, and maternal blood pressure. In the presence of an acute decrease in intravascular blood volume, progressive fetal acidosis occurs, with significant peripheral vasoconstriction, maternal tachycardia at rest and without pain (i.e, >105 beats per minute), drop in MAP of 10-15% (or <70 mm Hg), hematocrit less than 24%, or maternal oxygen saturation less than 92%. While maternal oxygenation requires adequate respiratory and cardiovascular function, the fetus relies entirely on cardiovascular function and placental transfer of oxygen. Understanding pregnancy changes in maternal cardiovascular physiology is critical to understanding the fetal response to trauma.

Cardiovascular Physiology

Hypervolemia, increased cardiac output, and positional hypotension are the major changes and risks of pregnancy-induced adaptations of the cardiovascular system. In healthy pregnancies, oxygen consumption (VO_2) is increased by a combination of increasing fetal metabolic requirements, maternal vasodilation, and arteriovenous shunting through the placenta. The full effects of vasodilation and arteriovenous shunting reach their maximum at 24-30 weeks' gestation, and a 30% reduction in both systolic and diastolic blood pressures is expected. Cardiac output rises rapidly until 30-32 weeks' gestation. This is accomplished by an increase in heart rate to 85 beats per minute and a lesser increase in stroke volume (Table 59.2).

In the course of anesthesia, surgery, and postoperative recovery, the obstetrician, surgeon, and anesthesiologist monitor and manipulate critical physiologic variables, such as blood pressure, heart rate, cardiac output, hematocrit, PaO_2, and $PaCO_2$ (Table 57.2).

The maternal cardiovascular system plays a key role in utero-placental physiology. Familiarity with the maternal cardiovascular response to surgical hemorrhage, trauma, and sepsis is critical in understanding the complications resulting from these abdominal disorders and their treatment (e.g., surgery, vasoactive drugs). Circulatory physiology in response to challenge in non pregnant animals and humans has been well described.

In summary, tissue perfusion and aerobic tissue metabolism are a reflection of overall circulatory function. Oxygen delivery (DO_2), defined as arterial oxygen content multiplied by cardiac index (CI), reflects circulatory function. VO_2, defined as arteriovenous oxygen content difference multiplied by CI, reflects the sum of all oxidative metabolic reactions plus arteriovenous shunting. The production of metabolic acids, especially lactate, indicates a failure of the circulatory system (i.e, DO_2) to meet the oxygen needs (i.e, VO_2) of the tissue.

Patients with shock associated with hemorrhage or cardiac dysfunction have greatly reduced DO_2 with moderately reduced VO_2. Increased oxygen extraction is the principal compensatory reaction when tissue perfusion is limited by reduced DO_2. In contrast, the

Table 59.2 Central hemodynamics in pregnancy

Hemodynamic Parameters	*Nonpregnant (± SD)*	*Pregnant (± SD)*	*Percent Change %*
Heart rate (beats per min)	71 (10)	83 (10)	+17
MAP (mm HG)	86.5 (7.5)	90.3 (5.8)	NS*
Cardiac output (L/min)	4.3 (0.9)	6.2 (1.0)	+43
SVR† (dyne sec/cm^5)	1520 (520)	1210 (266)	-21
LVSWI‡ (g m/m^2)	41 (8)	48 (6)	NS
Central venous pressure (mm Hg)	3.7 (2.6)	3.6 (2.5)	NS
PCWP (mm Hg)	6.3 (2.1)	7.5 (1.8)	NS
COP (mm Hg)	20.8 (1.0)	18 (1.5)	-14

* Not significant
† Systemic vascular resistance
‡ Left ventricular stroke work index

increased VO_2, which is provoked by increased metabolism from sepsis and trauma, is compensated by increased CI and DO_2. Therapeutically, management is directed at maintaining levels of VO_2 and DO_2 within the reference range rather than focusing on a specific cardiac profile (eg, blood pressure, wedge pressure).

The way uterine arteries (i.e, uterine blood flow) participate in the maternal compensatory response to hypovolemia and shock reflects fetal tolerance. Knowledge of uterine blood flow and response to hemorrhage, hypoxia, or vasoactive drugs is derived from data in anesthetized animal models, usually ovine. Data from animal experiments imply that the uterine vascular bed in pregnant organisms is a low-resistance system. The uterine vessels appear to be maximally dilated and, therefore, exhibit minimal autoregulation. More importantly, uterine blood flow reflects maternal arterial blood pressure in a linear fashion in pregnant organisms. When maternal blood volume is reduced by 30-35%, a minimal change in maternal mean arterial pressure occurs. As participants in the compensatory response, the uterine arteries constrict, and uterine blood flow is reduced by 10-20%.

Alpha-adrenergic compensatory vasoconstriction occurs in response to maternal hypoxia. Alpha-adrenergic blocking agents, such as phenoxybenzamine, limit this response. A decrease in uterine PaO_2 from 70 to 55 mm Hg was associated in one study with a 16% reduction in uterine blood flow; a decrease in PaO_2 from 96 to 28 mm Hg resulted in a 25% reduction in uterine blood flow.

These observations contribute considerable interpretative information to the clinician faced with a pregnant woman with an acute abdomen. Clinical evidence of alpha-adrenergic stimulation raises a concern regarding reduced uterine blood flow and subsequent fetal compromise, despite maternal blood pressures within the reference range. Alpha-adrenergic stimulation is manifested by marked peripheral vasoconstriction, cold and clammy extremities, a decrease in capillary refill in response to skin pressure, widened pulse pressure, decreased urinary output, and increased sweating.

In the third trimester, maternal position has a great impact on intravascular pressures and cardiac output. In the supine position, the uterus obstructs both the inferior vena cava and the aorta. Venous pressures in the lower leg can be as high as 20-25 mm Hg, and the caliber of the aortic lumen is reduced by 40%. Cardiac output in the supine position subsequently may be reduced as much as 25% compared with that in the left recumbent position. Approximately 10% of pregnant women in the third trimester have supine hypotensive syndrome, which is manifested by profound maternal hypotension and fetal hypoxia. Acute nausea is a common symptom. A key component in the treatment of a critically ill trauma patient is to place the patient with a left pelvic tilt via a wedge.

Respiratory Physiology

Hormonal and mechanical changes (e.g. enlarging uterus) combine to produce hyperventilation. Progesterone acts early to increase the respiratory rate by 15%. Minute ventilation and tidal volume are increased 50% and 40%, respectively. The relative hyperventilation is reflected by hypocapnia (i.e, $PaCO_2$ is 28-32 mm Hg). Anxiety and pain can cause a pregnant patient to increase her respiratory rate to the point of significant hypocapnia, which results in faintness and perioral numbness. A 5-minute episode of hyperventilation that drops the maternal $PaCO_2$ by 6 mm Hg results in a 4 mm Hg drop in fetal $PaCO_2$ and, more importantly, a 3.5 mm Hg drop in fetal PaO_2.

Baseline hyperventilation also reduces respiratory compensation for metabolic acidosis. Inhalation anesthesia has a more rapid onset in pregnant patients. After the first trimester, progressive anatomic changes reduce the functional residual capacity and residual volume by 20%. When these changes are coupled with an increase in oxygen consumption (15%), hypoventilation or apnea results in a more rapid onset of hypoxia. During pregnancy, the closing capacity is elevated in the first 48-72 hours after abdominal or thoracic surgery; the resultant arteriovenous shunting further hastens the onset of hypoxia.

Renal physiology

Changes in the cardiovascular system are reflected in the renal system. The 50% increase in blood volume during pregnancy results in an increased renal plasma flow and an increased glomerular filtration rate (GFR). As a result, an increase occurs in the excretion of metabolic products (eg, proteins, glucose) that may exceed the tubular reabsorption capability. In healthy pregnancy, BUN and creatinine levels are 10 mg/dL and 0.7 mg/dL, respectively. Glucosuria has been found on 2 or more occasions in 5-10% of women as a result of a reduction in the renal threshold between 140 and 160 mg/dL. Proteinuria levels as high as 300 mg/d are considered within the reference range. Hematuria is always abnormal during pregnancy.

Pregnancy-induced changes of the renal system include partial ureteral obstruction in the third trimester and increased glomerular clearance. A combination of smooth muscle relaxation by progesterone and compression by the enlarging uterus at the pelvic brim creates physiologic hydronephrosis of pregnancy. Changes occur before 12 weeks' gestation, and the obstruction is more pronounced on the right side. The anatomic changes revert to normal by 6 weeks postpartum. These normal changes must be recognized in the interpretation of intravenous pyelography during pregnancy and the puerperium.

While the exact pathophysiology is unknown, pregnant women are more susceptible to symptomatic urinary tract infections. The risk may be related to increased urinary stasis, or urinary human chorionic gonadotropin may enhance the attachment of pathologic organisms to the urinary mucosa. Approximately 5-10% of reproductive-aged women enter pregnancy with chronic, episodic, asymptomatic bacteriuria. If unidentified and untreated in the first trimester, asymptomatic bacteriuria leads to pyelonephritis in about one third of individuals. Because women who experience trauma often have Foley catheters, another risk factor for urinary tract infection, consider pyelonephritis when a trauma patient's fever spikes.

Coagulation Physiology

Pulmonary embolism is a major cause of maternal death, and the pregnant (or immediately postpartum) woman is at increased risk. Obesity (i.e, body mass index [BMI] >26) is an independent risk factor for deep venous thrombosis after trauma, and many women have a BMI greater than 26 in late pregnancy. In addition, changes in coagulation physiology place these patients at an even greater risk.

Thrombosis is more likely to occur in pregnancy because pregnant women have 2 of the components of Virchow triad, venous stasis and hypercoagulability. As occurs in the ureters, high progesterone levels relax the smooth muscle of maternal vasculature. A greater venous capacitance exists. The enlarged uterus compresses the vena cava and triples the venous pressure in the lower extremities (8-24 mm Hg).

Estrogen increases the hepatic production of coagulation factors, yielding a 30-50% increase in fibrinogen and factors VII, VIII, IX, and X. Fibrinolysis is decreased in the second and third trimesters. These changes increase the incidence of thrombophlebitis to 1:70.

Infection, general anesthesia, and surgery further exaggerate the risk when the third component of Virchow triad, vascular injury, is added. Postoperative bed rest increases the risk of stasis. Prevention is the cornerstone of management. Once high-risk patients are identified, prophylactic heparin (5000-7500 U q8-12h), intermittent pressure stockings, and early ambulation constitute standard therapy.

Gastrointestinal Physiology

Nausea and vomiting are common in pregnancy. In the first half of pregnancy, as many as 70% of pregnant women experience nausea and 40% report episodes of vomiting. Incidence is reduced considerably in the second half of pregnancy, but 15-20% of patients report persistence of symptoms throughout their pregnancy.

The diagnosis of nausea and vomiting in pregnancy (i.e., hyperemesis gravidarum) is a diagnosis of exclusion. Any patient with nausea and vomiting requires a history and physical examination performed in a timely and thorough manner. Gastroenteritis is the most common non obstetric diagnosis, but hepatitis, pancreatitis, and pyelonephritis also are frequent. Nausea and vomiting may be a component of appendicitis, but anorexia and pain usually are prominent. In a patient with previous pelvic and/or abdominal surgery, pelvic inflammatory disease, or endometriosis, intestinal obstruction is a consideration. In this case, the physical examination is very important in diagnosis and management.

Abdominal distention, with or without ascitic fluid, is best determined by the location of areas of dullness when the patient is turned from side to side. Peristaltic sounds characteristic of an obstruction are high-pitched, tinkling, and with rushes. Absence of peristalsis sounds is an important sign, often indicating an ileus or the presence of intraperitoneal fluid, pus, or blood. Between these 2 extremes, wide variations in the type and quality of peristaltic sounds may be noted, but these differences usually are not important. When intestinal obstruction is suspected, abdominal X-ray films (i.e, upright, flat plate, left lateral decubitus) are essential and should not be withheld for fear of fetal exposure to radiation.

Constipation is common in pregnancy because of the effects of progesterone on bowel mobility and the widespread use of hematinic agents; however, flatus always should be present. The combination of bed rest, pregnancy, iron supplements, and narcotics for pain after trauma during pregnancy poses an important management problem. Routine use of bulk stool softeners is recommended. Anorexia, constipation, and the failure to pass flatus are serious signs that could indicate appendicitis, bowel perforation, or intestinal obstruction. Diarrhea is seldom an indication of an acute surgical problem in the abdomen except as a symptom of recurrent ulcerative colitis.

Physiologic changes in the GI tract during pregnancy increase the risk of aspiration during surgery and anesthesia. Progesterone is a smooth muscle relaxant, and lower esophageal sphincter tone is decreased. One fourth of pregnant women have symptomatic lower esophageal reflux. Gastrin, the hormone that increases the volume of gastric secretion and lowers the pH of the stomach contents, increases considerably during pregnancy.

In addition, intragastric pressure is increased by the large uterus, the supine/lithotomy position, fundal pressure, and light anesthesia. Classic training has taught that approximately one fourth of pregnant women undergoing abdominal surgery after an overnight fast have gastric contents of sufficient volume and sufficiently low pH to place them at high risk of aspiration. More recent evidence demonstrates that pregnancy does not delay gastric emptying. Despite the latter finding, an 8-hour fast and metoclopramide or other histamine 2 (H2) antagonist should be prescribed as antacid prophylaxis before surgery.

When the patient is not allowed or cannot have oral intake, such as with prolonged ventilation, neurologic injury, and bowel injury, fetal intrauterine growth retardation may occur. Most patients with an acute abdomen are not permitted oral intake, at least for the acute phase, and intravenous dextrose and multivitamins are indicated. If a patient has had insufficient intake (i.e, <1500 kcal/d) for 72 hours, start parenteral nutrition.

If support is needed for less than 10 days, peripheral parenteral nutrition is indicated. An appropriate nutrient solution is the simultaneous use of 4.25% amino acid and 5% dextrose (1500 mL) with a fat emulsion (1500 mL of intralipid) through a Y-connector. This provides the patient with 3000 mL water, 64 g of protein, and 1950 calories in 24 hours. Electrolytes, trace elements, and vitamins can be added to the protein solution. If support is needed for more than 10 days or if a patient's condition is particularly severe, total parenteral nutrition through a central venous catheter is needed.

The specific problems of parenteral nutrition during pregnancy are the increased metabolic needs (i.e., increase to 40 kcal/kg/d, increase in protein by 30-50 g/d). Hyperglycemia can be a greater risk because pregnancy usually is a diabetogenic state. Treat mean blood glucose levels consistently greater than 105 mg/dL with insulin. Pregnancy is a hyperlipidemic state, and some theoretic caution exists about the use of lipid solutions (e.g., pancreatitis, preterm labor). However, hyperalimentation is a replacement rather than a supplementation, and this caution may not be applicable. The fetus is evaluated for growth and well-being. Nonstress tests are performed twice weekly, and serial ultrasonography for fetal growth should be obtained.

Central Nervous System

Pregnancy critically changes the need for several anesthetic drugs. The requirement for halogenated anesthetics (i.e., halothane) is reduced by 40% because of the increased minute volume. Serum pseudocholinesterase is decreased by 20% in late pregnancy; however, clinically significant increases in the duration of succinylcholine neuromuscular block are reported rarely. Venous distention increases the caliber of epidural veins. The dose of epidural anesthetic agents is reduced by 50%. The uterine vasculature is sensitive to alpha-adrenergic stimulation. Maternal stress response, maternal anxiety, or alpha-adrenergic vasopressors can result in fetal hypoxia and acidosis.

A General Approach to the Pregnant Trauma Patient

The primary initial goal in treating a pregnant trauma victim is to stabilize the mother's condition. The priorities for treatment of an injured pregnant patient remain the same as those for the non-pregnant patient.

Primary Survey

As with any other injured patient, the primary survey of the injured pregnant patient addresses the airway/cervical spine control, breathing and circulation (ABC; volume replacement/hemorrhage control), with the mother receiving treatment priority. Supplemental oxygen is essential to prevent maternal and fetal hypoxia. Severe trauma stimulates maternal catecholamine release, which causes uteroplacental vasoconstriction and compromised fetal circulation. Prevention of aortocaval compression is also essential to optimize maternal and fetal hemodynamics. Pregnant patients beyond 20 weeks' gestation should not be left supine during the initial assessment. Left uterine displacement should be used by tilting the backboard to the left or as a final measure, the uterus can be manually displaced.

Hypovolemia should be suspected before it becomes apparent because of the relative pregnancy induced hypervolemia and hemodilution that may mask significant blood losses. It's important to remember that even during pregnancy, the body never considers the uterus an essential organ. In a pregnant woman in shock, uterine perfusion will decrease before renal perfusion (or that of any other major organ). Although a pregnant woman might tolerate considerable blood loss with little consequence, a fetus inside a hypoperfused uterus will not. Because the signs of hypovolemia and shock are delayed in a pregnant woman, any signs of maternal hypovolemia indicate that the fetus is already compromised. Maternal blood and fluid replacement must be initiated immediately.

Aggressive volume resuscitation is encouraged even for normotensive patients. The pneumatic antishock garment (PASG/ MAST SUIT) may be used to stabilize lower extremity fractures and perhaps control hemorrhage. In the pregnant patient, inflation of the abdominal compartment of the PASG/ MAST SUIT should be avoided because it compromises uteroplacental blood flow.

Secondary Survey

The secondary survey consists of obtaining a complete history, including an obstetrical history, performing a physical examination, and evaluating and monitoring the fetus. The obstetrical history is important because the identification of comorbid factors may alter management decisions. A history of preterm labor or placental abruption puts the patient at increased risk for the recurrence of the condition. The obstetrical history should include the date of the last menstruation, expected date of delivery and any problems or complications of the current and previous pregnancies. Determination of the uterine size provides an approximation of gestational age, i.e., measurement of fundal height is a rapid method for estimating fetal age. Determination of fetal age and hence of fetal maturity is an important factor in the decision approach regarding early delivery.

The fetus is usually considered viable when it has a 50% chance of extra uterine survival. If neonatal facilities are available, this usually means at 25 to 26 weeks' gestation or an estimated weight of 750 g. More aggressive institutions use 24 weeks' gestation or an estimated weight of 500 to 600 g as the cut-off point, although chances of survival are then reduced to 20 to 30%. It should be noted that, even with the best of ultrasound dating criteria, unless the time of conception is known exactly, the assignment of gestational age is subject to 1 to 2 weeks of uncertainty. Decisions on fetal viability are made on the basis of the best gestational age available. When estimating the fetal age in the resuscitation area, a rough guide might be that when the fundus of the uterus extends beyond the umbilicus, the fetus is potentially viable.

Pelvic and rectal examinations should be performed. Aside from the usual secondary survey, assessment of the injured pregnant patient should rule out vaginal bleeding, ruptured membranes, a bulging perineum, the presence of contractions, and an abnormal fetal heart rate and rhythm.

Feto-Maternal Hemorrhage (FMH)

This is the transplacental hemorrhage of fetal blood into the normally separate maternal circulation, and is a unique complication of trauma during pregnancy. The reported incidence of FMH after trauma is 8 to 30%. There is no real correlation between severity of trauma, gestational age and frequency and volume of FMH. The total blood volume of the placental-fetal unit is about 120 mL per estimated fetal weight in grams and only 0.1 mL of Rhesus (Rh)-positive fetal blood into an unsensitized Rh-negative mother is required for Rh sensitization. Complications of FMH include Rh sensitization in the mother, fetal anemia, fetal paroxysmal atrial tachycardia or fetal death from exsanguination. In theory, FMH is possible by the 4th week of gestation; some say that FMH becomes a concern after 12 weeks gestation when the uterus rises above the pelvis and becomes an organ susceptible to direct trauma. FMH is detected by the *Kleihauer-Betke (KB)* acid elution technique on maternal blood. Upon examination, adult cells remain colorless while fetal red cells turn bright purple-pink. The ratio of fetal cells to maternal cells is recorded, enabling calculation of the volume of fetal blood leaked into the maternal circulation:

Most clinical laboratories will screen 1000 red blood cells taken from the mother. A maternal blood volume of 5 liters is commonly assumed in laboratory formulas so that one fetal cell per 1000 cells counted corresponds to a FMH of 5 ml. Unfortunately, the amount of FMH sufficient to sensitize most Rh-negative women is well below the 5-ml sensitivity level of the typical laboratory's KB test. As little as 1 ml of Rh-positive blood can sensitize 70% of Rh-negative women. Currently, several commercial kits expedite and simplify the test process. Unfortunately, the sensitivity of all the KB test is relatively low. Therefore, all Rh-negative mothers who present with a history of abdominal trauma should receive one 300 ug prophylactic dose of Rh immune globulin (anti-D immunoglobulin; Rhogam) within 72 hours of the traumatic event. Although controversial, we believe that the KB test should be reserved for Rh-negative women who are at risk for massive FMH that will exceed the efficacy of one dose of immune globulin, i.e. more than 30 ml. According to some studies, fewer than 1% of all trauma cases and only 3.1% of major trauma cases exceed the coverage of one 300-ug Rh immune globulin dose. As a general rule, 300 ug of Rh immune globulin should be given for every 30 ml of fetal blood found in the maternal circulation. The KB test is probably unnecessary before 16 weeks' gestation because the fetal blood volume is below 30 ml before this gestational age. For cases of documented FMH, some studies recommend repeating the KB test in 24 hours to check for increased bleeding. Given the imprecision of the Kleihauer-Betke test, the estimated fetal-maternal bleed must be reconciled with the estimated fetal blood volume. A large fetal-maternal hemorrhage may result in fetal anemia, chronic asphyxia, or fetal death. Pregnant women with trauma should have a serum alpha-fetoprotein determination and a Kleihauer-Betke test to estimate the volume of fetal-to-maternal transfusion. Serial fetal testing and ultrasonographic examinations are necessary when large bleeds are apparent. In-utero fetal transfusion may be considered when the fetus is very immature, 20-26 weeks' gestation

The Fetus in Trauma

The effect of trauma on pregnancy depends on the gestational age of the fetus, the type and severity of the trauma, and the extent of disruption of normal uterine and fetal physiology. The survival of the fetus depends on adequate uterine perfusion and delivery of oxygen. The uterine circulation has no autoregulation which implies that uterine blood flow is related directly to maternal systemic blood pressure, at least until the mother approaches hypovolemic shock. At that point, peripheral vasoconstriction will further compromise uterine perfusion. Once obvious shock develops in the mother, the chances of saving the fetus are about 20 %.

The most important surgical risk to the fetus is preterm delivery. Before 23 weeks' gestation, preterm delivery uniformly results in neonatal death. When delivery occurs at a hospital with a level 3 perinatal center, survival rates at 25, 26, 27, and 28 weeks' gestation would be 60%, 70%, 80% and 90%, respectively. Major long-term defects associated with delivery at 24, 25, 26 and 28 weeks can occur in 70%, 50%, 40%, and 20% of neonates, respectively. After 28 weeks' gestation, intact survival rates improves more slowly.

An infant born at term is better off than an infant born preterm. The key gestational age breakpoints in fetal outcome appear to be 25, 28, 32 and 36 weeks' gestation. Birth at hospitals without expertise in high-risk obstetrics and neonatology is associated with a significantly higher risk of perinatal death and a doubling or tripling of long-term handicap. Taking into consideration the transport time, resources, and maternal condition, in-utero transport is preferable to delivery and neonatal transport in most cases.

Factors Responsible for Fetal Morbidity and Mortality

Four factors in maternal trauma or surgery predict fetal morbidity and mortality—hypoxia, infection, drug effects, and preterm delivery. Fetal death can occur at any gestational age and usually results from fetal hypoxia. In particular, a decrease in maternal hematocrit greater than 50% and a decrease in maternal mean blood pressure of 20% or a maternal PaO_2 less than 60 mm Hg (oxygen saturation <90%) results in fetal hypoxia, acidosis, and compromise.

If fetal oxygenation or perfusion are compromised by trauma, the response of the fetus may include bradycardia or tachycardia, a decrease in the baseline variability of the heart rate, the absence of normal accelerations in the heart rate, or recurrent decelerations. It should be noted that an abnormal fetal heart rate may be the first indication of an important disruption in fetal homeostasis. During trauma resuscitation, evaluation of the fetus should begin with auscultation of heart tones and continuous recording of the heart rate.

Trauma to the uterus (direct or indirect) can also injure the myometrium and destabilize decidual lysosomes, releasing arachidonic acid that can cause uterine contractions, and perhaps inducing premature labor.

PRETERM LABOR

The most likely cause of preterm labor in a trauma patient is abruptio placentae; however, other etiologies are possible and must be considered. Preterm labor may be the cause of abdominal pain or a consequence of non obstetric disease, trauma, or infection. Diagnosis and treatment of preterm labor in pregnant patients are difficult perioperatively. Clear risks exist for preterm delivery; however, the intrauterine environment may not be ideal, and the treatment of preterm labor may exacerbate the effects of intra-abdominal disease. Before making a definitive diagnosis, consider the many obstetric conditions that pose greater fetal risk (e.g., chorio-amnionitis, abruptio placentae). These often mimic acute non obstetric conditions.

Tocolysis in the presence of these diseases is not indicated. The cardiovascular effects of beta-adrenergic drugs (e.g., terbutaline, ritodrine) can exacerbate those of sepsis (e.g.

vasodilatation, shock). For example, intravenous ritodrine poses a 5-10% risk of serious cardiopulmonary complications, such as pulmonary edema and significant subendocardial ischemia. Other tocolytic agents that involve calcium ion physiology (e.g., magnesium sulfate, calcium channel blockers) have less significant, but still disturbing, cardiovascular effects in the presence of sepsis. Prostaglandin synthetase inhibitors (e.g., indomethacin) are used cautiously for tocolysis because they mask the clinical signs of infection or cause maternal platelet dysfunction.

Keeping these problems in mind, the following management of preterm labor in trauma or after trauma surgery is suggested. First, uterine irritability is not considered labor until evidence of cervical effacement or dilatation exists. Prophylactic tocolysis is not indicated. Uterine contraction monitoring is appropriate only if the documentation of contractions changes management. In the acute phase, continuous uterine contraction monitoring is appropriate after 20-22 weeks' gestation with a normally formed fetus. Serial cervical examinations are essential for the diagnosis of preterm labor. Withhold tocolytic therapy until cervical change has taken place. If no uterine irritability exists, the patient's condition has stabilized, and she can recognize and report fetal movement and contractions, then continuous uterine contraction monitoring can be replaced by maternal perception and patient education about the signs of preterm labor.

Any decision to begin tocolysis requires demonstration of the following: cervical change, assurance that membranes have not ruptured via sterile examination using Nitrazine and fern tests, and the absence of the usual precautions against the use of tocolytics. Second, determine the presence of intrauterine disease by a thorough physical and ultrasonographic examination and, perhaps, amniocentesis. Amniocentesis under ultrasonographic guidance has many advantages. Bacteria or sheets of leukocytes on a high-power microscopic examination of an unspun specimen suggest chorioamnionitis. Fetal lung maturity studies can be performed rapidly in most institutions. Keep in mind the risks associated with third trimester amniocentesis, including fetal trauma (1%), ruptured membranes (1-2%), and preterm labor (1-2%). If peritonitis is present, amniotic fluid contamination is a special concern. In the presence of peritonitis, do not allow amniocentesis to delay an exploratory laparotomy. Localized peritoneal contamination over the amniocentesis site cannot always be predicted. Perform amniocentesis away from points of tenderness. An uncomfortable but acceptable alternative is to perform a suprapubic tap through a full bladder under ultrasonographic guidance. This approach avoids the peritoneum.

Once the diagnostic test or surgery has been performed and the mother's cardiovascular status is stable, the decision of whether or not to inhibit labor can be made. Magnesium sulfate is the therapy of choice. The dose is 4 g in 250 mL of isotonic sodium chloride adminis-tered intravenously during a period of 15 minutes, followed by 2 g/h by electronically monitored intravenous drip. Monitor the fetus continuously throughout diagnosis and management. Aggressively diagnose and treat fetal distress. Continue magnesium sulfate for 12-24 hours after the operation. At that point, patients are weaned off the medication.

Fetal Assessment

Fetal assessment in the recovery from trauma is always a concern for non obstetricians. At any gestational age, documentation of a live fetus by fetal heart auscultation is appropriate; however, continuous fetal monitoring for fetal heart rate changes is appropriate only if an obstetrician is willing to act on the information (e.g. a fetus >25 weeks gestation or with no lethal anomalies). In the recovery period, as a patient's condition becomes stable and consciousness is regained, continuous fetal assessment can be changed to a combination of recording 10 fetal movements every 12 hours and a non stress test twice a week. This scheme can be used until the patient has returned to the usual functional state but not necessarily for the duration of the pregnancy. The fetus is usually considered viable when it has a 50% chance of extra uterine survival. If neonatal facilities are available, this usually means at 25 to 26 weeks' gestation or an estimated weight of 750 g. More aggressive institutions use 24 weeks' gestation or an estimated weight of 500 to 600 g as the cut-off point, although chances of survival are then reduced to 20 to 30%. It should be noted that, even with the best of ultrasound dating criteria, unless the time of conception is known exactly, the assignment of gestational age is subject to 1 to 2 weeks of uncertainty. Decisions on fetal viability are made on the basis of the best gestational age available. When estimating the fetal age in the resuscitation area, a rough guide might be that when the fundus of the uterus extends beyond the umbilicus, the fetus is potentially viable. Reported direct fetal injuries include skull fractures, intracranial hemorrhage, and splenic rupture. As the largest abdominal organ, the fetal liver is also likely to sustain injury. Placental abruption-the detachment of the placenta from the uterine wall-is common after serious trauma and is a major cause of fetal death. Other causes include preterm labor, premature rupture of the membranes, placental lacerations, uterine rupture, and umbilical cord thrombosis. Emergent interventions for the treatment of fetal injuries are limited.

Cardio Tocography (CTG)

- Normal FHS 120-160 bpm.
- Beat to beat variability fluctuations in FHR between 3 to 20 bpm reflects metabolic status and autonomic control-loss means hypoxia or acidosis.

Decelerations:

- *Early:* Sustained decrease in FHR >15 bpm beginning at onset of uterine contraction, returning to baseline shortly thereafter. This is due to fetal head compression during uterine contraction.
- *Late:* >15 bpm drops near end of uterine contraction with slow resolution to baseline-signifying uteroplacental insufficiency, abruption, hypovolemia, hypotension.
- *Variable:* Changes in FHR with no relation to uterine contractions due to transient cord compression, abrupt increase in FHR and rapid return to baseline.
- During any maternal insult, changes occur in the fetal heart rate as loss of baseline variability, prolonged decelerations or late decelerations, occurs before maternal signs or symptoms appear.

Special Maternal Issues

- Abdominal pain and tenderness.
- Abdominal pain and/or tenderness in pregnant trauma patients raises the difficult question of whether the signs and symptoms are obstetric or non obstetric in origin. After the first trimester of pregnancy, the most common confusing obstetric diagnoses are preterm labor, intra-amniotic infection, or abruptio placentae. Unfortunately, these complications may be the consequence of maternal trauma, rather than the cause of the abdominal pain and tenderness.

The differentiation between non-obstetric and obstetric causes is critical to management.

The single most effective aid in diagnosis is an experienced obstetrician who has conducted a detailed history and physical examination. Subsequently, the results of serial pelvic examinations, electronic fetal monitoring, and ultrasonographic examinations are important in the diagnosis and management.

In selected cases, amniocentesis may provide useful information concerning amniotic fluid character (e.g., bloody, meconium stained), infection (obtain Gram stain and culture), and fetal lung maturity studies. When ultrasonography is not helpful, perform radiographic examinations in a calculated and focused manner. The fetal risks of diagnostic radiographs are minimal compared with the potential risk associated with delayed diagnosis or misdiagnosis of an acute abdomen.

When pain present, careful analysis of the location, type, intensity, and radiation is essential. Pain may be generalized or may be confined to the lower, middle, or upper abdomen. Generalized pain, when associated with rebound tenderness and guarding, is suggestive of severe irritation of the peritoneum, as found in pancreatitis, ruptured viscus, severe infection, or intra-abdominal hemorrhage. The presence of generalized pain and rebound tenderness subsequent to pain localized to one part of the abdomen suggests relatively sudden rupture of an organ, cyst, abscess, or tumor. With the rare exception of pancreatitis, early surgical exploration may be life saving for a mother and fetus. Central lower abdominal pain suggests a uterine origin.

Preterm labor may be the source or a consequence of the acute process. In either case, signs and symptoms of preterm labor must be evaluated. Preterm labor often is associated with one or more of the following signs or symptoms: waxing and waning central abdominal pain (similar to menstrual cramps), pelvic fullness, back pain, anterior thigh pain, groin pain, change in vaginal discharge, tenderness, urinary urgency, and vaginal bleeding or spotting. The diagnosis of preterm labor is based on evidence of effacement and dilation of the cervix. After confirmation of intact membranes and normal placental position, serial cervical examinations can be used to help diagnose preterm labor. The diagnosis of preterm labor is based on the presence of 3 contractions in 20 minutes plus cervical change or a cervix that is 2 cm dilated and less than 1 cm in length.

Steady central lower abdominal pain, especially when accompanied by point tenderness, is suggestive of an accident related to the uterus, such as uterine injury, torsion or infarction of a leiomyoma, abruptio placentae, or chorioamnionitis, each of which may be accompanied by localized tenderness or rebound tenderness. In rare cases, urinary disorders (e.g., cystitis) can cause pain levels sufficient to be confused with more serious and acute intra-abdominal problems.

Lateralized lower abdominal pain suggests an adnexal problem such as infection, torsion, rupture, or hemorrhage. The pain caused by ovarian disease often radiates to the anterior thigh. Extra peritoneal causes of lateralized pain include the intense, colicky pain of a ureteral stone, which may radiate to the groin or labia. The pain of pyelonephritis may be abdominal but is more often prominent in the flank area. Intraperitoneal causes include appendicitis on the right side. The pain may be higher than usual because of the upward displacement of the appendix by the growing uterus. As a result of displacement, the classic spread of pain from the umbilical area to the right lower quadrant of the abdomen may be absent in appendicitis.

Other rare causes of right lower abdominal pain include regional enteritis, diverticulitis of the cecum, and volvulus. Pain in the left lower abdomen may be due to disorders of the descending and sigmoid colon, such as ulcerative colitis, diverticulitis, or volvulus of the sigmoid.

Blunt Trauma

Although motor vehicle accidents are the most common cause of serious blunt trauma in pregnancy, assaults, abuse and falls are frequent. In addition to maternal mortality from blunt trauma, which is estimated to be about 7%, the fetus is at significant risk, especially if placental abruption, placenta previa, or uterine rupture occurs. Blunt trauma is a common denominator to many injuries during pregnancy. Motor vehicle accidents are a common source of blunt trauma. When the damage to the vehicle was severe, 7.2% died, and 13.5% had major injury.

Fetal death after 12 weeks' gestation occurs in 8% pregnant women surviving a severe collision. Except for cases of maternal death, first trimester loss could not be explained by trauma. The most common causes of fetal death after 12 weeks' gestation were maternal death, abruptio placentae, and maternal shock. Abruptio placentae occurred in 3.4% of pregnant women involved in severe accidents. Despite the recommendations of public health officials and obstetricians, the lay public, and, occasionally, misinformed physicians, 3-point restraints are safe for pregnant women in motor vehicles. Low birth weight and delivery within 48 hours were more common among unrestrained pregnant women (>20 weeks gestation) than among restrained pregnant women.[9] Regardless of the source or severity of trauma, the mother and her fetus benefit most by knowledge, planning, and protocols that reflect the physiologic differences between pregnant and non pregnant women and the special needs of the vulnerable fetus.

There are several important considerations when addressing blunt thoraco abdominal trauma in the pregnant patient. The physical examination may be unreliable because the enlarged uterus displaces the abdominal content and stretches the peritoneum thus perhaps diminishing the response to peritoneal irritation.

Evaluation

The evaluation of possible injury to the abdomen is different because of the presence of the gravid uterus. The preferred diagnostic modalities for evaluation during the first trimester of pregnancy are ultrasound, diagnostic peritoneal lavage (DPL), and CT-scan, in that order. Because the first trimester is the period of organogenesis, ultrasound is preferable for the detection of hemoperitoneum.

Because of its sensitivity especially in most trauma patients with multiple injuries or suspected intra-abdominal trauma, DPL can be used to evaluate the abdomen using the supraumbilical, open technique to avoid injury to the gravid uterus. The major disadvantage of DPL with respect to the pregnant patient is its invasiveness. The procedure can be used in all trimesters. In the first trimester, the abdomen can be catheterized through the midline subumbilical percutaneous route. In obese patients, a tap through the umbilicus may be easier. In the second or third trimester, a semi open technique is advised. The peritoneum is exposed under local anesthesia through a midline 3- to 4-cm incision. In either case, the abdominal cavity is entered with a peritoneal dialysis catheter. The catheter is gently advanced caudally, and, if no return of fluid occurs, 1000 mL of warm lactated Ringer solution is infused during a period of 5 minutes. The tubing and bottle then are placed on the floor, and the fluid is allowed to siphon back to the bottle. The average return is approximately 750 mL.

A positive finding on lavage is suggested by free aspiration of blood (>10 mL), an erythrocyte count greater than 100,000/mm^3, a leukocyte count greater than 175 cells/mm^3, or the presence of GI contents or an elevated amylase level (>175 mg/dL) in the effluent. A rapid negative test result can be achieved by the ability to read newsprint through the effluent. Even with a negative finding on lavage, significant injury can be present. The false-positive and false-negative rates are approximately 5%; however, a negative finding on lavage means that laparotomy does not need to be performed as long as bowel sounds are present and the abdomen remains soft and non tender.

If CT-scan is necessary, both oral and intravenous contrast media should be administered. During the second trimester, ultrasound or CT-scan may be used to evaluate the abdomen. DPL may be difficult to perform because the enlarged uterus may interfere with the dependent catheter position and return of fluid. On the other hand, several studies have shown its safety and usefulness. During the third trimester, the injured pregnant patient can best be assessed by ultrasound or CT-scan.

TREATMENT GUIDELINES

The following treatment guidelines are recommended. A pregnant trauma patient should be observed in a hospital ill equipped to diagnose and manage obstetric and neonatal emergencies. Transport the injured mother on her left side to avoid supine hypotension. Obtain a brief description of the severity of the accident and status of the patient from the ambulance attendant. Focus a brief physical examination on central nervous system function (neck injury), vital signs, chest wall motion, and movement of extremities.

At this point, perform diagnostic and monitoring studies. Before and during the screening physical examination, one or more large-bore intravenous catheters (16- to 18-gauge) are placed peripherally. If intra-abdominal trauma is suspected or if the patient is unconscious, place a central venous pressure line. Ringer lactate (2 mL/1 mL estimated blood loss) is transfused in a rapid fashion. The rate of subsequent transfusion is dependent on maternal vital signs and rate of continued blood loss. In most cases, early blood transfusion is preferable to massive crystalloid transfusion.

Obtain a complete blood count, urinalysis, serum electrolyte level, and blood for typing and cross-match. Administer tetanus toxoid (0.5 mL) to all patients. Perform endotracheal intubation on all patients in respiratory failure or who are unconscious. Place a 3-way Foley catheter in the bladder to monitor hourly urinary output and to identify hematuria. Insert a nasogastric tube to establish the integrity of the upper GI tract and to empty the stomach of its contents. In pregnancies after 24 weeks' gestation, apply an external fetal monitor as soon as possible. The presence of fetal heart accelerations (i.e, 2 accelerations of more than 15 beats per min for >15 s) is a good sign. During the placement of lines and monitors, obtain a more complete history and perform a complete physical examination.

Monitor the patient's vital signs frequently and have a trained attendant with her at all times, including when she is taken for diagnostic radiographic studies. Young healthy patients maintain their cardiovascular status to a point after which shock develops very quickly. Radiographic and obstetric ultrasonographic studies are important. No ordinarily indicated radiographic examination should be avoided during pregnancy. Irradiation of the fetus poses little risk compared with the dangers of undiagnosed maternal trauma. Focus standard studies on areas of injury.

The obstetric ultrasonogram should confirm gestational age and fetal and placental position. Fetal heart rate can act as a monitor of fetal well-being, adequacy of the pregnant woman's circulating blood volume, and her compensatory alpha-adrenergic response. Fetal bradycardia (i.e., heart rate <120 beats per min) or late decelerations may be due to maternal hypovolemia, maternal hypoxia, abruptio placentae, or uterine rupture.

In pregnancies of more than 25 weeks' gestation, consider cesarean delivery for fetal distress if the mother has been resuscitated and is stable. Continuous fetal monitoring should continue for 24 hours after major trauma because signs of fetal compromise can occur as long as 24 hours after injury. In patients with minimal non abdominal injury and no history of direct abdominal impact, continuous fetal monitoring can be limited to 8 hours if fewer than 6 contractions occur in an hour.

Indications for exploratory laparotomy in trauma are positive findings on lavage, free air under the diaphragm (before lavage), progressive abdominal distention with a declining hematocrit, or abdominal wall disruption or perforation. Intraoperative management of surgical trauma is specific to the type of injury involved.

Penetrating/Stab Wounds and Gunshot Wounds

As pregnancy progresses, intra-abdominal organs change position, with important implications. Because the bowel is pushed upward by the enlarged uterus, penetrating injury to the upper part of the abdomen is more likely to be associated with multiple gastrointestinal injuries. Organs involved in decreasing frequency are the small bowel, liver, colon, and stomach. During the third trimester, injuries to the lower quadrants of the abdomen almost exclusively involve the uterus. This may be advantageous to the mother because the uterus and amniotic fluid absorb most of the energy of the missile, resulting in less destruction to other organs. If the uterus is involved in penetrating trauma, fetal injury may occur in 60 to 90% of cases. Gunshot wounds to the uterus carry a maternal mortality of 7 to 9% and a fetal mortality of around 70%. Fetal mortality is higher if injury is caused before 37 weeks of gestation.

When evaluating the pathway of a bullet, radiographs (anteroposterior and lateral views) of the chest and abdomen, with the entrance and the exit wounds marked with paper clips may help the physicians. Some controversy exits but the prevailing opinion at this time is that pregnant women with gunshot wounds to the abdomen should generally undergo mandatory celiotomy. Stab wounds to the abdomen are managed similarly in pregnant and nonpregnant patients if signs of obvious intra-abdominal injury are present (shock, peritoneal signs, evisceration) or positive investigation.

A midline celiotomy should be performed, with exploration as in the nonpregnant state. If extrauterine intra-abdominal injuries are identified, organs are repaired or resected in the usual manner. Whenever the enlarged uterus interferes with adequate examination or repair, cesarean section is required. Celiotomy alone does not justify cesarean section because it prolongs the operation and increases blood loss by at least 1000 ml. Specific indications for cesarean section during celiotomy include maternal shock and pregnancy near term, threat to life from exsanguination from any cause, mechanical limitation for maternal repair, irreparable uterine injury, instability in a potentially viable fetus, unstable thoracolumbar spine injury, and maternal death.

Stab wounds and gunshot wounds are the most common major injuries to pregnant women other than those caused by automobile accidents or blunt trauma. Violence against pregnant women often focuses on the pregnant uterus. Seventy percent of fetuses are injured, whereas only 28% of mothers had extra uterine injuries. The perinatal mortality rate is around 64%, whereas only 3.2% of the mothers died. The extent of internal injury must be evaluated in all penetrating wounds to the torso even if a clear entrance and exit wound exists. Most stab wounds that enter the thoracic or abdominal cavity require an exploratory operation. Penetration of the cavities can be documented radiographically. A chest radiograph showing a pneumothorax and an upright radiograph of the abdomen showing free air are indications for exploration. If penetration cannot be determined by radiograph, a catheter is placed deep in the wound and held in place with a purse-string suture. Rapid injection of water-soluble contrast material with subsequent X-ray films demonstrates entry. If entry has occurred, exploration is required.unshot wounds require more aggressive management because debris often is carried deep into the wound. Removal of debris and debridement of necrotic tissue are essential to reduce infection. Anterior and posterior radiographs of the torso demonstrate the position of radiopaque debris (e.g., bullet fragments). If the mother's condition is stable, the fetus must be evaluated before exploration. After 24 weeks' gestation, an electronic fetal monitor is used to evaluate fetal health. Fetal heart rate accelerations (i.e., 2 accelerations >15 beats per min for >15 s) show the fetus to be healthy. In gunshot wounds to the torso, an amniocentesis under ultrasonographic guidance should be performed. Bloody amniotic fluid suggests fetal injury. If the fetus is at 30 weeks' gestation or greater, a rapid test (eg, optical density [OD] 650 or other rapid amniotic fluid test) of fetal lung maturity may be helpful in decision analysis. At the time of exploratory laparotomy, the uterus is examined for penetrating injury. If a penetrating injury to the uterus is present, if the fetus is older than 25 weeks' gestation, and if evidence of fetal compromise (e.g, bloody amniotic fluid, abnormal fetal testing) exist, cesarean delivery is indicated. A pediatrician who is experienced in the management of premature infants should attend preterm deliveries. If the fetal lungs show maturity, cesarean delivery is indicated for any penetrating injury to the uterus regardless of the results of fetal monitoring; however, if the amniotic fluid is clear but shows immature lungs and the monitor indicates fetal well-being, the uterus may be repaired and the fetus left alone. Labor may ensue after recovery from anesthesia. In the absence of vaginal bleeding or fetal distress, labor may be suppressed with indomethacin, intravenous ritodrine, or magnesium sulfate.Penetrating uterine injury at less than 25 weeks' gestation should be treated conservatively. Delivery means almost certain neonatal death from prematurity, and fetal fractures and stab or bullet wounds may heal in utero. The only reason for hysterotomy is maternal hemorrhage or fetal death in association with a uterine laceration that would preclude labor (e.g., a large fundal laceration). In general, vaginal delivery is preferable to hysterotomy in cases of fetal death, even if delivery occurs soon after exploration.

Burns

Pregnant women rarely are burned seriously, but when they are, they have unique medical problems. The mother and fetus are at great risk for fluid loss, hypoxemia, and sepsis. The overall fetal and neonatal mortality rate is greater than 50% when the mother is burned over more than 60% of her body. Fluid replacement, respiratory support, and initial wound care are the emergency management goals in pregnant burn patients. The loss of fluid through the denuded surface can be massive, and the amount often is underestimated in pregnant patients.On arrival to the hospital and after the vital signs of the mother and fetus (monitor) are evaluated, a large-bore (i.e, 18-gauge) intravenous line is started. In cases in which the burn covers more than 20% of the surface area, a central venous or Swan-Ganz catheter provides a better guide to fluid replacement. Lactated Ringer solution is started at 200 mL/h until the fluid replacement volume is calculated. Insert a nasogastric tube for burns involving more than 20% of body surface area.

Hospital admission is recommended for smoke inhalation, electrical burns, burns of both hands or both feet, partial-thickness burns that cover more than 10% of the surface area, or full-thickness burns on more than 2% of the surface area. The depth of the injury is estimated by appearance and sensation. Partial-thickness (i.e, intradermal) injury appears red or pink, with blister formation. Full-thickness injury may be charred or marble gray in color, dry, and anesthetic. Partial-thickness burns also may be anesthetic because of neurapraxias of skin nerve endings in the burn area. Thus, pain response to stimulation is valuable only to indicate a partial-thickness burn.

A general estimate of the body surface area involved by a burn is determined by the rule of nines: head and neck, 9%; upper extremities, 9% each; anterior torso, 18%; posterior trunk, 18%; lower extremities, 18% each; and genitalia, 1%. Another method is to equate the number of palmar surfaces the burn entails, each palmar surface being equal to 1.25% of body surface. During late pregnancy, 5% is added if the anterior abdomen is involved. The fluid requirements for the first 24 hours after a burn injury are calculated as follows: Body surface area burned (%) multiplied by 2-4 mL/kg body weight. For example, a 20% burn is calculated as 20 × 3 mL × 70 kg = 4200 mL.

Fluid requirements are met with lactated Ringer solution. The free-water requirement (i.e., 500 mL) is supplied with 5% dextrose in water. Fifty percent of the replacement fluid is administered in the first 8 hours and the remainder during the next 16 hours. In the second 24 hours, colloids (albumin) are administered to maintain the serum albumin greater than 3 g/100 mL.

Fluid replacement is monitored by clinical and laboratory means. Systolic blood pressure should be greater than 110 mm Hg, maternal heart rate less than 120 beats per minute, temperature less than 38°C, and respiratory rate should be 12-24 breaths per minute. Central venous pressure should be approximately 10 cm H_2O, and urine output should be greater than 0.5 mL/kg/h. The initial laboratory workup should include a complete blood count and determination of blood levels of electrolytes, glucose, albumin, urea nitrogen, and serum creatinine. Monitor these parameters on a serial basis (e.g., q4-8h). Smoke inhalation is a major cause of morbidity and mortality in burn patients. In pregnancy, the fetus is at special risk because of its relatively hypoxic state (i.e., normal umbilical vein PaO_2 = 27 mm Hg). The pathophysiology of inhalation injury relates to impaired maternal ventilation (e.g. upper airway obstruction from edema), increased diffusion distance (e.g., interstitial alveolar edema), and acute functional anemia from carbon monoxide poisoning. Carbon monoxide binds more efficiently to hemoglobin than does oxygen. In addition to displacing oxygen, carbon monoxide impairs the release of oxygen from oxyhemoglobin. Very little carbon monoxide is needed to cause serious hypoxia. One part carbon monoxide per 1500 parts air can result in blood concentrations of carboxyhemoglobin of 5-10%. Car exhaust is 5-7% carbon monoxide. Carboxyhemoglobin values less than 15% usually are well tolerated, whereas values greater than 30% cause severe maternal syncope and fetal death.

Inhalation injury should be suspected among patients who have a history of closed-space fire, facial injury, carbonaceous material in the oropharynx, or respiratory symptoms. Interstitial edema on chest X-ray film, a carboxyhemoglobin level greater than 10%, or abnormal arterial blood gas levels also aid in establishing the diagnosis of inhalation injury. Initial treatment of any burn patient should include an arterial blood sample for gases and carboxyhemoglobin, as well as a chest radiograph. Patients should be placed on 100% oxygen by mask for at least 3 hours or until the carboxyhemoglobin level is known. They should receive vigorous chest physiotherapy. Intubation and mechanical ventilation should be used early in the presence of upper airway obstruction or oxygenation failure.

Sepsis is another major risk for the fetus and mother. Initial wound care can be instrumental in the prevention of these complications. On admission, the wound is cleaned with bland soap and water, and all dirt and loose devitalized tissue are removed. Blisters should be left intact if they are smaller than 5 cm in diameter. When burns involve the scalp, axilla, or pubic area, the hair should be clipped short until an adequate margin of unburned skin is obtained. After cleaning and debridement, a topical agent is applied with a bulky dressing. Silver sulfadiazine cream is used most commonly, but the consideration in pregnant patients is that this drug can be absorbed. The sulfa derivative crosses the placenta and displaces bilirubin. Should delivery ensue, hyperbilirubinemia is a risk for the neonate. Silver nitrate (0.5%) also is used, but this agent requires continuous soaking (i.e., q2h) and a bulky dressing. Tetanus toxoid (0.5 mL) should be administered to all patients with burns.

After the initial management of a severely burned patient, her care requires a team approach with the obstetrician acting as a consultant. Pregnant women with severe burns are best cared for in centers geared both to managing severe burns and to the possibilities of early delivery. The major long-term problems are healing, sepsis prevention, scar complications, nutritional support, and rehabilitation.

Pelvic and rectal examinations should be performed. Aside from the usual secondary survey, assessment of the injured pregnant patient should rule out vaginal bleeding, ruptured membranes, a bulging perineum, the presence of contractions, and an abnormal fetal heart rate and rhythm.

Diagnostic Modalities/Radiation Exposure

Following maternal stabilization and assessment, and fetal evaluation, the extent of maternal and fetal injury is determined with the help of specific diagnostic modalities. Sensitivity to radiation is greater during intrauterine development than at any other time of life. Although there is much concern about radiation exposure, a diagnostic modality deemed necessary for maternal evaluation should not be withheld on the basis of its potential hazard to the fetus.

The fetal dose of radiation received in individual cases may vary by a factor of 50 or more, depending on the equipment used, technique used, number of radiographs done in a complete study, maternal size, and fetal/uterine size. In general, X-ray beams aimed more than 10 cm away from the fetus are not dangerous.

The major effects of exposure to the fetus include congenital malformations, growth retardation, postnatal neoplasia, and death. In the first week of life, before implantation, the embryo is very sensitive to lethal effects of radiation but has a low probability of sustaining teratogenic or growth-retarding effects if it is able to implant and grow. During major organogenesis of the 2nd to 7th weeks, the embryo is sensitive to the teratogenic, growth-retarding, lethal, and postnatal neoplastic effects of radiation. Organs are less sensitive to radiation teratogenesis in the 8th to 40th weeks, but growth retardation, central nervous system dysfunction, and postnatal neoplastic effects may occur. Studies show that exposure of the fetus to less than 5 to 10 rad (5000 to 10000 mrad) causes no significant increase in the risk of congenital malformations, intrauterine growth retardation, or miscarriage. Although this does not mean that there are definitely no risks in exposures less than 5 rad, it does mean that this level of radiation carries little risk for the fetus when compared to spontaneous risks. At a radiation dose of 15 rad, there is approximately a 6% chance that the child could develop severe mental retardation, a less than 3% chance of developing childhood cancer, and a 15% chance of having a small head size.

When performing radiographic evaluation of the mother, fetal irradiation should be minimized by shielding the abdomen when feasible with a lead apron. When many radiographs are required over a long period, a thermo luminescent dosimeter may be attached to the patient to serve as a guide to the dosage of radiation delivered. As a guide to physicians, reports from some studies indicate that the radiation dose from a plain AP chest X-ray is in general below 0.005 rad, a pelvic film below 0.4 rad, CT-scan of the head (1-cm slices) 0.05 rad, CT-scan of the upper abdomen (20 1 cm slices) below 3.0 rad and CT-scan of the lower abdomen (10 1-cm slices) 3.0 to 9.0 rad.

Cardiac Arrest and Perimortem Cesarean Delivery

In the event of maternal cardiac arrest, perform all standard life support interventions and maternal resuscitation like adequate oxygenation, fluid loading, and left lateral decubitus to see if maternal circulation can be improved followed by defibrillation and drug administrations. The only deviation is an added measure: manually move the gravid uterus off the vena cava to facilitate perfusion. Studies have shown that conventional external cardiac massage (ECM) becomes less effective as the patient approaches term because of mechanical factors. The only method of assessing adequacy of fetal oxygenation during CPR is to monitor fetal heart rate (FHR). Carotid pulse and end-tidal CO_2 monitoring should be used to monitor adequacy of maternal vital organ perfusion during CPR.

If maternal death appears imminent and if the fetus is alive with a gestational age of at least 24 weeks, case reports indicate that rapidly performing a perimortem cesarean section can improve the odds of survival for both patients, although one study found it was "rarely successful" for the fetus. Maternal survival after delivery of the fetus during unsuccessful cardiopulmonary resuscitation (CPR) has been reported. If there is no response to advanced cardiac life support within a few minutes (2 to 3 minutes), maternal cardiopulmonary resuscitation must be continued, anterior thoracotomy with open-chest cardiac massage (OCM) but without aortic cross-clamping should be considered, and emergency cesarean section for a viable fetus should be performed.

When the gestational age is less than 24 weeks, emergency cesarean delivery is usually not performed because the fetus is too small to survive and the birth is unlikely to have much effect on maternal hemodynamics. However, when gestational age is greater than 24-25 weeks, emergency cesarean birth probably will favorably affect maternal or fetal outcome. At a gestational age of 26 to 32 weeks, when external cardiac massage is not effective, as indicated by failure to generate a carotid pulse, inadequate end-tidal CO2 levels, or fetal bradycardia, OCM should be seriously considered before an emergency cesarean section is performed. If OCM prove successful, the delivery may be delayed so that chances of postnatal survival improve. Even slight prolongation of fetal intrauterine life will probably improve the chances of fetal survival, especially when gestational age is less than 28 weeks. If, however, OCM proves to be ineffective, the fetus must be delivered immediately. After 32 weeks gestation, when ECM is not effective, an emergency cesarean section must be performed immediately. Delivering the infant improves maternal cardiac filling, thereby improving the success of CPR. The longer the delay between the onset of cardiac arrest and delivery, the less are the chances of fetal and maternal survival. If, however, the ECM appears to be effective, ECM may be continued for 5 minutes. If a spontaneous circulation is not restored within 5 minutes, an emergency cesarean delivery must be performed. If this fails to revive the mother, OCM may be considered. Ideally, personnel trained in neonatal resuscitation should be available to attend the infant.

CONCLUSION

Trauma has become the most frequent cause of maternal death in many developed countries. The main principle guiding therapy must be that resuscitating the mother will resuscitate the fetus.

Many trauma patients require psychosocial intervention to help them cope with their injuries; when the patient is pregnant, she and her partner will also be worried about known or possible injuries to her fetus. Such parental anxiety should be continually addressed by the nurse. Short, frequent conversations relaying information about fetal status and explaining planned or likely procedures are helpful. If the fetus is not in distress, the mother will usually be allowed to deliver vaginally; if her condition is critical, a cesarean section may be performed. If the fetus has died, spontaneous vaginal delivery may be delayed by a few days. A bereavement protocol suggesting specific interventions to help the family cope with fetal loss is recommended. Nurses can provide referrals to social workers and help patients access community resources such as clergy or support groups. Victims of assault or domestic violence might need help finding a shelter, contacting the police, or obtaining legal representation.

Further Reading

1. Accidental Injury during Pregnancy. Shere, DM and Schenker JG. Obstetrical and Gynecological Survey, Williams Wilkins, 1989, Vol 44, No.5, p:330-337.
2. Trauma in pregnancy. Patterson,RM. Clin Obstet Gynecol,27:32,1984.
3. Trauma in pregnancy. Neufeld, JD, Moore, EE, Marx, JA. Emerg Med Clin North Am, 1987,5:623.
4. Trauma in late pregnancy. Golan,A, Sandbank,O, Teare,AJ. South Afr Med J, 1980, 57, 161.
5. Traumatic injuries during pregnancy. Crosby,WM. Clin Obstet Gynecol, 1983;26:902.
6. Pregnancy patients with burns. Schmitz,JT. Am J Obstet Gynecol,1971,110;57.
7. American College of Surgeons ATLS Student Course Manual, 1997).

60 Geriatric Trauma

INTRODUCTION

Trauma is the fifth common cause of death in the elderly. Trauma morbidity rises sharply between 45 to 55 years of age and doubles at 75 years and above. Age dependent survival decrement occurs at all Injury Severity Scores (ISS) for all injuries at all body regions. Resuscitation of the elderly must be done with special care as advanced age is a wll recognized risk factor for adverse outcomes folowing trauma. The elderly have compromised physiological reserves and ususally have a higher incidence of pre-existing medical conditions like chronic cardiac, respiratory and metabolic diseases that may reduce the ability to compensate for additional stresses imposed. Comorbid diseases like diabetes, coronary artery disease, congestive heart failure, liver disease, obstructive and restrictive lung disease, coagulopathies, osteoporosis and peripheral vascular disease are frequent in this age group. Also, the chronic use of medications can alter or blunt physiologic responses, resulting in a narrow therapeutic window in the elderly. Signs of raised inctracranial pressure develops slowly, due to cognitive deficits, the eldrely may forget an injury and not report it. Osteoporosis, reduced intervertebral disc space, narrow spinal canal, higher incidence of abdominal aortic aneurysms due to atherosclerosis, decreased ciliary clearance in airways and possibility of occult shock in the eldrely compound matters further. Prompt, aggressive resuscitation and early recognition of pre-existing medical conditions and medications is imperative to improve survival in the geriatric age group victims. Early institution of invasive monitoring is a valuable adjunct to management to avoid over or under resuscitation in this patient population. Pulmonary artery catheter monitoring has shown occult cardiac shock in 50% of geriatric trauma victims. In prehospital care of the geriatric age group, it is important that triage decisions are based on possible outcomes and appropriate destinations selected. UNDER-TRIAGE CAN BE LETHAL as the margin of error tolerated by the geriatric age group vicitms is really small. Hence, a stepwise evaluation of anatomic injuries and ensuring physiological stability is vital.Those aged > 65 years with GCS < 8 have dismal prognosis. Above 45 years of age ISS of 9-24 is associated with increased mortality. Those with trauma scores 12-14 have 25% mortality rate, those with scores between 9-12 have 65% mortality rate, while those with scores below 9 have very poor survival rates. Those with scores less than 7 may not reach the hospital alive. Also those with respiratory rate less than 10 have high mortality rate. Where ABG facilites are available, those with mild base deficit between -3 to-5 have 24% mortality, those with moderate deficits between -6 to -9 have 60% mortality and those with severe deficit of -10 and below have 80% mortality figures. Careful evaluation must be done in victims with systolic blood pressures less than 130 torr. Intravenous fluids in 250 ml aliquots is advisable to avoid fluid overload. With these considerations, it is advocated that those above 55 years are better off shifted to a trauma centre directly without regard for the severity of their injuries.

An Age-Related Approach to Patient Care

Age 55 to 64 Years

- Assume some mild decrease in physiologic reserve.
- Suspect the presence of diabetes mellitus, hypertension, previous surgery.
- Suspect the use of medications.
- Presume patient can provide accurate medical history.
- Look for organ dysfunction, ABG and ECG may be necessary.
- Presume a serious brain injury if loss of consciousness-order a CT Scan or MRI.

Age 65 to 74 Years

- Accept age-related disease-induced physiologic alteration of organ systems.
- Accept the presence of acquired disease and medications.
- Decide if the patient can give reliable medical history. Call patient relatives or personal physician for details.
- Aggressively monitor the patient to optimize cardiac performance and oxygen metabolism.
- Suspect brain injury if any alteration in mental status or cognitive or sensory function-imaging of the brain is mandatory.
- Undertake aggressive operative management.
- Be aware of poor outcome if CNS deterioriation.

Age 75 Years and Older

- As above.
- Assume a poor outcome if CNS injury or altered physiological function.
- Discuss appropriate care with family members.
- Be humane, consider early consultation with ethics and social services (Fig. 60.1).

SPINAL CORD INJURIES IN THE ELDERLY

There are many factors that predispose the elderly population to these injuries, including osteoporosis, changes in bone density, osteopenia, the development of spinal stenosis, the propensity to fall due to sensory deficits and medications, and an increased rate of motor vehicle crashes per miles driven. Chronic conditions in elderly patients can also contribute to risk factors. Some of these include: diabetes causing peripheral neuropathy; and osteoarthritis, which can contribute to immobility, difficulty maneuvering, and less core stability. Other neurologic disorders such as Parkinson disease can cause rigidity, decreased movement initiation, cognitive impairments, and impaired sensation. Many medications that elderly persons take can cause postural hypotension and impair coordination and sensation, all of which can contribute to a mechanism causing spinal injury. Older patients sustaining injury to the spinal column/cord tend to sustain incomplete neurologic injuries, as opposed to complete injuries. This is likely due to the less severe mechanism of injury. Upper cervical injuries are the most common location of fractures and SCIs in the elderly population. There are three types of injury that appear to be relatively specific to the elderly population: (1) central cord syndrome; (2) cervical extension/distraction injuries; and (3) odontoid fractures.

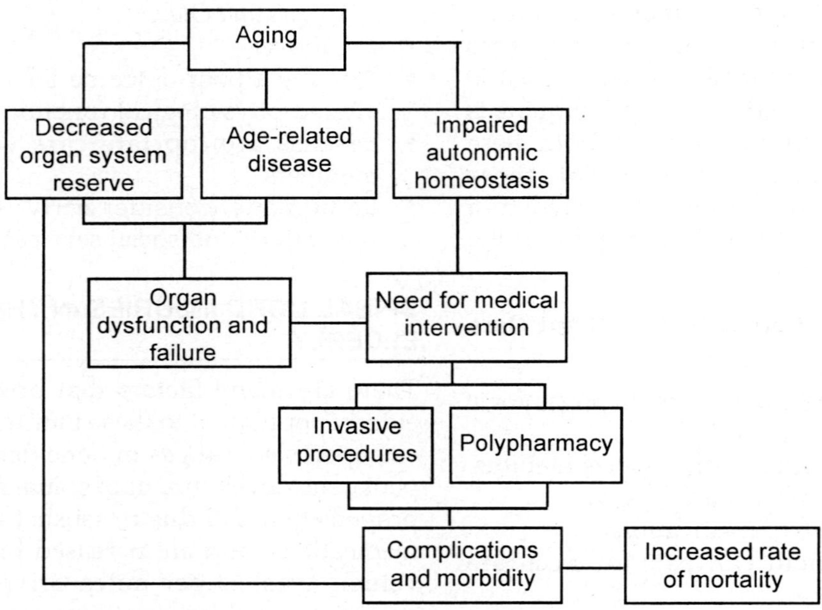

Fig. 60.1: Increased rate of complications and a greater likelihood of perioperative mortality in elderly subjects reflects the interactions of the effects of aging on organ system functional reserve and the consequences of age-related disease and its therapy. Polypharmacy and the need for medical intervention further amplify the likelihood of adverse outcome

Central Cord Syndrome

Central cord syndrome (CCS) is a disorder of the spinal cord that is thought to occur primarily in the elderly population. It is due to hyperextension of the neck. The elderly are more prone to this because of cervical spondylosis. Patients with CCS tend to have a disproportionate weakness in their upper extremities as compared to their lower extremities. Many of these patients do not have any associated fractures of their cervical vertebrae. Because these patients do not have any fractures and their mechanism is thought to be of low velocity, they are often initially misdiagnosed. Treatment of this injury may include surgical fixation or external immobilization. Risks and benefits of both must be evaluated before a decision is made. Some patients with CCS will have some recovery of function over time, but it is felt that surgical decompression of the spinal cord will maximize recovery and prevent repeated SCI.The surgery that is typically performed in patients with this injury is laminectomy, either with or without fusion.

Cervical Extension/Distraction Injuries

Cervical extension/distraction injury is another type that disproportionately affects the elderly population. This occurs because older individuals tend to have stiffness in their spinal column as their disc spaces collapse, and many have osteophyte formation as a result of degenerative spondylosis. All of this leads to decreased range of motion in the cervical spine. If an elderly patient presents with abrasions on his/her forehead or face and describes a hyperextensive injury, one should be highly suspicious of a cervical extension or distraction injury. These fractures are also referred to as "open book" fractures because they are associated with an opening or lengthening of the anterior column of the spine. Cervical extension or distractive fractures can often be overlooked because radiographs tend to display only minimal changes. Initial reads may indicate prevertebral soft-tissue swelling or distraction in a spondylitic disc space. If there is any question as to the presence of a fracture, a magnetic resonance imaging (MRI) scan should be obtained. An MRI can confirm the diagnosis because it tends to be more sensitive to soft tissue, ligament, and disc injury. An MRI will also demonstrate any injury to the spinal cord. These fractures are considered unstable, and most patients require surgical fixation and external immobilization. It is important to treat these patients with extreme care because any manipulation can worsen the fracture and potentially cause SCI.

Odontoid Fractures

Odontoid fractures are the third type of spine injury relatively unique to the elderly patient population. This is a fracture of the C2 vertebral body, specifically the odontoid process. These fractures usually occur from falling and hitting the head. Although these fractures can cause neurologic deficit, the majority of patients do not present with this. This is felt to be due to the generous width of the spinal column at this level, which allows for fracture displacement without spinal cord impingement. The goal in treating this injury is to protect the spinal cord while aligning the spinal column to promote stability and to decrease pain. Many of these patients are treated with external fixation in a rigid cervical collar or halo vest. A halo vest tends to cause significant mobility and respiratory issues in elderly patients, and therefore some surgeons will choose to do internal fixation in this population. In hospital mortality rates in patients with these types of fractures are disproportionately high, however, often due to the morbidity of immobilization in elderly patients.

Stabilization of Fractures

Definitive treatment for the elderly population with spine fractures is a matter of some debate in the literature. Halo vest immobilization and surgical repair each carry a significant risk of morbidity and has a less than 70% union rate. Additionally, halo vest immobilization has its own set of complications in the elderly population. Some of this complications include: mobility issues; respiratory issues such as atelectasis and pneumonia; skin breakdown; pressure sores; pin-site irritation (loosening of the pins or infection of the site itself); and swallowing issues, which can lead to decreased nutritional intake in a population that already is at high risk for malnutrition. They can also have high rates of cardiac and pulmonary morbidity and mortality than younger patients. Surgery or a hard collar are better options. In elderly patients with multiple trauma, neurologic deficit, and/or fractures that are more than six weeks old, operative internal fixation remains a viable option. Advanced age is well known to negatively influence fracture healing, despite optimal immobilization or surgical management.

Acute Management

Management of elderly patients with spinal injuries must take into account their preexisting conditions, pathophysiologic characteristics, and age-related disorders that affect the population. In the acute setting, the primary goal of treatment is to prevent secondary injury to the spinal cord. Primary injury occurs at the time of impact, and there is nothing that can be done to reverse that damage. The goal of caring for patients with acute cervical SCI is to stop the biochemical cascade of events that can cause "secondary injury", which causes additional insults to the spinal cord resulting in more neurologic deficit. Early establishment of adequate airway, oxygenation, and ventilation, early elective intubation is preferred, rather than waiting until loss of airway necessitates emergent intubation in a patient with an unstable cervical SCI. Local edema, parasympathetic stimulation causing an increase in secretions, decreased innervation of chest and abdominal muscles that inhibits generation of an adequate cough, and ventilation all contribute to airway compromise and respiratory failure. These difficulties are exaggerated in those with underlying medical disorders.Over 90% of patients with cervical SCI will require mechanical ventilation and those with complete SCI are more likely to require tracheostomy. It is well known that patients who are ventilated have an increased chance of developing pneumonia and atelectasis, as well as pleural effusions, pulmonary edema, and pulmonary embolism. Additionally, patients who are ventilated have a suppressed cough reflex, further compromising respiratory status.

The goal is to prevent respiratory complications and promote oxygenation and spinal cord perfusion in order to prevent secondary injury. Some of the ways in which this is accomplished is with early mobilization as soon as the spinal column is stabilized and the patient is cleared to get out of bed. Chest physiotherapy also helps in preventing atelectasis and promoting gas exchange. In the acute care setting, the goal is to maintain the arterial oxygen saturation rate of greater than 90%. Early tracheostomy also helps facilitate weaning patients from the ventilator if their level of injury allows liberation from mechanical ventilation.

Cardiovascular complications like hypotension can be due to neurogenic shock, the nature of traumatic injuries, or secondary to hemorrhage. The goal in must be to maintain a mean arterial pressure (MAP) of greater than 85 mm Hg to adequately perfuse the spinal cord. This strategy of intentional hypertension becomes more complicated in the elderly patients because many of them have pre-existing cardiac history and will not tolerate an increased MAP or the vasoactive drugs required to maintain this level of systemic perfusion. Bradycardia can also be a complication of SCI related to the interruption of the sympathetic nervous system. Due to unopposed vagal stimulation, even simple tracheal suctioning of patients may cause bradycardia. Many elderly patients are often on pre-injury beta blockers, calcium-channel blockers, or anti arrhythmic agents, which may further exacerbate bradycardia.

Other complications that occur frequently in patients with SCI include deep vein thrombosis (DVT) and gastrointestinal (GI) complications. Patients with SCI are at high risk of DVT due to immobility. If left untreated, fatal pulmonary embolism can occur. Patients should receive prophylaxis against DVT, with mechanical compression starting on admission and low-molecular-weight heparin as soon as it is deemed safe after injury or surgical stabilization. Prophylactic inferior vena caval filters are not recommended for prevention of DVT unless chemical prophylaxis is contraindicated. Low-molecular-weight heparin is initiated 72 hours after injury or surgery. Care must be taken to adjust dosing accordingly in elderly patients with renal insufficiency, or to use unfractionated subcutaneous heparin as an alternate regimen.

Frequent GI complications include paralytic ileus and gastric or duodenal ulceration or gastritis leading to GI bleeding. Early use of high-dose methylprednisolone may contribute to the risk of GI bleeding complications, sepsis and pneumonia. All patients with SCI must be given H2 receptor antagonists or proton pump inhibitors. They should have a naso-gastric tube placed initially to decompress the stomach. This reduces the risk for vomiting and aspiration. If an ileus develops, naso-gastric decompression should be continued until it is resolved, usually within 72 hours Tube feeding should be initiated as quickly as possible to help prevent ulcer formation and maximize nutritional status. Bowel function may also be compromised depending on the level of injury. This is important to keep in mind with the elderly population because many older patients have issues with chronic constipation prior to their injury. It is important to start these patients on an aggressive bowel regimen with stool softeners and prokinetic agents. Manual disimpaction should be performed as needed.

All patients with SCI should have an indwelling Foley catheter to promote bladder emptying. Urinary output should also be monitored. It is important to note that patients with SCI may have oliguria related to sympathetic inactivity during the acute phase. Fluid resuscitation should be done carefully to minimize the risk of pulmonary edema while maintaining normovolemia. Many elderly patients may have pre-existing renal or urinary dysfunction that may be complicated by SCI.

Skin breakdown is a huge concern in any immobilized patients. Integumentary issues such as pressure ulcers can occur as a result of immobility, decrease in sensation, and muscle atrophy. Patients' skin should be assessed frequently, and patients should be repositioned no less than every 2 hours.17 When patients are out of bed they should still be getting pressure relief by lifting or adjusting positioning. Heel protectors should be provided to relieve pressure. Some patients may also develop skin breakdown on their chin from cervical collars that may be needed for spinal immobilization. Collars should be removed and the area of skin under the collar should be assessed, cleansed, and dried before reapplication of the collar. Patients should remain flat in bed, or cervical immobilization should be applied when removing the collar. The back of the collar should remain intact when removing the front, and vice versa.

Long-Term Management

Some of the complications that are relatively unique to patients with SCI in the chronic phase of their injury include bladder dysfunction, GI dysfunction, and autonomic dysreflexia (AD). An indwelling catheter may be required for years. Depending on the level of injury and the dexterity of the patient, intermittent catheterization is often possible. It is important to monitor the intake and output of patients before initiating an intermittent catheterization program. Patients should be aware of their fluid status and expect to have an equal intake and output. Intermittent catheterization may be more difficult for the elderly patient because of decreased manual dexterity related to arthritis and compounded by SCI. Poor vision may also further exacerbate these difficulties. These patients are at high risk for urinary tract infections, nephrolithiasis, epididymo-orchitis, and urethral strictures.

Bowel dysfunction after SCI is exceptionally common. Many of these patients experience constipation, bloating, and fecal incontinence. Bowel distention can also occur in these patients but may not be associated with abdominal pain or discomfort due to lack of sensation from their SCI. It is important that these patients are maintained on an individualized bowel regimen and that it is reviewed frequently. Again, when caring for the elderly patient with SCI, a careful review of pre-injury bowel dysfunction should be discussed, as the symptomatology he/she previously experienced may be masked by his/her injury.

Autonomic Dysfunction (AD) is a life-threatening syndrome that can affect any patient with SCI at the level of T6 or above, triggered by noxious stimuli that occur below the level of injury. This stimulus produces severe vasoconstriction and increases blood pressure. Parasympathetic activity then produces vagal stimulation, bradycardia, and vessel dilatation. Patients may exhibit acute sweating and headache. AD can be caused by a wide variety of stimuli, most commonly, bladder distention, urinary tract infections, constipation, or pressure ulcers, and, less commonly, from acute illnesses such as fractures or appendicitis. The first-line therapy for AD is recognition of the inciting event and prompt treatment of the noxious stimuli like a kinked Foley catheter, loosening tight clothing, monitoring blood pressure every five minutes and administration of direct vasodilators. Beta blockers should be avoided to prevent unopposed alpha-receptor stimulation and worsening of hypertension. AD can be potentially life-threatening. If it is left untreated or unrecognized, patients may develop intracranial hemorrhage, encephalopathy, seizures, and/or cardiac dysrhythmias.

AXIOMS

- Elicit accurate history.
- Consider early intubation.
- Early and frank discussions with family members.
- Do not under estimate chest and head injuries.
- Consider invasive monitoring.
- Normal pulse, blood pressure and serum creatinine can be fallacious.

61 Trains and Rail Road Disasters

> The most important human factor in transportation is safety, and the safety record of high speed rail is perfect.
>
> —*(Former Amtrak President , before the ICE-train crash)*

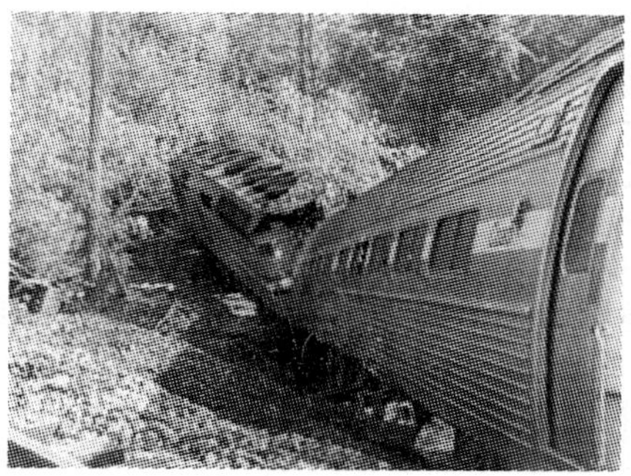

EVOLUTION OF TRAINS

Train transportation began in the late 1820s and it appeared to be a safe form of travel as they were slow and ran over short hauls with lower traffic density. Initial speeds were 15 mph and each carriage carried up to 36 passengers only. Train disasters began in 1853 and have continued ever since due to derailments, head-on or rear end collisions, level crossing collisions, collapse of weakened bridges, tunnels and tracks, human error, either due to faulty maintenance schedules or/ and gross negligence. Whatever the reason, train travel remains safer than other modes of ground transportation, with the risk of death in a one-way trip being close to 1 in 1million. But even this is not safe enough. Train accidents, very often, occur in areas that are virtually inaccessible to emergency vehicles, rescue squads and fire department personnel, especially at night or in extreme weather conditions. Response activities have to start with an organized search operation using helicopters fitted with high beam searchlights and even sniffer dogs. Goods and container carriages routinely transport hazardous and highly flammable chemicals. Accidents involving these add a further dimension to disaster containment services. With electric traction, train accidents can pose high-tension hazards to rescue workers. With a new chapter in high speed trains, bullet trains commenced plying in Japan in 1964 and France in 1981, attaining speeds of 175 to 190 mph. Trains can jump bridges and carriages can become submerged in rivers and waterways. In developing countries, train accidents invariably have high numbers of casualties as they are the only means of transportation and totally overcrowded, often combined with outdated safety devices and frequent human error ranging from momentary lapse in concentration to grave dereliction of duty. In high-speed rail accidents, the situation is often akin to an airplane crash with passenger cars totally destroyed and disintegrated during collision and survivors suffering extreme body mutilation. Bullet trains have pressurized windows that are virtually unbreakable even with sledge hammers and the highly polished exteriors causing extrication tools like saws and hydraulic devices to slip. Thus train accidents are an extreme challenge for any emergency service and the only way to meet the threat is awareness, pre planning and training.

ACCIDENT SCENE MANAGEMENT

A strong Incident Command System (ICS) structure is the on-scene key to contain hazards and undertake immediate rescue operations. The Chief of the ICS has to be at the site within minutes, appraise the situation and swing into action to prevent chaos, confusion and mounting casualties. Modern passenger trains can be more than 1000 feet long and, at high speeds, the train can travel upto 2 miles after applying emergency brakes.

Medical and rescue teams should not attempt to question train drivers and staff as to the cause of the accident, as these are the responsibility of investigating agencies. Additional security may be needed to protect these personnel from the media. Mass casualty scenes must be treated as a crime scene. Removal of accident related debris from the impact area must not be attempted without photodocumentation, as accident investigation is highly dependent on preservation of the accident scene. In case of fire outbreaks, fire suppression foam equipment must be made available expeditiously. In the event of chemical spills, arrangements for dousing chemical clouds with water mist sprays and covering contaminated ground site with mixture of sand and soda ash must be made. Personnel engaged in such activities must don level B protective suits with respirators and air tanks. Scene security is of extreme importance and double cordoning of the area and flood lighting must be undertaken to render it safe and accessible and also prevent disturbance of evidence and intrusion by looters and souvenir hunters. A traffic direction system has to be created expeditiously to ensure one-way-in and one-way out traffic movement for fire, ambulance and emergency vehicles like mobile Gottwald cranes, drills, sideboom Caterpillars, Bobcats, earth moving machines etc. Staging areas have to established for triage and a level piece of land identified, cleared and marked with a distinctive H using luminous paint to serve as an emergency helipad. Passenger lists have to be procured and communication lines established. Special arc cutting equipment, divers, floodlighting, sniffer dog squads, robots and video recorders may have to be mobilized in special situations. The ICS Commander has to draw upon help from local good Samaritans and emergency responders to extricate survivors and carry them into the triage area and also for fire fighting, traffic direction and security. Military units, Civil Defence and para military forces in the vicinity can also be inducted in quick time. Rescue, Accident Relief and special trains can bring in special equipment as well as essentials like food, water, medicines, emergency shelters and rescue personnel. V-SAT linking at accident site and assistance of amateur HAM operators can prove invaluable. If bodies have to be removed prior to the arrival of investigators, an attempt must be made to identify victims and mark the location and position in which the bodies are found. If photo documentation is not possible, spray paint can be used to create an outline of location and position and then numbered. Body bags must bear the same number and subsequent paperwork must be marked with an identical number too. All personal effects of victims must be placed inside the body bags. Any procedure to disentangle victims from wreckage by cutting metal etc must also be made note of to differentiate them from structural damage caused by the accident. Special care must be taken to provide up-to-date information to friends and family of victims. Temporary morgues may be set up in adjacent schools, sheds and other secure, preferably air conditioned buildings to prevent deterioration. The facility must be protected from public view and must have adequate waiting and rest rooms. A separate room must be established for interviews with individuals seeking missing persons and body identification. Enough personnel and communication infra structure to handle incoming and outgoing calls must be available, with separate working areas for press, clergy and counselors. Bodies must be segregated into male adults, female adults, male children, female children and those whose sex cannot be determined.

SAFETY CONSIDERATIONS IN PREVENTING RAILROAD MISHAPS

Historically, safety has been subjected to a fragmentary approach with every department having its own specific responsibilities towards factors like working conditions, internal and external safety, rescue and emergency etc. The worked out policies were then brought out as standing orders for everyone's compliance. The focus of safety has now shifted from just complying with orders towards interventions in primary operational processes, identifying and correcting deficiencies before they snowball into disasters, and a more integral assessment of safety in its societal context i.e. safety and security not being considered separately but as a holistic scientific interest, scanning the whole spectrum of engineering design, technological, social, behavioral, ergonomic, judicial and managerial disciplines, each with its own paradigms, notions, methodologies and techniques. Safety has become an interdisciplinary activity, but this integral notion is yet to acquire a worldwide harmonization, consensus and acceptance.

However, applying a systems engineering approach facilitates integration of both the accident investigation as well as the rescue and emergency efforts to meet the safety and emergency management strategies.

Safety in modern transportation systems has been discussed for the past 15 years. There are four points of views and schools of thought concerning safety.

The Law of Torts

It has its roots in the US railway industry since the end of the 19th century when safety-engineering design was introduced to standardize technical designs and issue of safety certification. Forensic engineering is an offshoot of this to detect technical failures like mechanical and structural failures to pinpoint liability in accidents. Lessons learned from train disasters have done more to advance engineering knowledge than discovery of successful machines or technical designs.

Reliability Engineering

This branch focuses on the problems of organizational aspects, maintenance, repairs and ergonomics to arrive at a probabilistic risk assessment (PRA), within a sophisticated and high risk service, targeting both mechanical and human reliability.

Systems Engineering

This adopts systems life-cycle safety analysis and hazard control actions from the conceptual phase of a system to design development, manufacturing, construction, modification and even demolition. Expanding scopes of the subject pays attention to higher order systems levels and post-event consequences dealing with rescue, emergency, crisis management, administrative responsibilities, policy management issues and institutional constraints.

System Deficiency and Change

This is based on the experiences over the past decade of transportation safety boards worldwide. These serve as safety ombudsmen and adopt the systems engineering approach to conduct an independent, unbiased, proactive investigative mission. They analyze their findings to remove inherent deficiencies and achieve safety enhancement by implementing sustainable safety changes within the system. These safety boards have evolved in five stages. Firstly, they are independent, with a permanent status to ensure the objectivity of their findings. Secondly, to determine cause of an accident, attribute responsibility and prevent similar accidents in the future. Thirdly, having multi modal implications, in that improvement of safety in one mode, e.g., railways improves safety standards in other modes and sectors, e.g., shipping or aviation. Fourthly keeping the investigation process specific and focus on deficiencies to improve safety. Fifthly, focus on safety studies of multiple events for identification of safety deficiencies rather than an exhaustive study of single events.

Accident investigation of a major accident must focus on technical investigations, human factors and operational practices to improve safety performance by following the principles of responsible care. It must also give an impression of being open and provide a temporary transparency and a confidence-building cohesive, coordinated image to the society and help democracy function properly. It must give an inside-out vision to identify oversights in design, development and manufacturing and also an outside-in vision to define risks based on a consensus of perception acceptable to the users and operators with a social-managerial focus. The goal being to:

1. Develop clear terms of reference with acceptable risks to society and uniformity in risk and safety assessments across projects and state boundaries.
2. Adopt a consistent procedure with respect to acceptable societal residual risk standards during the various phases of a project.
3. Achieve clear division of responsibilities across project phases and levels with reference to rescue and emergency tasks like fire fighting/containment, trauma care and public safety.

Trains must be equipped with crashworthy loco events recorders akin to the black boxes on planes. These event recorders contain details of train speed, direction, distance traveled, throttle positions and brake applications. High speed trains must have Positive Train Separation (PTS) and anti-collision control systems that automatically take over train operation when a driver does not comply with signals and operational rules. When investigating a train accident, investigators must obtain details of prevailing meteorological status to assess visibility conditions and sight distance at the time of the event. The engine crew must be subjected to blood, breath and urine testing for alcohol and drugs. Their past medical, performance and training records must be scrutinized. Pre and post accident track inspection records must be scrutinized, as well as the issue and confirmation of procedures along with audit of operational activities, track warrants, communications and work distribution workloads.

Driving a train is an activity in which human error can result in a catastrophic accident if, as is often the case, there are no technical protective systems which prevent the error or permit recovery from it. This is in marked contrast to other railway activities, such as the operation of signals where the equipment which is now provided almost eliminates the risk of serious harm arising from human error.

The existing automatic warning system sounds a warning to the driver at the approach to signals showing caution or danger; however if the driver acknowledges the warning but then fails to control the speed of the train, the system will do nothing further to prevent a possible disaster. It would be surprising if such errors did not occur from time to time. In fact, the majority of accidents which result from passing signals passed at danger happen in this way.

Thanks to technical advances such as improved signalling systems and the automatic warning system, major railway accidents have become less frequent over the years. Modern train design also means that accidents usually have less catastrophic consequences.The installation of train protection is a preventive measure; it helps to prevent collisions and derailments.and passengers will be protected by more crashworthy vehicles.

TRAIN PROTECTION SYSTEMS

Sophisticated systems which incorporate automatic braking as a primary rather than secondary feature, are installed on a highly selective basis.

Automatic Warning System

The most basic form of train protection is the Automatic Warning System (AWS). Magnets are fixed between the rails at a distance of about 200m before a signal.This activates a bell in the driver's cab if the signal show a clear line ahead, and sounds a warning if the signal indicates 'caution' (single or double yellow) or 'danger' (red). If the driver fails to acknowledge a warning within a few seconds by pressing a button, the brakes are automatically applied. The system is intended to keep drivers alert to adverse signal aspects, and to help maintain train speeds in poor visibility. Its effectiveness in preventing collisions is incomplete, because the warning can so easily be overriden. Particularly on busy lines and during peak periods where trains frequently proceed through successive yellow signals, the warning may sound so often that drivers may become desensitized to it and may occasionally fail to respond to signals correctly.

Driver Reminder Appliance

AWS is now being supplemented by a Driver Reminder Appliance (DRA).The DRA is set by the driver whenever he stops at a red signal. If the train has been standing, for example at a station, there is a risk of the driver forgetting to check the signal before departing. The device prevents the train from starting until the driver has reset it, which should remind him to check that the signal has cleared.

Automatic Train Protection

With the advent of technology a number of much more sophisticated train protection systems have been developed which give a very high level of protection against collisions due to failure to obey signals, derailments due to excessive speed, and buffer-stop collisions. Known collectively as Automatic Train Protection (ATP), these systems generally monitor the speed of the train, and compare the train's speed with a safe speed which the system calculates on the basis of the train's distance from red signals, the braking characteristics of the train and other factors. If this calculated speed, which is indicated on the cab display, is exceeded by more than a set margin, automatic braking is applied until the train slows down sufficiently. ATP should prevent the great majority of 'signals passed at danger' (SPADs). However if a train does pass a red signal, the system will initiate an emergency stop. The driver cannot override the system.

Automatic Train Control

Automatic train control (ATC) incorporates all the functionality of ATP. However it goes one step further by dispensing with the need for a driver, although there may be an operator who performs other tasks such as opening and closing doors a system which applies the brakes automatically when a train passes a red signal. The layout of signals and junctions, combined with low maximum speed and fast-acting brakes, are such that it should be possible to bring a train passing a red signal at full speed to a halt before it can cause a collision.

TBS is a new generation of signalling which uses radio transmissions and incorporates incorporates full ATP functionality.

Train Protection and Warning System (TPWS)

TPWS incorporates the existing AWS, but provides a higher degree of train protection. Transmission beacons are placed on the track which can initiate emergency braking to halt the train if it is either about to pass a red signal (the 'train stop' facility) or has exceeded a maximum permitted speed by more than a set margin (the 'speed trap' facility). Speed traps can be fitted at the approach to signals in order to slow down a train travelling at above the permitted speed sufficiently to avoid most of the more serious SPADs, where the train overshoots the signal by such a large distance as to cause an actual danger such as a collision or a derailment. They can also be fitted at any other location where a speed restriction is required, for example at the approach to buffer stops, sharp curves, or track under maintenance. Unlike AWS, the driver will not be able to override the system. TPWS has been designed to be simple to fit to existing track and trains.

Compared with AWS and DRA alone, the addition of TPWS should reduce the risk of collision or derailment significantly. However, because the system does not monitor the train continuously, it will give less complete protection than ATP. In particular, TPWS is unlikely to be totally effective if a train approaches a red signal at high speed. The extent to which TPWS is effective at high speeds will depend largely on the siting of the beacon relative to the signal, and the speed at which a train will be 'tripped' by the beacon. Generally, the further back the detector is placed from the signal, and the lower the permitted speed at that point, the more effective the system will be in preventing serious SPADs. Technically, it may even be possible to place two speed traps at different distances from a signal, each set to trip at different speeds, for example where the line speed on the approach to a signal is relatively high. A balance has to be struck between achieving maximum train protection and the need to operate an efficient railway.

Faulty wiring in the signalling system, and derailments caused by track conditions or obstructions are factors that make it difficult to quantify the reduction in risk which a general upgrade from AWS to TPWS would bring about, but it can reduce the current level of risk to passengers significantly and bring real benefit and reduce accidents by 50% and also reduce the risk of collisions and derailments by half. This will in turn make a major accident, and therefore major loss of life in a single accident, less likely to occur. TPWS is likely to achieve much of the benefit which would be provided by full ATP, at significantly lower cost. ATP and further developments such as TBS are advanced systems which offer a high degree of protection must be fitted to all new high-speed lines including freight trains which, although they do not carry passengers, can place passengers in other trains at risk.

Since TPWS is not a continuous monitoring system and is only effective where beacons are placed on the track, it is necessary to decide which locations should be fitted. Train protection should be fitted on the approach to, any signal where if a train passes a signal at red it could travel into the path of another train. This would exclude signals on plain line (i.e., not protecting junctions, cross-overs or stations) and also those where a train passing through at red would be automatically diverted onto another line and away from danger and also on any railway on which the line speed is 25 mph or less like heritage railways and other minor passenger trains. Any part of a railway in a factory, mine or quarry, harbour or harbourarea, unless used for the carriage of fare-paying passengers; any part of a railway used solely for the purpose of carrying out a building operation or work of engineering construction, or within a maintenance or goods depot. any parts of a railway which are laid along a street or other public place and are, therefore, to all intents and purposes sections of tramway where there will be no signalling and vehicles are driven 'by line of sight' (able to halt within the distance the driver can see ahead).

Crashworthiness of Chassis

Passenger rail vehicles, manufactured between 1951 and 1974 share certain characteristics like a steel frame and a steel-panelled body mounted on a steel underframe. These have few energy-absorbing properties and nearly all of the vehicle's structural strength is concentrated in the underframe. No safeguards are built in to prevent the underframe of one vehicle riding over the underframe of another in a collision. The relatively weak body and the absence of override protection means that in a collision, passengers are less well protected than they would be in more modern vehicles, increasing the risk of fatalities and serious injuries. Vehicles tend to be forced upwards and to slice into the passenger space of other vehicles, resulting many casualties. These 'bogies' also have 'slam' (hinged) doors without central locking which, though safe in normal use, can be opened by passengers while the train is in motion unlike that of later vehicles, which are of monocoque construction and offer much greater crash resistance because of their more rigid body, inbuilt crumple zones, and safeguards against overriding. More modern vehicles also provide better internal safety (for example fewer sharp edges), and higher levels of comfort and convenience. Hence it is necessary to withdraw the outdated compartments and replace them with new vehicles. The older models can also be rebodied with a new, stronger, body over the existing underframe to improve crashworthiness.

A "cup and cone" anti-override device. In a head-on or end-to-end collision, the "cones" lock into the "cups", effectively locking vehicles together and preventing one vehicle overriding another. Not only the two colliding vehicles but all vehicles within each modified train would lock together in this way. This would imply removal of buffers and alteration of couplings. The device is unlikely to be effective at collisions with closing speeds of over 35-40 mph and it will not improve resistance to damage from side impact or derailment, but reduce the likelihood of derailment following a head-on or end-to-end collision.

62 Aircraft Accidents

INTRODUCTION

Aircraft crashes, often with serious consequences, are an ever-present danger in air travel. This is because of the unforgiving nature of flight, where a relatively insubstantial medium, air, supports a significant mass through dynamically active technological means. Should this support fail, there is limited opportunity for remedial action. Because of this, aircraft are designed to minimize the chance of failure, and pilots are trained with safety as a primary consideration. Despite this, accidents still occur, though statistically flying is the safest form of transport. In fact, the relative rarity of incidents, coupled with the often dramatic outcome, is one reason why they still make headline news. Nevertheless, while the odds of being in a plane crash are nowadays distinctly low compared to other means of transportation, the chances of dying in such a disaster are notably higher.

Causes

Approximately 80 percent of all aviation accidents occur shortly before, after, or during takeoff or landing. An accident survey of aircraft accidents from 1950 through 2006 determined the causes to be as follows:

- 53%: Pilot error.
- 21%: Mechanical failure.
- 11%: Weather.
- 8%: Other human error (air traffic controller error, improper loading of aircraft, improper maintenance, fuel contamination, language miscommunication etc.).
- 6%: Sabotage (bombs, hijackings, shootdowns).
- 1%: Other cause bird hit, wind shear, defective parts.

The survey excluded military, private, and charter aircraft.

Aviation Safety

Has come a long way in over one hundred years of implementation. All aircraft manufacturers place huge emphasis on the use of aviation safety equipment, and made safety a major selling point as a poor safety record in the aviation industry is a threat to corporate survival. Some major safety devices now required in commercial aircraft involve:

- Evacuation slides – Aid rapid passenger exit from an aircraft in an emergency situation.
- Advanced avionics – Computerized autorecovery and alert systems.
- Turbine engines – Durability and failure containment improvements
- Landing gear that can be lowered even after loss of power and hydraulics.

It all depends on the yardstick used. When measured on a passenger-distance calculation, air travel is now the safest form of transportation available. When compared against all other modes of transport on a fatality per mile basis, air transport is once again the safest – six times safer than traveling by car and twice as safe as rail. However, when measured by fatalities per person transported, buses are the safest form of transportation and the number of air travel fatalities per person are surpassed only by bicycles and motorcycles. For every billion kilometers traveled, trains have a fatality rate 12 times larger than air travel, while automobiles have a fatality rate 62 times larger. On the other hand, for every billion journeys, buses are the safest form of transportation. By the last measure air transportation is three times more dangerous than car transportation and almost 30 times more dangerous than bus. Passengers sitting at the back of a plane are 40% more likely to survive a crash than those sitting in the front, although there is no such thing as the safest seat. The flight data recorder or the "black box" is usually mounted in the aircraft's empennage (tail section), where it is more likely to survive a severe crash.

Action at Scene of Crash

A major aircraft disaster presents a scene where wreckage, bodies and survivors can be strewn over a wide area. It can be further complicated by hazardous cargo. If the accident occurs near a school, housing area, or traffic area, the results can be catastrophic. Suggested action is as follows:

- SURVEY the scene for obvious hazards (Munitions, Fuel, Instability, etc.).
- RESCUE survivors. If possible, enter wreckage from UPWIND SIDE.
- MOVE survivors to safe place.
- OBTAIN emergency medical care as needed.
- SEARCH the wreckage for concealed survivors.
- PROTECT the environment from further damage (fuel or foam runoff, etc.).
- CONTROL additional property damage.
- NOTIFY the nearest military installation, Fire Chief or Command Post.
- PRESERVE the site as intact as possible for investigators.
- DO NOT MOVE anything not necessary for rescue or damage control.
- GUARD the wreckage.
- SEARCH for additional victims, parts or wreckage along the flight path.
- IDENTIFY witnesses for later interview.
- REPORT the accident to the Airport Control Tower or service center.
- DIAGRAM the scene or take official departmental photographs.
- REFER news media / photographers' requests to police/ military information officer.
- *STAY CLEAR FROM FRONT AND REAR OF EXTERNALLY CARRIED TANKS OR PODS* as these may contain missiles or rockets whose explosive wake is hazardous. Never disturb bullets, bombs or other armament thrown clear from the aircraft as they may explode. Heat, fire or shock may make munitions very unstable. If possible, put warning marker flags at munitions items when they are located.
- *SAFEST APPROACH TO THE CRASH IS GENERALLY FROM UPWIND, TO THE SIDE OF THE AIRCRAFT FUSELAGE* as ammunitions or fuel may be scattered along the crash path. Weapons may fire forward, or create a blast to the back. Concealed survivors may be tangled in debris behind the main wreckage.
- *ACCESS HATCHES, RESCUE POINTS, AIRCRAFT EXITS:* The location of escape hatches, doors, and exits on military aircraft are usually indicated by *Orange-Yellow markings* on the outside of the aircraft. On jet aircraft a *Red Rescue Arrow* will indicate the rescue points. Instructions are stenciled at this arrow for the jettisoning of canopies or hatches.

- *USE CARE IN JETTISONING CANOPIES OR HATCHES* as they are often blown away from the aircraft by explosive devices. When operating the jettison controls, always position yourself well to the side and clear of the canopy/hatch. A ***Red Rescue Arrow*** points to the canopy/hatch jettison controls. Follow all stenciled instructions at the arrow and in the ***Warning Triangle*** near it. If unreadable, the following steps generally apply. Near the warning triangle, you will find a small door with controls inside. Push a release button to open the small door. Inside is a "T" Handle, connected to a 10-foot cable. **Stand clear of hatch or canopy**. Pull the "T" Handle out all the way. Canopy or hatch will be blown off with explosive force.
- *EJECTION SEAT WARNING.* Always LOOK FOR WARNING MARKINGS ON THE AIRCRAFT, AND BEWARE HAZARDS OF EJECTION SEATS. Aircraft with ejection seats have ***Warning Triangles*** painted near crew rescue points. Use extreme care not to actuate the seat, before, during or after rescue. ***Do not raise, move, or tamper with the armrests of crew seats, or any controls painted YELLOW and BLACK.*** These controls fire the ejection seats.Do not move any controls, handles or levers in the cockpit unless you are thoroughly familiar with that particular aircraft. Ejection systems vary among models and types.
- Before removing survivors, always unfasten seatbelt, shoulder and/or parachute harness and oxygen mask as well as radio cords and oxygen tubes. Cut any wire, tube or harness if needed. Cutting will not actuate an ejection. Time permitting, "knot" the Oxygen line to reduce fire hazard.
- *DO NOT MOVE VICTIMS EXCEPT AS NEEDED TO PROTECT THEM FROM FIRE OR OTHER INJURY UNTIL **EMERGENCY MEDICAL PERSONNEL ARRIVE.*** If there is no military medical assistance nearby, request a civilian doctor and Emergency Medical Technicians/Paramedics be summoned to the scene. Have EMTs or other trained personnel prepare injured personnel for transport to a trauma center or nearest hospital. Notify the hospital of the number of inbound patients and apparent nature of injuries.
- ***AVOID DISTURBING THE WRECKAGE.*** Except as necessary for rescue, do not disturb the wreckage. An intact site is necessary for the crash investigation team.
- *KEEP BYSTANDERS AND UNAUTHORIZED PERSONNEL AWAY. NO SMOKING.*

Fire Fighting Guide

Fire and explosion are always possible at a crash scene. *Fuel sources* include residual aircraft fuel, cargo, structural materials and munitions, as well as materials on the ground. *Ignition sources* include hot metal, electrical systems, weapon fuses, flares and other pyrotechnic devices. *Oxygen sources* include high pressure cylinders, liquid oxygen tanks and ambient air. Other potential hazards include exploding oxygen bottles, nitrogen or CO_2 tanks, liquid oxygen containers, exotic fuels, ejection seats, canopy and hatch jettison systems, high pressure tyres and struts, magnesium components, munitions, and hazardous cargo. **PROHIBIT SMOKING.** Volatile materials may have been scattered over a very wide area. The crash may also be a HAZMAT incident. Evacuate not only for fire protection, but also for HAZMAT protection if indicated. As always, keep the public calm: Panic can be much more hazardous than any object carried aboard a military aircraft.

Use foam, high-pressure water fog, carbon dioxide, or dry chemical powder to attack aviation gasoline and jet fuel fires. Halon agents are most effective in these situations:

Bombs, missiles or rockets: If such a weapon is found in the wreckage, cool its entire surface with available fire extinguishing agents or water spray. ***Do not handle or move.***

Ammunition: Do not handle or move. Mark location for military disposal experts. If ammunition is scattered, cordon the entire area and keep spectators and souvenir seekers away.

Nuclear weapons: It is very unlikely that any nuclear device will be in the wreckage. By quickly reporting the crash to the nearest military base or the Air Force Center, you will get military assistance and procedural information about any weapons on board. ***If Nuclear Weapons are present,*** they present the same immediate hazard as any other high explosive. Fire will not cause a nuclear detonation. Some hazardous materials, including radioactive substances, may leak from the weapons if they are broken open, or be carried off as particles in smoke if the weapons burn, rupture, or explode. If nuclear weapons are burned, expect a high explosive, conventional explosion that may scatter radioactive debris. A nuclear reaction will not occur. Firefighter precautions are:

- Wear full protective gear, masks and SCBA for fire attack. Remain upwind.
- Declare HAZMAT Level "B" incident unless otherwise indicated.
- Avoid all physical contact with debris and immediately evacuate the plume area.
- Withdraw and take cover if weapons are engulfed in sustained fire.
- Instruct Emergency Management/Civil Defence to initiate radiological monitoring.
- Establish decontamination protocols for firefighters, survivors and other personnel in the area.

Searching the Wreckage

- If you are the first to arrive at a wreckage scene, you may find no one there. Several possibilities exist.
- Occupants may have parachuted, may have been thrown clear, or may have survived and gone off in search of help. You should.
- Sound the alarm for backup help. Do not enter the wreckage alone. You may become injured or trapped, engulfed in flames or caught in an explosion.
- Look around the crash path. Call out for survivors. They may not see you.
- Listen carefully for signs of life: Faint cries, groans, tapping or scratching.
- Survivors may be scattered over a very wide area, particularly if it was a large aircraft or a high altitude ejection was performed. If there is sign of inflight disintegration, you will need help in conducting a wide-area search.
- Survivors may be concealed in the wreckage itself, or scattered along many miles of the final flight path. Check voids in the wreckage, in ravines, in trees and in ponds or lakes along the final flight path and all around the wreckage.
- DO NOT TOUCH any bullet, missile, bomb or other ammunition. Fire, heat or shock may have made the ammunition unstable.
- TAKE COVER if bombs, rockets, or other munitions are engulfed in flames.
- BE CAREFUL of sharp, jagged metal, compressed gas cylinders, fuel or other liquids.

Reporting the Accident (Do Not Delay Reporting Because Some Information is Unknown)

Call the nearest military installation. If you do not know how to contact that military installation, give as accurate a geographical location as you can, and inform how to reach the crash site. If coordinates are not known, describe in terms of landmarks, distances from towns, or road features. Identify the aircraft if possible from any numbers or letters painted on the tail, any other numbers from the nose, the type of aircraft (Fighter, cargo, bomber, helicopter) or model if known.

Additional Information to Report

Sequences of what exactly happened? Number of people who parachuted from the aircraft, approximate number of victims at crash site, any injuries of people on the ground, scale of medical, fire fighting or rescue help needed, approximate number of fatalities or injuries, which hospital have injured been taken, summary of damage to private property or civilian injuries, nearest suitable helicopter landing area: A flat open field, clear of poles, wires and trees and any other information that can be of immediate value. Do not hang up until you are sure the information is understood, and you have answered any questions from the other end.

Medical Care for Survivors

Render first aid and provide all needed emergency medical care for survivors, with or without directions from the military. As needed, transport victims to hospitals/trauma centers. If anyone is concerned about payment for services, advise them that flight insurance/airline(s) involved will provide them with full and cooperative assistance in billing procedures, payment and claims processing. Do not remove remains from the wreckage unless absolutely essential prior to arrival of the emergency medical team.

Guarding the Wreckage

Evidence at the crash site must be preserved, consistent with the need to save lives, rescue survivors and control property or environmental damage. The entire wreckage area may represent an accident site, a crime scene, or both. Protecting the wreckage and any debris trail along the flight path is always essential. Establish a cordon and provide site security—or if the number of spectators presents a problem—local law enforcement officials should deploy enough police, contract guards to provide adequate protection. If necessary, request the Armed Forces through State radio/TV channels. Local law enforcement should stay on the scene and should attempt to isolate an area within a radius of 2,000 feet from the main wreckage or debris trail, in order to avoid bystanders being exposed to injury from fire, explosion, or contact with hazardous materials. Also, this secure cordon will prevent trampling important features, inadvertent contamination of the scene, or theft of evidence. Local law enforcement officials should rely on their own resources for site security until other arrangements are made. If nuclear devices or classified materials are involved, the military commander may declare a "National Defense Area" at the wreckage site, allowing the site to be temporarily protected as though it were a military reservation.

Duties of the Guard Force

Protect all civilian and military property, prohibit removal of deceased persons until properly identified by authorities. Laws of some jurisdictions may require that remains be taken into custody by local coroners. Comply with local law. Keep all spectators at a reasonable distance and admit only authorized personnel to the scene. Prevent handling or disturbance of the wreckage, theft of any parts, or compromising other evidence such as gauges or marks on the ground left by the crashed aircraft.

Preserving the Accident Site

Only admit crash, fire, rescue, military teams, medical examiners, local health, environmental or safety officials and accredited news personnel, the on-scene incident commander (normally a local Fire Chief) and incident command team. Each and every piece of the aircraft, its location, and its exact position is important to investigators in determining the sequence of events, causes of the accident, and injuries involved. The lives and safety of people on future flights and on the ground depend on a rapid and accurate determination of the accident cause. Lessons learned from each accident are used to prevent future aircraft accidents, and to improve aircraft and equipment design, and training of aircrews. Hence, nothing should be disturbed, other than that necessary to rescue survivors. If there are fatalities, the bodies should not be disturbed or moved until the medical examiner makes a positive identification, since the location of bodies may help determine significant facts about the accident.No aircraft part—not even a small fragment—should be moved or disturbed at all. The team of accident investigators needs to see everything just as it came to rest. The condition of light bulb filaments, watch dials, pointers on gauges, positions of switches and levers, condition of fluids, and scrapes and scratches can hold the clue to accidents. These clues are easy to destroy even by well-meaning responders. Touch or move nothing unless it is necessary to rescue a survivor.

Even marks on the ground are important clues. As such, the movement of people and equipment at the scene must be kept to the minimum needed to rescue survivors and control the spread of fire, environmental impact, or other property damage. Basic rule: Once the last survivor has been removed, withdraw all personnel to the security cordon and await the arrival of the investigating team. Souvenir hunters are often a serious problem. Unauthorized removal of crash debris is a violation of numerous state laws. Crash debris from a military aircraft is still federal government property. In addition, military aircraft are often equipped with ballistic cartridges, munitions, and other dangerous items and only trained experts should approach or handle these items. The military crash response team which comes to the scene will include specialists able to deal with every aspect of the crash: Identification and removal of human remains, safe collection and disposal of explosives and other haza-rdous materials, site security, and accident investigation. They will cooperate fully with local officials, and will make every effort to rapidly mitigate the hardship on the local community. The military team will probably request continued assistance with site security, fire protection, medical treatment and other support within the ability of the community.

Witnesses

Witnesses are extremely important in helping solve the cause of the accident. Names and addresses of all witnesses should be taken for subsequent interview by accident investigators. Likewise, anyone with film or video tape of the accident should be requested to furnish it to the accident investigation team. If possible, local law enforcement officials should take voluntary custody of this evidence as soon as they learn of its existence.

News Media and Military Aircraft Crashes

It is the policy of the Department of Defense to cooperate with legitimate news-gathering efforts at the scene of an accident, and to impose only those minimum restrictions on the news media that are necessary for safety, preservation of evidence, respect for victims and their families, and national security. The press has a job to do and is entitled to factual information about the event, and to photograph or televise the response efforts. For their own safety, the press should be advised to stay away from danger areas, and should be instructed not to interfere with rescue efforts or to disturb the scene in any way. Out of compassion for victim's families, the press should be requested not to photograph human remains, nor to release the names or any information about victims until their families have been properly notified. The military will furnish the press with complete information as soon as it is appropriate for publication. Do not use force to prevent media from taking photographs or televising the scene even if they are ignoring the above safety and decency guidelines, unless local laws are being violated. However, photographing classified equipment is a federal criminal offense as well as being detrimental to national security. Reasonable law enforcement actions may be taken should violations occur. Advise media representatives that a Military Public Information Officer will arrive with the service crash response team. The military PRO will assist all media reporters to establish facts and to interview service officials as needed.

Questions from witnesses regarding the weather conditions and other details at time of accident: The direction aircraft was headed, and what did the aircraft appear to be doing. What drew your attention to the aircraft, was it on fire in flight and if so, what was the color and direction of the flames. Was there an explosion in the air prior to the crash and what sounds did you hear before and after the crash (Engine sound, bangs or pops, etc.). Did you see any parachutes, people or other objects fall from the aircraft and who was first person to arrive at the wreckage scene. Do you know if anyone removed anything from the wreckage scene? If so, who did it and what did they take? What was the impact angle of the aircraft and position of bodies and survivors in the wreckage.

The "Black Box" Flight Data Recorder (ADR)

The flight data recorder (FDR) {also ADR, for accident data recorder} is a device used to record specific aircraft performance parameters. Another kind of flight recorder is the cockpit voice recorder (CVR), which records conversation in the cockpit, radio communications between the cockpit crew and others (including conversation with air traffic control personnel), as well as ambient sounds. In some cases, both functions have been combined into a single unit.

Popularly referred to as a "black box," the data recorded by the FDR is used for accident investigation, as well as for analyzing air safety issues, material degradation and engine performance. Following an accident, recovery of the "black boxes" is second in importance only to the rescue of survivors and recovery of human remains.

The design of today's FDR is governed by the internationally recognised standards and recommended practices relating to flight recorders which are contained in ICAO Annex 6 which makes reference to industry crashworthiness and fire protection specifications. Currently, EUROCAE specifies that a recorder must be able to withstand an acceleration of 3400 *g* (33 km/s^2) for 6.5 milliseconds. This is roughly equivalent to an impact velocity of 270 knots and a deceleration or crushing distance of 450 cm. Additionally, there are requirements for penetration resistance, static crush, high and low temperature fires, deep sea pressure, sea water immersion, and fluid immersion. Modern day FDRs receive inputs via specific data frames from the FDAU units. They record significant flight parameters, including the control and actuator positions, engine information and time of day. There are 88 parameters required as a minimum under current U.S. federal regulations (only 29 were required until 2002), but some systems monitor many more variables. Generally each parameter is recorded a few times per second, though some units store "bursts" of data at a much higher frequency if the data begins to change quickly. Most FDRs record approximately 17–25 hours worth of data in a continuous loop. It is required by regulations, that an FDR verification check (readout) is performed annually, in order to verify that all mandatory parameters are recorded.

This has also given rise to flight data monitoring programs, whereby flights are analyzed for optimum fuel consumption and dangerous flight crew habits. The data from the FDR is transferred, in situ, to a solid state recording device and then periodically analyzed with some of the same technology used for accident investigations.

Contrary to the "black box" reference, the exterior of the FDR is coated with heat-resistant bright orange paint for high visibility in wreckage, and the unit is usually mounted in the aircraft's empennage (tail section), where it is more likely to survive a severe crash as the entire front of the aircraft is expected to act as a "crush zone" to reduce the shock that reaches the recorder. Also, modern FDRs are typically double wrapped, in strong corrosion-resistant stainless steel or titanium, with high-temperature insulation inside. They are designed to emit a locator beacon for up to 30 days, and can operate immersed to a depth of up to 6,000 meters (20,000 ft).

Future Devices

Since the recorders can sometimes be crushed into unreadable pieces, or even located in deep water, some modern units are self-ejecting (taking advantage, of kinetic energy at impact to separate themselves from the aircraft) and also equipped with radio and sonar beacons to aid in their location. Alternatively, other aircraft such as the Space Shuttle Orbiter do not possess an FDR but instead use down-links to transfer such data. This modality could see wider use in aviation in modified form. The installation of a second cockpit voice recorder, digital flight data recorder system and emergency locator transmitter that utilizes combination deployable recorder technology in each commercial passenger aircraft that would be ejected from the rear of the aircraft at the moment of an accident has been mooted. One problem for the military is that these commercial devices offer no protection of the data that has been recorded. Therefore, they have the potential for exposing military secrets if the device is captured by non-friendly forces and exploited.

63 Identification of Victims During Aircraft and Other Disasters

INTRODUCTION

Disasters are characterized by a significant loss of human life and identification of the victims is a grim requirement for humane, investigative, legal and economic reasons. There is a natural human desire to claim ones own relative(s) for proper last rites and consignment. Proper identification of bodies affects payments of insurance policies, settling real estate ownership and partnerships as also proof of death of spouse before re-marriage of life partner. Discovery of an 'odd man out' not in the manifest and/or with autopsy findings different from the rest of the victims could be a pointer towards an illegal passenger, air piracy (hijacking) and sabotage. The physical condition of the crew members and the pattern of injuries sustained by the passengers may give valuable clues in the reconstruction of the sequence and circumstances of the accident including the final approach prior to impact. Usually there will be uniformity of injuries or a steady, logical gradation of their injuries. Marked deviation from the usual pattern would indicate an unusual type of accident. Discordant patterns of injury in the same accident indicates that different parts were subjected to differing stresses, like an explosion in one section and also the mode of the impact, e.g., nose or tail impact or multiple impacts. Examination of victims can also yield clues to willful sabotage and also methods to improve craft design and improve safety factors like modifications to the seating and safety equipment on board.

Identification of casualties in a mass disaster situation is usually applied in an irregular haphazard manner with an ad hoc flow of the identification process. This results in delays, conflicts, additional expense, errors and overall low efficiency. A flexible protocol for disaster victim identification has been evolved based on the experiences in a large number of aircrash accidents.

The Four Phases of Investigation

The 4 distinct phases in the process are:

1. Preliminary evaluation.
2. Data collection.
3. Data analysis.
4. Conclusion.

Preliminary Evaluation

In this process the location and nature of disaster, the approximate number of casualties and the availability of resources are evaluated. Appropriate personnel, equipment and a work site must often be selected on short notice and without direct knowledge of the nature and scope of the event. Extra attention given to evaluation at this point invariably simplifies subsequent tasks. Disruption of the disaster site is usually inevitable in the course of survivor rescue, but beyond this initial stage, it is vital that strict security measures be instituted to restrict access to the area. Only trained investigators and authorized personnel should be permitted entry into the area. Uncontrolled access can, by itself be disastrous. The number of casualties, the condition of the bodies as well as the environmental conditions will influence the selection of identification methods and personnel to assist in the identification process. Dental techniques proved to be a key factor in the B-747 disaster at Tenerife, while fingerprinting was conclusive in the Jonestown Guyana mass homicide/suicide episode. These factors also affect the choice of mortuary location. While there are many reasons for conducting the identification process as near the disaster site as possible, other factors like the availability of refrigeration, communications, hostile environment and various other facilities for the process may be overriding. It is always desirable to have a front man or a commander to deal with all outsiders and handling all enquiries from the press, family members, undertakers, lawyers etc to prevent distracting interruptions to the identification personnel. While it is desirable that he has expertise in identification techniques, he is not directly involved in the process. From a practical standpoint, the more rank and respect he commands in the community, the more effective he will be.

Data Collection

The second phase concentrates on data collection. This is a very intensive activity and overcoming initial inertia is one of the first hurdles when it seems that people are standing around waiting for something to happen, not realizing that they are the ones who must take the first step. Antemortem records must be obtained for comparison with post mortem observations. Immediate steps must be taken to obtain a list of the persons believed to be missing from flight manifests, passenger lists, reservation charts. The missing persons physician, dentist, employer, family and friends must be contacted for valuable sources of information and records. Details regarding clothing, personal effects, medical and dental records must be extracted on high priority. Before shifting of bodies to the mortuary, rescuers must mark body positions with tags, photographs and outlines on a diagram of the disaster site (terrain chart). Appropriate storage of the bodies must be arranged and each body must have a firmly attached identifying label that contains information obtained on site. Body bags, bed sheets, or crates may be used. Tough transparent plastic bags make excellent containers since they are moisture and tear resistant and will withstand extensive handling. Refrigeration of the bodies is particularly important in temperate and tropical climates. Refrigerated truck trailers can be used and each can accommodate approximately 50 bodies. An inventory procedure must be observed to keep track of each body and each investigator cannot be expected to keep track of more than 20 bodies at a time.

The organizational flow suggested is as follows: Clothing and personal effects must be removed, noted, photographed and labeled, all injuries must be documented. Small unburnt scraps of clothing can usually be found in the armpit and crotch areas and where the body has lain in contact with a hard surface and escaped the fire. The type, the cut, the material, the size, the brand labels and laundry marks can all prove invaluable and must be noted in detail. Clues to identity can also be obtained from cosmetics including lipstick, nailpolish, eye makeup, rouge, bleaches, dyes, blemish concealers and depilation practices must not be overlooked. The personal effects are then transferred to the personal effects group and details of these must be available to all other investigators. Specific identifying features on each body such as tattoos, scars, marks, deformities or abnormalities etc must be photographed as well as the face, hands and feet of victims. A polaroid or digital camera would be most ideal for this. Blood samples for analysis of carboxyhaemoglobin would suggest death by asphyxiation in a fire. Microscopic examination of lungs for features of fat and bone marrow embolism and plankton would also be useful in indicating sequence of death. Dental and fingerprint details are noted followed by full body X-rays. The value of complete X-ray views of all parts of the body has been clearly demonstrated. Whole body radiography on the remains demonstrates occult injury patterns, surgical artifacts, appliances and prosthesis, anomalies or unique skeletal features, dental structures, personal effects and foreign bodies, and should be a routine part of forensic autopsy. Fluoroscopy can be an alternative for rapid initial screening but it does not provide a hardcopy documentation and also causes undue radiation exposure. It is best to use only full size 14 × 17 inch sized radiographic film to avoid handling multiple sized film cassettes and finished films. Most human bodies can be radiographed with 3-4 such films in one frontal projection. An assembly-line type of operation is required and must precede pathologic examinations. Initial radiographs are taken with clothing still in place and additional radiographs taken after their removal to yield important clues in accident mechanism and personal identification. Jewelry and other items may be hidden in soot and char, eluding visual inspection and prove crucial in identification. Rings, hair ornaments, tiepins, lapel pins, nose rings, earrings, necklaces, watches, keys, bracelets, anklets will usually survive high impact forces and excessive temperatures with little damage (Fig. 63.1).

Careful note of these including which particular location they were worn, including right or left side must be noted. Serial number of watches, and initials, designs, inscriptions and dates on rings and lockets can prove very useful and the services of a professional jeweller can be requisitioned for a day to look into these details. Sex determination can be made based on the configuration of the pelvis and age from details of bone structure. Patterns of the frontal sinuses and degenerative changes of the spinal cord can clinch identification when compared with antemortem medical records. A through post mortem pathologic examination is then conducted and appropriate tissue specimens collected for toxicologic and serologic, blood grouping examination. Likewise, anthropologic and histologic procedures may also be required. Surgical and contraceptive devices recovered at post mortem must be tagged and stored.

Positive identification by fingerprinting depends on the antemortem database available. Fingerprinting is routinely done on a large scale in some countries while in others it bears a criminal stigma and not available except for those with police records. Fingerprints at employment, obtaining driving licence or ration cards can prove very useful in positive identification of victims. A positive identification can be made, in some instances, with a section of ridged skin no larger than the tip of a pencil eraser. Identification through fingerprints includes that through palm impressions and footprints. In some countries, there is a general practice to footprint and/or full palm print newborns together with finger impressions of the mother. These records when available can be extremely useful to facilitate identification. Expert knowledge and experience is necessary for preparation and recording of ridged skin.

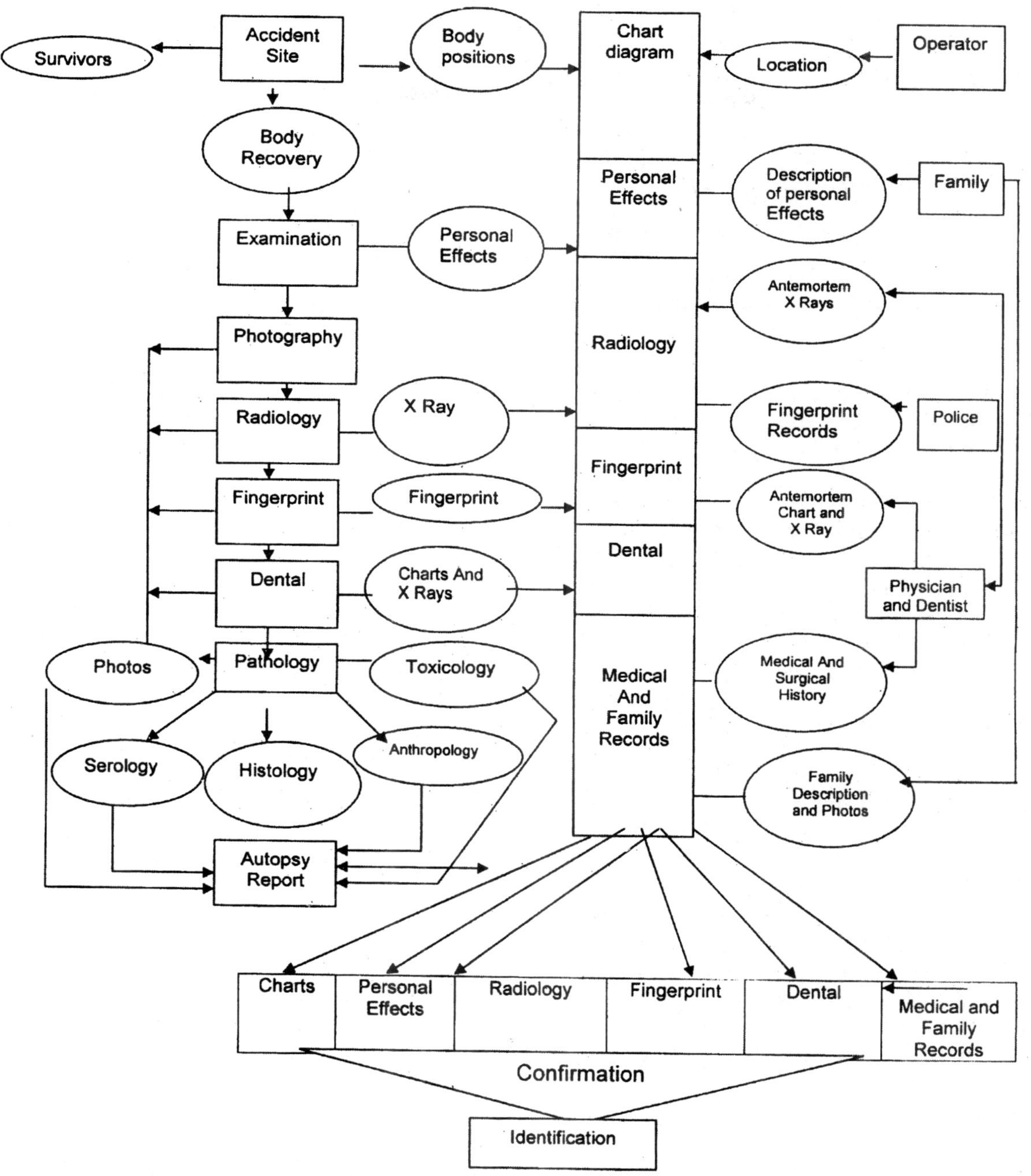

Fig. 63.1: Organizational flow concept for identifying casualties of a mass disaster

The second most valuable physical characteristic for identification are the teeth. The teeth present an infinite number of variations due to extractions, restoration works, dentures, prosthetic devices and abnormalities. They are highly indestructible in cases of incineration and injury since the tooth enamel is the hardest known biological tissue. Since the days of Nero, dental anomalies have been an important source of information. A forensic odontologist is best equipped to assist in this type of work with his or her considerable knowledge of cranio-facial anatomy and forensic training. Female victims are examined first as they more difficult to identify. The teeth are examined in situ and the jaws may be removed after radiography. On occasions, the heat generated can be so intense that the jaws become very brittle and break, even on gentle handling, and cause loss of valuable evidence. The maxillae can be removed after making a transverse saw cut perpendicular to the inferior nasal spine and extending as far back as the junction of the hard and soft palate. The mandible can be removed whole by dissection of the tempero-mandibular joints or by saw cuts through each vertical ramus. Teeth must then be cleaned with a toothbrush and hot soapy water and all blood rinsed off, over a sieve or a wicker basket to collect any material that may break off during the process. Thick carbon deposits can be removed by careful scaling. The dental findings are then recorded on colour coded dental charts for each sex. All fillings, extractions and prostheses must be filled described in intimate detail together with a description of any anatomical irregularities, pathological lesions and racial characteristics. Battery powered headlights, dissection instruments, bone saws, toothbrush, scalers, mirrors, probes, tweezers and cotton pledgets must be provided for this work. Dental identification must furnish the following details:

- The number of teeth present.
- The number of teeth extracted.
- The number of teeth filled and type of restoration used.
- The presence and type of prostheses.
- The presence of intra and extra-oral pathological lesions.
- Racial characteristics and tooth morphology.
- Age estimation.
- Sex estimation.
- Radiological appearances.
- Blood Group determination.

Some dentures may carry a coded mark to indicate place of manufacture and the year they were produced. Chinese, Eskimos, Mongoloid people and American Indians have distinctive shovel-shaped incisors and Negroes frequently have two lingual cusps on 4/4. Accurate age determinations to within +/ - 1 year will usually be possible in children from the stage of teeth eruption and mineralization. A lateral oblique view of a pantograph would be very useful. In adults the accuracy comes down to +/- 1year from the degree of enamel attrition, the amount of secondary dentine present and the amount of obliteration of the pulp chamber. Root translucency and colour density measurements using optical equipment can enhance accuracy to +/- 2 years. 67% positive identification can be made by this method, and that can increase greatly if antemortem dental records are made available. Proof is a matter of balancing the possibilities, but caution must be exercised in using fillings of the first permanent molars as the sole means, as these are very common, but porcelain jacket crowns and other unusual features can clinch an identity. Blood group identification from tooth pulp can also be made with 80-100% accuracy.

Data Analysis

Recognition of victims based on antemortem

records reveals several obvious identities. The second method used is the mix and match when logical manipulation of records into groups that have common characteristics are made to arrive at an identification. Personal effects such as watches, rings may be compared. The third method is by exclusion when, by a positive identification of one person, that of the second can be presumed so long as the list of the missing persons is accurate. Computers can be used to identify victims of mass disasters using image enhancement techniques in doubtful situations. A second opinion is taken before arriving at positive identification and the bodies may be handed over for burial so that subsequent exhumation can be done as additional information is obtained later on.

DNA PROFILING (FINGERPRINTING)

Like the fingerprints that came into use during the 1930's to identify individuals, each person has a unique DNA profile and, unlike the conventional fingerprints that can only be located on fingertips and can be altered by surgery, the DNA profile is the same for every cell, tissue (including bone) and organ of an individual. It cannot be altered by any known treatment methods. Developed by Professor Sir Alec Jeffreys in 1985, DNA fingerprinting or profiling has established itself as a powerful, efficient and highly accurate means of determining identities from whatever bodily traces that can be salvaged. The technology is so powerful that the DNA from the blood stained clothing of the late US president Abraham Lincoln could be analyzed to diagnose Marfans Syndrome hundreds of years later and likewise, the diseases afflicting the mummies in the pyramids. The characteristics and traits of all living organisms are essentially determined by information contained within the DNA inherited from their parents. The molecular structure of DNA can be compared to that of a zipper, with each tooth represented by one of four letters (A,C,G or T), and, with the opposite teeth forming one of the two pairs, either A-T or G-C. The letters A,C,G and T standing for the bases adenine, cytosine, guanine and thymine that constitute the building blocks of DNA. The basic genetic information is determined by the sequence of letters or the specific order in which these bases are arranged along the two DNA molecular strands e.g. the sequence ACGCT posting information different from another sequence AGTCC in the same way as the word Stop means different from the word Tops, though they both use the same letters. The DNA molecules are tightly wrapped, like bundles of rope into packages called chromosomes. The DNA molecules are very long and serve as very long instruction manuals whose words and sentences ar written using the letters A,T,G C. Most humans have 23 chromosomes collectively referred to as the human genome. Almost every cell in the body contains a copy of the individuals genome. Each genome has over three billion paired elements known as bases. Living organisms that look different or have different characteristics also have different DNA sequences. The more varied the organisms, the more varied the DNA sequences. This polymorphism of the DNA genome is seen as variations in molecular length. Because every organ or tissue of an individual contains the same DNA fingerprint, blood stains (the best source), hair, teeth, bone, sweat and saliva stains found at the scene of a disaster can be analyzed to identify victims, after comparing it with those of their biological parents. The process involves visualization of special segments of the human genome, unique to each individual. These special segments are called Standard Tandem Repeats (STR) that are cut out from the rest of the DNA by several processes like mapping Restriction Fragment Length Polymorphisms (RFLP), and Polymerase Chain Reaction (PCR). The STR segments obtained are then sorted by size using gel electrophoresis. These segments are then tagged with radioisotopes to produce a visual pattern known as an autoradiograph on x-ray film or by using automated DNA sequencing machines. A more refined method analyzes DNA segments for the number of repeats of bases at 13 specific DNA sites. The chance of misidentification by this method is one in several billion. The PCR method or Southern Blot is used to obtain multiple copies of segments from a very limited amount of DNA (as little as 5molecules). Even a flake of dandruff can serve to make a positive identification. Samples must not be contaminated and due precautions while handling the samples. DNA fingerprinting is expensive and, while a non match is conclusive, there is still less certainty when a match occurs.

Methodology of DNA Fingerprinting

DNA fingerprinting is a laboratory procedure that requires six steps:

1. *Isolation of DNA:* DNA must be recovered from the cells or tissues of the body. Only a small amount of blood, hair or skin is needed. An amount of DNA present at the root of one hair is usually sufficient for the test.

2,3,4. *Cutting, sizing and sorting:* Special enzymes called restriction enzymes are used to cut the DNA at specific places. An enzyme EcoR1 found in bacteria will cut DNA only when the sequence GAATTC occurs. The DNA pieces are sorted out according to size by a sieving technique called electrophoresis and then passed through a gel made from seaweed agarose.

5. *Transfer of DNA to nylon:* The distribution of DNA as per particle sizes is then transferred to a nylon sheet by placing the sheet on the gel and soaking them overnight.
6. *4-5:Probing:* Radioactive or coloured probes are added to the nylon sheet to get a pattern – the DNA fingerprint.

The DNA fingerprint: The final DNA fingerprint is built by using several probes (5-10 or more) simultaneously, resembling the bar codes used by supermarket store scanners.

Further Reading

1. An organizational concept for pathologic identification in mass disasters- Colonel Robert R McMeekin, Chief of Aerospace Pathology, Armed Forces Institute of pathology, Washington D.C. J of Aviation,Space and Environmental Medicine. Sept 1980, Vol 51, No.9, Section II,:999-1003.
2. Role of radiology in aviation accident investigation. Joel E.Licenstein, John E Madewell, Robert R McMeekin, David S Feigin and John H Wolcott. Dept of Radiologic Pathology, Armed Forces Institute of Pathology, Washington D.C. J of Aviation, Space and Environmental Medicine, Sept 1980, Vol 51, No. 9, Section II, p1004-1014.
3. Medical investigation of fatalities from aircraft accident burns. Dunne MJ Jr and McMeekin, RR. J of Aviation, Space and Environmental Medicine, 1977, 48:964-968.
4. Pathology patterns in aircraft accident investigations. Gable, WD. J of Aerospace Medicine, 1968, 39:638-640.
5. Diaghnostic patterns of injury and death in USAF aviation accidents. Smelsey,SO. J of Aerospace Medicine, 1970, 41:790-793.
6. Fingerprint identification and the disaster victim. Francis M Leapley, Latent Fingerprint Section, F.B.I., Washington D.C. J of Aviation, Space and Environmental Medicine. Sept 1980, Vol 51, No.9, Section II, p1015-1018.
7. Use of personal effects in the Canary Island accident investigation. John H Wolcott, Robert Menzies, Edmund Donahue and Norman Hoffa,

Aerospace Pathology Division, Armed Forces Institute of Pathology, Washington, D.C. J of Aviation, Space and Environmental Medicine, Sept 1980, Vol 51, No.9, Section II, p1019-1025.

8. Dental identification in fatal aircraft accidents. Hill,IR, Royal Air Force Institute of Pathology, Halton, Aylesbury, Bucks, U.K. J of Aviation, Space and Environmental Medicine, 1980, 51(9):1021-1025.
9. Dental identification in the Stockport air disaster. Haines,DH. British Dental Journal, 1967,123:336.
10. Identification of mass casualties: Experience in four civil air disasters. Stevens,PJ and Tarlton, SW. J of Med. Sci.Law,1963,3:154.
11. Blood group determination from teeth. Higginson, AG and Hill,IR. J of Aviat Space Environ Med, 1980, 51 (9):1026-1029.
12. Administrative organization and function during the identification process for mass disasters-Canary Islands crash. Wolcott,JH, Hanson,CA, Menzies,R, Ballo J, Donahue E and Hoffa,N. J of Aviat Space and Environ Med, 1980, 51(9):1030-1033).

64 Military Medicine

> "Tell the surgeon to get his instruments ready. I know my arm must come off, and the sooner it is done, the better."
>
> —*Captain Horatio Nelson*
> *(Aboard Santa Cruz, Espana, 1797)*

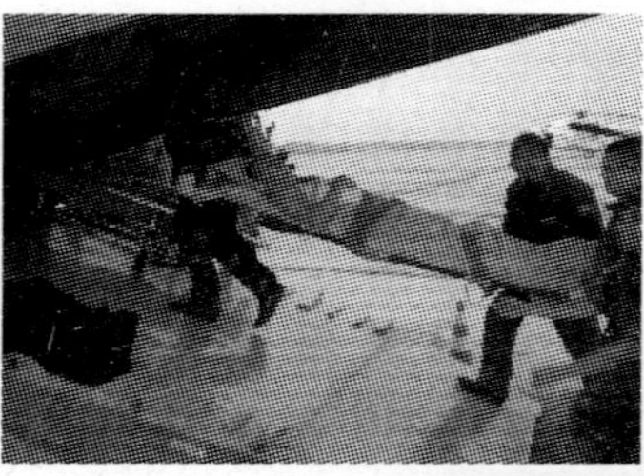

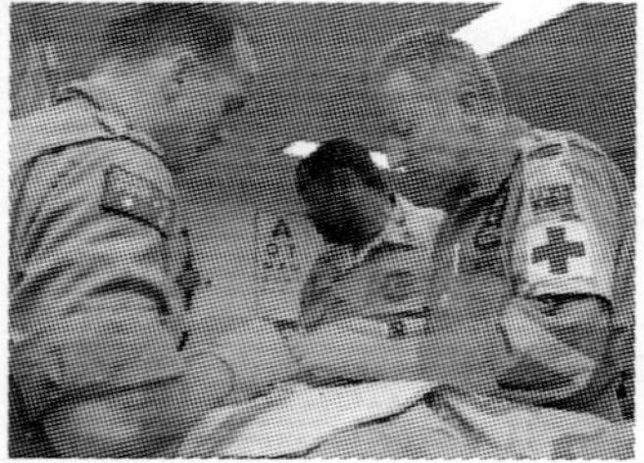

Fig. 64.1

INTRODUCTION

War is the greatest disaster known to man. In addition, as wars often erupt with little or no warning, they also can be classed as "emergencies". Because of the ever-changing nature and increasing sophistication of modern weaponry, it is vital that defence medical planning is aware of these changes and reacts accordingly. Modern warfare has moved away from the concept of large set piece battles involving large numbers of troops, to smaller conflicts, that erupt often at long distances from the area in which the troops are based. These so-called "Fire Brigade" actions require the ability for rapid deployment of highly mobile troops, often over long distances. In addition, although the number of casualties are likely to be less because the number of troops deployed is reduced, the severity of the wounds is greater due to the increased fire power of modern weapons.

The military is frequently identified as a provider of services to disaster-stricken populations. Their quick response facilitated by the clear-cut chain of command, excellent communication and logistic infra structure, discipline and skills in operational medicine are major attributes that automatically make them the first choice as a primary resource for disaster relief.

BATTLEFIELD CASUALTY MANAGEMENT

In Homers' Iliad, wounded soldiers were carried from the line of battle, laid beneath a tree and given a refreshing drink. The surgeon would then make a visitation and cleanse the wounds with cold water, rub herbs in them to relieve pain, extract the arrows heads, and dress the wounds with woolen bandages. The wounded soldiers were then carried to their tents to recover or die.

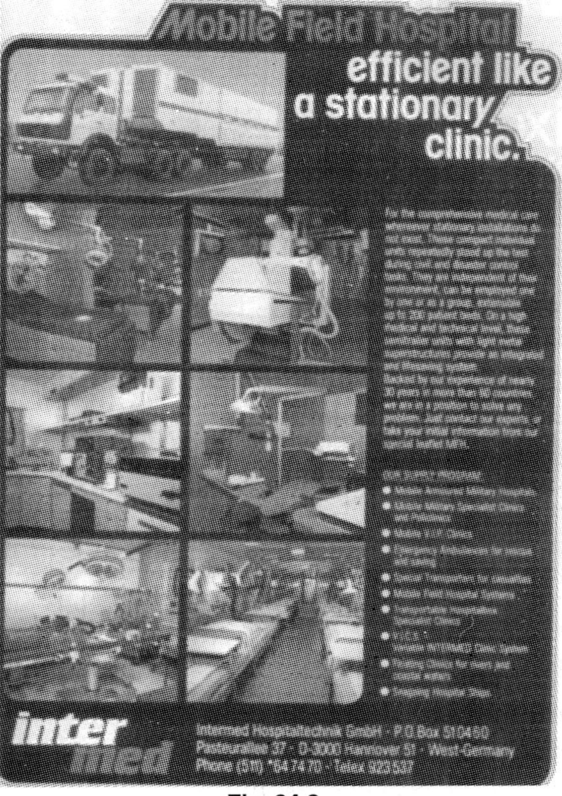

Fig. 64.2

In the history of warfare, it is probable that more servicemen have died as a result of inadequate and delayed medical treatment following trauma than as a direct result of the trauma itself. The percentage of combat casualties killed in action which was 40% during the Revolutionary War of 1775-1783, dropped to 35% during the civil war of 1861-1865 and even lower to 25% during the Vietnam War of 1961-1973 and just 10% during Op Enduring Freedom in 2001. This amply reflects improvements in combat casualty care especially in the far forward trauma resucitation and surgery. It is estimated that 10%of battle casualties will end up as missing, 20% killed in action, 70% wounded of which 20% will need sugery within 2 h and 80% within 6 h. Almost 50% or more of battle casualties will require surgical treatment and the central aim of battlefield casualty management would be to keep the interval between wounding and surgery less than 8 h.

It has been argued that the nature of wounds is getting increasingly severe due to sophisticated weaponry. Rapid casevac is only part of the solution, and should not always be seen as an effective alternative to immediate treatment. The link between effective triage, early treatment and survival rates is no longer disputed; what is, however, is the type and extent of treatment that can be taken forward into the battle area. Some maintain that forward surgical centres are needed, while others question the practicality of this. All however emphasize the importance for well-trained unit-level medics being able to reach the casualties in the important minutes after a soldier is wounded. The concept of the Golden Hour following wounding is well established and during this time, not only can life-threatening symptoms be treated, but the onset of other potentially fatal problems can be pre-empted. The traditional concept of first-aid is essentially reactive and does little more than address the most obvious symp-toms. No consideration is given to standardizing treatment, partly on the grounds that, in the stress of battle, a soldier is doing well if he receives even the most basic treatment. During the 1970s, the Israeli army, considered by many as having the best field medical care in the world, recognized the value of forward trauma teams able to resuscitate and stabilize casualties who could not be immediately evacuated to field hospitals. By the mid-

1980s, some NATO forces accepted that the traditional methods of casualty handling would not be adequate in a major European war. The British began to apply the lessons of the 1982 Falklands war despite the relatively limited numbers of casualties in that theatre. Terrorist-inflicted wounds have subsequently influenced trauma care the world over and especially in the Northern Ireland experience of the 1980s.

BATTLEFIELD MEDICAL EQUIPMENT

The US College of Surgeons Committee on Trauma put together the Pre-Hospital trauma Life Support (PHTLS) and the Advanced Trauma Life Support (ATLS) systems and provided a didactic approach to trauma management, both before and after a casualty is evacuated to a hospital. Under the ATLS system, casualties are inspected and treated by doctors according to a set of strict guidelines, where a limited number of responses are permitted for a given set of symptoms. Some have criticized the rigidity of this approach and consider it too simplistic assuming that a trained doctor would be on site with the back up of a well equipped medical infra structure. The imposition of treatment protocols or drills, however, has a positive benefit amidst the chaos of battle. Standardized treatments simplify equipment holdings and the problems of replenishment. They also enable the military doctors to work effectively outside an established medical infrastructure. The U.K. Register of Emergency Technicians (REMT) was also a national initiative aimed at standardizing treatment. The extension of the ATLS-type training below physician level is limited, but nine-day casualty care courses are available in the U.S. for medics and nurses. The first specific battlefield system to have been developed from ATLS is the British Army Trauma Life Support (BATLS) course developed in 1985 taking on the principle of rapid and disciplined intervention, aimed specifically at battle casualties. It is based on the knowledge that treatment will be carried out in poor conditions and extreme stress by unit medical orderlies, medical officers, and medical corps specialists. Students are assessed for aptitude and technical skills and ability to work under stress. The qualification is valid for 4 years only and revalidated based on attendance at update courses. BATLS equipment has been reduced to a sensible minimum and designed to fit into portable backpacks. Maximal use of disposables has been made, replacing steel with plastic. The Howmedicas external fixator device is now widely used and is a simple and effective bone stabilizer. Malleable metal-based splints (SAM) are lightweight, multifunctional field splints permitting wound access features suitable for Level 1 care. The inflatable air splints are useful devices but they do not prevent rotation of limb or telescoping of fractured ends and need to be constantly supervised for loss of air pressure. They also turn brittle and crack in cold or extreme tropical environments. Pre-padded Plaster of Paris slabs remain a useful alternative because of its conforming characteristics, strength, ease of application and safety, but is perhaps better left for Level 2 and 3 care, as availability of water and buckets on the field may not always be assured. Traction splints such as the Thomas splint needs special training for their application and needs more than one operator to apply. It is bulky and awkward for a medical corpsman to carry and precludes patient positioning on a standard litter. While suited for single femoral fractures, they are unsuitable for proximal femur fractures and combined femur-tibial fractures and bilateral femoral fractures. Excessive traction force can produce ischaemic changes and pressure sores at the level of the ring and nerve palsies from excessive pressure of the fibular head against the lateral bar. It also precludes positioning a comatose patient in a lateral position and application of a MAST suit. A modification of the Liston Splint is suitable for fractures of both upper and lower segments of the same limb as it immoblizes a joint above and below the fracture and suited for proximal femoral fractures. The Australian invention, the Collite Splint, has been specifically developed for military application. It consists of three extendible rods of high tensile aluminium adjustable from 400mm to 1555 mm and 6 neoprene straps with aluminium stay pegs weighing just 1 kg. The rods can be adjusted by breaking down the 400mm units to accommodate the size of the limb being immobilized and the carry pack itself serves as an effective cervical collar. The kit is bouyant, corrosion and temperature resistant and compatible with application of a MAST suit. The neoprene straps have good gripping features and can also serve as tourniquets or compression bandages. A BATLS medic would be adept at restoring an airway, inserting chest drains and capable of improvisation by using his common sense to overcome equipment shortages and thereby save lives on the field.

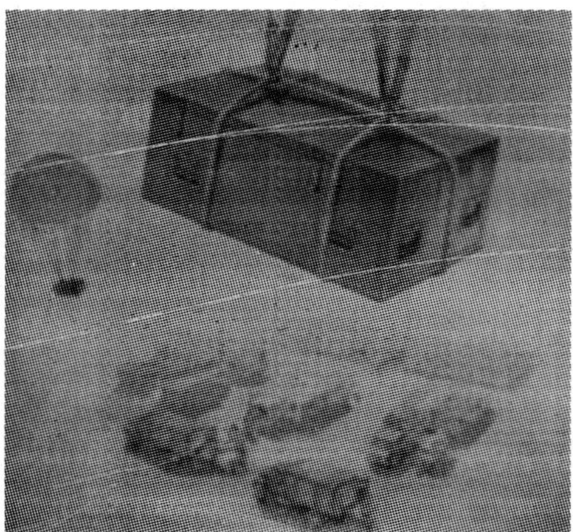

Fig. 64.3

The National Acute Spinal Cord Injury Study Groups (NASCIS 1 and 2) has endorsed pulse therapy with methylprednisolone sodium succinate in neurological injuries. A 30mg/kg bolus followed by a 23 hour infusion of 5.4 mg/kg/hour showed maximum benefits IF STARTED WITHIN 3 HOURS OF INJURY. For those between 3 to 8 hours of injury, the infusion has to be given for 48 hours. Spinal cord injury triggers a cascade of metabolic changes including ion release and formation of free radicals that promote lipid peroxidation. This damages cell membranes and can directly harm the myelin and axons, causing secondary microvascular damage and ishemic insult that can result in permanent neurological deficits. Methylprednisolone is lipid soluble and scavenges superoxides and lipid peroxides and also inhibits lipid peroxidation.It also has anti inflammatory and immunosuppressive activities that are definitely neuroprotective. The drug must, therefore, be incorporated into all field first aid kits. Naloxone does not affect neurologic recovery.

There is an appreciation to provide medics with greater knowledge and training to execute advanced life support procedures such as insertion of chest drains, as it reduces the fear of the unknown and the accompanying stress. These courses are now being incorporated by Belgian and Dutch armies. The combination of professional and legal limitations upon the use of such procedures by staff below the status of doctor does pose limitations in some countries. Austrian law, for example, prohibits paramedics from insertion of intravenous lines. In Germany, paramedics are authorized to perform advanced life support under supervision of a doctor. The status regarding self-aid is still nebulous, especially on aspects of self administered morphine-based analgesics and antibiotics. These are presently restricted to high echelon troops and special forces.

General Principles of Wound Management

Shell and bomb splinter wounds will far outnumber those caused by bullets, hand grenades and bayonets. Incidence of flame burns will also be high due to deployment of incendiary explosives like napalm bombs and flame throwers. Limb wounds will constitute 50% of all injuries. Wounds of head and neck, chest and abdomen are often rapidly fatal and, unless air evacuated, a surgeon will seldom deal with these.

The principles of wound management in the field is as follows:

- Resuscitate traumatic shock. ATLS recommendations are for two large bore (16 gauge or larger) cannulae into a femoral vein and an arm vein to ensure I/V access above and below the diaphragm. This will ensure adequate preload even if the IVC or SVC has been disrupted. Ringers lactate is the initial fluid of choice for resuscitation, given as a fluid bolus of 1 to 2 litres for an adult. Give 3 ml to replace each ml of blood lost – the 3-for-1 rule.
- Saline pre warmed to 45°C can be added to packed cell units to reduce blood viscosity, improve platelet function and prevent hypothermia. All wounds must be considered contaminated and can be expected to be the nidus for an invasive infection in 6 hours time. Wounds must be attended to within this period.
- A 2-stage procedure must be adopted in tackling war injuries. First, an immediate primary wound debridement followed by a delayed primary closure after 4 to 5 days. If the wound is still oedematous and infected, with slough and skin loss, it is considered for secondary suturing and skin defect closure later on.
- Avoid frequent wound inspection during triage as this will aggravate pain, blood loss and introduce infection.
- Wound debridement must be thorough, excising all devitalised tissue to prevent anaerobic infections setting in. Nerve and vascular repair is best left to tertiary centres and extreme care must be taken to avoid overzealous skin excision.
- Bandages must be firm, not tight, permitting a finger to slip underneath.
- Tourniquets if applied, must be endorsed in case sheets/triage tags or as a T-Time with skin marker on the victims forehead.
- Wounds must be cleansed with hydrogen peroxide and saline and dressed with gauze soaked with povidone iodine solution. If chemical contamination is suspected, the wound is irrigated with alkaline sodium hypochlorite solution.
- Damaged subcutaneous fat is excised. Incision is made into the deep fascia to expose damaged muscle. All muscle that looks mushy, discoloured and is non contractile to a pinch with forceps and not bleeding is excised. Do not remove large bone pieces or delve for foreign bodies/ fragments.
- Splint wounds after dressing.
- Administer a booster dose of Tetanus globulin, tetanus toxoid and intravenous antibiotic like a third generation cephalosporin and an aminoglycoside provided renal function is normal.
- In crush syndromes, prophylactic wide spectrum antibiotic cover and intravenous mannitol would be indicated to prevent sepsis and acute renal failure due to myoglobinuria.

Ballistic Penetrating Injuries

Objects that penetrate the human body lacerate, disrupt, destroy and contuse tissues. When a projectile is fired from a weapon, it is retarded by air resistance. This decreases the velocity and kinetic energy of the projectile, reducing its wounding potential. Bullets have spin and fin stabilization (rifling twist) incorporated to reduce the angle between the projectile axis and its trajectory (yaw angle) and improve its accuracy. The behavior of the projectile in a dense medium will depend on the projectiles mass and caliber, moments of inertia, position of its centre of gravity and pressure, fracture strength of its core/jacket, its shape and structure, angle of yaw and rotational velocity at impact (Fig. 64.4).

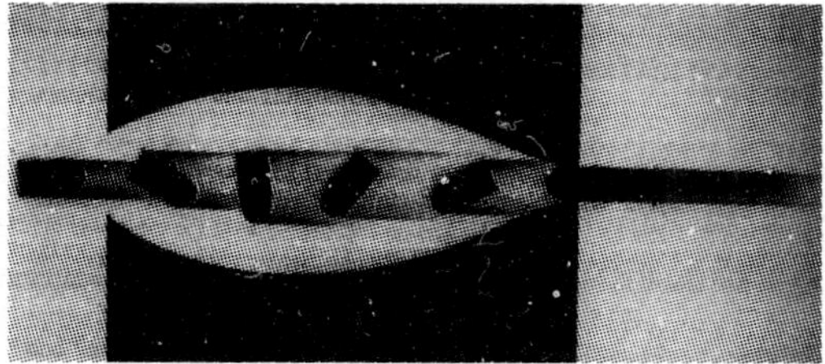

Fig. 64.4: Ballistics tumble and yaw

The factors affecting tissue damage connected with ballistic trauma depends upon tissue density and elasticity, rupture strength of skin, fascia, ligaments, bone and viscera. Fragmenting bullets will create secondary projectiles on impact and larger cavitation and tissue damage. The amount of damage caused by a missile is related to the amount of energy transferred by a missile to the tissues. The greatest damage is done by high energy transfer, related to the retardation of the missile. The more rapidly a missile is retarded, the greater the energy release and consequent tissue damage. In wartime, fragments account for 44-92% of all surgical cases. These fragments from military munitions are small, numerous and fairly regular in shape. Tertiary blast injuries caused by blast wind occurs in 25% of victims in a confined space.

Wounds from tracers, incendiary or HE bullets are complicated by their high phosphorus content that cause considerable tissue destruction, early and progressive shock and a risk of fatal hepatic and renal necrosis if not removed early. These types of missiles also produce more severe wounds because of their comparative lack of stability. Military surgeons must be aware of the tissue damaging properties of projectiles to objectively evaluate ballistic wounds. At times, they may be required to extricate impaled unexploded projectiles from live victims. The nature of entry and exit wounds of projectiles would be useful in assessing and managing war injuries. As regards combat deaths, head wounds accounts for the highest incidence followed by wounds of the thorax and abdomen. Penetrating wounds to these sites are associated with a significantly higher mortality rate than non penetrating wounds. Extremity wounds account for more than half of all injuries in a confrontation and lower extremity wounds account for 40% of all admissions. Use of flak vests and helmets afford some degree of protection.

Management decisions of penetrating injuries are based on wound location, trajectory, tissue injury, ballistic and anatomical considerations. Trajectory determination often defines anatomical injuries. The biomechanics of tissue damage is often based on the kinetic energy of the projectile and density and elasticity of the victims tissues. The greater the tissue density, more the energy transferred. As the projectile moves through body tissues, it creates a cavity along its tract corresponding to the cross sectional area of the projectile. This is referred to as the permanent cavity. Dissipation of the kinetic energy creates lateral displacement depending upon local tissue elasticity is termed temporary cavity. Cavitation within solid organs such as liver, spleen and kidney results in shattering of tissues and is associated with high morbidity and mortality (Fig. 64.5).

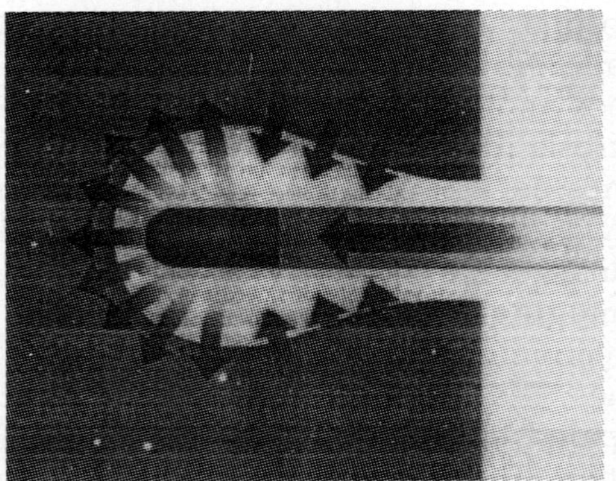

Fig. 64.5: Cavitation

Firearms are weapons capable of firing a projectile, using an explosive charge as propellant, e.g., pistols and rifles. Ballistics refers to the science of powder-propelled projectiles in motion or a study of the wounding of the body by a projectile.

Internal ballistics refers to motion within the weapon. This, in turn, depends upon the diameter of the gun barrel or bullet, known as the caliber and conventionally designated as decimal fractions of an inch. Bullet caliber does not correlate to wound size. The velocity of the bullet as it leaves the gun barrel is termed muzzle velocity and approximates the velocity of the projectile as it impacts its target. This may vary from 200-500m/sec for handguns and 500-1000m/sec for shotguns and rifles. Muzzle velocity increases with length of the gun barrel. Riflings are spiral grooves milled into the barrel of a firearm to stabilize the flight of its projectile and improve accuracy. The bullet cartridge is composed of its casing, propellant powder, primer, wads and projectile (Table 64.1).

External ballistics refers to the motion of the projectile in air. The deviation of the bullet from the longitudinal axis of flight is called yaw or wobble. Rifling imparts spin and discourages wobble by improving flight stability.

Table 64.1: Comparison of bullet weight, velocity, kinetic energy, and maximal temporary cavitation

Cartridge/bullent	*Weight (grains)*	*Velocity*		*Kinetic*	*Maximal tempo-*
		(m/sec)	*(ft/sec)*	*energy (joules)*	*rary cavity (cm)*
Handguns					
–.38	82-188	214-384	693-1.244	200-390	4.0-8.3
–9 mm	82-115	372-430	1.205-1.393	500-700	4.0-8.3
–.46	140-255	241-421	781-1364	480-800	4.0-12.3
–.357	110-325	425-479	1,377-1,552	730-810	9.4-11.0
Shotguns					
–12g, #4 shot (27 pallets) @ 3m	540	412	1,335	2m970	12.0
–12g rifled slug	437	461	1,191	3,.018	11.0
Rifles					
–.22 long rifle	37-40	342-388	1,122,1,272	152-181	4.0-5.0
–30-30	170	615	2,017	2,089	18.0
–30 carshing	110	619	2,030	1,370	14.0
–223 center-fire	50-55	943-960	3,094-3,150	1,475-1,500	13.0-14.0
Military rifles					
–5.56 mm (M16)	50-55	853-1,000	2,800-3,250	1,350-1,670	13.0-14.0
–5.45 mm (AK-47)	53	935	3,029	1,486	14.0
–7.62 mm (AK-47)	150-170	615-891	1,993,2,887	2,010-3,850	14.0-23.0

Terminal ballistics refers to motion and effect of a projectile on striking a solid or liquid target.

Tissue damage on impact depends on its kinetic energy and less on its mass.

Kinetic Energy (KE) in Joules = ½ of its mass (in grams) x (velocity^2 in feet /sec).

From the above equation it is obvious that increasing the velocity of a projectile has a much greater effect on the kinetic energy than increasing its mass.

KE varies from 200-700 joules that cause low energy transfer wounds as with handguns to 1000-3000 joules for shotguns and rifles resulting in high energy transfer wounds. As far as the target is concerned, the greater its density of the tissue, more energy is transferred. The low energy transfer wounds are characterized by injury confined to the wound track=the permanent cavity corresponding to the cross sectional area of the projectile that is also influenced by its deformation, yaw and fragmentation. The high-energy transfer wounds have local laceration and crush injury features as well as injuries remote from the wound track caused by temporary cavitation resulting from lateral displacement of the missile tract from dissipation of its kinetic energy (Figs 64.6 and 64.7).

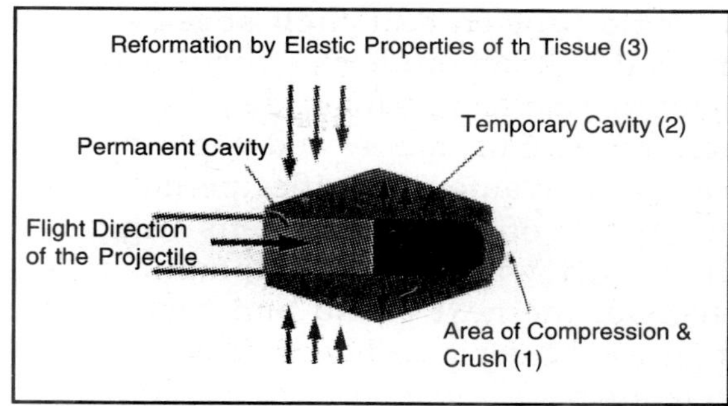

Fig. 64.6: Conceptual and graphic representation of the wound profile. As the projectile passes through the tissue, the permanent cavity is created by crushing (1) The cavitation is created around the permanent cavity by stretching of the surrounding tissue (2) This elastic property of the tissue recoils and closes the temporary cavity (3) All this occurs in microseconds. (Modified from McSwain NE, Basslistics. In: Ivatury R, Cayton C, eds. Textbook of penetrating trauma. Philadelphia; WIlliams and WIlkins 10996:105-120.

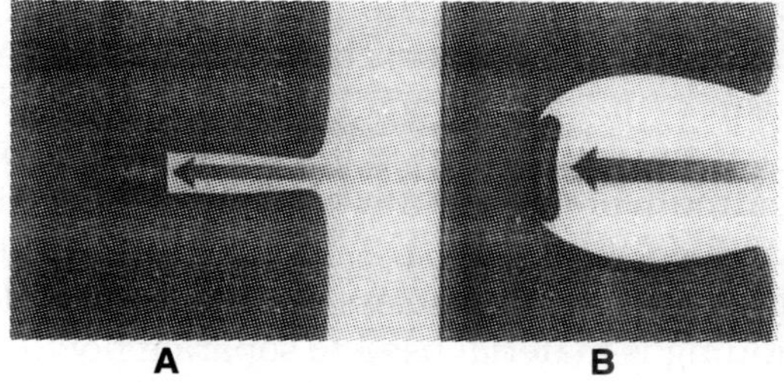

Fig. 64.7A and B: Cavitation results (A) Sharp missiles with small, cross-sectional fronts slow with tissue impact, resulting in little injury or cavitation (B) Misslies with large, cross-sectional fronts, e.g., hollow-point bullets that expand or muschroom on impact, cause more injury or cavitation.

WEAPONS

Handguns refer to weapons that can be fired with only one hand, the barrel length being usually less than 8 inches and the weapon devoid of a shoulder stock. Revolvers are handguns with a revolving cylinder to advance cartridges into line with the barrel for firing. Pistols are semiautomatic handguns with spring-loaded magazine to chamber cartridges that position the next round into the firing chamber. This permits rapid firing of sequential rounds. Magnum guns have additional explosive in the bullet cartridge to increase muzzle velocity and KE. Shotguns are long guns that fire shells containing multiple projectiles. Each shell has 8-20 shots or spherical pellets that result in massive soft tissue destruction with minimal bony injury. They may be single or double-barreled, shortening of barrel-length increases the shot spread at close quarters. Cartridges are loaded by manual means, pump action or by semi automatic loading mechanisms. Rifles are long guns with rifled barrel, usually discharging a single projectile at high speeds using manual bolt action, lever, pump or semi-automatic mechanism for loading. They cause deep penetrating injuries and fragment bone easily. Fully automatic rifles permit continuous fire of bullets while its trigger is depressed while semi automatic rifles chamber the next round and require the trigger to be depressed each time a round is to be fired.

A single round of ammunition is termed a cartridge. Its casing is of metal and houses the propellant, primer and bullet. The cartridge jacket is a hard metal coating to facilitate feeding into the firearm and prevent the bullet from deforming as it strikes its target. Hollow or soft point bullets allow the projectile to flatten or mushroom as its hits its target and also deliberately allow the jacket to peel away from the tip, forming talons on the outer edge of the bullet on impact. The core of the bullet is usually made of lead. The bullet diameter or caliber is connoted in millimeters or hundredth or thousandth of an inch, with mm bullet equating to a 0.35 caliber bullet. Propellants are smokeless gunpowder while wadding is material used to separate powder from the projectile. Air guns use compressed air, gas (CO_2) or springs to discharge the projectile. Tracers, incendiary or HE bullets contain phosphorus and this causes chemical destruction of body tissues, early and progressive shock and risk of fatal hepatic and renal damage if not extracted early.

The differentiation between entrance and exit wounds is very difficult and not relevant to the care of the victim. It is best left to forensic experts and documentation is best limited to the location and appearance of the wounds, organs injured and an assessment of the direction and trajectory as discerned during dissection at surgery.

X-rays can determine trajectory, but not the caliber or the age of a bullet. Bullets are best extracted using rubber-shod instruments to prevent scratches and alteration of the bullets signature and all special and strange characteristics noted.

Management of Missile Injuries

Soft tissue wounds are first photographed, cleaned with an antiseptic and generous longitudinal incisions made through the skin and deep fascia to allow visualization and access to deeper structures and also decompress underlying edematous muscle. A minimal amount of contaminated skin edge is excised around entrance and exit wounds and scrubbed vigorously to dislodge indriven debris. Neurovascular bundles along the wound track are identified, examined and nerves considered injured must not be dissected out but marked with a non-absorbable suture for subsequent identification. Dead muscle that does not bleed or contract is excised. Tattered tendon edges are trimmed but nor repaired. Major arterial and venous damage can be repaired with a vein graft and covered with healthy muscle or temporarily shunted. Rest of the wound is left open after haemostasis for delayed primary closure 4-6 days later. Avoid synthetic grafts. Contaminated bone is cleaned with a curette, saving all fragments attached to periosteum or muscle and thoroughly irrigated with saline to remove organic matter. Exposed articular cartilage must be covered by synovium, muscle or skin. Fractures must be reduced and immobilized using an external fixator or traction splint. Third generation cephalosporins and metronidazole must be administered for five days in proper dosage and/or 1mega unit of penicillin G I/V daily after test dose. Amputations must be completed at the lowest level possible and left open. Administer 25 units of anti-tetanus gamma globulin subcutaneously for those not previously immunized and 0.5 ml of tetanous toxoid booster dose for those who have had a full initial course of tetanus toxoid earlier.

In case of abdominal injury, pass nasogastric tube and bladder catheter and perform a digital rectal examination. Complete all relevant investigations, stabilize the patients condition and open abdomen by a full midline incision from xiphisternum to pubis. Gunshot wounds most commonly involve the small bowel (50%), colon (40%), liver (30%) and abdominal vascular structures (25%).This incision allows rapid access and extension laterally or into the chest when required. Control haemorrhage and inspect all abdominal contents, including the lesser sac to examine the posterior gastric wall. Small intestinal perforations are either excised and closed transversely, or the damaged section resected if multiple holes over a short length. Injuries along right side of colon can be repaired or resected primarily. If wounding is severe with extensive contamination, a vented ileotransverse anastomosis is warranted. For left side, injured colon is resected and proximal end brought out as a colostomy and distal end as a mucus fistula, or closed off in low sigmoid/rectal injuries.

Renal injuries are treated conservatively and divided ureter may be repaired over a pigtail stent. Bladder and urethral injuries are treated by suprapubic cystostomy. For hepatic injuries, manual compression and perihepatic packing is done, generous drainage followed by formal resection in a more sophisticated surgical facility is recommended. Damage to spleen and tail of pancreas will require resection.

Perform warm saline peritoneal toilet and close abdomen by mass closure method. 80% of chest wounds can be treated by bilateral tube thoracostomy, urgent angiography to visualize the thoracic aorta and its main branches, water soluble contrast esophagography with complementary esophagoscopy, bronchoscopy, thoracoscopy, cardiac echo and CT scan followed by measures to arrest of hemorrhage, staple or oversew holes in the lung followed by elective ventilation. Thoracotomy will be required for the rest after resuscitation.The overall mortality rate for mediastinal penetrating wounds is about 20%, and almost double this if the victim is haemodynamically unstable.

Victims with head injuries must be ventilated, resuscitated and subject to CT scan before planning surgical exploration. Gentle irrigation and suction is used to remove devitalized brain and bony fragments and dura closed using temporalis fascia or fascia lata. ICP must be monitored post operatively.

All penetrating injuries of the neck are open and exsanguination is the major initial consideration, with morbidity and mortality being related to arterial injury and displacement and obstruction of the airway. The management is facilitated by dividing the neck into three zones:

- Zone 1 below the sternal notch.
- Zone 2 sternal notch to the angle of the mandible.
- Zone 3 angle of the mandible to the base of the skull.

After initial resuscitation, nature of vessel injury in Zone 1 3 is delineated by arteriography, as surgical exploration is very difficult due to anatomical factors, unlike Zone 2. Also Zone 1 2 penetrating injuries are more likely to be associated with pleural damage, haemopneumothorax and venous air embolism. Chest imaging must be done and measures like IPPV and digital compression over wound may be life saving. Suspect laryngeal injury if there is hoarseness, noisy breathing like gurgling, crowing or snoring, subcutaneous emphysema, palpable fracture, shift of trachea from midline, extreme agitation or depressed level of consciousness.

DOS AND DONTS OF MISSILE INJURIES

DO

- Incise skin generously.
- Incise fascia widely.
- Identify neurovascular bundles.
- Excise all devitalized tissues.
- Remove all indriven clothing and debris.
- Leave wound open after surgery.
- Dress with absorbent gauze.
- Record all injuries in notes and photograph wounds.

DONT

- Excise too much skin.
- Practice key hole surgery.
- Repair tendons or nerves.
- Remove attached pieces of bone.
- Close the deep fascia.
- Insert synthetic prosthesis.
- Pack the wound.
- Close the skin.

Further Reading

1. Accident and emergency surgery. Chapter 19, Bailey and Loves Short Practice of Surgery, 23rd Edn, 2000, Arnold Publishers, p280-286.
2. Hamilton Baileys emergency surgery, 13th Edn, 2000, Arnold, London, P:97-137.
3. MaxillofacialInjuries. Rowe and Williams, 1994, 2nd Edn, Churchill Livingstone.
4. The Trauma Manual. AB Peitzman,M Rhodes, CW Schwab, DM Yealy, TC Fabian. 2002, 2nd Edn. Lippincott Williams and Wilkins.
5. Indian Disasters Report. S Parasuraman and PV Unnikrishnan, Oxford University Press, 2001.
6. American College of Surgeons Committee on Trauma, 1982.

STANDARDIZATION OF FIELD MEDICAL EQUIPMENT

The relationship between civilian and military medicine has always been somewhat adversarial. Military surgeons believe that war-surgery tends to lead rather than follow civilian practices, often snubbing those who demand purple sutures. Civilian surgeons counter that their desire for excellence is rarely matched on the battlefield. While the latter were more adept at handling blunt trauma and low velocity ballistic injuries, the rising incidence of sophistication in the armamentarium of drug cartels, terrorists and mass casualties in urban disasters seems to have restored the balance considerably. Management of high-energy transfer wounds in soldiers would differ from urban settings in that soldiers would have high levels of bacterial flora on their skin. Penetrating wounds would be so much more contaminated, requiring wide exposure and radical excision that would be managed by scrubbing, irrigation, dressing and some 'wondercillin' by the civilian counterpart. Field surgeons are now able to close gut injuries with skin staplers in a matter of minutes a procedure that would take hours for civilian surgeons. Versatility, flexibility, speed, good clinical skills and the ability to work under stress are the hallmark of field surgeons. Documentation is also kept to minimum and perhaps replaced by computer controlled systems to keep a better track of casualties. The echelon-based system observed in the field, where casualties are being rapidly evacuated from the front backwards to the next level of care, demands some such sophistication.

Further Reading

1. The Cutting Edge Battlefield Casualty Management. Murray Hammick, International Defense Review, 1992, Vol 25/3, 243-251.
2. Hall, ED. The neuroprotective pharmacology of methylprednisolone. J Neurosurg 1992;76:13-22.
3. A Field Hospital in Tents. Dr Hubert Fischer. Medical Corps International1987, Vol 2, No 2, 35).

Mobility in Field Medicare

In an attempt to bridge the gap between frontline and second-echelon care, some armies have opted for mobile treatment centres. The basic ingredient of these centres is a standard 20 feet or 40 feet ISO container that can be can be easily provided with an environmentally controlled workspace against NBC threats and also the noise and distractions of battlefield. Sophisticated mobile medical systems are now available, such as the mobile hospital manufactured by EWK Intermed, MAN and Clinomobil Hospitalwerk of Germany, French Sante Diffusions SEH 600 expandable modular shelter, EMMIR (lelement medical de intervention rapide) and COFRAS Advanced Mobile Surgical Unit (ACP 80), Piaggio and Aermarelli of Italy, Lenoir turn-key mobile hospitals of Switzerland, Deployable Rapid Assembly Surgical Hospital (DRASH) of U.S.A.F. and Automotive Engineering Mobile Field Hospital of Singapore. They can provide comprehensive medical care wherever static installations do not exist. They can function independent of their environment and can be employed one by one or as a group to cater to a maximum of 200 patient beds. The semi-trailer units with light metal superstructures can provide an integrated system and assembled within 2 hours from kits trans-ported by airlift (CH 47 helicopter or C130 Hercules/ C222/C160 Transall aircraft) or lorry mounting. They can also be linked to form a good sized hospital with a wide range of treatment facilities. Containers can also be bullet proofed using armour plating but this provides only partial protection against sand ingression The Swedes utilise the Trell (Trelleborg) tents consisting of PVC covered synthetic fabric canopy with inflatable air-filled supporting arches. Each tent is 7.25 metres long, 5.20 wide and 2.60 high (2.25 under the supporting arches weighing 220 to 250 kilograms each, capable of being carried by six men. Each tent takes 10 minutes to set up and the assembled tent hospital can withstand rough handling and is immune to extremes of climate. The tents can be interconnected and a full field hospital has 37 square metres of floor surface, a transport volume of 1,200 cubic metres weighing about 200 tons. The Italians use the RSA (Reparto di Sanita Aviotransportabile) modular field hospitals of pneumatic tents. A typical installation would consist of two surgical and two resuscitation theatres supported by four units specialising in burns, radiology, blood storage and laboratory work. Each module has a floor area of 24 sq metre and has enough stocks for 48 hours of autonomous operation. They are equipped with two ceramic molecular sieve adsorbers working in tandem to remove nitrogen and deliver medical grade oxygen (95% purity) to a surge tank. Oxygen exits the tank via pressure regulators, flow control valves, bacterial filters and on to the flowmeter. Transportable high intensity halogen light source working on mains or batteries like the Martin Chromophare B 48SNM operating lamp provide high luminous, shadowless cold light and these are fitted with polygonal reflectors to ensure good depth of illumination. The batteries are fully encapsulated and maintenance free and provide for 5 hours of continuous operation. Where light source is unavailable, jeep headlights have been mobilized to create ad hoc OT lights. Rough terrain detachable mobile X Ray units (MXMs, MXT-MS, MXT-CS and Siemens SIREMOBIL) as well as computed tomography units are now available from Picker International. These are backed by self-contained generator units, mobile field darkrooms and special film processing units. The Picker Polaroid

Processor (MPS-P) uses polaroid film for instant imaging without the need for chemical developers.

Further Reading

EWK-Intermed Hospitaltechnik GMBH, product brochure on medical container systems, floating clinics, Armoured Units and systems, Mobile units and systems and transportable units.

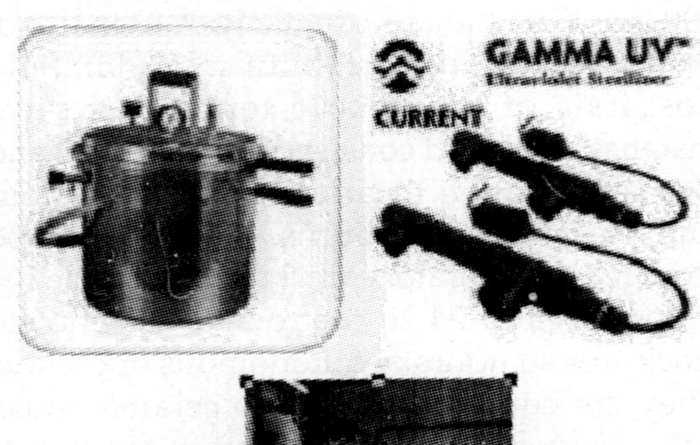

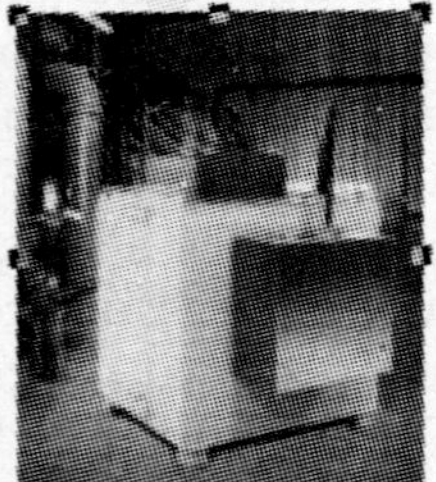

Fig. 64.8

STERILISATION UNDER FIELD CONDITIONS

Sterilisers have to be extremely robust, easy to operate and lightweight. It should have low water consumption, fully automated in operating sequence, incorporate push-button program selection and have warning and instruction signals for defects and troubles hooting. The facility must work independently without the need for further external operating equipments and auxiliary units. The facility must be capable of working at extremes of environmental temperature. A choice of six programs is desirable. Laundry (134ºC), instruments (134ºC), rubber articles (120ºC), heating, emergency and short laundry programs as well as vacuum and sterility testing. It must have an air-cooled or water-cooled condensate recovery feature. The Technomara AG 334 D 86 and D 86 models are transportable semi-stationary sterilizers incorporating all these desirable standards. Sterilizer trailers by Sauter-Sulgen of Switzerland is a comprehensive mobile unit fitted with sterilizers, vacuum pumps, electric steam generator, water pressure pump, water softener, reverse osmosis unit, washing machines, packing table with drawers, compressed air facility, room heating, sterile and unsterile stowage cabinets and detachable hose units. It is mobile, autonomous, has a low degree of maintenance and meets stringent standards with a high degree of safety even in aggravated conditions.

Further Reading

Sterilisation under field conditions. Hans C Reiman Medical Corps International, 1986, Vol 3:49-53.

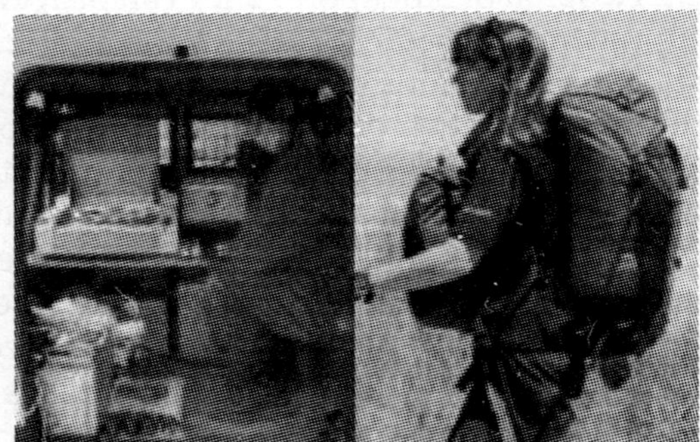

Fig. 64.9

FIELD LABORATORIES

Though modern clinical chemistry is just over 100 years old, its foundation dates back to about 200 B.C. Arab physicians applied their alchemical know-how to the art of healing by 1300A.D. The first textbook of alchemy was issued by A Librarius in 1595. In the 17th century, the alchemistical approach developed into a study of chemistry as a science and pioneered by Johann Baptista von Helmont, H Boerhaave and Paracelsus. The actual breakthroughs to modern laboratory diagnostics took place in the 18th and 19th centuries and the first medical laboratory was founded by Christoph Wilhelm Hufeland in the Berlin University in 1810. The development and improvements of the miscroscope by R Hooke and Ernst von Abbe, the ultramicrsocope by Siebentopf and Zsiymondy, the ultracentrifuge by Theodor Svedberg and photocolorimetry led to refinements and accuracy of clinical biochemistry.

In the field, it is essential that both qualitative and quantitative examinations be carried out for optimal patient care and immediate feedback to the treating physicians. All equipment must be robust, light and easy to operate. Level I labs are equipped with equipment limited to test strips and dipsticks only. Level II labs are only capable of performing qualitative examining methods. Level III labs are capable of all tests and will have the basic equipment for clinical chemistry, a refrigerator, blood gas machine, a coagulometer, centrifuge, hot air sterilizer, bacteriological incubator, microprocessor based photocolorimeter, suspended thermostat laboratory boiler, monocular/binocular microscope, stop watch and calculator. Dry chemistry has revolutionized lab techniques and uses the reflection photometer for quantitative determination of clinical-chemical parameters from blood, plasma and serum without the need for centrifugation. Results are accurate, taking just 2 to 4 minutes, and incorporates signals for errors, trouble-shooting, has in-built autocalibration and these units are easy to operate and moderately priced. These can be a closed system for cuvette test with a pre-programmed course of analysis or an open system using reagents of all manufacturers. Dry chemistry analyzers have even been used aboard space flights in zero gravity situations with 95% efficiency.

Imaging in the Field

The combat theatre imposes unique diagnostic imaging requirements. Between 1838 and 1940 Picker X-ray company designed and developed a radiographic fluoroscopic device and a compact portable x ray unit. WWI and II drove the development of highly reliable medical imaging devices as commercial imaging devices cannot match the demands of modern military scenarios. Until 1960, traditional diagnostic imaging was confined to the use of ionizing radiation with flexible photofilms and acqueous developing solutions to process the recoded images. After 1960s a spate of developments occurred with CRT, diagnostic ultrasound, CT and MRI revolutionizing imaging techniques and methodology. However combat military imaging confines itself to traditional plain radiography and ultrasound for immediate evaluation of the injured soldier. The condition of the patient and the specific type of injury determines the most appropriate imaging modality. Other matters like location of the imaging facility and availability of expertise to interpret images is also important. Plain radiography remains an essential component for the immediate evaluation of the injured soldier.

Echelon Based Imaging Availability

1st echelon: The immediate combat point in the front would have facilities for first aid by medics and buddy care. No imaging methods would be available.

2nd echelon: Combat area emergency care and resuscitation at field hospitals can be expected to have a portable low capacity mobile imaging device, single display, filmless system or fluoroscopy. This facility receives wounded soldiers within 30 min of injury, initiates triage and evacuates.

3rd echelon combat area surgical capable hospital, MASH, combat support hospital (CSH) would be capable of surgery and holding the wounded troopers for 24-36 h. This facility will not have a radiologist or neurosurgeon but conventional radiography and portable ultrasound for handling abdominal and chest emergencies can be expected.

4th echelon-major hospital will have a radiologist and all imaging facilities.

Plain Radiography

Trauma victims will need to be monitored, supported by a trauma team during the course of these diagnostic interventions. For those seriously injured, it is advisable to have the films exposed in the resuscitation room itself-the cervical spine and chest AP and lateral views must form part of the initial evaluation. Take care to get a C1 to T1 view in lateral C-spine films and an erect frontal PA chest radiograph where possible. AP pelvic film may be avoided in an alert asymptomatic patient without distracting injuries. Posturing may be postponed in hemodynamically unstable patients and further films ordered after secondary assessments. Radio opaque markers placed over entry and exit wounds will give an idea of the missile trajectory and identify retained fragments. On table IVP may be ordered during surgical exploration.

Chest X-ray suggestions

Abnormal findings	*Diagnoses to consider*
Any rib fracture	Pneumothorax
Fracture, first 3 ribs	Airway or great vessel injury
Lower ribs, 9 to 12	Abdominal injury
Two or more rib fractures in two or more places	Flail chest, pulmonary contusion
GI gas pattern in the chest (loculated air)	Diaphragmatic rupture
Gastric tube in chest	Diaphragmatic or esophageal rupture
Air fluid level in chest	Hemothorax or diaphragmatic rupture
Loss of diaphragmatic contour	Diaphragmatic rupture
Sternal fracture	Myocardial contusion, head injury, c-spine or thoracic spine injury
Mediastinal hematoma	Great vessel injury, sternal fracture
Disrupted diaphragm	Prompt celiotomy
Respiratory distress without X-ray findings	CNS injury, aspiration
Persistent large pneumothorax after chest tube insertion	Bronchial tear, esophageal disruption
Mediastinal air	Esophageal disruption, pneumoperitoneum tracheal injury
Scapular fracture	Airway or great vessel injury, or pulmonary contusion
Free air under the diaphragm	Ruptured hollow abdominal viscus

The Picker mobile (MXM) military X-ray mobile is a lightweight, rugged, shock resistant radiological unit, designed for performance under extreme environmental conditions, manouverable, self propelled with oversize tyres and maximum ground clearance. It can travel 8 km and climb 25° incline on a single battery charge. It is easily disassembled, transportable in containers, quick and easy to operate and quickly set up at field hospitals. Also available are the transportable MXT-MS and MXT-CS units. The Picker Polaroid processor can provide instant images without the need for chemicals to develop films. For ships, X-ray unit must be pitch,yaw and torque-hardened, with self-contained autoprocessors, collapsible darkrooms and digital imaging. The Clinix-RM. Auto Universix F-8 is transportable in light metal containers and assembled in less than 1 h without special tools is one such unit for hospital ships. Its basic frame can be adjusted to uneven floors and comes with a 35 kW generator. Another rugged, light-weight system is the Siemens-Transport-able Radiographic system (TRS) with Vertix B stand and Mobilett high frequency x-ray generator with separate control console and radiation protection screen. The Siremobil 3.2kW rated system comes with a mobile stand, C arm, generator and monitor packed in 4 boxes and capable of being assembled/disassembled without tools (Fig. 64.10).

The Kodak-portable table top processor is ideal for high quality radiographic processing, and a fully automated room light film handling system without need for darkrooms. Helium-neon laser printers produce high quality images.

The LIXI imaging scope is a hand-held x-ray unit for real time imaging.

Ultrasound

Physicians in Germany and Japan began using routine bedside ultrasound for trauma patients in the 1970's. In the United States emergency physicians started using this tool in the 1980's and it has now become the initial imaging test of choice for trauma care in the United States and is part of the Advanced Trauma Life Support (ATLS) protocol developed by the American College of Surgeons.

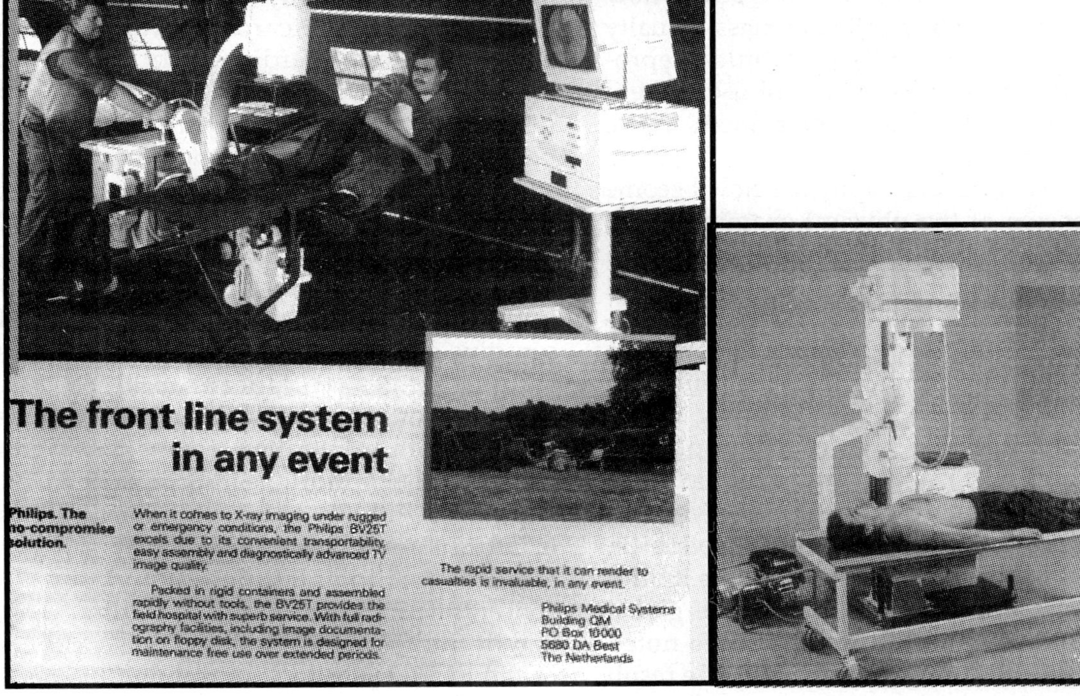

Fig. 64.10

Even body armor doesn't protect soldiers from getting wounded on the battlefield and blood loss from such wounds is ranked the No. 1 cause of preventable battlefield death. Therefore, accurate assessment and rapid decision-making are essential to save lives and many trauma patients have injuries that are not apparent on the initial physical exam. Patients can present with distracting injuries or altered mental status. Significant bleeding into the peritoneal, pleural, or pericardial spaces may occur without obvious warning signs. Real-time point-of-care ultrasound has become an invaluable adjunct to the clinical evaluation of critically ill and injured patients in field situations and has become. the initial imaging test of choice in trauma care. The numerous advantages of ultrasonography make it an ideal triage tool for rapidly screening patients Wireless and satellite transmission of ultrasound images is now feasible and may be applied to mass-casualty situations. Ultrasound's portability, reproducibility, accuracy, and ease of use make it an important diagnostic instrument in the field.

Focused ultrasonography has now become an extension of the physical examination of the trauma patient. Performed in the trauma room by properly trained and credentialed staff, it allows the timely diagnosis of potentially life-threatening haemorrhage and is a decision-making tool to help determine the need for transfer to the operating room. Focused Assessment with Sonography for Trauma (FAST) is a limited ultrasound examination directed solely at identifying the presence of free fluid in the chest or abdomen. In the context of traumatic injury, free fluid is usually due to haemorrhage. Severe global ventricular dysfunction may also be noted during the FAST exam, more likely the result of severe acidosis from hypovolemic shock. The importance of prompt cardiac ultrasound in all patients with significant blunt chest trauma having associated hypotension needs no elaboration.

Many patients with penetrating shrapnel wounds to the heart don't suffer significant blood loss because the wound in the pericardium seals. Cardiac tamponade will usually develop, but may be delayed by several minutes or even hours. Prior to the development of tamponade patients will be relatively asymptomatic. When symptoms eventually develop, clinical decompensation occurs rapidly resulting in shock and then cardiac arrest. The "classic" signs of Beck's triad are not commonly present and are difficult to appreciate by physical exam alone. The key to managing penetrating chest trauma is to identify a developing pericardial effusion as early as possible, before tamponade and cardiac arrest occurs. All patients with penetrating chest injury should be "screened" for a potential pericardial effusion. If an effusion is present cardiac injury is assumed until proven otherwise and the patient should go directly to the operating room for a pericardial window or sternotomy.

In blunt abdominal injury, spleen or liver trauma is difficult to diagnose on physical exam. The FAST exam is an ideal initial screening modality for early recognition of intraperitoneal blood since it is rapid, safe and sensitive and can be repeated if the patient's status changes. It appears to be equally sensitive for detecting hemoperitoneum in patients with penetrating trauma and it can be used to help prioritize initial management in patients with multiple penetrating injuries or an unknown missile trajectory. Within minutes it allows clinicians to know to concentrate initial efforts on a cardiac, chest and or intraperitoneal injury. The sensitivity of the FAST exam for determining the need for laparotomy is only about 50% as bowel injuries are very common in penetrating trauma and the FAST exam does not detect most of these injuries.

Hemothorax, is common in both blunt and penetrating trauma. It can usually be managed with placement of a simple chest tube. About 200 ml of pleural fluid is required before it can be detected with a plain CXR. Ultrasound is much more sensitive for detecting pleural fluid and can identify as little as 20 mL in the pleural space. It was found to be equivalent to CXR in detecting hemothoraces in trauma and also showed to be a much quicker procedure, taking about 1 minute versus 15 minutes for chest radiography. Chest radiographs are still necessary in trauma patients to evaluate the mediastinum, lung parenchyma and several other anatomic features. Ultrasound can be used during the initial minutes of the trauma evaluation to determine if urgent chest tube placement is necessary. A chest radiograph can then be obtained after chest tube placement. This approach saves valuable time when managing an unstable multiple-trauma patient. Pneumothoraces are common in trauma and more than half are missed on a supine chest radiograph. Bedside ultrasound has been shown to be equal or more sensitive than CXR for detecting this lung injury.Using ultrasound to look for occult pneumothoraces is most important in situations where missing one could result in significant deterioration, especially patients requiring positive pressure ventilation or helicopter transport.

A handheld device is now available for imaging soft tissue as well as blood flow with high quality in real time. Four component ASICs for digital beamforming, signal processing and scan conversion are designed and integrated with a convex array scanhead in this device. The device can be either battery driven or AC powered with image storage and cineloop playback capability. It weighs less than five pounds. In addition to diagnosing trauma in the combat battlefield, this device can also be used in a variety of mobile diagnostic applications, bringing quality medical imaging to the bedside, areas of natural disaster, or remote areas that do not have access to medical imaging.

MUSTPAC is a highly portable ultrasound system offering three-dimensional scanning and images. The data, stored in the computer for transmission via telephone line or satellite. This enables on-site technicians to perform ultrasound imaging scans and transmit the data anywhere in the world for interpretation. a highly portable ultrasound system for the rapid diagnosis and treatment of wounded soldiers.

Ultrasound Vs CT Scan

CT of the abdomen is better than ultrasound for showing parenchymal injury and the source of intraperitoneal bleeding. CT is useful to differentiate solid organ injury from bowel injury or other causes of hemoperitoneum and it is far superior demonstrating retroperitoneal bleeding. Modern CT scanners can also use abdominal/pelvic images to reconstruct bone windows and rule-out fractures of the spine and pelvis. Unfortunately, CT is very expensive, exposes patients to radiation and usually requires a bolus of IV contrast material. Because of these problems ultrasound will always have certain advantages over CT. Since CT has better accuracy for diagnosing torso injuries, the FAST exam is most useful in situations where CT is not practical due to time constraints or when CT scan can be reasonably avoided. Maxillofacial fractures are also better evaluated by CT scan. The accuracy and speed of CT imaging has increased with the development of spiral and multislice units.

MRI

Does not need contrast administration and can obtain images in saggital, coronal and oblique planes and useful to diagnose shear injuries to the brain, spinal column and cord, or vascular abnormalities. It is time consuming and offers minimal access to the victim during the procedure and has limited application in trauma situations in the field.

Field Blood Banks

'We few, we happy few, we band of brothers:
For he today that sheds his blood with me
Shall be my brother.'

—*Shakespeare: Henry V (act 4, scene3)*

Historical Aspects

Wars were a good motive for the developments of blood transfusion.

*1818:*The first blood transfusion on the battlefield was performed in 1818 by the Prussians (Germans) directly from one patient to another.

1901: Discovery of blood groups by Karl Landsteiner.

*1914:*The first transfusion of citrated blood was performed by Professor L. Agote of Buenos Aires on November 14th 1914, but despite this, transfusion of blood was considered to be too difficult and unsuited for the stress of war conditions.

1914–18: During the war surgeon's were often confronted by a problem when soldiers would arrive in relatively stable condition and suddenly, and for no immediately apparent reason, their pulses would become rapid and thready, their blood pressure would plummet, their faces would become pale, and their bodies would be cold and clammy. Many would die of this mysterious condition. At the time, doctors considered the collapse without evident blood loss to be "pure" shock also termed "wound shock" was thought to result from the cold, damp, dehydrated, sleep-deprived existence imposed by trench life, in combination with injury, further exposure, and painful transport. Hemorrhage was seen further to complicate the condition. British surgeons, unaware or unconvinced by American experiments with blood transfusion, infused these patients with saline solution with little success as shocked soldiers proved to be poor candidates for operations. They were sent to "moribund wards," where many died. It was in the summer of 1916, during the bloody Battle of the Somme, that the problem became more urgent as the number of healthy young reserves back home was dwindling. Something had to be done. The Canadian surgeon Edward Archibald believed citrate transfusion to be suited for easy adoption in Army work as donors could be bled by a junior medical officer with the instruments at hand in any clearing hospital and the surgeon could then perform the transfusion by himself, with blood at hand when he needed it without fear that clots would clog syringes or the paraffin-coated tubes, Many lives were saved and Archibald's article was published in the 16 Sep 1916 issue of The Lancet and a more detailed account in the Journal of the Royal Army Medical Corps. The Royal Army Medical Corps was reinforced by doctors from the United States of America and the knowledge that blood could be safely transfused and blood transfusion was used during the first world war, when it was transported to the battlefront in modified, clean, sterilized milk bottles. At this time German researchers studied the relative blood group distribution among different races. The development of blood banking and transfusion was indeed the most important medical advance of that war.

1926: The British Red Cross instituted the first human blood transfusion service in the world.

1930: The first mobile blood bank was set up in the 1930s during the Spanish civil war

1932: The first facility functioning as a Blood bank was established in a Leningrad Russia hospital.

1934: The first blood bank in Chicago by Seed and Fantus. Their unique contribution was twofold: Development of a facility to store blood and the use of live human donors.

1936: During the Spanish Civil War, from Aug 1936 to Jan 1939, the Barcelona Blood transfusion Service collected more than 9000 litres of blood, maintaining a list of 28,900 donors.Citrated blood was stored in heat insulated wooden or canvas boxes.

1941: The onset of World War II created the need for modernization in transfusion delivery as well the need for a suitable substitute. Cohn's discovery of blood fractionation led to human albumin and freeze dried plasma being extensively used for the management of shock and 13 million units of blood and blood products were contributed by United States citizens for use by the Armed Forces between 1941 and 1945.

During the Nazi rule in Germany, blood groups acquired racial overtones and blood group B was attributed to Slavic and Jewish race, while blood group to persons of "aryan" race and linked to positive attributes like intelligence and racial superiority.The German army accepted blood only from ascertained Aryan donors. In parallel, the US Red Cross was gathering blood only from the same race, and considered that donors' blood from black race could be used for albumin production only. By the end of 1950 a law passed in Louisiana which forbade doctors to administer blood from a black donor to a white patient without his consent.

Lessons learned in World War II were described by White and Weinstein in their book on current transfusion practices. Topics in the book included the use of human plasma in treating shock on the battlefield.

1950: Carl Walter and W. P. Murphy, Jr., introduced the plastic bag for Blood collection. This replaced breakable glass bottles with rugged plastic bags. This technical development enabled the evolution of a collection system capable of safer and easier preparation of multiple blood components from a single unit of whole blood. Baxter and Terumo pioneered closed circuit blood collection systems.

1953: Development of the refrigerated centrifuge began to further expedite blood component therapy.

1961: After many clinical trials, CPD solution (citrate-phosphate-dextrose) was consolidated as an anticoagulant by Gibson for blood preservation up to 28 days.

1966: The first reports regarding to the production of devices for intraoperative collection and autologous blood retransfusion were presented In 1969, researchers assembled a centrifuge device with continuous flow that had the potential to separate and concentrate red blood cells.

1967: The role of DPG (diphosphoglycerase) was discovered by Chantin, Curnish and Benesches.

1970: Autotransfusion was widely used in the Vietnam War and the first article appeared in 1975 with a detailed description of the experience on 71 patients, who received a mean volume of 4000 ml autotransfused blood collected in a reservoir containing of crystalloids with 3 IU heparin/ml.

1974: Haemonetics Corporation introduced the Cell Saver, a system that washed and concentrated red blood cells before their re administration.

1979: A new anticoagulant preservative, CPD with adenine extended the shelf life of whole blood and red blood cells to 35 days facilitated resource sharing among blood banks.

2007: Battlefield attacks that resulted in mass casualties or severe injuries often overtaxed the military's blood supply system until 2007, when medics collected fresh blood from those on site for emergency treatment of the wounded. But the emergency transfusions meant "wounded service members may survive the acute event only to suffer from potentially fatal or chronically debilitating transfusion-associated infectious diseases in the future. The U.S. Army Institute of Surgical Research tested 2,831 units of unscreened blood transfused in Iraq and Afghanistan between May 2003 and February 2006. Testing showed three units were tainted with hepatitis C and two were positive for human T-cell lymphotropic virus. None of the samples tested positive for hepatitis B or human immunodeficiency virus. The use of uncreened blood has dropped by about 80 percent since 2007, when facility upgrades and new high-tech storage facilities allowed the military to provide regulated blood. The vast majority of the military's blood supply is collected, tested and supplied by the Armed Services Blood Program under the same U.S. Food and Drug Administration blood safety standards adhered to by the Red Cross and other civilian blood banks. The emergency unscreened transfusions on the battlefield are used only when ASBP blood is unavailable. With the advent of blood substitutes, the military often overstocked blood, and it would often expire before it could be used and only 2 percent of the blood stocked in the first year of the Iraq war was used. Instant testing kits for HIV and hepatitis that are more than 90 percent accurate are now supplied in combat zones to provide safer emergency transfusions when necessary. However, sporadic large-scale attacks could quickly deplete locally stored blood supplies, driving up the need for the emergency transfusions. The latest generation of cell salvage machines are so compact as to be easily deployed in a field role and cell salvage is a practical technique, even when the wound potentially is infected, as would occur in a missile injury to the abdomen.

Problems of BT in the Field

- Unsanitary field conditions.
- Testing of the blood is usually unavailable.
- Unreliable donor information. It was seen that "dog tags" were wrong 2-11% of the time.
- Requires blood banking/lab support.
- Logistical re-supply problems.
- Refrigeration problems.

Concept of a walking blood bank: Unit members pre-screened prior to deployment and roster of non combatant volunteer donors kept e.g. Cooks, mechanics, housekeepers etc after cross verifying donor's blood type and screening for HBsAg and HIV I and II. Almost 50% of the population would be type "O". Bleeding of donors done after cleaning the donors arm for at least a minute with povidone iodine and using a closed circuit collection system with CPDA bags, drawing off approximately 450cc of whole blood per individual donor. Single unit transfusions are to be discouraged. These cases can be managed with:

6% Hexastarch 500ml I/V =3 liters of Ringer Lactate (Hartmann's). Rate of administration is calculated as amount to be infused/ 4 × time period over which to be infused. E.g. if 500 ml is to be infused in 1 h, 500/4 × 1=125 drops/min.

3.5% Polygeline (Haemaccel) Has to be stored between +2°C to +25°C. If kept at higher temperatures, shelf life is reduced by 2 years.

Estimated fluid and blood losses' based on patient's initial presentation

	Class I	*Class II*	*Class III*	*Class IV*
Blood Loss (mL)	Up to 750	750-1500	1500-2000	>2000
Blood Loss (% Blood Volume)	Up to 15%	15%-30%	30%-40%	>40%
Pulse Rate	<100	>100	>120	>140
Blood Pressure	Normal	Normal	Decreased	Decreased
Pulse Pressure (mm Hg)	Normal or Increased	Decreased	Decreased	Decreased
Respiratory Rate	14-20	20-30	30-40	>35
Urine Output (mUhr)	>30	20-30	5-15	Negligible
CNS/Mental Status	Slightly anxious	Mildly anxious	Anxious, confused	Confused, lethargic
Fluid Replacement (3:1 Rule)	Crystalloid	Crystalloid	Crystalloid and blood	Crystalloid and blood

Differences in composition of major blood products

	Normal whole blood (in vivo)	*Citrated whole blood (2 wk old) ACD/GDP*	*Citrated packed red blood cells***	*Frozen packed red blood cells*	*FFP*
PH	7.4	6.6-6.9	6.6-6.9	6.6-7.2	6.6-6.9
pCO_2	35-45	180-210	180-210	0-10	I 80-210
Base deficit (mEq/l)	0	9-15	9-15		9-15
Potassium <mEq/l)	3.5-5.0	18-26	18-26 mEq/l	1-2 mEq/l	4-8
Citrate	None	+++1	++	None	++++
Factors V and VIII	Normal	20-50%	20-50%	None	85-100%
Fibrinogen	Normal	Normal	Normal	None	Normal
Platelets	240,000-100,000	None	None	None	None
2-3 DPG	Normal	3% of normal	3% of normal	Nearly normal	–
Hematocrit	35-45	35-45	60-70	50-95	–
Temperature	37°C	4-6°C	4-6°C	4-6°C	Cold

Modified from Miller RD:Refresher Courses in Anesthesiologv 1:101. 1973)

*Cltraied whole biood and citrated PRBCs have the same chemical cornposition, but citrated PRBCs have considerably less plasma volume

Field Blood Bank Aids

- *Storage:* Range from thermoinsulated glass fibre and polysterene containers capable of storing blood for 1-2 days to highly reliable, heavy duty blood chain thermostabilizers (Electrolux) with forced air CFC free refrigeration, built in temperature monitoring and alarm unit for safe transportation of blood under arctical and tropical conditions. The RCB25 S and RCB 42 P maintain safe temperature for blood storage upto 8 days with external temperatures below 43°C without external energy supply.
- Solcotrans sterile hand held disposable device for intra op collection and reinfusion of autologous blood.
- MTM IV-PUSH (Canada) pressure infusors—with a constant pressure spring. No batteries required and device can be rested on the patient's cot itself and adaptable to all iv apparatus. It accommo-

THERMOSTABILIZER

Safe storage and transport of blood under arctical and tropical condition

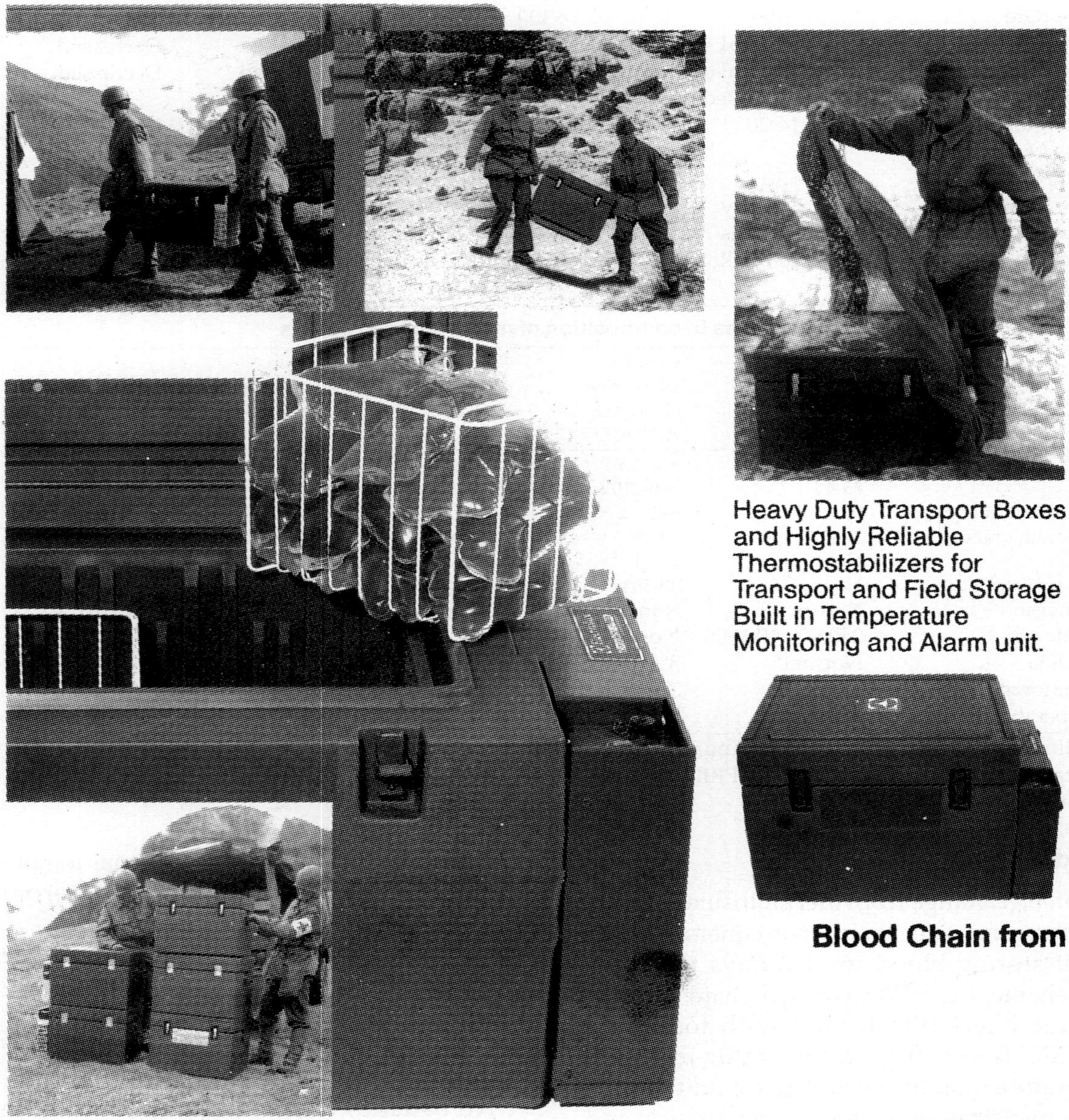

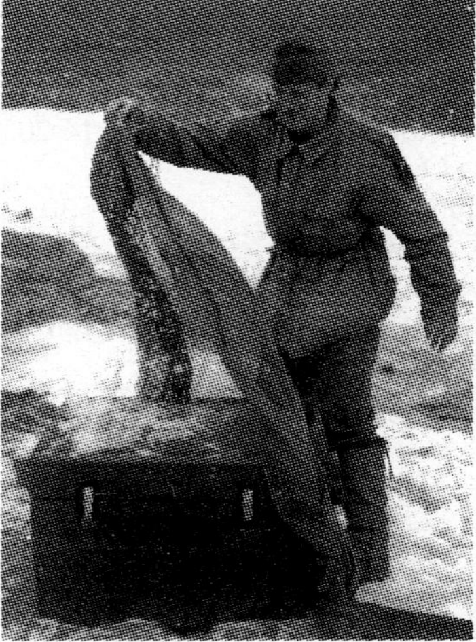

Heavy Duty Transport Boxes and Highly Reliable Thermostabilizers for Transport and Field Storage Built in Temperature Monitoring and Alarm unit.

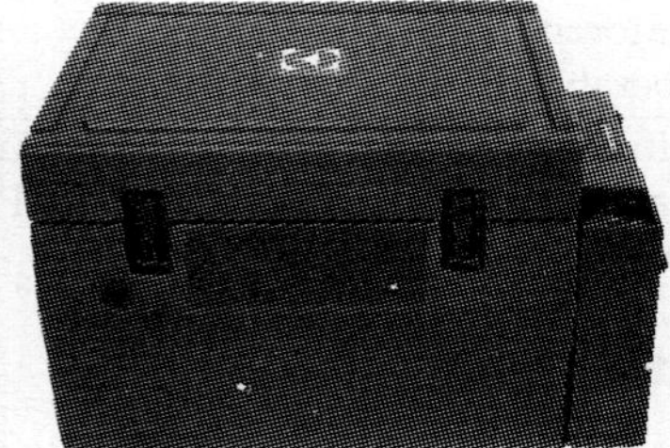

Blood Chain from

Fig. 64.11

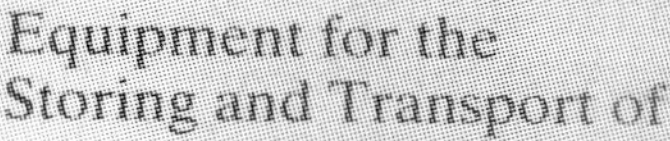

Equipment for the Storing and Transport of BLOOD and Blood Components

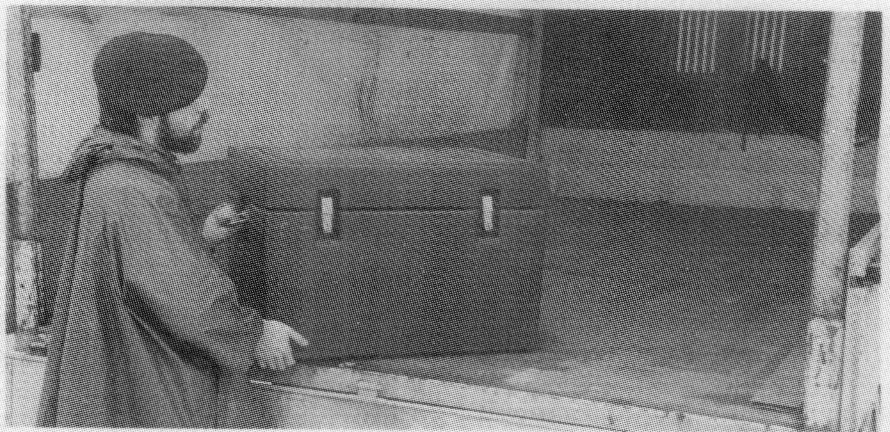

BLOOD FIELD REFRIGERATORS AND TRANSPORT BOXES

Electrolux has developed a range of refrigerators and transport boxes for safe storage of blood under military field conditions.

Different models are available for hot or cold climates and some models accept very big variations in ambient temperatures.

Examples:

Blood transport box RCB25 S maintains a safe temperature for blood in 8 days at a constant ambient temperature of +43°C or in 3 days at an ambient of -25°C without supply of outside energy.

Blood refrigerator RCB 42 P maintains a safe temperature for blood automatically within a range of ambient temperatures from -40°C to +38°C. It also accepts different voltages from 240 V a.c. to 12 V d.c. automatically.

All refrigerators and transport boxes can be supplied with alarmsystem FCU 200.

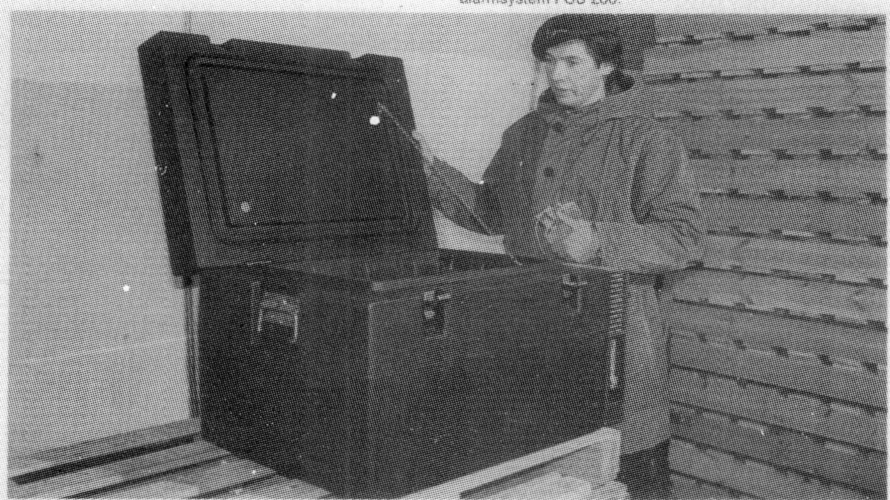

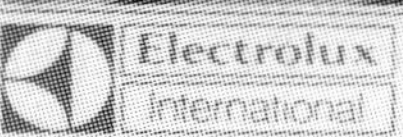

Electrolux s.a.r.l.
4-rue de la Frontiere
L-9412 Vianden
Tel.: 84595, Telex 2949 frelux lu

Fig. 64.12

dates 500 and 1000 ml blood bags and can administer flows from 75 to 350 ml/h. It has a fail safe function once the spring is engaged and obviates the need for I/V stands or blood bag suspension.

- Blood must be warmed prior to administration. This can be effectively done by the addition of normal saline prewarmed to 45°C in a water bath or in a microwave oven (one litre crystalloid can be warmed to 39°C in 2 min in a 600W microwave oven). Closed flow, single-channel counter-current heat exchangers with large-bore tubings like Thermal Angel are now available and capable of warming blood and fluids to 38°C at flow rates of 500 ml/min without red cell damage. Centrifugal and roller pumps can increase transfusion rate to 750 ml/min, but these are expensive, complex, labour intensive and take 5 to 8 min to set up.

Future Trends

1. The Defense Advanced Research Projects Agency, known as DARPA, is starting a "blood pharming" program aimed at developing a system that can make red blood cells from progenitor cells on the battlefield. Human embryos left over from IVF treatment are being genetically programmed to develop into the "O-negative" blood group, which is the universal donor group that can be transfused into anyone without fear of tissue rejection blood and free of infections that is seen with donated blood. They have generated 10 billion to 100 billion red cells starting from a single plate of human embryonic stem cells. Incidentally, a pint of blood contains more than one trillion cells The red cells produced from embryonic stem cells so far tend to resemble embryonic or fetal red cells more than adult ones. They tend to be larger and often contain nuclei, which could impede their passage through the body. And they have a different form of the globin molecule, which carries oxygen. With the expensive growth factors needed to develop red cells from embryonic cells, the costs could be thousands of dollars per unit issue of cost whereas people donate for free, and free is a difficult price point to compete with. Red cells can also be derived from so-called induced pluripotent stem cells, which are made from adult skin cells. These cells are becoming popular for research because they avoid the ethically controversial destruction of embryos needed to create embryonic stem cells. Other cells, like those from bone marrow orcord blood, can also be used to make red blood cells, but those cells cannot reproduce indefinitely in culture like embryonic stem cells.
2. By using genetic engineering techniques, researchers have created artificial hemoglobin that could someday alleviate perennial blood bank shortages. Cell-free, oxygen carrying resuscitation fluids (CFOCRFs) can be stored at room temperature and have a shelf life in excess of two years.
3. Perfluorocarbons in dose of 5 ml/kg of were introduced into clinical trials in the early 1980's with the hope that these products would develop into acceptable blood substitutes. Unfortunately, the limited potency, short half-life, and potential toxicity of these early formulations coupled with unrealistic expectations for efficacy prevented the perfluorocarbons from playing a significant role in transfusion medicine. Recent changes in formulation to improve efficacy and eliminate toxicity have stimulated renewed interest in perfluorocarbons as

alternatives to allogeneic transfusion. Perfluoroctylbromide (PFOB), a second generation perfluorocarbon is now being tried as an adjunct to autologous transfusion and acute normovolemic hemodilution (ANH), rather than as a total blood substitute. Small doses of PFOB has been observed to maintain oxygen delivery without the need for blood transfusion in the setting of hemodilution and is expected to have a significant role in the future as one of several, additive alternatives to blood transfusion.

4. Recombinant human erythropoietin (rhEPO) takes 2–6 weeks to raise hemoglobin from 6 g/dl to over 10 g/dl by stimulating erythropoiesis. Suggested dose is 700 IU/kg to elicit greater effect or 3 doses of rhEPO at 24,000 IU over a week.
5. Experience form the Gulf War showed that it is feasible to deploy the latest compact apheresis machines and produce platelets in the field. These machines also can provide fresh plasma, thus, obviating the need for freezers in which to store fresh frozen plasma.
6. The US Army recently has developed a fibrin bandage, that can be used to pack wounds and arrests bleeding almost instantaneously. Once this becomes available commercially, it may have a dramatic effect on blood requirements.
7. New additive solutions (QASs) are being developed that will extend the shelf life of concentrated red cells (RBCs) to longer than 3 months. These will reduce the demand for blood during the build-up phase of an operation, with a consequent reduction in wastage.
8. Compact, mobile thermoregulated blood banks are available, with capacities varying from 40 to 3,000 units of blood. Blood donation and processing now is carried out in the home blood transfusion centres, where the degree of quality control is much higher than would be possible under field conditions.
9. Whole blood cryopreservation is a cost-effective approach to large-scale storage of viable cells in resilient thermoplastic film bags with flat transfusion port tab inserts. Freezing red blood cells using 11.5% hydroxyethyl starch (HES) to -130°C liquid nitrogen results in 90% red cell viability at 20 months of storage.
10. Resuscitative fluids production system (REFLUPS) is a device to manufacture all commonly used range of sterile pyrogen free I/V solutions in a field environment without the aid of laminar airflow hoods.

FIELD CASEVAC

Whatever the method of casualty evacuation (casevac) adopted, the chain of critical care must be a continuum and not be broken at any stage, if therapeutic gains are to be maintained in transit. Behind every small improvement in a severely ill patient, there is often a whole-hearted effort based on patience, knowledge, experience and untiring observation, supported by high technology hardware. It is so very important to maintain the therapeutic progress during transportation so that there is no let up during critical minutes. Hours and days of dedicated work can receive a setback and require great efforts to reconstruct. Transportation of Priority-1 patients poses a threat to their clinical stability and every interruption carries a serious risk. Uncompromising and continuous monitoring and medical care must be ensured throughout. With the right method, however, there is no patient who is unfit for transportation. Specially trained rescue services must oversee this. It may be preferable to take time and make careful preparations to ensure casevac

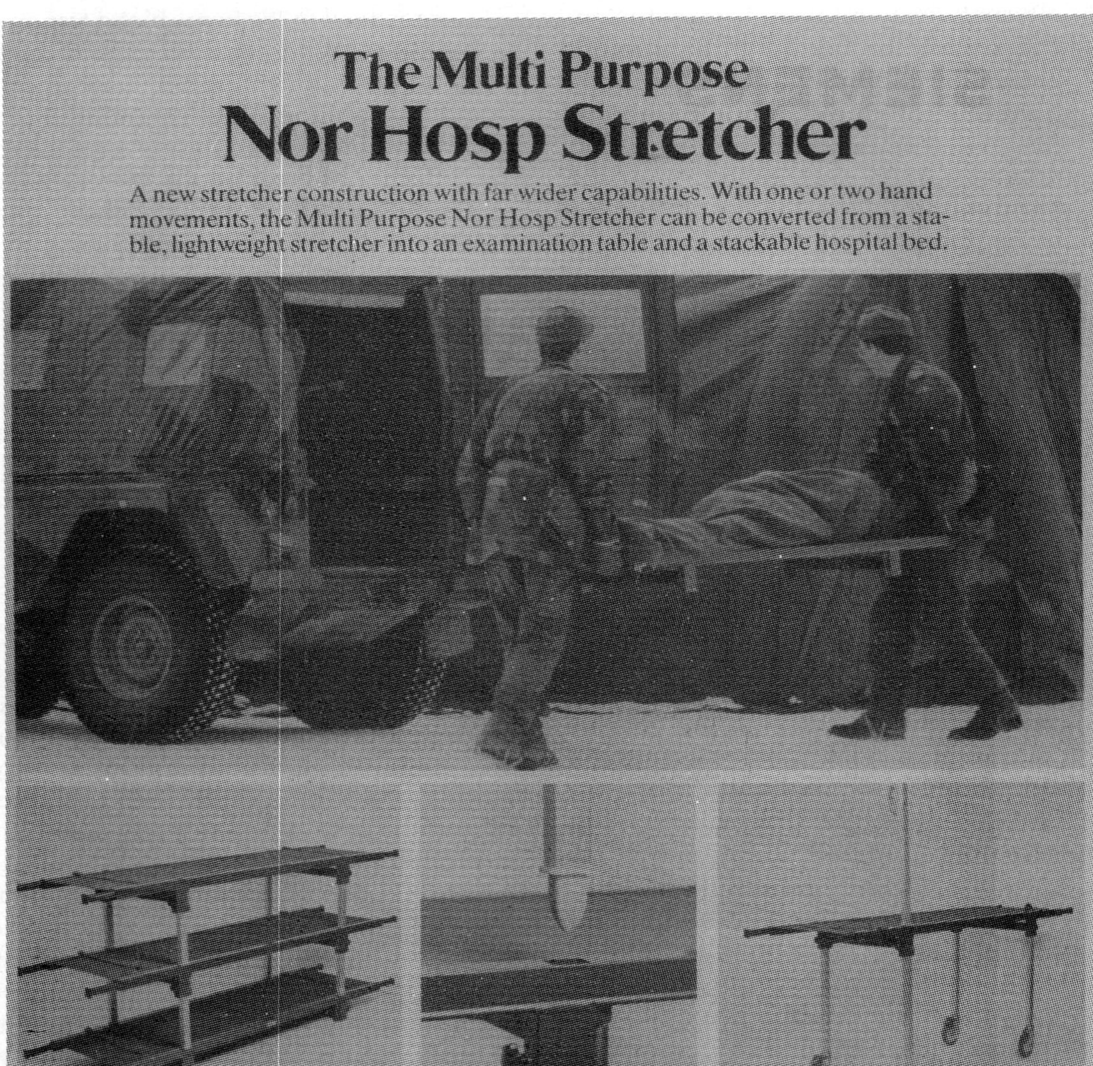

The Multi Purpose
Nor Hosp Stretcher

A new stretcher construction with far wider capabilities. With one or two hand movements, the Multi Purpose Nor Hosp Stretcher can be converted from a stable, lightweight stretcher into an examination table and a stackable hospital bed.

The support stand poles (the legs) give the stretcher flexibility. The poles can be fixed at height with a retaining screw and it can tolerate a load of some 450 kg on each leg.

The support stand poles come in two lengths. The shorter legs are ideally used in the stacking of stretcher. There is a plug of tough plastic fixed at one end of each leg.

When stacking the stretchers, the poles are mounted with the plugs facing downwards so that they then fit directly into the holes in the side arms of the stretcher beneath.

Fig. 64.13

rather than concentrating on speed of such transfers. Every patient must be ensured maximal therapy to improve outcome.

The bulk of casevac from the front would remain vehicular, either tracked or wheeled and over distances. These transports must be equipped with radio and all supply vehicles returning empty from the front would have to be utilized to transport the walking-wounded rather than utilizing specialized vehicles for their evacuation. Standardization must ensure that there is no incompatability between the various stretchers and the rescue/ambulance vehicles. Over long distances, helicopters may be better suited to transport casualties. Their resonant frequencies can however rupture recently sutured structures by inducing whole body oscillation. Journeys over 3 minutes in helicopters are therefore prohibited for those recently operated and their evacuation must be by fixed-wing aircraft. Here too, considerations of shift of body fluids during take off, ascent and descent can cause cardiac overload, making constant supervision a necessity. Medical evacuation by train is another option and dates back to the Crimean War when railway freight cars were utilized for the purpose. Faster, better equipped and more stable than road transportation, they can evacuate large numbers of lying and seated wounded personnel in relative comfort. The disadvantage is easy spotting and straffing by enemy aircraft. The traditional ambulance will continue to be a part of any casevac system for some time to come.

BURNS

Tissue damage by thermal energy in any form is termed as a burn. Both in peace and war, the incidence of burn injuries is on the rise. Fire has been used as a weapon since ancient times. Flame-throwers, pitch, boiling oil, napalm bombs, chemical blistering agents like mustard gas, phosphorus and arsine and the thermonuclear weapons are all based on inflicting thermal injury on their target population. 35% of the energy of an atomic device occurs in the form of thermal radiation. In disaster situations, many people can sustain burns of all grades. The skin is the largest organ of the human body and forms the first line defense against the environment. Burns damage this protective envelope and can also involve deeper structures like muscles, nerves, bone and blood vessels, the eye and the airway. A large number of superficial skin cells and capillaries are destroyed by the high temperature insult causing release of vasoactive and toxic substances like bradykinins, histamine, serotonin, prostaglandins, leukotrienes and free radicals. These increase capillary permeability and allow leakage of large molecular weight intravascular proteins and thereby change the water distribution within the body spaces. This fluid movement into the interstitial space reaches a peak within 6 to 8 hours after injury and then slowly declines. During this period, hypovolemia develops and the extravasated fluid manifests as tissue swelling and formation of blisters. The body responds to this loss of fluid by releasing endogenous catecholamines that cause vasoconstriction and decreased blood flow to the gut and kidneys in order to maintain blood flow to the brain and heart. This compensatory mechanism gets overwhelmed if untreated and a state of shock ensues. In massive burn injury, this vascular hyperpermeability can occur in the brain and lungs also, causing cerebral edema and ARDS. Hemolysis or red blood cell lysis upto 0.5 to 1.% of total erythrocyte weight per BSA percentage is seen in 3rd degree burns situations. After a primary phase of 48 to 72 hours, bacterial invasion compounds the situation further. Burns are life threatening if they involve over 20% of the Body Surface Area (BSA) in adults or 10% in children. While handling burns, it is important to consider the cause and the severity of the burnt surface. Agents causing burns can be:

- Thermal–flame, radiation, steam, hot liquids and objects.
- Chemical–acids, bases and caustics.
- Electrical–AC, DC and lightning.
- Light–sunlight, laser, flash and arc welding.
- Radiation–nuclear and ultraviolet.

Burns are classified into 3 degrees. First degree is superficial burn involving only the epidermis and characterized by pain, redness and local swelling. This type heals without scarring. Second degree burns involves the deeper dermis also and characterized by intense pain, reddening, blistering and mottling. These too heal with minimal scarring. Third degree burns also called full thickness burns involve all layers of the skin and deeper layers and characterized by charred or white and dry surface. Pain is usually minimal due to damage to underlying nerves. These heal with dense scarring and will require skin grafting. All burn injuries can pose a serious medical and logistical problem in a disaster situation.

Assessment of burns is by the Rule of Nines. Each of the following areas of the body surface is allotted 9% area for an adult. The head and neck combined, each upper limb, chest, abdomen, the upper back, the lower back and buttocks, the front of each lower limb and the back of each lower limb to make up 99%. The remaining 1% is assigned to the genital region. In infants and children, the head and neck is assessed at 18% (twice that of an adult), each upper limb 9%, chest and abdomen 18%, the entire back 18%, each lower limb 14% and genitals as 1% of body surface area. As a general rule, the palm (not including the fingers) of the victims hand approximates 1% of the victims body surface area.

Infants and elderly tolerate burns poorly and need extra care. So do those with burns of the respiratory tract and smoke inhalation and burns in patients with poor general health.

The severity of burns is assessed as critical as per following criteria:

- All burns complicated by injury to the respiratory tract.
- Third degree burns involving more than 10% of BSA.
- Second degree burns involving 30% of BSA.

Electrical Burns

Electrical burns result from electric current flowing through tissues or bone. The type and voltage of the circuit, the pathway through the body, the duration and the resistance of the body will determine the severity of damage. A key characteristic of electrical burns is that there is an exit wound. This is the location where the electricity leaves the body. A person with an electrical burn in his or her arm may have another wound in the leg. Because the electricity runs through the body, it is important to know the effects the burn had on the muscles, veins, arteries, and nerves between the entry point and the exit point of the electricity. Entry points are most commonly in the hand. If the exit point is the opposite hand, it may be likely that the electricity ran through the heart. At levels of current flow exceeding 1/10 of an amp or 100 milliamps, the heart stops and experiences fibrillation. A person may survive an electrocution if his or her heart can be started again. This is why CPR is such an important skill in the electrical industry. Remember, Electrical burns are one of the most serious injuries you can receive and should be given immediate attention.

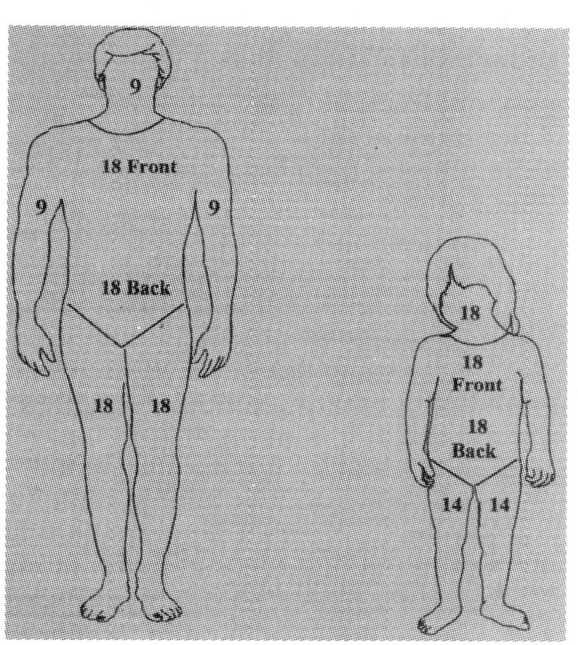

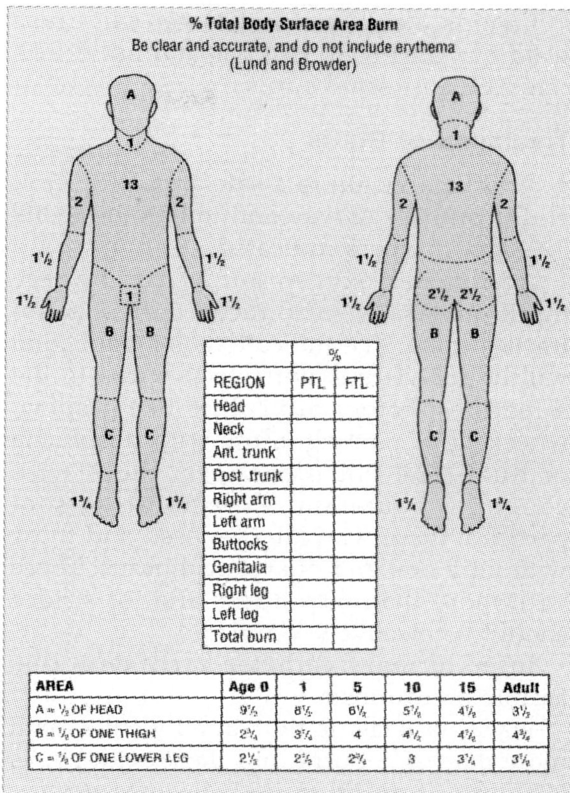

REGION	% PTL	% FTL
Head		
Neck		
Ant. trunk		
Post. trunk		
Right arm		
Left arm		
Buttocks		
Genitalia		
Right leg		
Left leg		
Total burn		

AREA	Age 0	1	5	10	15	Adult
A = ½ OF HEAD	9½	8½	6½	5½	4½	3½
B = ½ OF ONE THIGH	2¾	3¼	4	4½	4½	4¾
C = ½ OF ONE LOWER LEG	2½	2½	2¾	3	3¼	3½

Fig. 64.14: Rule of nines

Chemical Burns

Household chemicals that cause burns include acids, bleach, boric acid, paint thinner, and plumbing decloggers such as Drano or Liquid Plumber. While many chemical burns occur in the home, they are also common in the workplace in certain industries. Occupational agents such as liquid concrete in the road construction and paving industry are also the source of chemical burns. The extent of damage depends on how long the skin is exposed to the chemical. The chemical will continue to 'eat' its way through the skin and deeper layers until it is washed away. It is important to wash away the chemical burn as soon as possible and remove clothing and jewellery that may have the chemical on them.

Scalds

"Hot water can burn like fire". Yet setting the water heater higher than 120 degrees is common and because many homeowners, landlords and apartment dwellers keep their hot water between 140 and 160 degrees, unnecessary pain, suffering and even death occur. Scald injury is responsible for two-thirds of all visits to hospital emergency rooms and more than one-third of all admissions to burn centers. Hot water is particularly harmful for young children. Because their skin is thinner than adult's, it burns deeply and at lower temperatures. A child will suffer a severe burn if exposed to 140^0 water for just three seconds. Elderly people are more vulnerable, as well, due to less sensitive skin and slower reaction times.

Liquids other than hot water can cause scald burns as well. Hot oils and hot drinks can also cause scald burns.

Treatment of Burns

- Evacuate victim to a safe area.
- Do primary survey and initiate basic life support where indicated.

Administer oxygen 4-6 L/min by face mask or nasally introduced cuffed endotracheal tube. The indications for intubation will be for victims with deep burns to the throat, respiratory difficulties like gasping, wheezing or panting, those with dysphonia or dual-tone voice changes, those with coughing bouts and expectorating soot particles, those who are cyanosed and those with intra oral and pharyngeal burns. Those with more than 60% burns and/or stridor should be electively ventilated.

Insert urinary catheter early with due aseptic precautions.

Insert nasogastric tube in all victims with more than 25% burns and those with above 20% burns scheduled for helicopter evacuation to prevent distension and ileus.

Treat shock with analgesics and intravenous fluids to ensure adequate urinary output of more than 1 ml/kg/h for those weighing 3kg or less and 30-50 ml of urine per hour for adults. All victims with more than 20% BSA (include only 2nd and 3rd degree burnt surface) burns need circulatory volume support. Do not follow any of the various formulae for volume replacement therapy blindly. During the first 12 hours, it is advisable to administer 2/3rd of fluid as Ringer Lactate and 1/3rd as a macromolecular solution. Avoid 5% dextrose and start with non glucose containing crystalloids (RL preferred). Calculate fluids as 4 ml/kg/%BSA/24 h-give half in first 8 hours (from time of sustaining burns) to obtain a minimum of 0.5ml/kg/h urine output. Insert a central line and monitor central venous pressure in all patients with burns above 40% of BSA. Avoid subclavian vein in all blast injuries and respiratory burns because of the danger of pneumothorax during cannulation.

Order a Chest X-ray Film

- Always maintain good asepsis and barrier nursing methods.
- Prophylactic antibiotics are not indicated in the early post burn period and should be reserved for the treatment of infections.
- Administer balanced salt solutions orally to quench thirst and electrolyte losses
- Administer booster dose of tetanus toxoid or tetanus globulin.
- Obtain a baseline carboxyhemoglobin level and, if it is above 20%, ensure high oxygen flows via a non rebreathing mask/circuit.
- Clean burnt surface with gentle flowing sterile water for several minutes.
- Then wash area affected with mild soap and water after removing contaminated clothing and artifacts in the involved area.
- Immerse in cold water for 2 to 5 minutes. Avoid if burns are extensive.
- Cover entire burnt surface area with sterile dressing.
- Apply moist gauze pads to cover eyelids.
- Monitor victims condition closely and evacuate to hospital when condition is stable.
- In chemical burns, brush away powder residues and flush with copious amount of water for 20-30 minutes. Alkali burns require continuous irrigation for the first 8 hours after the burn.
- In electric burns, monitor ecg and check urine for hemochromogens when a urine output of at least 10 ml/h must be ensured with I/V fluids and mannitol 25 gm stat and 12.5 g per litre of parenteral fluids.

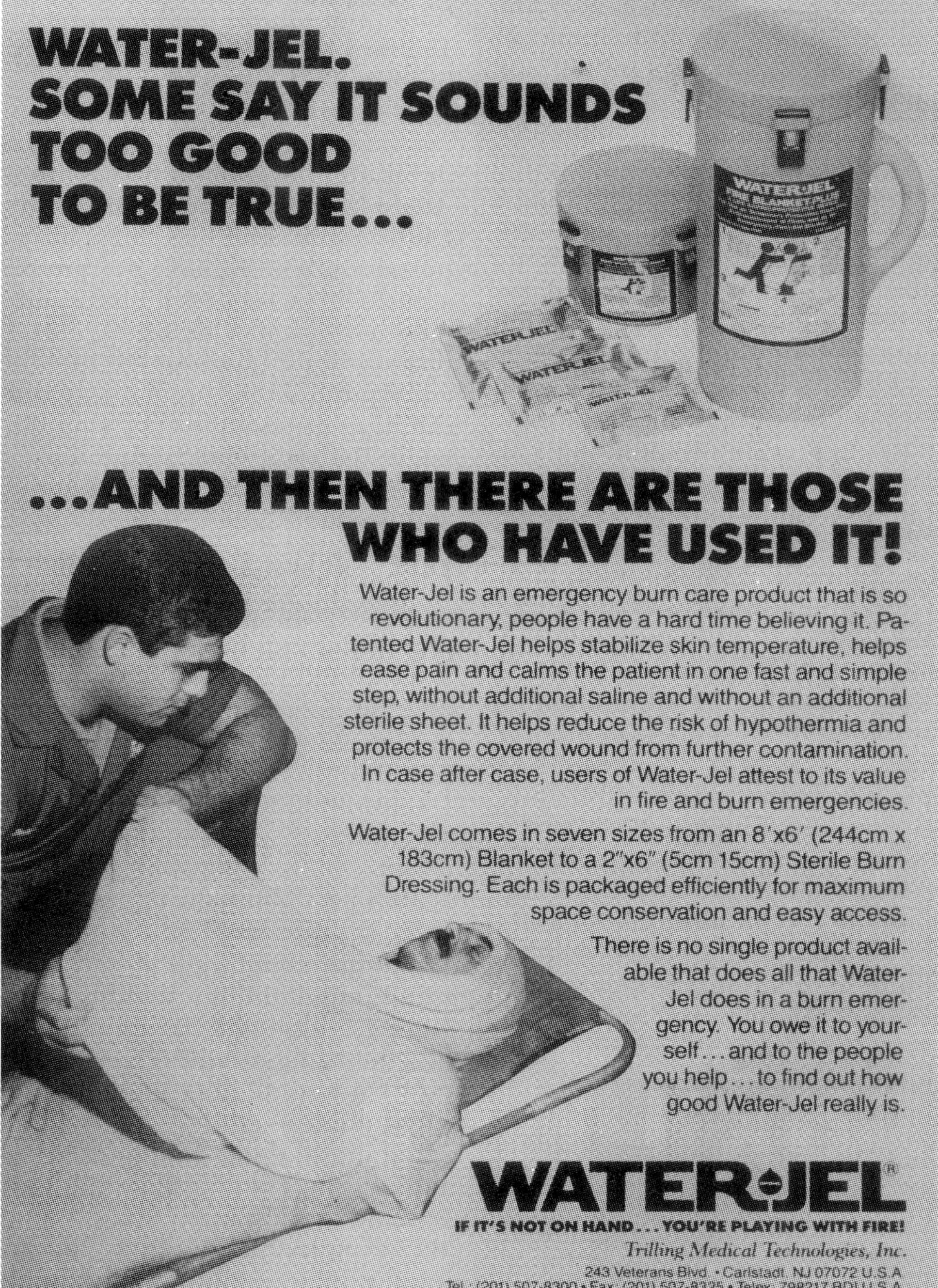
WATER-JEL.
SOME SAY IT SOUNDS
TOO GOOD
TO BE TRUE...
...AND THEN THERE ARE THOSE
WHO HAVE USED IT!
Water-Jel is an emergency burn care product that is so revolutionary, people have a hard time believing it. Patented Water-Jel helps stabilize skin temperature, helps ease pain and calms the patient in one fast and simple step, without additional saline and without an additional sterile sheet. It helps reduce the risk of hypothermia and protects the covered wound from further contamination. In case after case, users of Water-Jel attest to its value in fire and burn emergencies.
Water-Jel comes in seven sizes from an 8'x6' (244cm x 183cm) Blanket to a 2"x6" (5cm 15cm) Sterile Burn Dressing. Each is packaged efficiently for maximum space conservation and easy access.
There is no single product available that does all that Water-Jel does in a burn emergency. You owe it to yourself... and to the people you help... to find out how good Water-Jel really is.
WATER-JEL®
IF IT'S NOT ON HAND... YOU'RE PLAYING WITH FIRE!
Trilling Medical Technologies, Inc.
243 Veterans Blvd. • Carlstadt, NJ 07072 U.S.A.
Tel.: (201) 507-8300 • Fax: (201) 507-8325 • Telex: 798217 BDI U.S.A.

Fig. 64.15

The Stephan UMC system machines are capable of rapid and problem-free manufacture of topical preparations for surface application in mass casualty scenarios. They ensure careful processing, finest grinding and equal mixing of ingredients, optimal gelatinisation of finished products, homogenization of dispersed material, tangential, axial and radial fluid movement, a vacuum environment of 10mbar to prevent bacterial contamination, robust heavy-duty motors and production capacity from 0.2 to 6litres at a time. The DuoDerm hydroactive waterproof sterile dressings can be cut and moulded over burnt surfaces to provide non adherent and biological gel dressing that can be left in place for up to seven days without signs of clinical infection. Patients can also have a bath with these dressings in place. Waterjel sterile burn dressings from Trilling Medical Technologies are also very useful in such situations and the dressings come in sizes ranging from 5 cm × 15 cm for small area application to blanket size for full body draping in size 244 cm × 183 cm.

The Epigard synthetic skin substitute, Sorbalgon, Hydrocoll, Hydrosorb etc can be also used as a temporary covering over deeply burnt surfaces. Pelnac burn dressing made with silicone and porcine atherocollagen can be used as a bilayer artifical dermis in treating skin loss due to third degree burns. It is available in sizes 82 ×60 mm, 82 × 9 mm and 82 × 12 mm.

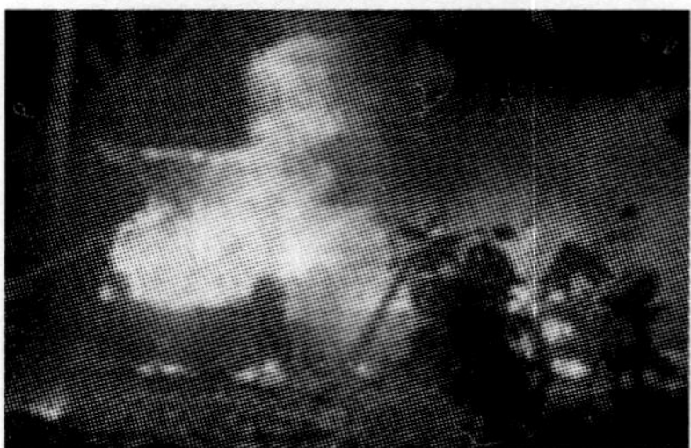

Fig. 64.16

BLASTS AND EXPLOSIONS

The explosive pressure that accompanies the bursting of bombs and shells ruptures their casing and imparts high velocity to the resulting fragments. These can cause more devastating injuries to tissues than bullets. All explosives are accompanied by a complex blast wave having two components, a blast pressure wave (dynamic overpressure) with a positive and negative phase and another mass movement of air (blast wind). The blast pressure wave travels at the speed of sound and flows over and around obstructions and can have devastating effects on the human body. The blast wind is supersonic, disrupts the environment and buildings, hurling debris and people.

Most of the damage is done as a result of the shock wave that is generated outwards in all directions at speeds in excess of 3 km/sec creating two types of pressures. The first is the OVERPRESSURE i.e. pressure increase over the normal atmospheric pressure and surrounds the object as the shock wave hits it and crushes it inwards. Next, the DYNAMIC PRESSURE strikes each object like a wind force, with the shock wave, moving objects outwards, toppling and tearing them apart. Injury is usually directly proportional to the distance from the point of detonation. The primary blast wave injures the tympanic membrane, middle ear, lungs and bowel while the blast wind gives can cause grave penetrating injuries. This results in deafness, post blast respiratory insufficiency (PBRI) consequent to pulmonary contusion and perforations of the stomach, small intestine and caecum. The eyes must also be carefully examined for distortion of iris, hyphema and blast energized debris or fragments Typical injuries include ruptured internal organs, lung contusions, burns, lacerations, impaled objects, fractures and crushing injuries. Explosions often produce superheated air that can cause thermal burns of the surface as well as of the respiratory system. Blast shock waves travel more rapidly through liquid media. Hence injuries sustained from a blast when immersed in water cause more severe deafness, post blast respiratory insufficiency (PBRI) consequent to pulmonary contusion and perforations of the stomach, small intestine and caecum. The eyes must also be carefully examined for distortion of iris, hyphema and blast energized debris or fragments. Blast victims will also frequently have thermal burns and inhalation of toxic gases and smoke An explosion is defined as a rapid release of energy and its magnitude depends upon on the type of explosive detonated, the space in which the blast occurs and the degree of confinement of the explosion. Most of the damage is done as a result of the shock wave that is generated outwards in all directions at speeds in excess of 3 km/sec creating two types of pressures. The first is the OVERPRESSURE, i.e., pressure increase over the normal atmospheric pressure and surrounds the object as the shock wave hits it and crushes it inwards. Next, the DYNAMIC PRESSURE strikes each object like a wind force, with the shock wave, moving objects outwards, toppling and tearing them apart. Injury is usually directly proportional to the distance from the point of detonation. Typical injuries include ruptured eardrums and internal organs, lung contusions, burns, lacerations, impaled objects, fractures and crushing injuries. Explosions often produce superheated air that can cause thermal burns of the surface as well as of the respiratory system. Blast shock waves travel more rapidly through liquid media. Hence injuries sustained from a blast when immersed in water are more severe.

INHALATIONAL INJURY AND LUNG BAROTRAUMA

Exposure to fire and smoke is a common occurrence in conflagarations and may require emergency respiratory care. Events such as carbon monoxide poisoning, chemical tracheobronchitis caused by inhalation of incomplete products of combustion and toxic fumes as well as the direct effect of thermal injury can cause airway obstruction, mucosal sloughing, bronchorrhoea and pulmonary oedema. Presence of progressive hoarseness or stridor appearing 2 hours after inhalation, associated with deteriorating consciousness, needs careful evaluation and follow up. Burns of the tongue are most hazardous and tissue edema could be aggravated further by administration of large volumes of i/v fluids for large surface-area burns. Oxygen therapy and airway management by endotracheal intubation, emergency tracheostomy or cricothyroidotomy accomplished expeditiously and as atraumatically as possible may be life saving.

Toxic products of combustion

Substance burned	*Toxic products*
Wood, cotton, paper	Acrolein, acetaldehyde, formaldehyde, acetic acid, formic acid
Petroleum products	Acrolein, acetiuc acid, formic acid
Melamine resins	Ammonia, hydrogen cyanide
Nitrocellulose film	Oxides of nitrogen, acetic acid, formic acid
Polyvinyl chloride	Hydrogen chloride, phosgene, chlorine
Polyurethane	Isocyante, hydrogen cyanide
Polyfluorocarbons	Octafluoroisobutylene
Fire retarded mate	Fluorides, bromides and iodides

Inhalational injury can occur from direct inhalation of flames, inhalation of hot air, steam, smoke, toxic gases or by aspiration. The larynx represents a natural barrier, shielding against noxious agents from outside. Burn injuries of lower airway are nearly always associated with upper respiratory involvement. The direct pathological sequelae include hyperaemia, exudation, oedema and necrosis of affected mucous membranes. From the clinical point of view, notable manifestations include reddening, swelling and blistering. In the vicinity of the glottis, this may present an acute danger by airway obstruction and asphyxiation. In the lower respiratory tract, intra alveolar and/or interstitial oedema, necrotic mucoparticles can cause atelectasis, proceeding to infections (bronchopneumonia, interstitial pneumonia, pulmonary abscess) and acute respiratory failure especially if the pulmonary situation is complicated by general burn injuries. Pulmonary barotrauma often occurs in blast injured victims. The varying pressure of waves created by the blast and their propagation in air and fluid results in interfaces of mediums of varying densities often called the 'spalling effect'. The pulmonary membrane system represents the anatomically largest interface between air and tissue. Underwater pressure waves, say from torpedo detonation results in pressure waves with less attenuation than an air blast because of low compressibility of fluids in comparison with air. This often affects other large parenchymatous organs of the body like the liver and spleen, in addition to the lung. The blast effect on the lungs is rupture of tissue and vessels, resulting in pneumothorax, haemothorax, subcutaneous emphysema, diffuse pulmonary contusions and respiratory failure. Rapid assessment for signs of hypoxia like cyanosis, restlessness, irrelevant talk and falling oxygen saturations must be made. Do not miss evidence of tension pneumothorax like shock, signs of mediastinal shift and rapidly progressing dyspnea. Insert a needle into the pleural space at the 2nd intercostal space anteriorly and aspirate. If it is positive for air, insert a chest drain and connect to a water-seal drainage system. Assess the extent and degree of facial and chest burns and subcutaneous emphysema. Look for subcostal indrawing, chest wall deformities and flail movements. Chest is percussed to detect changes in air entry in both lungs to evaluate pneumo-haemothorax. Laryngoscopic evaluation must be done to detect airway burns and a CXR ordered (look for broken ribs, subcutaneous emphysema, mediastinal shift, haemo-pneumothorax and changes in diaphragm orientation or movements). Order for an ABG analysis and decide on the need for artificial ventilation. This will often be merited in the presence of inspiratory stridor, progressive desaturation/coma especially when associated with maxillofacial and /or cranio-cerebral trauma. Blast lung cases have the dual problem of parenchymal contusion impairing diffusion and parenchymal broncho-pleural fistulae affecting ventilation (leaks are in the vicinity of 15 to 20% of tidal volume). Insert large diameter apical and basal pleural closed/water-seal drainage. This may often have to be done through a burn-injured chest wall surface. If patients circulatory condition does not improve after relief of tension pneumothorax or if the shock index is more than 1, suspect internal bleeding, concomitant abdominal trauma/limb fractures. Anticipate difficult intubation and ventilation. This is best done in a tertiary level trauma centre, so consider an urgent evacuation. Do not air-evacuate victim without insertion of chest drains. Crash induction with ketamine and vecuronium and insertion of double lumen endotracheal tube is preferable. Apply PEEP judiciously. Consider inverse-ratio (duration of inspiration phase to that of the expiration phase = 4:1) ventilation to provide sufficient gas exchange and enable the fistula to closure spontaneously. Pressure Regulated Volume Control (Siemens) PRVC mode is a definite choice. Also order endoscopy with a flexible bronchoscope to detect bronchial rupture and mucosal hyperemia of segmental bronchi. Bronchial lavage is performed to flush out necrotic mucosa and spray topical corticosteriods. Cover with broad spectrum third and fourth generation antibiotics. Administer blood transfusion when indicated and assess progress. Good ventilatory management, early circulatory volume correction with hexastarch/pentastarch and blood together with prophylactic mannitol 30ml/h to prevent multi organ dysfunction. Consider bolus dose of methylprednisolone 3 mg/kg.

CARBON MONOXIDE POISONING

The hemoglobin molecule has 24 to 25 times more affinity for CO than for O_2. CO also binds to myoglobin and decreases its oxygen carrying capacity. The molecule binds with the cytochrome oxidase enzyme inhibiting cellular respiration. The net effect being profound hypoxia, anaerobic metabolism and lactic acidosis. Dissociation of HbCO is very slow, the half life of COHb when breathing room air is 4 hours, which reduces to 40 minutes when breathing 100% oxygen at one atmosphere and 15 minutes while breathing 100% oxygen in a hyperbaric environment. Clinical symptoms of CO poisoning manifest when COHb levels exceed 15%. A COHb level above 20% is considered as a toxic level and that above 40% as severe exposure and likely to produce neurologic sequelae like ataxia, cortical blindness and behavioural disturbances. Levels in excess of 50% produce

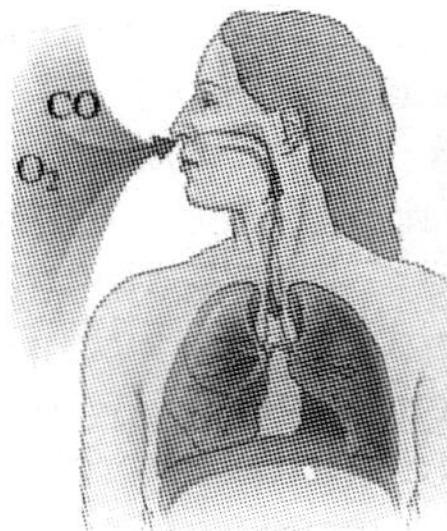

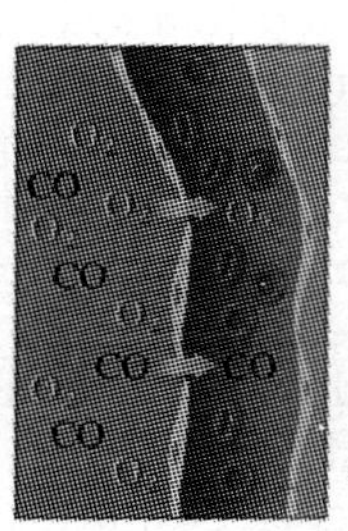

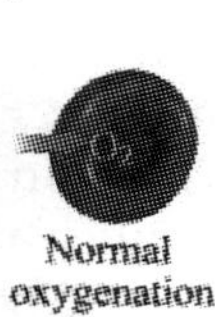

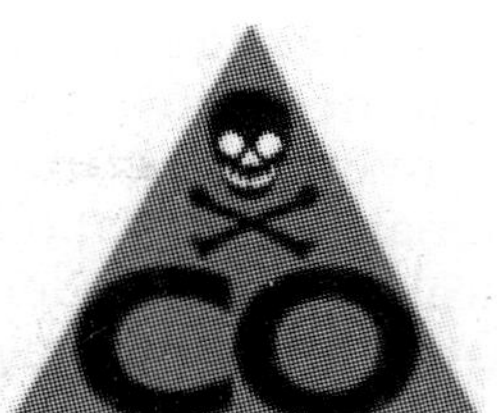

Fig. 64.17

irreversible neurologic damage. Detection of poisoning by multiple band spectrophotometer such as the IL 232 CO-oximeter is advisable. Treatment of CO poisoning is by administering 100% oxygen at 10 litres/min flow by face mask until COHb levels fall below 5%. Infants and pregnant women will require longer duration of oxygen therapy as fetal hemoglobin has even greater affinity for CO when compared to adult hemoglobin. When available, hyperbaric oxygen at 2-3 atmospheres is therapeutic and life saving.

Further Reading

1. War Surgery Field Manual. Hans Husum.Third World Network.
2. Oxford Handbook of Clinical Specialties. Judith Collier, Murray Longmore, Peter Scally. 6th Edn,2003, Oxford University Press).

FIELD ANALGESIA

"He who would become a surgeon should join the army and follow it."

—*Hippocrates*

Introduction

The history of warfare parallels the history of medical advances. Provision of adequate pain relief in the field setting was ignored for long due to serious misconceptions and frank ignorance or fears that it would complicate in-hospital management and confuse diagnosis. The subject got a boost in the 1970safter experiences with the use of various analgesics in heart attack and obstetric patients. The testimonies of patients who have suffered the agony of being trapped in the wreckage of roadside accidents and bounced around with a fractured femur over roads and ditches brought humanitarian considerations to out-of-hospital medical care and redefined the goals and priorities with respect of pain management. In the field of anesthesia, wars have resulted in marked technical, chemical, and procedural advances, including the first battlefield use of inhalational anesthesia (Mexican-American War), first widespread use of anesthetics and inhalers for the application of inhaled anesthetics (Methoxyflurane by the self administered "whistle" apparatus during the US Civil War), use of the eye signs chart for safe monitoring by lay practitioners (World War I), development of specific short course training centers for predeployment anesthesia training (World War II), and the establishment of military anesthesia residency programs in response to shortages of specialty trained doctors (Korean War). The current wars in Iraq and Afghanistan are no exception to this historical trend, and perhaps the most significant advance resulting from these conflicts is the Military Advanced Regional Anesthesia and Analgesia Initiative (MARAA)—the collaborative effort of like-minded anesthesiologists who perceived a need for improvement in battlefield pain management. Deployed military anesthesiologists recognized a disparity between battlefield and civilian analgesic care that needed to be bridged. Colonel (Retired) John Chiles was the first to voice the potential benefit of increasing the use of regional anesthesia in the Iraq war. With Lieutenant Colonel Chester Buckenmaier, Chiles started the Army Regional Anesthesia and Pain Management Initiative in 2000. Dr Buckenmaier administered the first continuous peripheral nerve block in Iraq on October 7, 2003. Upon his return, Buckenmaier, Chiles, Lieutenant Colonel Todd Carter, and Colonel (Retired) Ann Virtis created MARAA, following in the tradition of the Anesthesia Travel Club created by John Lundy to rapidly disseminate research advances to practitioners. MARAA's purpose is to develop consensus recommendations to implement improvements in medical practice and technology that will promote regional anesthesia and analgesia in the care of military beneficiaries. The organization also serves as an advisory board to the individual service anesthesia consultants and to the Surgeon General. Initial support was provided indirectly by the public's demand for better pain control for wounded soldiers and directly via American Congressional funding that obtained sanction for the use of the Stryker Pain Pump 2 on Air Force military aircraft and patient-controlled analgesia (PCA) pumps on the battlefield and on evacuation aircraft. In this era of rediscovery and refinement, pain relief is being reexamined as an important element of pre hospital care. Interest is being focused not only on the agents that have been previously used in the field, but also on newer drugs and routes of administration that may prove to be safe and effective for use in emergency situations. Basic measures like gentle handling, splinting and a compassionate and caring rapport with the patient and also the use of imagery to distract the patient continue to play an important role in the field setting. Morphine sulfate has been in use since the early 1970s, but its long duration of action, ability to depress the respiration, cause hypotension and dull the protective airway reflexes has led to a search for newer narcotic agents. Fentanyl citrate with its shorter duration of action and cardiovascular stability allows for greater safety and control when given in incremental bolus dosing. Nalbuphine, the newer agonist-antagonist analgesic does not induce adverse hemodynamic changes and minimal psychomimetic effects. Self administered "Entonox" through a demand valve apparatus is safe, a good anxiolytic and effective in mild to moderate pain states. It is, however, ineffective when pain is severe in nature. Use of low dose regimens of the d-stereoisomer of the racemic mixture of ketamine is also encouraging in field settings, especially when combined with midazolam to reduce side effects like vivid dreaming and hallucinations. The availability of its antagonist flumazenil has also encouraged its use further. Newer routes like transmucosal and intranasal spray delivery when vascular access is limited is an exciting development.

Battlefield Analgesia Protocol

The aim is to produce an advanced battlefield analgesia protocol that provides the maximum benefit for the greatest number of patients using the minimum of resources considering aspects of logistics, drug pharmacology, safety, etiology of the pain and the experience of the medics. Analgesia is only considered after the "ABCD" criteria of the Primary Survey are satisfied.

Logistic Factors

The availability of drugs and medical expertise would depend upon the military threat and supply line, so the protocol should only rely on those resources that are likely to be commonly available.

Pharmacological Factors

The drugs used must be effective and familiar with minimal morbidity associated with their use.

a. Morphine or pethidine has been the most widely used opioid drug with the intramuscular route being favoured because of its familiarity and simplicity, but it is accepted that patient-controlled analgesia may be appropriate in some circumstances. The latter is likely to be limited by availability of equipment and expertise. Fentanyl in a dose of 0.5 to 1.0 mcg/kg is now the preferred narcotic as it does not cause vasodilatation and has a shorter duration of action.
b. Non-steroidal anti-inflammatory drugs are included for their opioid-sparing effects but are not recommended until adequate cardio-respiratory stability has been established in order to minimise the potential adverse renal effects.
c. Local anaesthetics, such as lignocaine or bupivacaine, may be useful in some circumstances by those, with the appropriate training, to perform nerve blocks (local infiltration, digital nerve, femoral nerve).The intercostal nerve block is not included as there is a potential for morbidity outweighing the potential advantage.
d. Other drugs such as ketamine (0.25-0.5 mg/kg intravenously or 1-2 mg/kg intramuscularly) or Entonox (50% oxygen in 50% nitrous oxide) could be used for short painful procedures or for the extrication of trapped victims.

Personnel Factors

This protocol is for use by combat medical technicians, nurses and doctors. The latter may have experience or training in more sophisticated methods of providing analgesia which are outside the scope of this protocol.

Safety Measures

The provision of analgesia follows only if the A. B. C. D. approach is satisfactory and the opiod antidote naloxone or nalmephene is available.

Chronological Factors

The protocol is designed around the intensity of pain as measured by the VAS. This means that the same protocol could be applied at any point throughout the patient's illness, from admission to discharge.

Aetiological Factors

The protocol should be equally applicable to 'medical' pain (e.g., myocardial infarction), 'surgical' pain or that from an injury.

Analgesic Protocol Elaboration:

1. Analgesia is administered to those servicemen who are cardio-respiratory stable, are alert or are verbally responsive and who say they are in pain.
2. Naloxone protocol is an additional safety feature: 400 micrograms of naloxone is diluted in 4 ml normal saline and 1ml is given intravenously every minute to ensure a respiratory rate of at least 8 breaths per minute or a sedation score of alert or verbally responsive. By careful titration one can reverse overdosage whilst preserving as much analgesia as possible. Since the plasma half life of naloxone (60 min.) is less than that of morphine (150-180 min.) or pethidine (180 min.) it is important to be aware of the possible need for further doses of naloxone. This protocol permits the intravenous administration of opioids for a more controlled analgesia and this circumvents the potential problem of intramuscular injections in a shocked patient. Nalmefene 0.5-1.5 mg I/V is another option as this has a longer duration of action with a half life of 10 h.
3. The cause of the pain may not always be initially obvious, and servicemen who had previously been well controlled could become worse due to other problems like infection, compartment syndrome, haematoma and muscle cramps/stiffness and other medical or surgical causes for pain. This has to be looked into and excluded before opioid administration.
4. The Visual Analogue Score (VAS) is based on an eleven point scale from 0 to 10 where 0 is no pain and 10 is the worst possible pain imaginable by the given patient.
5. Analgesic therapy is then based on the severity of the pain, starting from oral analgesics at one end to titrated intravenous opioids at the other. Since the VAS scale is a continuum, the final choice will depend on the trend of serial VAS observations: (is the pain getting better or worse?), and whether the oral route is feasible. The choice of therapy must be dynamic and reflect the changes in pain severity. For example, if a patient has a VAS score of 9 and is given intravenous opioid titrated to response and his next score is 3; it may be more appropriate to use an intramuscular or subcutaneous opioid rather than oral analgesics. If the oral route is not possible, and the pain score is in the lower range it would be preferable to use an intramuscular or subcutaneous opioid.
6. Enteral medication should be given regularly if possible, by the clock, to maintain a sustained-analgesic effect.
7. Opioids are equally effective when given intramuscularly or subcutaneously. The latter is preferred as it is less painful for the patient and repeated doses may be given through an indwelling-subcutaneous cannula/butterfly needle.
8. Provided there is autonomic homeostasis (particularly intravascular volume) and that the urine output is at least greater than 0.5 ml/kg/hr then consideration should be given to the co-administration of a non-steroidal anti-inflammatory drug such as diclofenac or ketorolac.
9. A safe anti-emetic like ondansetron/granisetron and other 5HT3 antagonists may be included to offset the increased likelihood of nausea and vomiting after the administration of opioids. Choice to drugs is limited to those that are commonly available and the advantages that each drug of those drugs may have over the others in particular cases.

The Stryker Pain Pumps are infusion devices designed to deliver controlled amounts of local anesthetics to the patient for post-operative pain management. Medication is delivered directly to the surgical wound site or in close proximity to the nerves associated with the surgical area. The pump infuses the medication at an hourly flow rate or combination of an hourly flow rate and controlled bolus doses. It is a programmable, portable, and disposable pain management device for optimal management of continuous peripheral nerve blocks and its use has been clinically proven to significantly reduce pain and length of stay in orthopaedic surgery. The advantages include improved pain relief. And patient satisfaction levels as the mechanically driven pump ensures a consistent and accurate infusion of medication. The device is simple to set-up with two-button controlled programming, that is easy to understand, and comfortable to wear. Its digital screen clearly displays settings and medication delivered and the device has the ability to reprogram flow rate and bolus options with lock-out times using a security code to ensure patient safety. It is also refillable and contains a 400ml fluid reservoir with a refill port that can be used up to 1000 ml. Local anesthetics do not induce the negative side effects often associated with narcotics and the device does not restrict patient mobility during post-operative activity and rehabilitation. The Stryker pump also contains silent visual warnings including a tube blockage sensor warning.

CONCLUSION

"Pain begets pain", probably secondary to peripheral and central neuromodulation after major trauma and early treatment with analgesics can decrease the overall requirement of these drugs, besides improving patient satisfaction. Effective analgesia in the battlefield attenuates the adverse pathophysiological responses to pain, aids evacuation and maintains morale. While the efficacy of self-administered, opioid-based analgesia by the serviceman prior to arrival at a medical facility will continue, the newer protocol will assist those healthcare workers who may not have been trained in acute pain management but are called to administer analgesics to the serviceman in pain.

Suggested Reading

1. Hocking G, De M Ello Wf. Battlefield Analgesia —A Basic Approach. *JR Army Med Corps* 1996; 142: 101-102.
2. Battlefield Advanced Trauma Life Support handbook. Chapter 14. Army Code 63726.
3. S Emple Tj, U Pton Rn, M Acintyre Pe, R Unciman Wb, M Ather Le. Morphine blood concentrations in elderly postoperative patients following administration via an indwelling subcutaneous cannula. *Anaesthesia* 1997; 52(4): 318-23.
4. J Affe Jh, M Artin Wr. Opioid analgesics and antagonists. In: Gilman AG, Goodman LS, Rall TW, Murad F, eds. The pharmacological Basis of Therapeutics. New York: MacMillan Publishing Co, 1992: 485-521.
5. Analgesia in the field. Stewart,RD. Medical Corps International, 1990. Vol 5,No.3:7-10.

65 Aeromedical Evacuation Procedures During Disasters

"Every attempt to make war easy and safe will result in humiliation and disaster."

—*William Tecumseh Sherman*

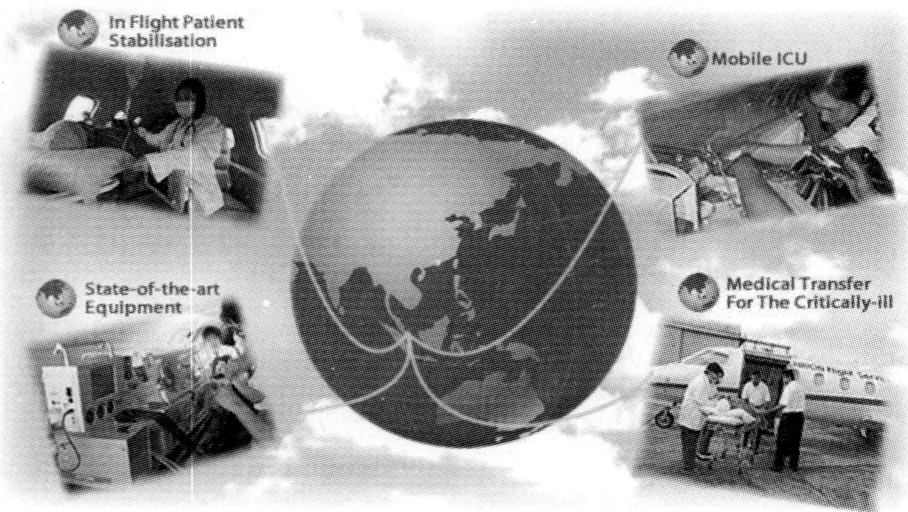

Fig. 65.1

INTRODUCTION

The first balloon evacuation of patients was conducted during the Prussian siege of Paris in 1870. During the siege of Paris in 1870-71, a total of 160 patients were evacuated from the city by manned balloons. The Germans pioneered this effort from Kiel-Holtenau on 01 Jun 1913 for rescue operations in the Baltic. Later their 2nd Naval Aircraft Division at Wilelmshaven operated in the North Sea area. During World War 1 in 1917, a young military physician Lieutenant Chassaing was inspired to transform a military plane for medical use, but the experiment was considered too risky and was limited to simulatory exercises using dummies. Actual air evacuation of casualties took place during the colonial wars in Lebanon and Morocco in the 1920s.It was only towards the end of the Second World War that successful search and rescue (SAR) missions were flown over the Baltic. Then the French, Dutch and Americans flew ambulance planes with Red Cross symbols to ferry injured soldiers. Both the Geneva Convention of 1906 and the Hague Convention of 1907 did not consider immunity for air ambulances. In 1925 France put forward a proposal for immunity of air ambulances from attack and a broadening of the Geneva Conventions. But, because of the outbreak of World War 2 in 1940, the meeting did not take place. The concept of airlifting patients was first introduced in the military in 1912, but it was dismissed as too hazardous for transporting sick and injured soldiers. It was in 1942, during the course of World War II that aeromedical evacuation was widely utilized to transport a total of 1,338,717 sick and wounded servicemen. During this period, the concept of the Flight Nurse began to emerge and the first flight nurses were members of the Army Air Corps, the first batch of 4 students attending the first flight-nurse course at Bowman Field, Kentucky in Feb 1943. Risky aeromedical evacuations were conducted in the theatre of war all through the Korean, Vietnam and Granada conflicts and also during peacetime during the U.S. hostage situation in Iran; Lebanon bombing of US Marines and the devastating earthquakes in Armenia. During the Chernobyl nuclear disaster, aircrew risked their lives by flying into contaminated zones, suffering the consequences of radiation exposure in the process. Tremendous progress has been made in aviation medicine and aeromedical aircraft since then.

The requirement for rapid deployment has also increased the use of air transport and air transportation of battle casualties has made it possible for all but the most immediate surgery to be performed outside the battle zone, often in the soldier's own country. However, if large numbers of wounded are to be brought home, it is essential that adequate liaison is established with the civil medical authorities, so that the civilian population is not put at risk.

Aeromedical evacuation aims at transporting patients rapidly, comfortably and safely to areas of definite medical care or appropriate echelons of medical care. Aircrafts used for the purpose have been the McDonnel-Douglas MD-80, C-9, C-17 and C-130 Hercules, the tactical workhorse for frontline airlifts, the long haul C-141 Starfighter, Boeing B-767. The French German C-16 Transalls medical version carries 61 litters with an additional 20-25 stretcher capacity on the deck in an emergency situation, while the B-767 carries 111 litters and MD-80 accomodates 45 litters.The C-9A Nightingale is the only aircraft built specifically for aeromedical evacuation with specialized medical equipment, ICU, piped oxygen and the capability to carry 40 litter patients. The Hercules and the giant AN-225 have also been appropriated for large scale casevac in special situations.The Cessna 340 is a popular and versatile aircraft for airevac. Rotary wing aircraft are more versatile and efficient and the PUMA, Sikorsky, BK 117 rescue helicopter also known as the airborne ICU have been converted for exclusive casualty evacuation purposes. Elevated four blade rotor systems reduce vibration levels and provision of two rear doors ease the process of loading/unloading of casualties, even when rotors are running. Built in latest generation emergency equipment has enabled rescue teams to administer quality inflight prehospital care to casualties. Smaller helicopters like the Alloutte and Gazelle are commonly employed to transport two lying casualties at a time in scoop and run type of evacuation. The system of aeromedical evacuation permits movement of casualties with periodic check-points/staging stations to support patient needs and monitor safe patient transfer within the golden-hour following injury. The first echelon of transfer aims at scoop and run after initial quick triage at the disaster site, stabilizing the patient enroute like performing life-saving procedures, arrest of hemorrhage, resuscitation and intravenous fluid administration. The second echelon moves stabilized victims between medical treatment facilities. Use of a rescue helicopter shortens the interval in which the victim is without medical attention. This modality is unaffected by traffic snarls, provides maximum flexibility when integrated by a radio network with land-based rescue services, covers more territory than a ground based system, ensures the shortest transport time of victims to the most suitable/tertiary care hospitals and maximises the efficiency of tertiary hospital infra structure. In 85% cases of battle injuries, victims were still alive within 5 minutes of the accident. If medical care could be provided within 10 minutes of injury, death rate can be reduced by 20 percent. Incidence of wound infection is 3.5% in those transported by helicopter against 12% in those evacuated by surface transport. Preliminary medical care at the scene of accident reduces hospital mortality by 7%. In situations of cranio-cerebral trauma, mortality among those evacuated by conventional transportation is 47% against 32% in those evacuated by air. The operating cost of a rescue helicopter is compensated by the five-fold benefit of shorter hospital stays, lower infection rates and significantly lower morbidity/mortality.

THE STRESSES OF FLIGHT

As one travels higher, the amount of available oxygen in the atmosphere is reduced in accordance with Dalton's law. Exsanguinated, anemic patients are affected by hypoxic hypoxia above 4000 feet altitudes in uncompressed aircrafts. Also, as per Boyles law, the volume of gas increases with

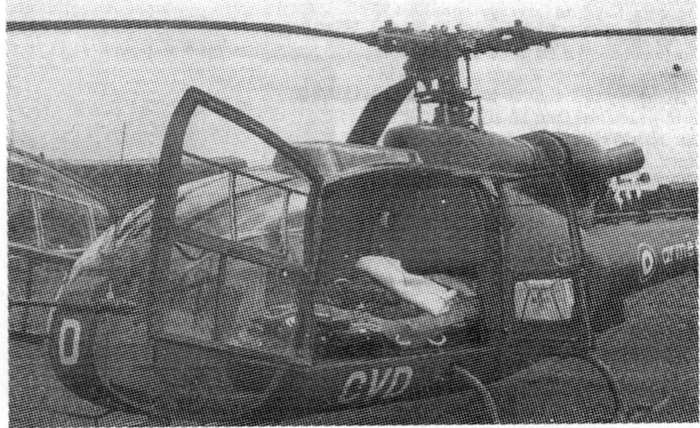

Fig. 65.2

decrease in barometric pressure when temperature is constant. Patients with air-trapping as in gastric distension states will suffer further distension with splinting of their diaphragm and suffer respiratory embarrassment. Those with pneumothorax can have mediastinal shift and progress into shock states and those with open eye injuries can develop vitreous prolapse. The temperature also drops with altitude, and patients with hypothermia, burns and shock states need special attention. Humidity decreases with altitude and humidified air/ oxygen must be provided to all patients in flight and detailed attention paid to their hydration. Aircraft engine noise can create auditory fatigue, affecting communication and vital sign monitoring such as auscultation during flight. Auditory protection must be provided in transit to minimise this stress. Acceleration, deceleration and vibration can add to the stresses. Altitude restriction or transport by compressed aircraft would be required for patients with air embolism, lung cavities, angina pectoris and acute myocardial infarction, open eye injuries, anemia with hemoglobin less than 7 gm/dl, free air in body cavities such as ileus, pneumothorax, gangrene, sinusitis, otitis media and those with effusions. Altitude restriction will involve added flight time and increased turbulence and this factor needs to be considered prior to planning air-evac. Patients with wired jaws can develop air sickness and vomit in flight and hence wire cutters must be provided for quick release and suction kept at hand. Tracheostomy tubes must be changed before flight and high volume low pressure cuffs preferred as the cuff volume expands with increasing altitude. Ventilators for transit ventilation must be discrete, compact, noise free and have a simple maintenance schedule. It must incorporate microblower technology with preset invasive and non invasive modes, intuitive and user friendly interface, dedicated alarm menu and 4 h battery backup. The ResMed Elisee 150 comes close to this requirement. Orthopedic plaster casts must be dry or be bivalved prior to flight as sudden limb swelling might result in vascular insult.

OPERATIONAL REQUIREMENTS

Missions must be planned considering the weather, aircraft limitations, patients condition, number of casualties, crew duty schedules and orders of the treating doctors. Daytime visual flight rules may insist on a one mile visibility and 500 feet ceiling in the presence of mountains and foggy weather conditions. There is always the possibility of a flight diversion to pick up another serious patient en route. The in flight medical personnel must have superior nursing skills and capable of exercising independent judgement in times of crisis. Flight medical equipments must be designed or adapted for airborne environments and be compatible with various aircraft systems and ground transport vehicles.

LANDING AREAS FOR HELICOPTERS

Circle minimum 10 metres diameter-Ideal 10-20 m with no obstruction in approach and take off areas 25 m in all directions with minimum obstructions like trees, chimneys, spires, pylons, power lines. No dust/sand or loose objects like litter, paper, cardboard or clothing in the landing area. Grass and tarmac are OK. The optimum approach angle is 7′ and the approach path must have a gradient of 1 in 8 or less and should be at least 30 m wide. Slope must not exceed 5′ at landing and take off areas. The distance of the helicopter from any unavoidable obstruction should be three times the height of that obstruction. A windsock and fire extinguisher must be available. Clothing must be secure-especially headgear. Personnel are advised to kneel within an area 3 to 9 o clock position in front of aircraft and stoop low while approaching the aircraft. Remember that as the engines shut down the rotor blades dip even lower as they slow to a stop. The tail rotor may not be visible and is another danger especially when sliding open clam shell doors or during a tail side approach to a rotary wing aircraft.

There are no absolute contra indications for air transport of casualties and safe practice for aeromedical evacuation involves stabilizing the patient prior to the flight, a thorough medical evaluation, a planned care protocol based on the patients condition in relation to the stresses of flight. When a patients basic needs are ignored, problems of great urgency are bound to occur down the line (Fig. 65.3).

Helicopters must not be approached unless signaled clear to approach by a flight team member. Be alert to rotor blade clearance and always approach the helicopter from the front of the aircraft and move away in the same direction. An exception is a downhill approach if the helicopter has landed on a slope as main rotor clearance is always greater in the rear. Never walk around the tail rotor area and always hold long objects like I/V stands parallel to the ground. No unauthorized personnel must be allowed on the tarmac within 10 feet of the aircraft (Fig. 65.4).

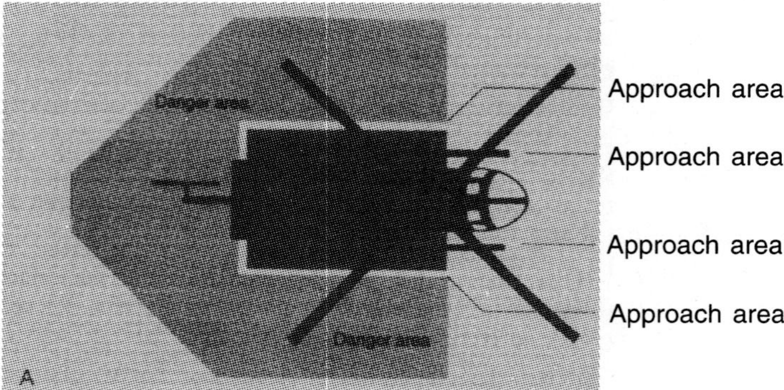

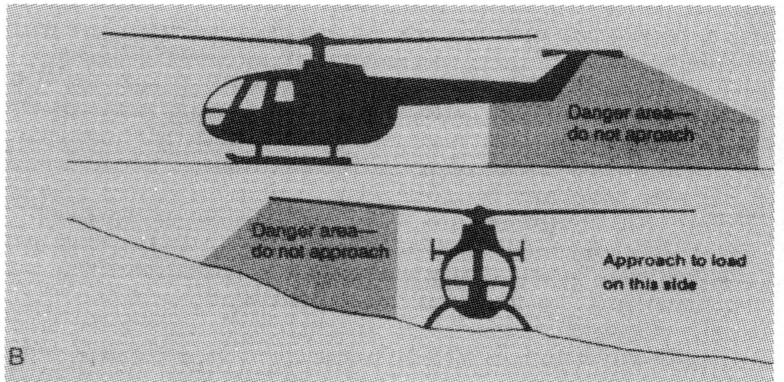

Fig. 65.3: Air view (A) and ground view(B) of safe approaches

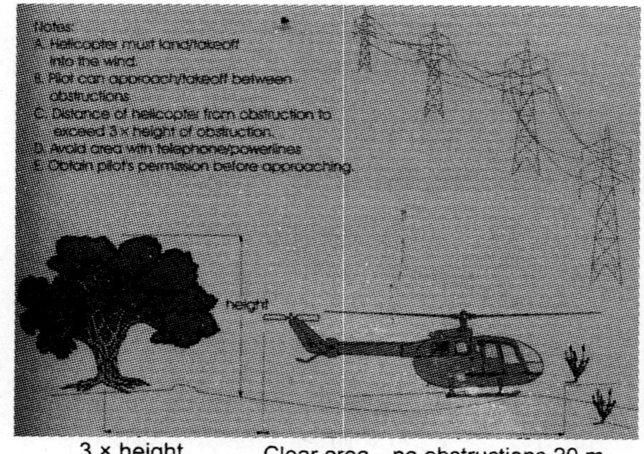

Fig. 65.4: Helicoper lending area

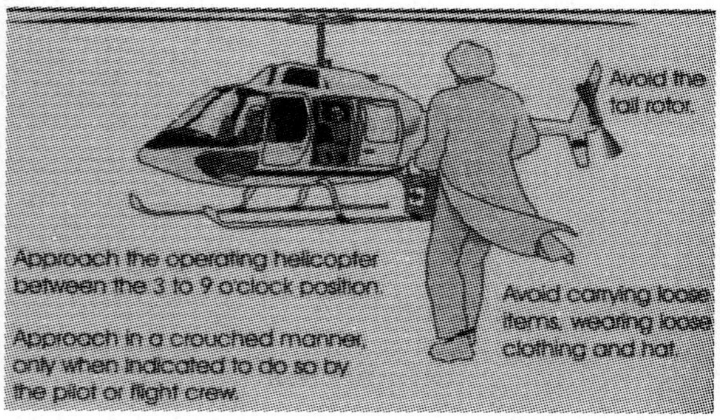

Fig. 65.5: Aircraft safety

Further Reading

1. Safepractice for our aeromedical evacuation patients.Lt Col Phyllis J Hansen,USAF. Military Medicine, 1987, Vol 152, No 6 ,p:281-283.
2. Air transport for the man who needs everything. PJ Hansen, Aviat Space Environ Med, 1980,51,p:725-728.
3. Flight Nursing.Proud past, demanding present, exciting future. Major Richard Smith Captain Danny L Addison,USAF. Medical Corps International,1990,Vol 5,No 3,18-21).

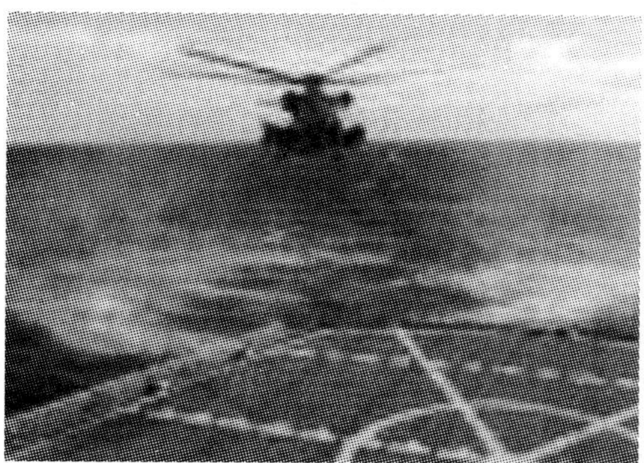

Fig. 65.6

AERIAL RESCUE AT SEA

Rescue at sea by mean of aircraft enables faster surveying, a birds eye view of a larger area and quicker evacuation of victims to the nearest treatment facility. Weather conditions pose the most severe restriction to SAR (Search and Rescue) efforts. Rescue at sea is characterized by the difficulty of locating victims and rescuing them from heavy choppy seas.

HISTORY

Air Force Commander Goering of the Third Reich used his influence with Adolph Hitler to set up a seaplane salvage unit to rescue crew who had ditched their aircraft. On April 12,193a Sea Rescue Squadron was established at Bad Zwischenahn headed by Karl Born and they operated in the North Sea and Baltic sea and divided into five sea-rescue districts for SAR purposes. The Heinkel 5W was specially designed for long distance reconnaissance and sea rescue by Reinhold Mewes. It served this function well until 1942 as it had ample space, signaling devices, electric blankets and a folding down ladder that reached down to the surface of the sea after the plane alighted. Above this ladder port, a winding tackle could be fastened to hoist on board even unconscious and exhausted victims. The JU 52 aircraft were also utilized for SAR over the sea and they ejected pneumatic lifeboats and sea rescue equipment to victims located from the air. Later the amphibious Dornier 24 with its greater action radius of 100 km, 1hour cruising range, higher speed of 255 kmph and planned capacity for 18 persons became the most dependable sea rescue aircraft of the Great War. Their stub-wing design enabled them to start and land even in heavy sea conditions and helped rescue approximately 12,000 victims during the course of the War. The Second Accord of 12 Aug 194and supplementary protocols of 1974 and 1977 drew up protection to sea rescue units.

AEROSPACE DISASTERS

The space environment is absolutely adverse to life. The vacuum, the extremes of temperature and the radiation exposure (ultraviolet and other forms) are all factors that are totally alien to life on earth. .Manned space flights below the Van Allen radiation belts at altitudes between 30and 50 kilometres do not pose serious radiation problems. Dosimeter measurements reflect an absorbed dose between 0.5 to 5.rem (over a 7 months space flight) that are far below the permissible dose of 15 rem per mission. During inter-planetary space missions, galactic cosmic radiation consisting primarily of chemical nuclei with relativistic velocity

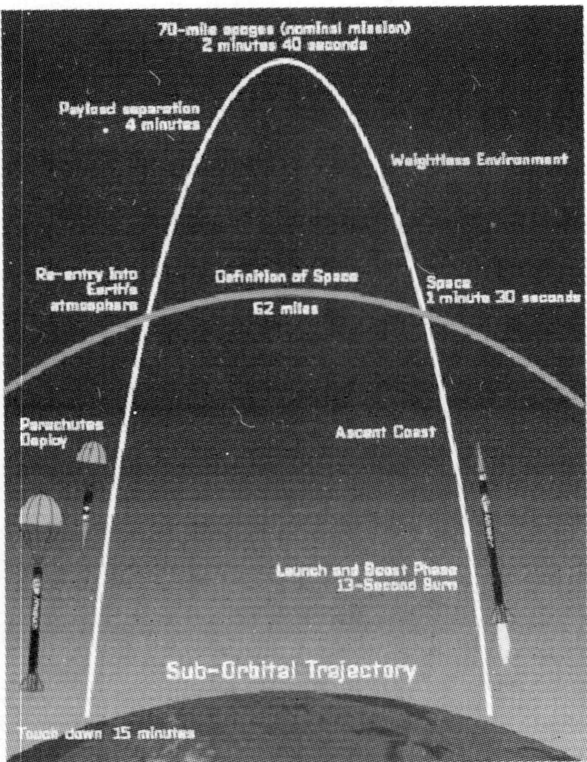

Fig. 65.7

can have adverse biologic effects, especially if the track of a heavy particle passes through an agglomeration of nerve cells forming an important neuronal centre in the brain. The effects of such radiation under conditions of weightlessness is yet to be evaluated. Weightlessness in space causes fluid shift from lower extremities to the thorax and head areas. This redistribution of upto 2000ml of blood and body fluid causes mucosal congestion in upper nasal and throat regions and space sickness. Negative water balance and loss of muscle mass results in weight loss. Suppression of erthyropoiesis and decalcification of bone by upto 8% can occur. Co ordination between the eye and the vestibular system is affected (viseo-vestibular incoordination) and information mismatch between the two can cause dizziness, irritability and vomiting The natural circadian rhythm is lost and this impairs performance and well being. Space travel and exploitation of the space environment for manufacture of extremely pure grade drugs like erythropoetin by electrophoresis operations in space (EOS programs), space stations, spacelabs, space astronomy etc will see more manned space missions in the near future. The problem of a disaster in space will have to bear in mind the problems mentioned. Special space suits, work-rest cycles, hard muscle training using treadmill, restriction of head and body movement and methods to enhance immunity would have to be addressed.

Further Reading

Medicine in aerospace. Dr Edward C Burchard. Medical Corps International 1987;Vol2(2):36-48.

66 Hospital Ships in Disasters

Any blue-water Navy must aim to provide medical cover at the right place, at the right time and in an uninterrupted manner. Hospital ships are vessels constructed, equipped and manned solely for the treatment and transportation of the wounded, sick and the shipwrecked in accordance with the 2nd Geneva Convention. These floating hospitals lend a vital and mobile capability to the fleet and serve to impart flexibility to operations, and also as a morale booster to the troops in changing tactical scenarios.

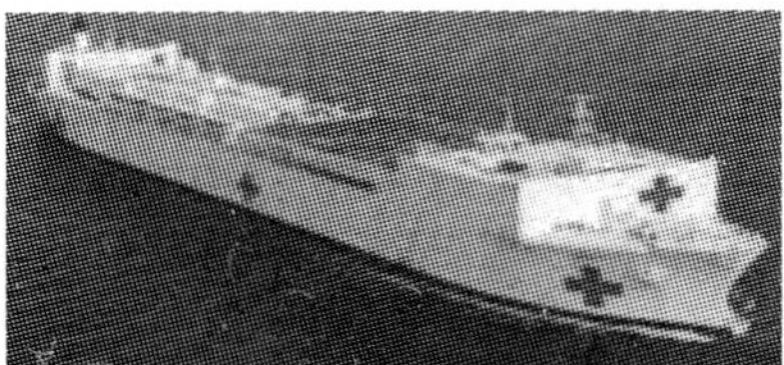

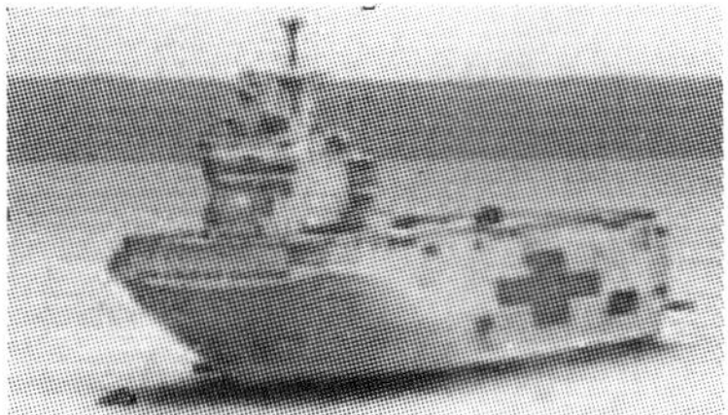

Fig. 66.1

History

The first account of a hospital ship dates back to the year 1588 when the Spanish Armada set sail to vanquish the British fleet. During the First World War, several hospital ships like Haven, Benevolence, Consolation and Tranquility were deployed, escorted by paddle boats to allow their early identification by enemy sonar and avoid being attacked. In the Second World War, the International Red Cross chartered 43 ships to transport patients and medical stores. In 1966, during the Vietnam War, the United States deployed the 560 bedded hospital ships USS Repose and USS Sanctuary when shore based units came under heavy enemy attack. During the Falklands War of 1982, a total of 6 hospital ships were deployed. The British deployed 4 vessels including the 110 bedded MV Uganda which served as the mother ship to 3 other smaller hospital ships RMS Hecla, Hydra and Herald. The 25,581 tonne former aviation training ship RFA Argus was refitted in under three weeks to create a 100-bedded gas proof ward created in one of its huge helicopter hangars. She did not carry a red-cross emblem which allowed it to operate outside the box stipulated under the Geneva Conventions and allowed to sail under escort with the British and US battle groups. She was fitted with light anti-aircraft guns and 45 Portakabins were used to form a hospital complex, each with its own power supply and self-generating citadel pressure to counter gas-warfare. A brainchild of Surgeon Commander Paxton Dewar, the converted ship was thus able to overcome the requirement that a casualty admitted on board had to return to his unit via a neutral country and avoid its inspection by the enemy forces. The ship was designated as a Primary Casualty Receiving Ship or PCRS as opposed to the old style hospital ship.The Argentinians deployed the Hospital Ship A.R.A. Bahia Paraiso and Almirante Irizar, a modified ice-breaker and a troop ship respectively, as hospital ships in the same theatre. The Indian Navy deployed the hydrographic ships INS Sandhayak, Nirdeshak and the training ship INS Tir as hospital ships during combat and exercise. During the Gulf War, the 1000 bedded hospital ships USS Mercy and Comfort were anchored off Dubai with 500 medical staff, 400 support personnel and 300 nurses, capable of operating for 30 days at a time without any replenishment of supplies or equipment. High speed amphibious hover-crafts are being tried as hospital ships for the future and several companies now offer turnkey-fitted, small versatile hospital ships with facilities for deployment in nuclear, chemical and biological warfare scenarios.

Geneva Conventions and Hospital Ships

Under the Second Geneva Maritime Convention of August 1949, hospital ships command protection and immunity from attack subject to their adhering to the following:

That they provide medical cover to casualties and shipwrecked irrespective of the country of their origin.

That they are deployed in a theatre of operations after intimating details of silhouette, radio codes, manpower, stores, modifications, aircraft etc to the parties in conflict a full ten days before their actual deployment.

That the hospital ships anchor and function from specified locations termed Red Cross Box and refrain from communicating directly with any man-of-war.

That they restrict all their radio transmissions to the standard international distress frequencies and in the clear i.e. refrain from all coded transmissions.

Radio regulations permit frequencies for radiotelegraphy as 500KHz(MF), 2182 KHz for radiotelephony (MF) and 156.8 MHz (VHF).

That they carry no weapons. Casualties admitted on board have to surrender their personal arms too.

That they are distinctively marked to be identifiable with the following recommended features:

- They must be painted white with prominent red cross or red crescent symbols all round and on the decks in the largest size possible and with a black border for better infra red identification. These must be flood-lit at night.
- They must fly a red cross/red crescent flag on the main mast of minimum size 2 × 2 metres.
- All life boats the prefix used is PAN-PAN-PAN pronounced as the French word panne followed by the term MAY-DEE-CAL pronounced as medical.
- Ships can transmit their call signs underwater on frequencies 5KHz and 5.1 KHz to enable submarines identify hospital ships.
- Since 1982, the International Maritime Satellite Organisation (IMMARSAT) has been operating a worldwide satellite radio-communication system. Satellites positioned in geostationary orbits some 36,000 kilometres above the equator over the Atlantic, Pacific and Indian oceans enables telephone, telex, fax, low, medium, high and very high speed (upto 1 megabit/second) data transmission, and CTV imaging. The system provides an instantaneous, high standard mobile communication service.

- Upon discharge from the hospital ship, battle casualties can return to their units via a neutral country only.

Construction Details of Hospital Ships

The ships are required to be fitted with dynamic stabilisers to minimise roll. Lloyds criteria for hospital ship design specifies a maximum permissible roll of 5 in sea states 5-6. Inputs from the gyro and ships speed are fed to a microprocessor comparator which computes error correction and activates fins or righting levers (2-4 numbers) to counter the roll. The actifins work on the Bernoulli principle and lift the ship, decreasing its draught and decrease the period of roll. This electro-hydraulic-servo system is based on sensors actualising the fins in a continuous, dynamic manner. The ships Captain can alter the ships head (course) and steer to calmer waters to minimize the roll further, if required. Much also depends on the propulsion. Diesel and turbine propelled ships emit greater noise, vibration and pollution when compared to steam and nuclear propelled ships. The latter have the additional advantage of providing feed water for medical use, steam for autoclaves and an engine room that can function as a citadel in an NBC situation. Smaller floating clinics adopt the twin-hulled catamaran design based on the principle of small waterplane area twin hull (SWATH) concept that imparts stability in treacherous sea conditions and at high speeds. Both hulls are adjusted using gyroscopes and servomechanism to counter pitch, coupled with two adjustable canards to counter roll. Newer hull designs, hydrofoils (hydrofoil small waterplane area ships or HYWAS), water jet concepts and ship geometry hold promise of crafts with less than 3 degrees of roll and pitch. Hospital ships must be fully air conditioned with fitted with NBC filters. Casualties are received from helicopters landing on the flight deck and also on the quarter deck by boats. A hydraulic lift must connect the two decks. Triage is usually conducted on the quarter deck. The radiology services (including ultrasound), laboratory and blood bank must necessarily be located in the vicinity. Operation theatres are best located amidships in the lower decks for best stability, one in each water tight compartment. Wards are routinely fitted with two-tiered bunk beds and the intensive care is confined to cubicle type rooms in the proximity of the triage area. The mortuary is best located in the forward area and must have a large sized deep freezer. There may be a need to duplicate facilities to cater for each water tight compartment of the ship. The future will see the emergence of hydrofoil small waterplane area ships (HYSWAS) that have the ability to operate at high speeds over long distances in heavy sea conditions. Subsurface crafts that can exploit the calm conditions just a short distance below the waves can also be expected in the near future.

Equipment

All equipment fitted must be necessarily lightweight, sturdy, reliable, simple to operate with minimum moving parts and maintenance free. Standard inventories have been drawn up and careful planning of consumables must be made based on realistic appreciation of casualties. Medical gases is likely to be a problem and use of oxygen concentrators in the central supply using ceramic molecular sieves to adsorb atmospheric nitrogen would be preferred. These units supply oxygen of 85 to 95% purity depending on flows. Unsupplemented air was used in the Falklands war where the Tri-Service anaesthetic apparatus comprising of an Oxford Miniature Vaporiser, Laerdal resuscitator and a Houtonox valve was used successfully without any adverse effects.

Maximal use of total intravenous techniques and circle absorbers must be made. All theatre equipment must be riveted to the deck plate or clamped to the bulkheads and all flammable anesthetics avoided. Regional techniques will continue to have a place in field conditions. A recompression chamber would be required to handle subsunk survivors and bends among divers. The Picker International Clinix-RM seagoing radiographic unit and CT units were constructed to overcome gyroscopic effects and are exclusively designed for use on board hospital ships.

Manpower

A senior medical administrator must work with the captain of the ship to co ordinate ships speed, course etc. All medical personnel must be physically fit and mentally stoic to work under cramped conditions and in all sea states. Surgical teams comprising of a general surgeon, an anesthesiologist and a maxillofacial surgeon must be assigned at each theatre. Paramedics must comprise of OR technicians, laboratory assistants, radiographers, blood transfusion assistants and dental technicians. The ships crew must be trained in casualty transportation using conventional as well as the Neil-Robertson type of stretchers.

Planning Considerations for Casualties

Casualty figures for a Naval engagement is estimated at 10% maximum for a landing operation in which the ratio of killed to wounded is taken as 1:4. Of the 80% wounded, Priority 1 cases would be estimated at 10-15%, Priority 2 at 15-20% and Priority 3 as 60-70% of total. Lying patients would be 40% of total wounded figures and sitting/walking casualties would be account for approximately 60%. A single surgical team can be expected to handle 10-12 surgeries over a 24 hours period.

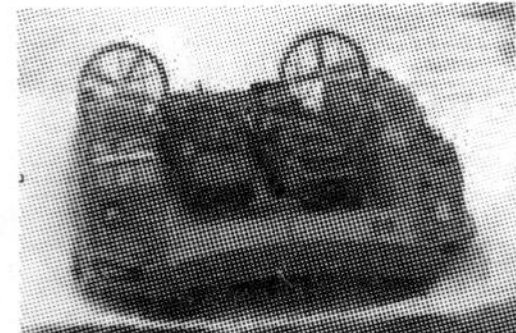

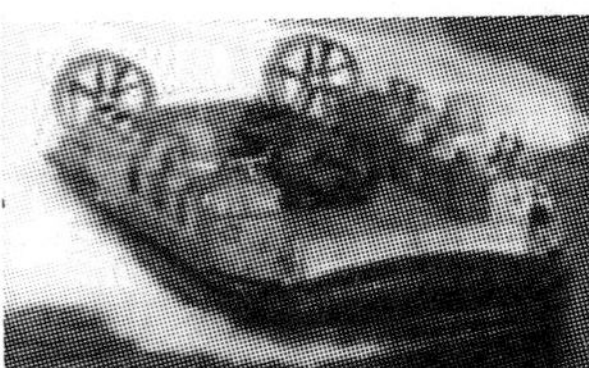

Fig. 66.2

LCAC MEDEVAC CONSIDERATIONS

The Air Cushion Landing Craft (LCAC) has added a new dimension to amphibious operations. It lends speed to the transportation logistics of battle casualties and can improve survival rates thereby. In the Vietnam War, 98% of all casualties who safely reached field medical facilities were saved due their rapid transportation by helicopters. The battlefields of the future would be too lethal for such evacuation and alternative evacuation methods would have to be worked out. Despite its drawbacks, such as low capacity, excessive noise and high winds from propellers and exposure to cold weathers, the casualty evacuation using M997 type of armoured ambulances mounted on the deck of such vessels, placement of an enclosed air conditioned container or a rigid expeditionary shelter system as used by the Marine Corps, offer alternatives in overcoming such drawbacks. The LVTP-7 amphibian tractor which can be driven onto LCACs can also be considered as each can be fitted with six stretchers each and two such tractors can be housed on the decks of LCACs and then rapidly driven to the beach medical post/evacuation station or the nearest hospital ship. The normal LCAC can carry 24 sitting passengers and this can be modified with wider hatches and stretcher-securing devices. Its speed, versatility and mobility make the LCAC an ideal vehicle for rapid evacuation of combat casualties.

67 Marine Disasters

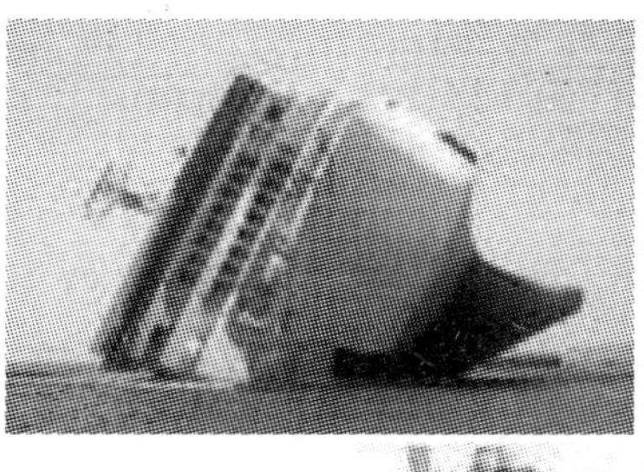

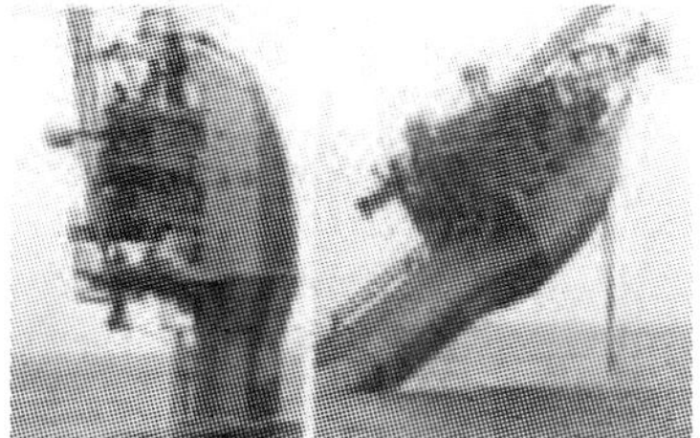

Fig. 67.1

INTRODUCTION

Marine accidents remain a possibility as eliminating all of the hazards to human health and life is still impossible. After fire, sinking or capsizing is the other main risk on any ship. This could result from many reasons like collision with another ship or floating object, grounding, failure in seawater piping or losing stability by inadequate ballasting of the vessel, catastrophic weather events or navigational errors. In the event something happens, a "Titanic-like" slow sinking in upright position might not be the case: in heavy seas the vessel could capsize in an early stage of the distress, making evacuation all but impossible. Lifeboats are provided for at least 75% of the persons onboard, the remaining using life rafts. As lifeboats can be very difficult and dangerous to board in heavy weather, some consider life rafts accessed by chutes or slides a better solution. In bad conditions successfully abandoning even a smaller ship can be very dangerous, if not impossible. Due to this, the safest way is always to make the ships so safe that abandoning ship does not become necessary. In this respect ships are very similar to aircraft: everything must be done to prevent an accident happening. Today the number of persons onboard has only a small effect in the stability requirements of the vessel. However, the new damage stability regulations, which will come into force in 2009, define a required damage stability index, which is affected by the number of persons onboard. As an example, a vessel with 7,000 persons onboard needs to have 5% higher damage stability index than a vessel with 4,000 persons onboard. In the other words, the fewer persons there are onboard, the less safe the vessel needs to be against sinking or capsizing. Most ships today are only built to withstand waves up to 50 feet tall—while freak waves have been calculated to reach heights of up to 198 feet. Technically, a freak wave is defined as a wave that is twice the "significant wave height", which is the mean of the largest third of waves in an area The basic reason for the occurrence of freak waves seems to be what is known as nonlinear wave interactions—by a certain mechanism there is an energy exchange between the waves resulting in a large growth in wave amplitude, much larger than what would be possible through ordinary linear superposition of waves.

Simulation is a new development for ship evacuation in emergencies. The University of Greenwich software package, EXODUS, has most of the features required to implement a ship evacuation simulator. It has abandonment models to cover the entry of personnel into lifeboats, human performance data to account for the effect of motion and the list angle of a sinking ship, database for evacuating a passenger ship and the degree to which the evacuation will meet standards set by national and international authorities. It can also support research in evacuation situations and technologies. The software accounts not only for ship layout and equipment locations, but also for human behaviour, the effect of hazards such as smoke or flooding, and ship heel and motions:

Indicators of Imminent Sinking

Increasing heel or list of the ship and increasing sea water sloshing over the decks.

Abandon Ship Drill

- *General alarm:* Seven short horn blasts followed by a long one.
- *Emergency communication:* Over VHF or single-sideband radio employ the appropriate levels of priority communications: distress, urgent, and safety, identified by MAYDAY, PAN-PAN, and SECURITE. Panicked radio communications can confuse a rescue effort. Learn the proper procedures and remain calm.
- Use the acceptable distress signals as outlined in the Navigation Rules. Flares are fast and effective—red for distress.
- Avoid panic as this leads to pushing, shoving and trampling, which can lead to other injuries, like broken bones or concussion. Studies have shown that 70 percent of victims of a maritime accident are bewildered and have impaired reasoning, 15 percent exhibit irrational behaviors and only 15 percent stay calm and alert. Larger boats take longer to sink, so there should be plenty of time to get everyone into the lifeboats. Modern lifeboats are large, often fully covered and sometimes come equipped with motors. Once full, they're lowered into the water mechanically by large davits that hang over the edge of the ship. The International Maritime Organization's guidelines require that all cruise ships be able to get passengers lowered into the ocean in lifeboats within 30 minutes of passengers being gathered on deck.
- When a large ship sinks it will probably tilt, making it difficult to make your way to the deck. Hold handrails and go slowly to avoid slipping. Also keep an eye out for objects that could be sliding around. The last thing you want is to be near evacuation and get plowed by a grand piano. Try to stay behind large, fixed objects for pro-tection. The crew of the ship should be the last ones off the boat and assist each passenger in getting to their preassigned lifeboat.
- At least one life vest per passenger is required by law on board passenger ships. Keep the vests handy but secure so they don't get lost overboard during a capsize situation. Have a buddy assist you in wearing a life jackets/immersion suits in 60 seconds time. At least one life vest per passenger is required by law. Keep the vests handy but secure so they don't have an opportunity to go overboard. Flotation suits are a little more advanced than your average life vest. They're full body suits, with built-in shoes that keep you afloat and insulated—even in icy waters. In any case, put on all available waterproof clothing, including gloves and headgear.

- Locate your slot in the ship's muster and station bill and proceed to emergency/ assembly station. Collect your survival kit and try to enter life raft directly from the boat. If impossible, use minimal swimming effort to get on board.
- The crew of the ship should be the last ones off the boat and assist each passenger in getting to their preassigned lifeboat.
- Get to a safe distance from the sinking vessel. Ships sink with a large supply of air left aboard. The air forms bubbles and, together with implosions forming a drag or vortex that can drag down survivors floating within 10-30 meters depending on how big the ship is or how bouyant you are. Collect all available flotsam. The most unlikely articles can be adapted for use under survival conditions. Once in the water the life jacket should be adjusted down around the body as much as possible. Relax and take it as easy as possible in order not to overexert in order to conserve energy as you may have to remain in the water for a long time. The breast stroke and side stroke are considered the better ones to use as these assist in clearing the water ahead of any oil or vortex. The breast stroke is best for clearing a path through flaming oil. If any enemy bombing operations are in progress you should float on their backs or swim the back stroke for it has been found that survivors swimming on their stomachs and treading water have sustained serious internal injuries. If there is much oil on the water surface, a handkerchief tied over the mouth will help you to keep the oil out of the lungs and stomach. By pulling your shirt over the head, you can safely swim through an area of burning gasoline on top of the water. In the water, you must attempt to stay close to other survivors for mutual protection, easy identification from the air and rescue. Whistles and Boatswain's pipes are useful in attracting attention. You must realize that it is your life jackets that will help you survive in the water - not the life raft. The life raft can take in not more than ten adults. If there is no space for you, remember that there are short lines on the periphery of the raft. You must tie yourself to this trailing line so that you will not have to exert yourself continually to keep close to the drifting raft.

SURVIVAL AT SEA

In any major disaster occurring at sea, crew and passengers on board ships are lowered by life boats as part of an abandon ship drill. Where time precludes such orderly procedures, crew and passengers don life jackets and jump overboard and attempt to swim clear of the sinking vessel in order to avoid being sucked in by the vortex formed by a sinking ship. Life rafts are released overboard and these are self inflating and capable of accommodating 25 survivors. Where a distress message has been transmitted before going down, rescue can be expected within 48 hours in favourable weather conditions and position of the mishap. Where the SOS message is not possible, rescue can take five days or longer. Life rafts afford a high degree of protection from the elements and have succeeded in saving many lives in marine accidents. Life rafts must preferably stay in proximity of the location of the place of wreck as drifting off course would impede their being spotted by search and rescue parties zeroing in on the site of the disaster. Lookout must be kept for other survivors and the floating injured and exhausted should be pulled in on board the life raft from the lee (non wind facing side). All other life rafts must attempt to link up using 1 metre nylon lines provided in each raft and survivors must be divided equally among all the rafts. Unmanned life rafts must be salvaged and secured. Other flotsam and jetsam like clothing, containers of any type must be picked up as these may prove useful later on. The life raft is made of air-tight rubber-proofed high strength fabric. It has four major parts– the twin buoyancy rings, the floor, the arch or column supporting the canopy and the canopy itself. The buoyancy chambers and the central columns are inflated automatically with a mixture of carbon dioxide and nitrogen gases stored in cylinders on board. Provision exists for topping up pressures using the bellows provided. The floor is double layered to provide cushioning against the swell and also insulate against the cold. The canopy has a provision for collection of rainwater. The raft has two entrances provided with ladders for hauling oneself on board and a grab line to provide a hand-hold. Stability of the craft is ensured by water pockets and a sea anchor. Two paddles are provided. All sharp objects must be safely secured to avoid accidental puncture to the floatation chamber of the raft. If the inflation pressures exceeds normal, venting of excess gas occurs through the safety valve with a hissing/whistling sound which is quite normal. Immediately after boarding a raft, a careful inspection must be made for leaks and damage and leak-stoppers used to close small tears and punctures. Even if one of the buoyancy rings is damaged, a life raft can carry its full complement. Accessories provided on the raft must be inventoried. Bailers are essential to scoop out flooded water and sponges used to wipe the inner surface dry. The marker light on top of the life raft canopy and the interior light are lit as soon as the battery is activated on contact with seawater. It has a life of ten hours and the terminals can be disconnected during day time and shaking out the water within. A spare battery is sometimes included in the survival pack. The contents of the survival pack vary on international liners and other inland, coastal, short haul vessels. Their usual provisions are:

- Drinking water in plastic containers at a scale of 1 litres per person.
- Desalination tablets are also provided for preparing potable water from sea water with detailed instructions on the package.
- Barley sugar, glucose, chocolates, biscuits are provided to allow for 2500 calories per person per day.
- A calibrated drinking mug to allow measured intake of water.
- Can openers for opening water and food cans.
- Pyrotechnics:Two parachute rocket signals and six hand fired red flare cartridges.
- A signaling torch with spare cells and bulbs.
- A signaling whistle.
- A fishing tackle with adequate line and hooks.
- A comprehensive first aid kit.
- Anti seasickness tablets.

One energetic and prudent person on board must be nominated to handle the safety aspects of the craft and his or her directions must receive implicit obedience by others. He must establish a daily routine and be responsible for maintaining a detailed log book of the events of the day, commencing from the date, time and site of the accident, to include details of survivors, weather conditions, stock of rations available etc. Later entries must cover all details of the stay on the raft, rations issued, weather, sighting of ships/planes, morale of survivors etc. The survival packs must be in his charge and he must personally distribute water, rations, medicines etc. Smoking must not be permitted on board at any time.

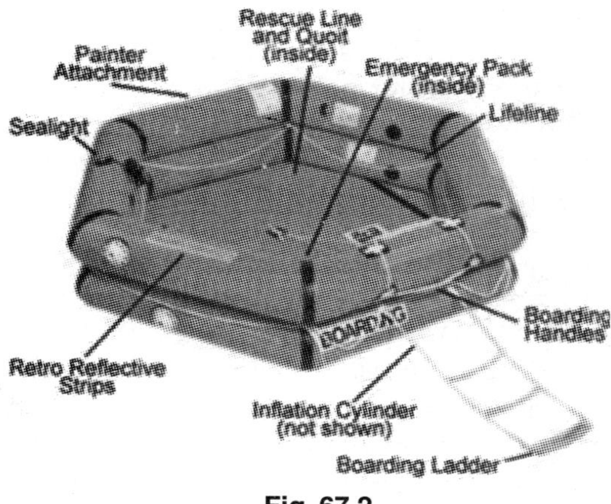

Fig. 67.2

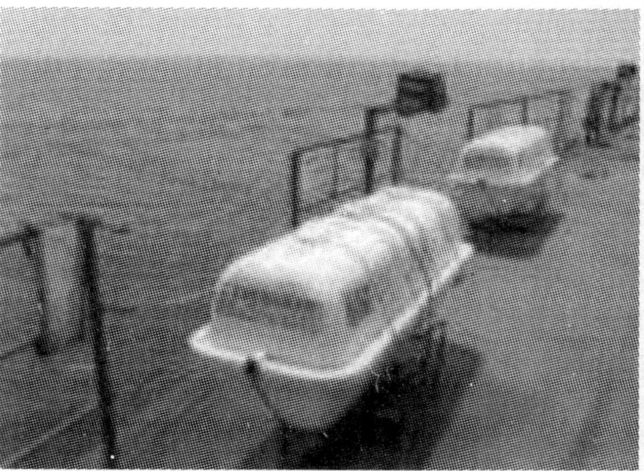

Fig. 67.3

Topping up of air in the buoyancy chambers and the arches/columns must be done periodically using bellows through valves marked Inflate Here or Safety Topping Up. The stoppers must be plugged tight after inflation.

Leaks must be repaired by patches large enough to overlap the hole/tear by 25 mm (1 inch). The site is thoroughly dried, roughened with sand paper provided and a layer of rubber solution applied and allowed to nearly dry. The same is applied to the patch and then a second layer of solution applied to both areas and pressed firmly into apposition using the provided wooden spatula. Inflation is commenced after a 2 minute waiting period.

A lookout must be kept through the day and night by watch-keepers keeping the torch and flares at hand. Unnecessary firing of flares must be avoided. Two persons keeping watch over a 2 hour period is recommended, one to serve as a lookout, and the other to check for leaks and collecting rainwater. Others must huddle together to prevent hypothermia and the entrance flaps must never be kept fully closed. In hot weather, the flaps can be kept fully open and outer canopy kept damp.

One of the most difficult aspects of being adrift at sea in a small life raft is the psychological toll it takes. Seeing nothing but open water everywhere can cause a lot of mental distress. This feeling of hopelessness can increase when boats and aircraft come nearby without seeing you. Survivors must occupy their time by playing word games or talking about future plans. This will help keep their mind off the situation and give them something to look forward to once you get rescued.

In rough seas, all survivors must wear life jackets and keep them inflated. If the raft capsizes it will continue to float upside down and survivors can exit via either of the entrances and cling on so that the raft does not drift away. The raft must be righted and boarded, then bailed and sponged dry. Righting can be done by one person and, in cold inclement weather by two persons. This is done by holding on to the righting strap, pushing down on the raft with the feet and throwing the bodyweight backwards at the same time. Survivors must be prepared to be submerged for a few seconds before swimming out from under the righted raft.

Diet: No water must be drunk by anyone, except for the sick and the injured during the first 24 hours. Consumption of water must be limited to 500ml per day thereafter. The lips must be moistened and the water taken in small sips and swilled in the mouth before swallowing. Empty cans can be used to store rainwater, even if in very small quantities. Plastic bags in the survival kit are also provided for this purpose. During rains, the canopy exterior must be cleaned to remove traces of salt and rationing must be adhered to even if collections are abundant. Excess intake after long period of fast can cause vomiting. Sea water, even if diluted with fresh water must not be drunk even in small quantities. Desalination tablets must be used as per instructions. Food rations must be distributed sparingly from the second day only. If water is in short supply, food must also be curtailed. Some types of seaweeds are edible. Fresh good seaweed is odorless and feels smooth and firm. Algae on the surface must be removed prior to consumption. Angling must be done by watch-keepers and generally all sea fish are edible. Excess fish may be dried and preserved for later use. Fish with spikes and which swell or bloat must be avoided. Fish skin or entrails can be used as bait. Sea birds can be safely eaten.

The body must be kept as dry as possible and survivors must remain in the shade to avoid sunburns and loss of body water by perspiration. Bathing overboard in seawater must be avoided as some of it may be swallowed and also, tropical waters may be frequented by sharks and predators. Skin inflammations must be covered with ointment or Vaseline. All survivors must take anti seasickness tablets as per instructions for the first 48 hours whether or not he or she feels seasick. Once accustomed to the raft movements, only those who still experience nausea should continue with the medications to prevent sea sickness and dehydration. Those prone to sea sickness must swallow one anti sea sickness tablet as early as possible and one every day in rough swell. The tablets make the mouth dry, and can cause drowsiness and blurred vision.

ATTRACTING ATTENTION

The life raft is fitted with a single or double unit Sarbe locator beacon or a flashing beacon. The locator beacon is a lightweight radio that transmits distress signals automatically on the international aviation UHF frequency of 243 Megahertz and also equipped with a transceiver on this frequency. The controls are easy to operate with Press to transmit and Press to Receive buttons on the beacon unit. The transceiver must only be used when in visual contact with an aircraft or a passing vessel as this will drain the battery significantly. When transmitting or receiving, the automatic distress signals are interrupted. The battery is water activated and connected to the beacon unit after the two nylon sealing plugs are removed. The black ring from the speech unit is removed to extend the aerial skywards and then mount the beacon and speech unit on the outside of the canopy in the pocket marked SARBE and into the sleeve on the canopy arch respectively. Under normal conditions, a life raft can be spotted at a distance of 4 nautical miles with the naked eye and by radar at 2 nautical miles. An empty water can attached to the highest point of the canopy improves detection by radar. Pyrotechnic signals can be seen at a distance of 25 nautical miles in good weather. Distress signals must be fired only when one is sure of these distances and when the ship or aircraft is veering away from your location. Sighting can be expected when the super structure of a ship or the flashing port and starboard lights on the wings of the aircraft can be made out by the naked eye. Flares must be fired strictly following the instructions on each signal pack. Careless handling can have disastrous results. Flares are fired into the wind from the lee side of the craft, holding it out as far away from the craft as possible. Mirror reflectors can be used in daytime and can be seen upto 2 nautical miles away. At night the water proof signaling torch can be used to transmit blink signals or by Morse code. When spotted, a plane will usually circle around to indicate that the raft has been noticed and its location radioed to other ships in the area. Some SAR planes carry rescue supply kits that will be air-dropped in the vicinity to provide essentials until final rescue. These are in the form of a string of containers containing food, water, clothes, medicines and comforts. To mark the location of the life raft, the SAR plane may drop a smoke flare. Rescue ships will approach the raft, keeping it on its lee side and then throw a line that must be made fast and then a life-boat may be lowered or some other rescue action instituted to pick up survivors. Rescue by helicopter is made, one survivor at a time by winch, net, rescue-sling or cradle. The weakest and women and children must be allowed first. The downward air draught from the hovering helicopter can be intense and destabilise the raft. Survivors must avoid abrupt movements or movement altogether to one area to avoid capsizing. Survivors must wear their life jackets at all times.

Further Reading

BR 1329, Handbook for Survivors in a 25 man inflatable liferaft, 1980).

THE PROBLEMS OF IMMERSION

Immersion in cold water <15°C stimulates the sympathetic system causing increases in heart rate and blood pressure. Victims find themselves incapacitated and even experienced swimmers cannot swim for very long in cold waters. Some may develop cramps or tetany. The vestigeal diving reflex is activated causing reduction in peripheral blood flow, breath holding and bradycardia. This response is exaggerated by fear. The pressure of the water surrounding the victim produces a hydrostatic squeeze that increases venous return and cardiac output by 25 to 35%. The same squeeze moves the diaphragm upwards and reduces FRC by 30-60%. These changes can prove disastrous in elderly patients and those with poor cardio respiratory reserve.

Also, rescue of submerged victims can reverse the effects of the hydrostatic squeeze and cause post rescue collapse. An after-drop in core temperature can also occur and precipitate ventricular fibrillation. ECG trace may show the Osborn 'J' wave at core temperatures below 35°C.

Management

Monitor ABG, base deficit, ECG, core temperature, urine output, CXR, TC, DC, urea, creatinine and sputum for culture, urine: plasma osmolality ratio. Treatment is aimed at restoration of adequate ventilation and circulation, prevention of further heat loss and slow rewarming, correction of acid-base status, treatment of bradycardia and arrhythmias. A broad spectrum antibiotic cover is advisable. Victims may have swallowed water and a full stomach situation must be presumed. Pulmonary edema is treated with diuretics and ventilation and cerebral oedema must be suspected where response to treatment is delayed. Role of corticosteroids is doubtful.

Treatment of Hypothermia

Hypothermia is classified as mild when a victim's core temperature is between 32° to 35°C (95°F), moderate when it is between 26°C (78.8°F) to 32° C and severe when it is below 26°C.

- Handle the patient gently.
- Prevent further heat loss.
- Evaluate ABC.
- For the patient in coma, consider Dextrose 50, Naloxone and Thiamine.

Options For Rewarming

Passive external rewarming, Insulating blanket, warm room, active external rewarming, heating blanket (Bair Hugger/Convective air warmers), heating lamps, hot water immersion,active internal rewarming, warm intravenous fluids, warm, humidified oxygen, Water's to and fro soda lime cannister, gastric, colonic, bladder, lavage, peritoneal, pleural, mediastinal lavage, continuous arteriovenous rewarming (CAVR), hemodialysis and cardio-pulmonary bypass.

Rewarming rates:

Passive external rewarming	-	0.5 to 2.0º C/hour
Shivering	-	2.0 to 3.0º C/hour
Warm gases	-	1.0 to 2.5º C/hour
Peritoneal dialysis	-	1.0 to 2.5º C/hour
CAVR	-	2.0 to 3.0º C/hour
CPB	-	10º C/hour

The diving reflex: Sea mammals can remain submerged for more than half an hour by shutting down their peripheral circulation and slowing the heart rate to as low as 2-3 beats/min. This reflex, mediated by the trigeminal nerve, independent of either the chemoreceptor or baroreceptor function, decreases cardiac output and prevents associated rise in blood pressure.In man, there is a vestigial diving reflex, more marked in children and exaggerated by cold and fear. This can cause severe bradycardia or asystole and result in dry drowning.

Poor prognosis is indicated by deterioration in level of consciousness after an initial improvement.

Further Reading

Problems of Immersion. Golden, FSC. J of Applied Medicine 1980:939-942).

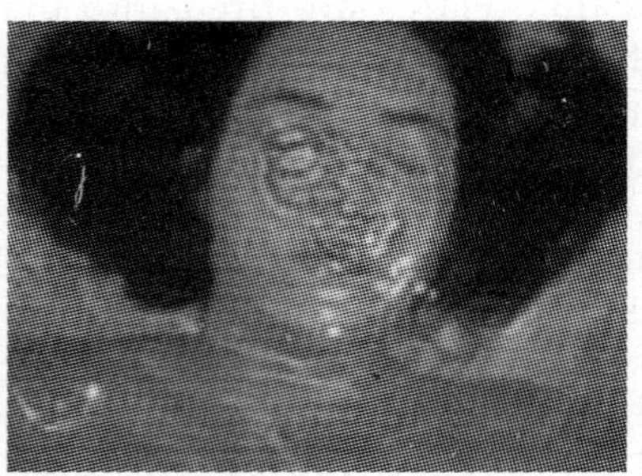

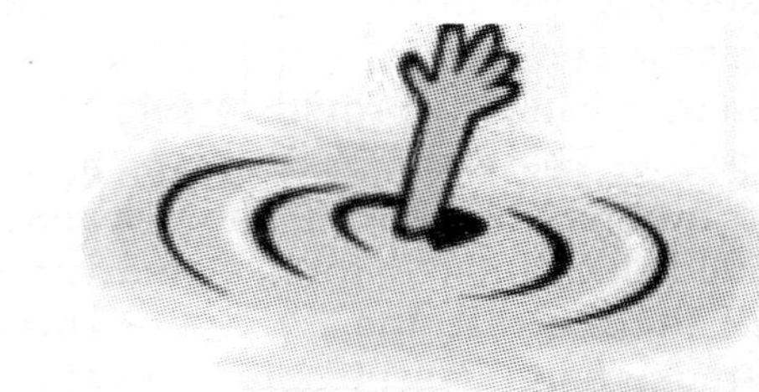

Fig. 67.4

DROWNING

Annually, approximately 150,000 deaths are reported worldwide from drowning, with an annual incidence probably closer to 500,000. Several of the most densely populated nations in the world fail to report near-drowning incidents. The adult mortality rate is difficult to quantify because of poor reporting and inconsistent record keeping. Thirty-five percent of immersion episodes in children are fatal; 33% result in some degree of neurologic impairment and 11% in severe neurologic sequelae. Male-to-female ratios are approximately 12:1 for boat-related drownings and 4:1 for non–boat-related drownings. Only in bathtub incidents do girls predominate in incidence. Peak incidences of submersion injury occur in the following 2 age groups: Children younger than 4 years and young adults aged 15-24 years. A high risk of death exists secondary to the development of adult respiratory distress syndrome (ARDS), which has been termed postimmersion syndrome or secondary drowning. Morbidity is due to neurologic insult as well as to multiple organ system failure.

DEFINITION

Drowning is a process resulting in primary respiratory impairment from submersion in a liquid medium. Implicit to this definition, is that a liquid-air.interface is present at the victim's airway. Outcome may include delayed morbidity or death, death, or life without morbidity. The terms wet drowning, dry drowning, active or passive drowning, near-drowning, secondary drowning, and silent drowning are now discarded.

Pathophysiology

Thermal conduction of water is 25-30 times that of air. The temperature of thermally neutral water, in which a nude individual's heat production balances heat loss, is 33°C. Physical exertion increases heat loss secondary to convection/conduction up to 35-50% faster. A significant risk of hypothermia usually develops in water temperatures less than 25°C, which is the temperature found in most natural waters during the majority of the year. During immersion in ice water, a subject will become hypothermic in approximately 30 minutes. Cooling at this temperature becomes life-threatening in approximately 60 minutes.

The principal physiologic consequences of drowning are prolonged hypoxemia and acidosis and the multiorgan effects of these processes. After initial gasping and possible aspiration, immersion stimulates hyperventilation, followed by voluntary apnea and a variable degree and duration of laryngospasm. This leads to hypoxemia. As the level of oxygen in the blood decreases, and the level of carbon dioxide increases. Increasing carbon dioxide levels lead to a stronger and stronger breathing reflex, up to the breath-hold breakpoint, at which the victim can no longer voluntarily hold his or her breath. This typically occurs at an arterial partial pressure of carbon dioxide of 55 mm Hg, but may differ significantly from individual to individual and can be increased through training. The breath-hold break point can be suppressed or delayed either intentionally or unintentionally. Hyperventilation before any dive, deep or shallow, flushes out carbon dioxide in the blood resulting in a dive commencing with an abnormally low carbon dioxide level; a potentially dangerous condition known as hypocapnia. The level of carbon dioxide in the blood after hyperventilation may then be insufficient to trigger the breathing reflex later in the dive and a blackout may occur without warning and before the diver feels any urgent need to breathe. This can occur at any depth and is common in distance breath-hold divers in swimming pools.

Depending upon the degree of hypoxemia and resultant acidosis, the person may develop myocardial dysfunction and electrical instability, cardiac arrest, and central nervous system (CNS) ischemia. Asphyxia leads to relaxation of the airway, which permits the lungs to take in water in many individuals (previously referred to as "wet drowning"), although most patients aspirate less than 4 mL/kg of fluid. Approximately 10-20% of individuals maintain tight laryngospasm until cardiac arrest occurs and inspiratory efforts have ceased. These victims do not aspirate any appreciable fluid (previously referred to as "dry drowning"). Most individuals are found after having been submerged in liquid for an unobserved period of time. Ingestion of large volumes of fresh-water, rather than aspiration, is the likely cause of clinically significant electrolyte disturbances, such as hyponatremia, in children after drowning.

The target organ of submersion injury is the lung. Aspiration of 1-3 mL/kg fluid leads to significantly impaired gas exchange. Injury to other systems is largely secondary to hypoxia and ischemic acidosis. Additional CNS insult may result from concomitant head or spinal cord injury. Fluid aspirated into the lungs produces vagally mediated pulmonary vasoconstriction and hypertension. Fresh water moves rapidly across the alveolar-capillary membrane into the microcirculation. Surfactant is destroyed, producing alveolar instability, atelectasis, and decreased compliance with marked ventilation/perfusion (V/Q) mismatching. As much as 75% of blood flow may circulate through hypoventilated lungs.

In salt water drowning, surfactant washout occurs, and protein-rich fluid exudates rapidly into the alveoli and pulmonary interstitium. Compliance is reduced, alveolar-capillary basement membrane is damaged directly, and shunting occurs. This results in rapid induction of serious hypoxia. Fluid-induced bronchospasm also may contribute to hypoxia. The distinction between fluid type is somewhat academic, as other than epidem-iologic importance, the initial treatment is similar.

Pulmonary hypertension may occur secondary to inflammatory mediator release. In a minor percentage of patients, aspiration of vomitus, sand, silt, stagnant water, and sewage may result in occlusion of bronchi, bronchospasm, pneumonia, abscess formation, and inflammatory damage to alveolar capillary membranes. Postobstructive pulmonary edema following laryngeal spasm and hypoxic neuronal injury with resultant neurogenic pulmonary edema may also play roles. Adult respiratory distress syndrome (ARDS) from altered surfactant effect and neurogenic pulmonary edema commonly complicate drowning in survivors. Commonly, these edematous, noncompliant lungs may be further compromised by ventilator-associated lung injury (VALI).

Primary CNS injury is a function of tissue hypoxia and ischemia. CNS injury has proven to be a major determinant of subsequent outcome. The brain will die after approximately six minutes without oxygen but special conditions may prolong this ('cold water drowning'). Freshwater contains less salt than blood and will therefore be absorbed into the blood stream by osmosis. In animal experiments this was shown to change the blood chemistry and led to cardiac arrest in 2 to 3 minutes. Sea water is much saltier than blood. Through osmosis water will leave the blood stream and enter the lungs thickening the blood. In animal experiments the thicker blood requires more work from the heart leading to cardiac arrest in 8 to 10 minutes. However, autopsies on human drowning victims show no indications of these effects and there appears to be little difference between drowning in salt water and fresh water. After death, rigor mortis will set in and remains for about two days, depending on many factors including water temperature.

If the period of ischemia is limited or the individual rapidly develops core hypothermia, injury may be limited and the individual may recover with minor neurologic sequelae. Prolonged hypoxia and ischemia may lead to primary and secondary injury from sustained acidosis, edema, hyperglycemia, hypotension, reperfusion, release of excitatory neurotransmitters, impaired cerebral autoregulation, and seizures.

Resultant autonomic instability (so-called diencephalic/hypothalamic storm) is common in severe hypoxic and ischemic brain injury and traumatic brain injury. It may lead to hypertension, tachycardia, diaphoresis, agitation, and muscle rigidity. More recently, it has also been found to present as takotsubo stress-induced cardiomyopathy, with associated ECG changes, apical ballooning on echocardiogram, and elevated serum troponin levels. Rhabdomyolysis and acute tubular necrosis are also well-recognized sequelae of drowning.

In young children sudden submerging the face in water colder than about 21 °C (70 °F) triggers the mammalian diving reflex, found in all mammals, and especially in marine mammals such as whales and seals. This reflex protects the body by putting it into *energy saving* mode to maximize the time it can stay under water. The strength of this reflex is greater in colder water and has three principal effects:

- *Bradycardia*, a slowing of the heart rate of up to 50% in humans.
- *Peripheral vasoconstriction*, the restriction of the blood flow to the extremities to increase the blood and oxygen supply to the vital organs, especially the brain.
- *Blood shift*, the shifting of blood to the thoracic cavity, the region of the chest between the diaphragm and the neck, to avoid the collapse of the lungs under higher pressure during deeper dives.

The reflex action is automatic and allows both a conscious and an unconscious person to survive longer without oxygen under water than in a comparable situation on dry land. The exact mechanism for this effect has been debated and may be a result of brain cooling similar to the protective effects seen in patients treated with deep hypothermia.

After death, rigor mortis will set in and remains for about two days, depending on many factors including water temperature.

SECONDARY DROWNING

Water, regardless of its salt content, will damage the inside surface of the lung, collapse the alveoli and cause pulmonary edema with a reduced ability to exchange air. This may cause death up to 72 hours after a near drowning incident. This is called secondary drowning. Inhaling certain poisonous vapors or gases will have a similar effect.

Freshwater can be more dangerous than salt water in secondary drowning. When fresh water enters the lungs it is pulled into the pulmonary circulation via the alveoli because of the low capillary hydrostatic pressure and high colloid osmotic pressure. Consequently, the plasma is diluted and the hypotonic environment causes red blood cells to burst (hemolysis). The resulting elevation of plasma K^+ level and depression of Na^+ level, due to the hemolysis, alter the electrical activity of the heart. Ventricular fibrilation often occurs as a result of these electrolyte changes. Additionally, if drowning occurs in very cold water (<10° C), the uptake of cold water into the vascular system can stop the heart. In open heart surgery, the technique of pouring cold saline solution over the heart is used to slow down enzymes in destroying the cells of the heart. If the victim is resuscitated death can occur hours later due to renal failure. During hemolysis, hemoglobin is also released into the plasma which can accumulate in the kidneys leading to acute renal failure. In contrast, salt-water drowning does not lead to uptake of inspired water into the vascular system because it is hypertonic to blood. Therefore, no hemolysis occurs and the cause of death is asphyxia.

Management

The first step in rescuing a drowning victim is to ensure your own safety. Then bring the victim's mouth and nose above the water surface. For further treatment it is advisable to remove the victim from the water. Conscious victims may panic and thus hinder rescue efforts. Often, a victim will cling to the rescuer and try to pull himself out of the water, submerging the rescuer in the process. To avoid this, it is recommended that the rescuer approach the panicking victim with a buoyant object, or from behind, twisting the victim's arm on the back to restrict movement. If the victim pushes the rescuer under water, the rescuer should dive downwards to escape the victim.

Actively drowning victims do not usually call out for help simply because they lack the air to do so. It is necessary to breathe to yell. Human physiology does not allow the body to waste any air when starving for it. They rarely raise their hands out of the water. They use the surface of the water to push themselves up in an attempt to get their mouths out of the water. Lifting arms out of the water always pushes the head down. Head low in the water, occasionally bobbing up and down is another common sign of active drowning.

There can be splashing involved during drowning, usually a butterfly like stroke where the hands barely clear the waters surface, and sometimes victims can look like they are climbing an invisible ladder in the water.

Extenuating factors such as increased levels of stress, secondary injuries, and environmental factors can increase the likelihood of distress and/or drowning in persons who end up overboard. It is important that you recognize the behaviors associated with aquatic distress and drowning, so you can make informed decisions during emergencies.

Signs or behaviors associated with drowning or near-drowning:

- Head low in the water, mouth at water level.
- Head tilted back with mouth open.
- Eyes glassy and empty, unable to focus.
- Eyes open, with fear evident on the face.
- Hair over forehead or eyes.
- Hyperventilating or gasping.
- Trying to swim in a particular direction but not making headway.
- Trying to roll over on the back to float.
- Uncontrollable movement of arms and legs, rarely out of the water.

After successfully approaching the victim, negatively buoyant objects such as a weight belt are removed. The priority is then to transport the victim to the water's edge in preparation for removal from the water. The victim is turned on his or her back. A secure grip is used to tow panicking victims from behind, with both rescuer and victim lying on their backs, and the rescuer swimming a breaststroke kick. A cooperative victim may be towed in a similar fashion held at the armpits, and the victim may assist with a breaststroke kick. An unconscious victim may be pulled in a similar fashion held at the chin and cheeks, ensuring that the mouth and nose are well above the water.

There is also the option of pushing a cooperative victim lying on his or her back with the rescuer swimming on his or her belly and pushing the feet of the victim, or both victim and rescuer lying on the belly, with the victim hanging from the shoulders of the rescuers. This has the advantage that the rescuer can use both arms and legs to swim breaststroke, but if the victim pushes his or her head above the water, the rescuer may get pushed down. This method is often used to retrieve tired swimmers. If the victim wears lifejacket, buoyancy compensator, or other flotation device that stabilizes his or her position with the face up, only one hand of the rescuer is needed to pull the victim, and the other hand may provide forward movement or may help in rescue breathing while swimming, using for example a snorkel.

Special care has to be taken for victims with suspected spinal injuries, and a back board (spinal board) may be needed for the rescue. In water, CPR is ineffective, and the goal should be to bring the victim to a stable ground quickly and then to start CPR.

If the approach to a stable ground includes the edge of a pool without steps or the edge of a boat, special techniques have been developed for moving the victim over the obstacle. For pools, the rescuer stands outside, holds the victim by his or her hands, with the victim's back to the edge. The rescuer then dips the victim into the water quickly to achieve an upward speed of the body, aiding with the lifting of the body over the edge. Lifting a victim over the side of a boat may require more than one person. Special techniques are also used by the coast guard and military for helicopter rescues.

After reaching dry ground, all victims should be referred to medical assistance, especially if unconscious or if even small amounts of water have entered the lungs. An unconscious victim may need artificial respiration or CPR. If this is the case, it is recommended that the patient be positioned on their back with the head level to the body. The goal should be to perform chest compressions if the patient is pulseless, and if the patient isn't breathing to push air into the lungs even though the lungs may be filled with some amount of water.

The Heimlich maneuver is not recommended; the technique may have relevance in situations where airways are obstructed by solids but not fluids. Performing the manoeuver on drowning victims not only delays ventilation but may induce vomiting, which if aspirated will place the patient in a far worse situation. Oxygen may be administered and treatment for hypothermia may also be necessary. Water in the stomach need not be removed, except in the case of paediatric drownings, as a gastric distension can limit movement of the lungs. Other injuries should also be treated. Victims that are alert, awake, and intact have a nearly 100% survival rate.

Drowning victims should be treated even if they have been submerged for a long time. The rule "no patient should be pronounced dead until warm and dead" applies. Children in particular have a good chance of survival in water up to 3 minutes, or 10 minutes in cold water (10 to 15 °C or 50 to 60 °F). Submersion in cold water can slow the metabolism drastically. There are rare but documented cases of survivable submersion for extreme lengths of time.

Prehospital Care

The focus is on the following important points:

- Optimal prehospital care is a significant determinant of outcome in the management of immersion victims. The victim should be removed from the water at the earliest opportunity. Rescue breathing should be performed while the individual is still in water, but chest compressions are inadequate because of buoyancy issues. The patient should be removed from the water with attention to cervical spine precautions. If possible, the individual should be lifted out in a prone position. Theoretically, hypotension may follow lifting the individual out in an upright manner because of the relative change in pressure surrounding the body from water to air. Management of the ABCs is the priority, with particular attention to securing the earliest possible airway and providing adequate oxygenation and ventilation.
- In the patient with an altered mental status, the airway should be checked for foreign material and vomitus.
- Intrinsic compressions to remove water from the lungs is not recommended, as they have proven not to remove fluid, delay the start of resuscitation, risk causing the patient to vomit and aspirate, and ventilation is achieved even if fluid is present in the lung. If the rescuer is unable to ventilate the patient, then an airway clearing method should be attempted.
- Immediately place the patient on 100% oxygen by mask. If available, continuous noninvasive pulse oximetry is optimal. If

the patient remains dyspneic on 100% oxygen, or manifests a low oxygen saturation, use CPAP if available. If it is not available, consider early intubation, with appropriate use of positive end-expiratory pressure (PEEP).

- Immobilize the neck if the patient has facial or head injury, is unable to give an adequate history, or may have been involved in a diving accident or MVA.
- More traditional literature proposes that prehospital care providers should begin rewarming. Wet clothing is ideally removed before the victim is wrapped in warming blankets. More recent studies suggest that therapeutic cooling may actually be beneficial in patients to reduce ischemic brain injury. This area needs additional vigorous clinical research to determine the most efficacious treatment strategy.

Emergency Department Care

Initial management of near drowning should place emphasis on immediate resuscitation and treatment of respiratory failure. Evaluate associated injuries early, as a cervical spine injury may complicate airway management. Provide all victims of a submersion injury with supplemental oxygen during their evaluations.

- *ET intubation:* Intubation may be required in order to provide adequate oxygenation in a patient unable to maintain a pO_2 of greater than 60-70 mm Hg (>80 mm Hg in children) on 100% oxygen by face mask.
- In the alert, cooperative patient, use a trial of bilevel positive airway pressure (BiPAP)/CPAP, if available, to provide adequate oxygenation before intubation is performed.
- **Other criteria for ET intubation include the following:**
  - Altered level of consciousness and inability to protect airway or handle secretions.
  - High alveolar-arterial (A-a) gradient—PaO_2 of 60-80 mm Hg or less on 15 L oxygen nonrebreathing mask.
  - Respiratory failure—$PaCO_2$ >45 mm Hg
  - Worsening ABG results.
- Intubated victims of submersion injury may require PEEP with mechanical ventilation to maintain adequate oxygenation. PEEP has been shown to improve ventilation patterns in the noncompliant lung in several ways, including. (1) shifting interstitial pulmonary water into the capillaries, (2) increasing lung volume via prevention of expiratory airway collapse, (3) providing better alveolar ventilation and decreasing capillary blood flow, and (4) increasing the diameter of both small and large airways to improve distribution of ventilation.
- ECMO has been shown to be helpful in individuals who remain hypoxic despite aggressive mechanical ventilation.
- Bronchoscopy may be needed to remove foreign material, such as aspirated debris or vomitus plugs from the airway.
- *Temperature management:* Optimal temperature management in drowning patients is a current topic of significant research and clinical interest. Hypothermic patients with core temperatures less than 86°F, who have undergone sudden, rapid immersion, may display slowing of metabolism and preferential shunting of blood to the heart, brain, and lungs, which may exert a protective effect during submersion. This is not, however, the case with most immersion victims, who have become hypothermic gradually and are at risk for ventricular fibrillation and neurologic injury. As such, traditional studies

would suggest vigorous rewarming of hypothermic patients to normothermia. In order to rewarm, a number of modalities may be used.

- Place a nasogastric tube to assist in rewarming efforts and urinary catheter to assess urine output.
- Core rewarming with warmed oxygen, continuous bladder lavage with fluid at 40°C, and intravenous (IV) infusion of isotonic fluids at 40°C should be initiated during resuscitation.
- Warm peritoneal lavage may be required for core rewarming in patients with severe hypothermia.
- A cascade unit on the ventilator provides warm inspired air.
- Thoracotomy with open heart massage and warm mediastinal lavage may be effective. The hypothermic heart is typically unresponsive to pharmacotherapy and countershock.
- Extracorporeal blood rewarming may be used in patients with severe hypothermia who do not respond to lavage/thoracotomy or who are in arrest.
- Attempt central venous access cautiously in these patients in order to avoid stimulation of the hypothermic atrium and resultant dysrhythmias.
- Do not abandon resuscitation of a submersion victim until the patient has been warmed to a minimum of 30°C.
- Newer literature, however, suggests that therapeutic hypothermia may be effective in reducing ischemic brain injury.
- Therapeutic hypothermia (TH) improves oxygen supply to ischemic brain areas, decreases cerebral metabolic demand, and decreases increased intracranial pressure and confers neuroprotection.
- Initiate appropriate treatment of hypoglycemia and other electrolyte imbalances; seizures; bronchospasm; and cold-induced bronchorrhea, dysrhythmias, and hypotension as necessary.

Patient disposition depends on the history, presence of associated injuries, and degree of immersion injury.

- Patients able to relay a good history of minor immersion injury, without evidence of significant injury and without evidence of bronchospasm, tachypnea/dyspnea, or inadequate oxygenation (by ABG analysis and pulse oximetry) can be safely discharged from the ED after 6-8 hours of observation. However, be aware that these studies did not include older individuals or in those with underlying medical conditions that might place them at increased risk of hypoxic injury and acidosis.
- Victims of mild to moderately severe submersion, who only have mild symptoms that improve during observation and have no abnormalities on ABG analysis or pulse oximetry and chest radiograph, should be observed for a more prolonged period of time in the ED or observation unit.
- Certain patients may display mild to moderately severe hypoxemia that is corrected easily with oxygen. Admit these patients to the hospital for observation. They can be discharged after resolution of hypoxemia if they have no further complications.
- Admit patients who require intubation and mechanical ventilation to the ICU. Varying degrees of neurologic as well as pulmonary insults typically complicate their courses.

Consultations

- Neurosurgical, orthopedic, or trauma consultation (institution dependent) is required for patients with concomitant significant head or neck trauma.

- Early consultation with the intensivist or admitting physician is wise for patients who exhibit pulmonary or CNS insult in order to coordinate ongoing ICU care.
- Cardiovascular, intensivist, or trauma surgical consultation may be necessary for patients who require bypass for rewarming or ECMO.

Medication

Cold-induced bronchorrhea or irritation of the tracheobronchial tree by inhaled water or particulate material can produce cough and bronchospasm. Manage these aggressively because they may worsen hypoxia. The DOC is an inhaled beta-agonist bronchodilator. Sympathomimetic agents like Albuterol relax bronchial smooth muscle during bronchospasm with little effect on cardiac muscle contractility. For adults it is nebulized: 1.25-2.5 mg diluted in 2-5 mL sterile saline or water and for children <5 years: 1.25-2.5 mg q4-6h prn.

Further Inpatient Care

- The primary management goals are good pulmonary care and preservation of CNS perfusion and function.
- Certain patients may display mild to moderately severe hypoxemia that is corrected easily with oxygen. Admit these patients to the hospital for observation. They can be discharged after resolution of hypoxemia if they have no further complications.
- Admit patients who require intubation and mechanical ventilation to the ICU. Varying degrees of neurologic as well as pulmonary insults typically complicate their course. Pulmonary hypertension may result from the release of inflammatory mediators, increasing right ventricular afterload, and decreasing left ventricular preload and pulmonary perfusion. Newer ventilatory modes, including airway pressure release ventilation and high frequency oscillatory ventilation can decrease the risk of VALI.
- In patients with significant lung disease but a reasonable likelihood of neurologic recovery, ECMO has been used successfully to treat pulmonary insufficiency.
- Myocardial dysfunction may result from PEA, dysrhythmias due to hypoxemia, acidosis, electrolyte disturbances, or hypothermia. These are usually transient in nature.
- Look for evidence of ARDS; multiple organ system failure; nosocomial infection, especially pneumonia; and/or gastric stress ulceration.
- Management of ARDS due to submersion is similar to that of ARDS from other causes.
- Use of permissive hypercapnia to decrease barotrauma in many patients with ARDS may not be appropriate in this setting of hypoxic ischemic CNS injury.
- The extent of invasive monitoring needed (e.g., arterial catheter, pulmonary artery catheter, central venous pressure catheter) is determined by the degree of hemodynamic or respiratory instability and the presence of renal failure.
- Invasive monitoring of intracranial pressure has been shown in both human and animal studies to be neither useful nor necessary.
- Watch for evidence of pneumonia and CNS infection. Uncommon infections may present late and unusually. Prophylactic antimicrobial therapy has not proven beneficial.
- Begin early and aggressive rehabilitation to prevent disuse injury.

Further Outpatient Care

- Outpatient care is dictated by the nature and degree of residual functional impairment. With severe neurologic impairment, the patient may benefit from admission to a rehabilitation facility and aggressive rehabilitation. In one case report, neuropsychological testing delineated problems with memory, visuo-spatial performance, executive function, verbal fluency, flexibility, planning, and abstraction. Visuo-spatial testing, verbal learning, recall, and logical reasoning showed improvement during their 3-year follow-up period.

- Patients able to relay a good history of minor immersion injury, without evidence of significant injury and without evidence of bronchospasm, tachypnea/dyspnea, or inadequate oxygenation (by ABG analysis and pulse oximetry) can be discharged from the ED after 6-8 hours of observation.
- Be aware that early ED discharge has not been studied in older individuals or in those with underlying medical conditions that might place them at increased risk of hypoxic injury. As such, these factors should be taken into consideration during discharge planning.
- Victims of mild to moderately severe submersion, who have only mild symptoms that improve during observation and have no abnormalities on ABG analysis or chest radiograph, can be discharged after a longer period of observation in the ED or observation unit.
- Tell discharged patients to return immediately if they develop dyspnea, cough, and/or fever.

Transfer

- Patients who exhibit significant hypoxia that requires intubation, worsening dyspnea with the potential for intubation, evidence of hypoxic cerebral injury, evidence of renal insufficiency, evidence of hemolysis, or severe hypothermia requiring cardiopulmonary bypass must be in a facility capable of providing appropriate, age-related intensive care.
- Manage patients who require care for significant cervical spine or head trauma in a facility capable of sophisticated neurologic monitoring and neurosurgical intervention.

Laboratory Studies

- *Arterial blood gas analysis*
  Arterial blood gas (ABG) analysis is probably the most reliable clinical parameter in patients who are asymptomatic or mildly symptomatic. A surprising degree of hypoxia can exist without clinical signs.
- Obtain blood for a rapid glucose determination, CBC count, electrolyte levels, lactate level, and coagulation profile, if indicated. Collect urine for urinalysis, if indicated.
- If initial test results show elevated serum creatinine level, marked metabolic acidosis, abnormal urinalysis, or significant lymphocytosis, serial estimations of serum creatinine should be performed.
- Acute renal impairment is known to occur frequently in near drowning, and, while usually mild (serum creatinine level <0.3 mmol/L or 3.4 mg/dL), severe renal impairment requiring dialysis may occur.
- Consider a blood alcohol level and urine toxicology screen for use of drugs.

Imaging Studies

- Chest radiography.
- For evidence of aspiration, pulmonary edema, or segmental atelectasis suggesting foreign body(s) (eg, silt or sand aspiration).
- For evaluation of endotracheal (ET) tube placement.
- Cervical spine radiograph or computed tomography (CT) scanning in individuals

with an appropriate history, neck pain, or if doubt exists about the circumstances surrounding the submersion injury.
- Non-contrast head CT scanning in an individual with altered mental status and a suggestive or unclear history.

Other Tests

- Continuous pulse oximetry.
- Electrocardiography if evidence of significant tachycardia, bradycardia, or dysrhythmia or risk of underlying cardiac disease.

Prevention

Children have drowned in buckets and toilets. The reduction of drowning through education and basic prevention steps has become a necessity. In order to avoid drowning, emphasis should be made in the following areas:

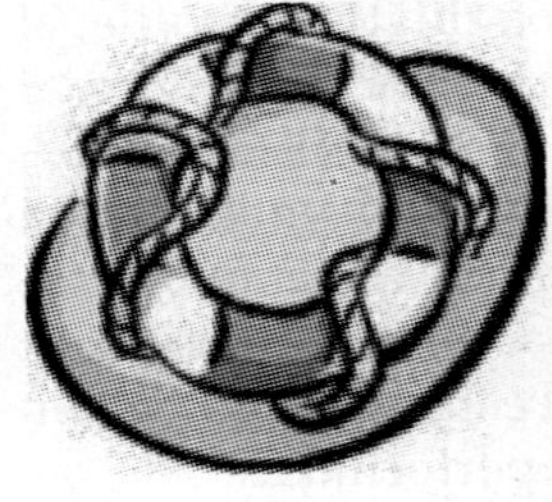

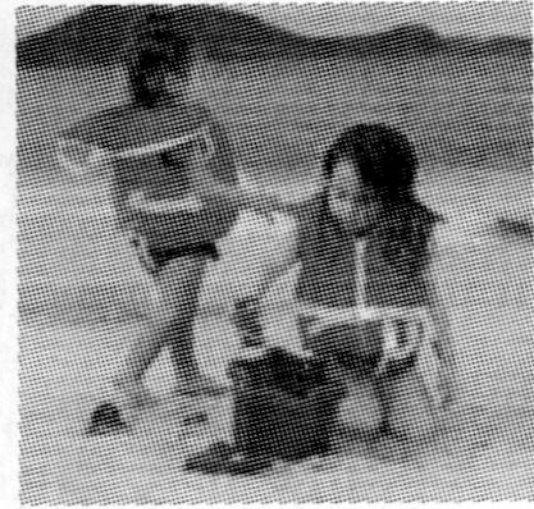

Fig. 67.5

Training

- Learn how to swim.
- Learn basic water rescue and basic life support.

Practices to be considered:

- Children, especially toddlers, should be supervised at all times when they are around water, including a bathtub or bucket full of water. Household buckets should be immediately emptied after use and left empty when not in use. Water containing objects, such as water tanks and cisterns, should have childproof fastenings and solid tops. They should not have items adjacent that afford children easy access.
- All pools should be fenced appropriately, with the gate to the area locked when not in use under adult supervision. These fences should be at least 4-5 ft tall. Pools not in use may be made safer with appropriately fitted and maintained pool covers and alarms, but these have not been shown to prevent drowning. Any windows with access to the pool area should remain closed and locked. Parents who own pools or who take their children to pools are encouraged to learn CPR. Children should wear personal flotation devices in pool areas, but these do not obviate the need for constant supervision. Children should be taught to swim, but these lessons should not provide parents with a false sense of security.
- All individuals involved in boating activities should be able to swim, should use personal flotation devices when on the boat or in the water, and should avoid the use of alcohol or other recreational drugs. Boaters should be taught to anticipate wind, waves, and water temperature, and to use protective suits and other insulating garments in cold weather.
- All children should be taught to check the water carefully for depth and possible injurious objects before diving in. Children should also be taught their swimming limitations and to not play dangerously in natural water areas, pools, or on the decks surrounding pools.
- All individuals should be taught not to drink alcohol or use other recreational drugs when swimming.
- Individuals with underlying medical illnesses that may place them at risk when

swimming, such as seizure disorders, diabetes mellitus, significant coronary artery disease, severe arthritis, and disorders of neuromuscular function, should swim under the observation of another adult who can rescue them should they get into trouble.

- Individuals should not swim alone.
- Keep a watch out for others.
- Keep children under full view.
- Swim only in areas where adequate supervision is present (i.e., a trained and certified Lifeguard).
- Have a locked fence around swimming pools.
- Bring a cordless telephone to the pool, so children are not left unsupervised while answering a phone call.
- Have cold-acclimatisation training prior to swimming in very cold waters.
- Ensure that boats that are in use are reliable, properly loaded and that functional emergency equipment is onboard.
- Wear a properly fitting lifejacket while enjoying water sports such as sailing, surfing or canoeing.
- Pay attention to the weather, tides and water conditions, and especially currents. Currents are usually perceived from the outside as weaker than they actually are.
- Be aware of your personal limits.

Practices to be avoided:

- Diving into water where the bottom cannot clearly be seen or the depth determined.
- Swimming alone.
- Swimming at night.
- Swimming while under the influence of drugs or alcohol.
- Using hyperventilation in an attempt to extend a breath-hold dive. See deep and shallow water blackout.
- Relying wholly on swimming aids, as they may fail.
- Playing games that will put your life, or others' at risk.
- Walking on ice, unless it is known in absolute certainty that the ice is thick enough over the entire route.

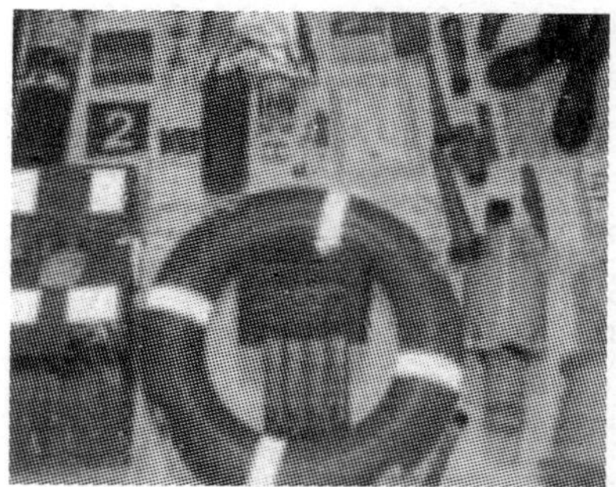

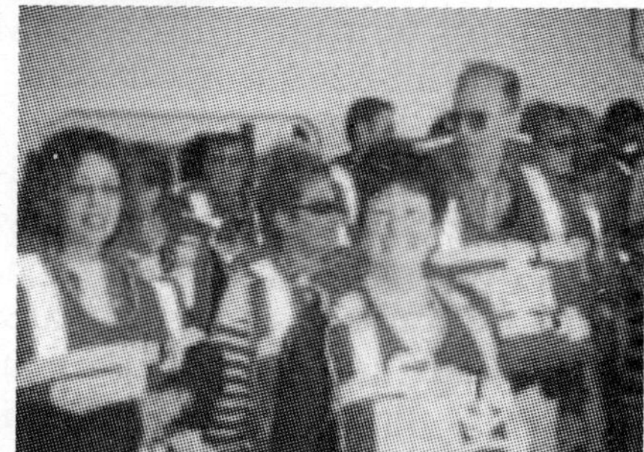

Fig. 67.6

SAFETY ASPECTS ON BOARD SHIPS

Construction

Basic principles and goals for goal-based standards (GBS) for new ship construction were agreed in principle by IMO's Maritime Safety Committee (MSC) when it met for its 80th session from 11 to 20 May 2005. The Tier I goals are based on the premise that ships are to be designed and constructed for a specified design life and to be safe and environmentally friendly, when properly operated and maintained under the specified operating and environmental conditions throughout their life of 25 years or less in accordance with relevant long-term sea state scatter diagrams relating to structural strength, fatigue life, residual strength and protection against corrosion. Ship safety has to be verified at design and construction stages and during the ship's operational period so that it remains safe for its entire economic life. The standards would also have to ensure that all parts of a ship can be easily accessed to permit proper inspection and ease of maintenance. the International Code for the Construction and Equipment of Ships Carrying Dangerous Chemicals in Bulk (IBC Code), ordains specifics related to fire protection, fire extinction, including the fitting of a system for continuous monitoring of the concentration of flammable vapors on ships of 500 gross tonnage. Resolution MSC.81(70) deals with life-saving appliances, including revisions and prototype tests for lifebuoys, lifejackets, immersion suits, anti-exposure suits and thermal protective aids, pyrotechnics such as rocket parachute flares, hand flares and buoyant smoke signals, life rafts, lifeboats, rescue boats and fast rescue boats. It also details on launching and embarkation appliances, position-indicating lights for life-saving appliances and hydrostatic release units; and revisions to production and installation tests for survival craft, and its launching and stowage arrangements. International Life-Saving Appliance Code (LSA Code), also deals with matters related to life rafts, life boats and rescue boats, particularly in relation to stowage and release mechanisms testing and calculations for buoyancy, stability. The MSC and its Working Group on Goal-based Standards (GBS) for New Ship Construction has adopted a prescriptive approach on GBS for hull construction of bulk carriers and oil tankers and a safety level approach for all other ship types and agreed on a five-tier system, consisting of goals (Tier I), functional requirements (Tier II), verification of compliance criteria (Tier III), technical procedures and guidelines, classification rules and industry standards (Tier IV) and codes of practice and safety and quality systems for shipbuilding, ship operation, maintenance, training, manning, etc. (Tier V). The MSC has finalized the technical specifications of the components of the Long-Range Identification and Tracking (LRIT) System and its wider applications for safety, especially search and rescue. LRIT has been made mandatory on board ships on international voyages, passenger liners, high-speed craft, and cargo ships of 300 gross tonnage and upwards and including and mobile offshore drilling units.

Ship design and construction is the use of defensive engineering and defensive design that analyzes alternatives to proposed design steps, and then assesses the relative safety, cost, functionability and repairability of the alternatives, prior to making a design decision. Engineers have to strive and work beyond the specifications or standards given by authorities and then clearly spell out the basis for their design decisions. This involves the ship owner, the owner's naval architect, the shipyard, and its subcontracting naval architects who produce the working drawings. The in-place foremen of the shipyard work force, as well as the owner's construction supervisors, must be in a position to identify potential sources of equipment failures, inoperability or injury and undertake modifications to enhance the safety of the vessel without going back to the owner's home office for approval. These change-order procedures for the sake of safety should be more readily accomplishable and more easily justified to ensure it is fulfilled. The cost overruns would be negligible if implemented at the outset of contract development between the shipyard and the yard's naval architects by added design effort. The owner could also advise his naval architect to identify such areas during the course of development of contracts, plans as well as during the construction supervision phase. The contracts between vessel owner and shipyard could be augmented by a provision requiring the shipyard to advise the owner of possible added safety measures, obtainable through defensive engineering. Component suppliers can also benefit from the feedbacks from the purchaser as to the use and maintenance of the supplied equipment to have a more thorough knowledge of the on-going use and life of his product. Then, as in the aircraft industry, component manufacturers could send notices to the users for suggested overhauls, modifications, or withdrawals from service of that particular piece of equipment. All this will certainly add to the cost of contracting, the cost of doing business and the cost of acquiring the vessel, but if it permeates all aspects of contract management, that cost would be small and worthwhile.

A double hull is a design and construction method where the bottom and sides of the ship have two complete layers of watertight hull surface: one outer layer forming the normal hull of the ship, and a second inner hull which is somewhat further into the ship, perhaps a few feet, which forms a redundant barrier to seawater in case the outer hull is damaged and leaks.The space in between the two hull layers is often used as storage tanks for fuel or ballast water.Double hulls are a more extensive safety measure than double bottoms, which have two hull layers only in the bottom of the ship and not the sides. In low energy casualties, double hulls can prevent flooding beyond the penetrated compartment. Watertight compartments, or hull divisions, are another safety feature. If a puncture occurs on a shipside, the incoming water is contained and isolated to keep the ship afloat until rescue or repair. The Joint MSC/MEPC Working Group on Human Element considers the human element issues, including the report of the Group of Independent Experts established by the Secretary-General and its impact and effectiveness in the enhancement of safety of life at sea and protection of the marine environment. It also considers the report of the Inter-Industry Working Group (IIWG), established to study the reported incidents of explosions on chemical and product carriers and evolve guidelines for abandonment of ships alongside in port and aspects of human element research related to ship safety.

Fire Protection

Fires on board ships are one of the most serious risks to property and persons, as well as for the surrounding environment. A ship is evidently subject to the same risks with regard to fire as a civil or industrial land structure. On board ship there are tons of liquid fuel, electrical equipment, air-conditioning plants, engines, boilers, stores of flammable material and crew accommodation areas (kitchens, mess rooms, lounges, cabins, WCs). To all this we must add the load, which in cargo vessels consists of a high percentage of solid and liquid goods that are flammable or at least combustible, and often of a dangerous nature. In passenger ships the load consists of accommodation and entertainment facilities for the passengers and, in ferries, of a large garage spaces for motor vehicles. Offshore rigs and tanker storage ships are essentially oil plants. There is a requirement for fixed fire detection and alarm systems, including requirements for fire detectors and manually operated call points capable of being remotely and individually identified.

Enhanced fire safety of atriums, the means of escape in case of fire, orderly evacuation and abandonment, including requirements for the essential systems to remain operational in case any one main vertical zone is unserviceable due to fire has to be ensured on board all ships. The International Code for Fire Safety Systems (FSS Code) oversees the fire protection arrangements in relation to cabin balconies on passenger vessels, deployment of free-fall lifeboats during abandon-ship drills, either by only the required operating crew on board, or even without the operating crew on board. Fire extinguishers, specifically portable foam applicators, fixed foam fire-extinguishing systems, fixed-pressure water-spraying and water-mist fire-extinguishing systems are mandatory.

All passenger ships are today required to be equipped with ship-wide sprinkler system, which greatly reduces the risk of fire spreading uncontrollably. In addition, the requirements for structural fire protection, or fire insulation, are such that, at least in theory, the vessel would survive a fire for one hour even without sprinklers, giving time for passenger and crew to abandon the vessel. The fire protection especially on new ships is at a very high level, and older passengers vessels are also today retroactively fitted with sprinkler systems. Thus the main risk does not usually come from inadequate fire protection, but from a non-working sprinkler system: it is possible that the ship's only sprinkler pump unit is destroyed in a collision. This risk is avoided on many new ships by dividing the sprinkler system between two or three redundant pump units. Another risk is always an installation or user failure: if a section valve is accidentally left closed after maintenance, the sprinkler system will not work as planned. When the systems get larger and more complicated, possibility of different failures normally increases. A recent example of balcony fires has caused a rapid change in rules. However, there are also other spaces onboard that by rules are not required to, and thus usually do not have sprinklers: examples are the bathrooms, both in cabins and in public spaces and ship's air conditioning rooms. A fire is of course not so likely to start from these spaces, but so was the case with balconies as well.

Freefall lifeboats have become more prevalent, and mandatory on bulk carriers. Ships crews are able to board and launch a freefall lifeboat quicker than a conventional lifeboat, which usually means a quicker evacuation in an emergency. Some of these lifeboats can be launched from heights of over 30 metres. Regular inspections, tests and services by manufacturer-trained and approved technicians are now mandatory for all SOLAS ships. These rules require regular tests and inspections of lifeboats, release gear and davit winches, and specify that whilst weekly and monthly work can be carried out by on board personnel, they must be done to the standards set down by the manufacturer. The guidelines require owners to use correct spares and technicians approved by the original equipment manufacturer. The annual and five-yearly tests and service have to be done by personnel trained and authorised by the manufacturer. Where the manufacturer's own engineers are not available, there are a number of authorised service companies whose engineers must be trained by the lifeboat manufacturers.

Some of the problems that service engineers have found include:

- Excessive paint or rust.
- Indicator showing unsafe situation.
- No grease on wire falls.
- No records on board of maintenance.
- No pendant eyes on davit, making it harder to inspect.

The irony here is that a chief engineer is able to operate and maintain the engine and machinery on a supertanker or large container ship, but seemingly incapable of maintaining a lifeboat.

Maritime Safety Committee in 2002, identified the following causes of lifeboat accidents:

- Failure of on-load release mechanism.
- Inadvertent operation of on-load release mechanism.
- Inadequate maintenance of lifeboats, davits and launching equipment.
- Communication failure.
- Lack of familiarity with lifeboats, davits equipment and associated controls.
- Unsafe practices during lifeboat drills and inspections; and
- Design faults other than on-load release.

Hence, improvements were needed in existing escape, evacuation and rescue (EER) systems employed on offshore petroleum facilities. The Ocean Ranger and Piper Alpha marine disasters initiated extensive inquiries into the adequacy of marine EER systems. These inquiries were the Public Inquiry into the Piper Alpha disaster, and the Royal Commission on the Ocean Ranger marine disaster (1984). Common to the results of both inquiries was the recommendation for improvements in existing escape, evacuation and rescue (EER) systems employed on offshore petroleum facilities and also to develop performance-based standards for EER systems for offshore installations, rather than a prescriptive regulatory framework. Development for such a framework, for both open and ice populated waters, requires supporting development work on EER performance evaluation and appropriate technologies The rescue component of EER entails the survival of the evacuees and their transfer to a safe haven.

TEMPSC

The totally-enclosed motor-propelled survival craft (TEMPSC) permits human survival for many hours in severe seas where immediate rescue is not possible until the weather and sea conditions improve. The TEMPSC is a form of lifeboat typically installed on seagoing vessels, oil platforms or floating installations (Floating Production Storage and Offloading) related to the oil and gas industry for the evacuation of passengers or personnel on board. In most offshore installation emergencies TEMPSC are relied upon as the secondary means for mass evacuation, the primary method being bridge systems and helicopter or in situations where the primary method could not operate because of the nature of the incident, the environmental conditions, or due to insufficient capacity to evacuate everyone in the time available. The design of lifeboats/TEMPSC and their launching systems have changed gradually over the years, in response to the demands for larger capacity, greater protection for those using them, ease of operation and enhanced safety. The force for change has tended to be accidents resulting in large loss of life such as the passenger vessel *Titanic* in 1912 and semi-submersible accommodation unit *Alexander Keilland* in 1980. There are a number of types of TEMPSC as follows:

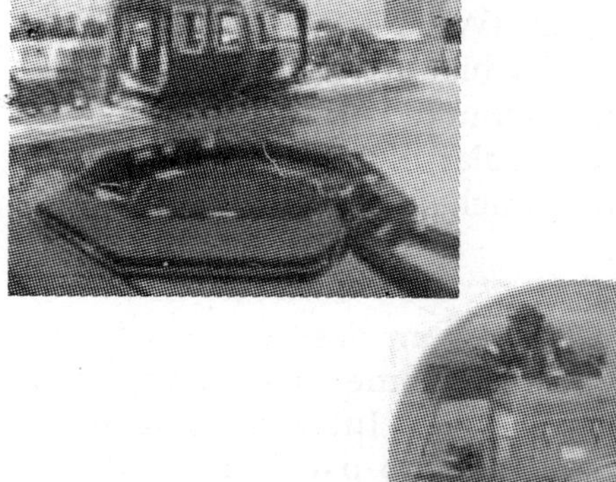

Fig. 67.7

- Davit Launched:
  - Single fall (Whittaker type).
  - Twin fall which can be.
    - Parallel mounted; or
    - Perpendicular mounted.
- Freefall Launched:
  - Skid.
  - Drop.

Most are made from glass reinforced plastic (GRP), though some are made from aluminium or steel. International marine standards (IMO) are used in the design, manufacture, testing, inspection and maintenance of lifeboats. Adherence to these standards ensures a minimum and universally accepted expectation of performance and to some extent consistency of operation across all TEMPSC, However, the standards are based entirely on the equipment being used on vessels and the needs unique to that environment. Though the IMO standards for design, manufacture, testing, inspection and maintenance of lifeboats are broad in scope and highly detailed, there is an absence of weather parameters under which the tests should be carried out.

Performance Standards of TEMPSC: 'Fitness for Purpose'.

- *Functionality:* TEMPSC system should provide safe evacuation for 'reasonably foreseeable' events and conditions when its likely to be needed. Care should be taken not to create new hazards.
- *Survivability:* TEMPSC system should provide protection from hazards and ensure that the risks during evacuation are ALARP. Account should be taken of all threats to successful evacuation (Setback, Washback, Release Hooks malfunction, Fire).
- *Reliability:* The design of the TEMPSC system should have high reliability and facilitate maintenance to ensure functionality (Engine, On-Load Release Hooks).
- *Availability:* The design of TEMPSC evacuation systems should enable a high level of availability; taking account of those conditions (fire, explosion, weather) that may effect its availability. TEMPSC are ready for immediate use.

Adherence to these standards ensures a minimum and universally accepted expectation of performance and to some extent consistency of operation across all TEMPSC.

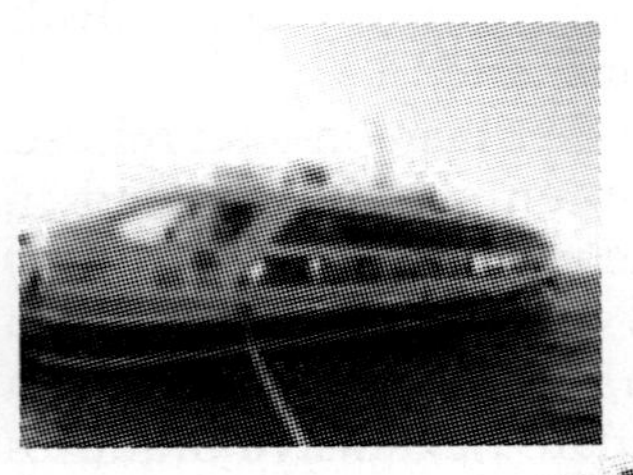

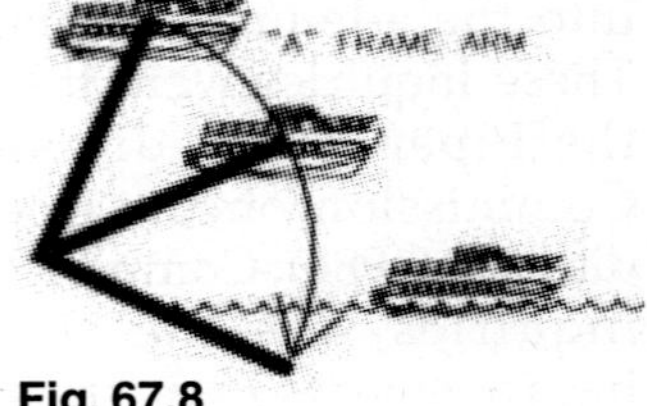

Fig. 67.8

THE SEASCAPE SYSTEM OF EVACUATION (SSE)

The SSE comprises a specially designed TEMPSC, termed the 'Life-Rescue Craft (LRC)', along with a launching davit and ancillary equipment. The Seascape Life-Rescue Craft (LRC) as now configured is a state-of-the-art life support and rescue craft that will give offshore workers a chance for survival in the icy waters of the Atlantic. It is approximately 12.8m long with a width of 3.6m and constructed in aluminium. It is powered by twin 150 turbo diesels, giving a range of 300 kilometres and a maximum speed of 10.5 knots for 24 hours. Accommodation is suitable for 70 people wearing survival suits and the craft has already demonstrated its ability to cope with ice conditions. Its operation has been tested in arctic pack ice and harbour/sheet ice when the LRC has functioned well in ice up to 4.25 m thick. The LRC has also undertaken extensive sea-trials in 60-knot winds with 10.6 m seas. Other manoeuvers have included operations with the new EH 101 search and rescue helicopter, known as the Cormorant by SAR National Defense Canada. Based on a very extensive and strict set of performance standards, the LRC and the entire Seascape System of Evacuation exceed SOLAS in every aspect and will be, it is claimed, the only lifeboat to obtain Lloyd's Register ice notation.

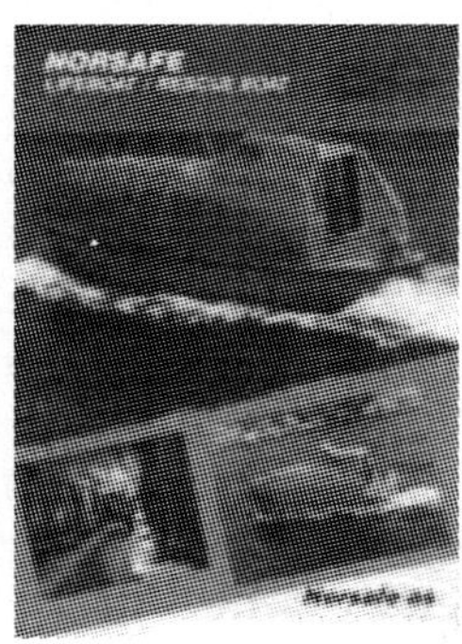

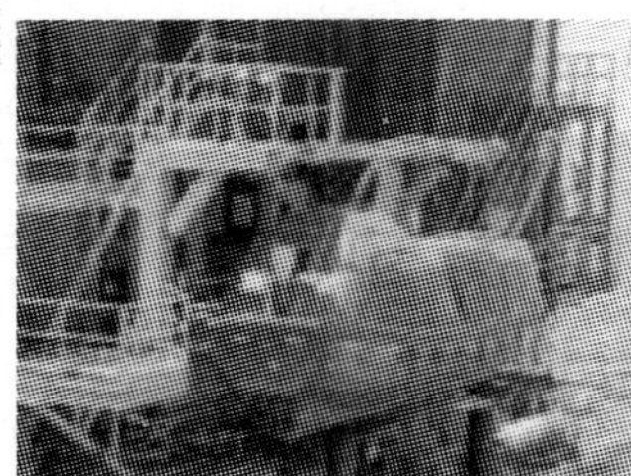

Fig. 67.9

THE NORSAFE RESCUBE

It is a 'dry shod' evacuation system that has a large capacity and is capable of launching quickly. Norsafe, previously known as Jorgensen and Vik AS, began building lifeboats in Grimstad on the south coast of Norway in 1903 and since then has supplied more than 17,000 lifeboats to the global ship and offshore markets. With a staff of over 140 skilled personnel, Norsafe has built a tradition for developing innovative systems and the company remains committed to quality control and is one of the leading providers of evacuation systems to the maritime and rescue offshore industries. Indeed, in 2005, Norsafe announced the launch of the rescube lifeboat – an evacuation system specifically designed as a safe, effective and practical evacuation solution in accordance with SOLAS 1983/96 and subsequent amendments.

Most of the large passenger vessels capable of carrying 5000 passengers or more are still equipped with conventional davit-launched lifeboats, arranged in open-air on deck. From a safety perspective, these aging systems involve significant risk potential, such as congestion, lengthy travel time to the water's surface and extending evacuation time due to overcrowding on deck, amongst others. To manage these safety issues, the Norsafe Rescube lifeboat has been designed to act in a safe area, reduce congestion and deploy quickly. Because Rescube is an integrated part of the ship superstructure, designed for a vertical installation in a recess in the shipside or on the aft end of the vessel and placed into the fire bulkhead between rescue zones, passengers can make their way to the lifeboats from up to six decks in parallel. This configuration even reduces the deck space occupied by lifeboats by up to 30 per cent. The Rescube allows evacuation from more than one deck level at the same time and employs a free fall system to enable quick escape. The free fall principle will provide for a quicker release from the ship. Rescube is designed for 350-400 persons with a typical construction size will be 20 × 7 × 6 m and estimated weight is approx. 70 tons when fully loaded.

Surveys

Implementation of the revised STCW Convention: The updated provisions of the International Convention on Standards of Training, Certification and Watchkeeping for Seafarers (STCW) keeps a watch over various independent evaluations and ship surveys.

It mandates that:

1. The structure, machinery and equipment of a ship shall be subject to an initial survey before the ship is put in service or before a cargo ship safety construction certificate is issued in respect of the ship for the first time.
2. The initial survey shall include a complete inspection of the structure, machinery and equipment, including an inspection of the outside of the ship's bottom. The survey shall ensure that the arrangements, materials, scantlings and workmanship of the structure, boilers and other pressure vessels, their appurtenances, main and auxiliary machinery including steering gear and associated control systems, electrical installations and other equipment comply with the requirements of these regulations, are in satisfactory condition and are fit for the service for which the ship is intended. In the case of tankers, the survey shall also include an inspection of the pump rooms, cargo spaces, bunker and ventilation piping systems and associated safety devices.
3. Upon completion of an initial survey of a ship, and on the application of the owner, agent or master of the ship, if the Director is satisfied that the ship complies with the requirements of these regulations, he may issue in respect of the ship a cargo ship safety construction certificate. The certificate shall be valid for 5 years from the date of issue or for such shorter period as may be specified in the certificate.

Renewal Survey Requirements:

1. The structure, machinery and equipment of a ship shall be subject to a renewal survey at intervals specified by the Director which shall not exceed 5 years for the renewal of a cargo ship safety construction certificate.
2. The renewal survey shall include an inspection of the structure, machinery and equipment as referred to in regulation 74A(2) to ensure that they comply with the requirements of these regulations, are in satisfactory condition and are fit for the service for which the ship is intended.
3. Upon completion of a renewal survey of a ship, and on the application of the owner, agent or master of the ship, if the Director is satisfied that the ship complies with the requirements of these regulations, he may issue in respect of the ship a cargo ship safety construction certificate. The certificate shall be valid for 5 years from the date of issue or for such shorter period as may be specified in the certificate.
4. Where a renewal survey of a ship in respect of which an extension of a cargo ship safety construction certificate is granted under regulation 74G is completed, the new cargo ship safety construction certificate issued in consequence of the survey shall be valid for 5 years from the date of expiry of the existing certificate before the extension was granted or for such shorter period as may be specified in the certificate or, if the Director considers it is appropriate in the special circumstances of the case, valid for 5 years from the date of completion of the survey or for such shorter period as may be specified in the certificate.

74C. Intermediate Surveys

1. The structure, machinery and equipment of a ship in respect of which a cargo ship

safety construction certificate has been issued shall be subject to an intermediate survey within 3 months before or after the second anniversary date or within 3 months before or after the third anniversary date of the certificate, which shall take the place of an annual survey to be carried out in the same year in which the intermediate survey is carried out.

2. The intermediate survey shall include an inspection of the structure, boilers and other pressure vessels, machinery and equipment, the steering gear and associated control systems and electrical installations to ensure that they remain in satisfactory condition and are fit for the service for which the ship is intended. In the case of tankers, the survey shall also include an inspection of the pump rooms, cargo spaces, bunker and ventilation piping systems and associated safety devices and the testing of insulation resistance of electrical installations in dangerous zones.
3. If an intermediate survey is completed before the period specified in subregulation:
   a. Then a new date, which shall not be more than 3 months after the date on which the survey was completed, shall be endorsed by the surveyor on the cargo ship safety construction certificate to be the date for ascertaining sub-sequent anniversary dates.
   b. The subsequent annual survey required under regulation 74D shall be carried out at the intervals prescribed by that regulation using the new date in paragraph as the anniversary date; and the expiry date of the certificate may remain unchanged provided one or more annual surveys are carried out so that the maximum intervals between the surveys prescribed by regulation 74D(1) are not exceeded.
4. If the ship is not surveyed in accordance with this regulation, the Director may cancel its cargo ship safety construction certificate. The Director shall notify the owner of the ship in writing of the cancellation specifying the grounds therefore and the date on which it takes effect.

74D. Annual Surveys

1. The structure, machinery and equipment of a ship in respect of which a cargo ship safety construction certificate has been issued shall be subject to an annual survey within 3 months before or after each anniversary date of the certificate.
2. The annual survey shall include a general inspection of the structure, machinery and equipment as referred to in regulation 74A(2) to ensure that they have been maintained in accordance with the requirements of these regulations, and that they remain in satisfactory condition and are fit for the service for which the ship is intended, and to ensure that the ship in all respects remains fit to proceed to sea without danger to the ship or persons on board.
3. If the ship is not surveyed in accordance with this regulation, the Director may cancel its cargo ship safety construction certificate. The Director shall notify the owner of the ship in writing of the cancellation specifying the grounds therefore and the date on which it takes effect.

Bottom Inspections

The outside of a ship's bottom including the sea connections, overboard discharge valves, and other ship side fittings and the rudder shall be subject to a minimum of 2 inspections during any 5-year period, and the interval between any 2 inspections shall not exceed 36 months.

UNDERWATER DISASTERS AND ACCIDENTS

Diving accidents as well as rescue of crew trapped in submarines is a highly specialised field that calls for a sound understanding of underwater physiology. As a person descends, the pressure around increases with depth, causing his or her lungs to collapse, unless air is supplied at high pressures, or the working atmosphere is kept at one atmosphere. A column of fresh water 34 feet high or sea water 33 feet high (10 metres) exerts a pressure of one atmosphere, i.e., the pressure exerted on a diver at that depth would be one plus one i.e., two atmospheres. At further depths, the pressures would be as following:

Depth	*Pressure in atmospheres*
Sea level	1
33ft (10m)	2
66ft (20m)	3
100ft (30m)	4
133ft (40m)	5
166ft (50m)	6
200ft (60m)	7
300ft (90m)	10
400ft (120m)	13
500ft (150m)	16

With increase in depth, gases get compressed so that a volume of 10 litres becomes 1 litre at a depth of 300 feet. Lung squeeze occurs at 100 feet unless air is pumped to the diver. While breathing air, high partial pressures of nitrogen in the blood causes nitrogen narcosis at about 120 feet depth, causing euphoria and carelessness initially, and then drowsiness at 150-200 feet depths and then extreme weakness at 200-250 feet depth. Beyond 300 feet, a diver cannot perform at all. These stages are akin to alcohol intoxication and hence termed 'rapture of the depths'. Oxygen behaves in a similar fashion and, as its partial pressure increases, the dissolved oxygen in the plasma increases and, at 3 atmospheres pressure, oxygen pressures of 2280 mmHg against 100 mmHg at sea level, causes oxygen toxicity. This manifests as nausea, muscle twitching, dizziness, visual disturbances, irritability, and reduced cerebral blood flow terminating in fatal coma. As the time spent at depths increases, the body becomes saturated with nitrogen and, if the diver surfaces too rapidly, the dissolved nitrogen forms bubbles in tissues producing decompression sickness, also known as bends. In the nervous system, these bubbles produce severe neuritic pain, paralysis, mental disturbances and unconsciousness. In the gut, air distends to produce colic and even rupture of viscera. Expansion of air in a carious tooth can produce excruciating toothache. In the lungs, bubble formation can block the pulmonary circulation producing the chokes, breathlessness, pulmonary edema and air embolism It takes nearly one hour for two-third of the dissolved nitrogen to be liberated and almost 6 hours for its 90 percent elimination, and the diver may not be totally safe for 9-12 hours after surfacing. Diving decompression tables have been worked out correlating duration of a dive and depth to the safe method of surfacing to prevent decompression sickness. Where surfacing has to be expedited, the diver is placed in a decom-pression tank within 5 minutes of surfacing and compressed to his last working depth pressures and then decompressed as per the schedules.

Diving apparatus can be self-contained (SCUBA) not requiring connections with the surface with either demand type open circuit or a closed circuit system. One or more tanks of compressed air with a first stage reducing valve (approximately tenfold) brings down the working pressure to 100 psi by incorporating a diaphragm-type demand valve, an expiratory valve and a mask-tubing system. In closed circuit systems, tanks are filled with pure oxygen and incorporates rubber bellows, a valve system between the tank and bellows, a soda lime cannister and a mask-tubing system fitted with one-way flap valves. Helium-oxygen mixtures are now used for deep dives (more than 100feet depths) as helium lacks narcotic effect, dissolves poorly and diffuses out 2.5 times quicker than nitrogen because of its lesser molecular size.

Saturation Diving

The time required for decompression after deep dives is gross and uneconomical. At 15 metres, it takes 6 hours of decompression after spending just 150 minutes at that pressure and 20 hours decompression time after spending 1 hour at that depth. The concept of saturation diving was introduced for commercial diving to abbreviate such prolonged decompression periods. Once an inhaled mixture of gases at a given pressure totally replaces the normal body gases, the time required for decompression remains the same. Based on this principle, the diver is compressed to the working pressure and after his task, he is shifted to the pressure chamber within the diving bell lowered to the working depth at the end of the shift. The diver spends 2-10 days in this manner, and the cycle is continued till the task is completed. He is then decompressed to the atmospheric pressure over the next few days depending on his working depth. At 100 metres depth, it takes 3 days for decompression, at 200 metres 5 days and at 300 metres it can take nearly one week.

THE SUBMARINE ENVIRONMENT

When a submarine is submerged, its crew is completely cut off from the outside world, in particular, from the normal atmosphere. Modern nuclear submarines remain underwater for 2-3 months at a time and the artificial microclimate within is maintained near normal throughout. Oxygen is generated by hydrolysis of water, by release of oxygen from compressed gas cylinders or from a O_3 patented substance. The expired CO_2 from the crew substance is absorbed by chalk filters to maintain its concentration between 0.5 to 1.0% by volume in the ambient air.

SUBMARINE ESCAPE AND RESCUE

Over the past 100 years, over 200 submarines have been lost by accident or error, usually with a disastrous loss of life. Seven submarines have been lost in the past 20 years (The KURSK being the most recent) and there have been a large number of near-misses. Material failure was the usual cause of accidents in the early period, however, in the past 30years, the cause has been normally a collision or a navigational error as a result of a human error. If an accident does occur and a submarine sinks (SUBSUNK) those on board who survive the initial accident are faced with threats of CO_2 poisoning and oxygen depletion inside the submarine, and pressure and cold from the outside. The crew would attempt to blow ballast tanks to lighten displacement and attempt to surface. If the surrounding water pressure exceeds the hull strength, it will crumble and the crew will die quickly. If the hull remains intact, the crew is faced with the option of escape by buoyant ascent or await rescue from outside. Surface indicators of such disasters are by fire locator rockets, communication bouys, flotsam and jetsam from distressed submarines. The buoyant ascent developed in the early 1950s, uses an air lock permitting 1-2 crew to escape at a time and has been successfully used from depths as great as 180 metres. A prerequisite for this method is that the internal pressure of the disabled submarine (DISSUB) is not too high and that the ambient air within has not been tainted. Noxious fumes or excessive CO_2 greatly increase the risks of decompression sickness. The Mansen's rescue chamber is an example. An improperly conducted ascent can cause barotraumas, air embolism and the bends. Without immediate recompression, these events are rapidly fatal. Escape training drills in escape towers is vital to ensure better survival of crew under such situations. Descent and ascent rates are a part of planned decompression. Descent must not normally exceed 30 metres a minute while ascent must be limited to 15 metres a minute to avoid problem of decompression sickness. The BSAC/Royal Navy Physiological Laboratory table gives detailed instructions to divers about this drill. The facility at HMAS Stirling in Western Australia is the worlds most modern. A number of diving bells and McCann submarine rescue chambers were developed in the 1930s and successfully deployed to rescue crew of USS Squalus in Sep 1939. It has its limitations in the presence of strong currents and when dealing with a submarine lying at extreme angles of tilt. Free-swimming submersibles were the next generation of rescue vehicles and carried on board some of the submarines. External rescue is preferably done by submersible crafts. These are, however, are very expensive and beyond the scope of all but the wealthiest of nations. Deep Submergence Rescue Vehicles (DSRVs) are capable of recovering a maximum of 24 survivors at a time and flown by transport aircraft to a convenient embarkation port and then piggy-backed on a specially modified nuclear submarine and transported to the site of the accident. Rescued crew are then transferred to a mother ship / diving support vessel with recompression chambers (RCC) facilities or to another submarine whose forward compartment is modified to serve as a recompression chamber (RCC). Alternatively, a rescue vessel capable of mating with the disabled submarine and using an articulated interface (skirt) to transfer crew under pressure into adjacent RCCs can be attempted. The Australian REMORA is one such Submarine Rescue Vehicle (SRV) built about a diving bell capable of operating at depths of 500 metres in a current of 3 knots and mating with submarines lying at angles of upto 60º from the vertical. Rescue and transfer is by a Transfer Under Pressure Chamber (TUPC). It utilises underwater telephone and the IMMARSAT for communication and is housed in ISO containers for total mobility.

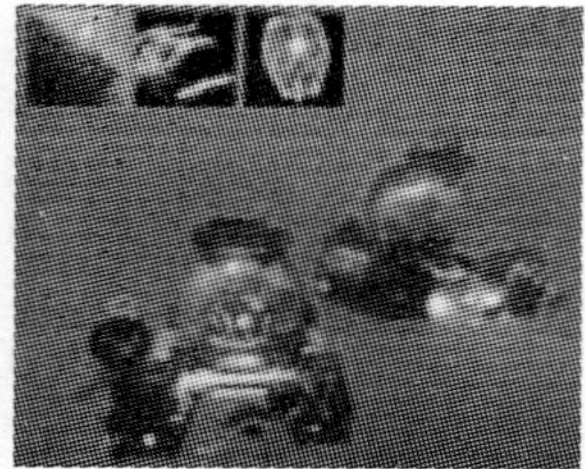

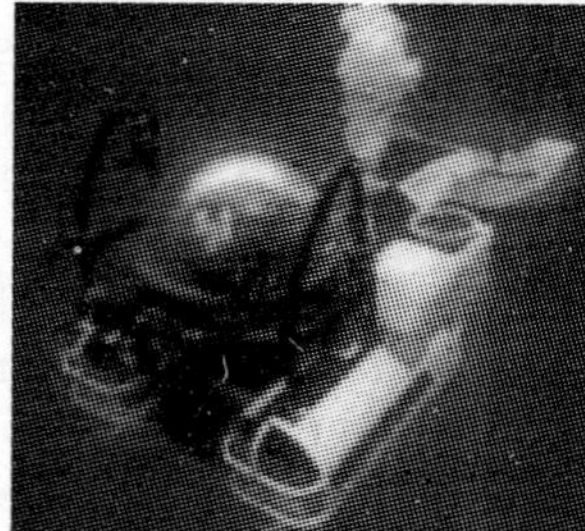

Fig. 67.10

SUBMERSIBLES

The commercial and scientific utilisation of submersibles was very popular in the 1960s and 1970s. General Dynamics, Rockwell, General Motors, Westinghouse, Perry, Comex, Rauma Oceanics, JP KennyIntershelf,

Kharax Company Ltd., Krylov Shipbuilding Research Institute have all been very active in designing and manufacturing a variety of submersibles. Over the last decade, Remote Operated Vehicles (ROVs) and AUVs with long umbilicals have largely supplanted manned submersibles for many work-related tasks, principally because of cost issues related to insurance, manning requirements and vehicle handling system complexity. Manned vehicles are still popular, as there is no substitute for direct, in situ observation of the marine environment. The most recent boost to manned submersibles has been the advent of the purpose-built tourist submersibles. Constructed to accommodate 28 to 48 passengers, they take tourists undersea on hour-long excursions to depths of 50 to 150metres. An estimated 140 commercial and scientific manned sub-mersibles have been built in the last 40 years of which approximately 30% are still operating.

Endurance and Developments in Submersible Technology

Submersibles are rated by their depth capability. The Mir I and II are 6000 metre capable. The Japanese Shinkai 6500 has a 6500 metre depth rating and Deep Flight ceramic version would be capable of exploring Challenger Deep, the deepest spot in the ocean floor. The development of transparent plastic acrylic (polymethyl methacrylate) for viewports and complete pressure hulls upto metres thick and rated from 600 to 1000 metres has permitted better all round underwater viewing. Another notable development has been the utilisation of computers for control and monitoring functions that effectively reduce pilot workload, clutter and reduce manning requirements. Touch sensitive screens with multi-level animated graphics, servo sensors that provide automatic alarms and even maintenance reminders are available. Very accurate doppler (sonar) velocity systems provide pinpoint submerged navigation data. Improvements in battery technology to propel the pressure compensated electric thruster motors that drive the main propulsion axial motor and auxilliary propulsion (lateral, vertical and horizontal thrusters) have imparted these vehicles excellent manouverability, speed and endurance. Advances in silver-zinc and silver-iron batteries as well as the lithium-aluminium-iron sulphide cells using metal hydride hydrogen and liquid oxygen (proton exchange membrane fuel cell technology) have shown great promise. Advances in systems engineering and workable closed-cycle diesel systems by Kockums of Sweden have proven reliability in underwater operations. Titanium is being largely replaced by graphite-based composites and hybrid-ceramic variants that include metal/fibre components. These have excellent reliability, permit deeper diving with lightweight hulls and weight-to-displacement-ratios approaching 0.6. Of the newer hull designs, the Subcat 7.5 with a catamaran configuration has several advantages over its monohull counterparts. It has excellent surface stability, better than even those fitted with active stabilisers. It has more deck space and 100% more speed aided by lateral aileron between the hulls. Laser-aimed, broadcast quality underwater cameras fitted with xenon arc lights, approximating sunlight in intensity, helps illuminate underwater scenes in true colour even in the darkest seas. The rigorous classification standards of the American Bureau of Shipping and its international counterparts has ensured a perfect safety record of tourist submersibles, enabling them to make over 3000 dives a year. For underwater rescue using submersibles and submarines, a mixed gas diver lock-out and a deep diving docking manned facility have been developed.

OPERATIONAL CAPABILITIES OF SUBMERSIBLES

- Long-term observations of underwater objects under both stationary and dynamic conditions.
- Controls over the construction and technical state and servicing of underwater pipelines, cable routes and other hydrotechnical structures.
- Search, discovery and marking on the ground of sunken objects, as well as providing for their recovery. Upto 100 ton loads can be salvaged.
- Data acquisition and mapping of sea floor scapes on a shelf.
- Light diving operations, ensuring entering and egress to depths of 100metres and onboard RCC.
- Support to accomplish emergency and rescue operations.
- Research in underwater fields.
- Submarine teleshooting, filming and photography.
- Research in marine flora and fauna like estimation and prediction of their stock, effects of pollution, study of man-made reefs, plantation of mussels etc.
- Studies of hydrobiont behaviour and distribution against marine environment.
- Sampling of water, gas, soil, icthyofauna, mineral deposits using a titanium alloy electrohydraulic telemanipulated gripping and manipulator arm with 7 degrees of freedom or more and a kit of renewable instrument spares. It can also make initial processing of the samples on board.
- Analysis of hydrological parameters like salinity, temperature etc.
- Conduct of EPRON type operations like underwater electric welding, cutting hydraulic washout using pressurised water jets.

68 Robots in Disasters

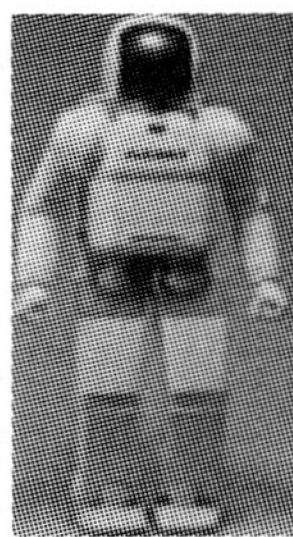
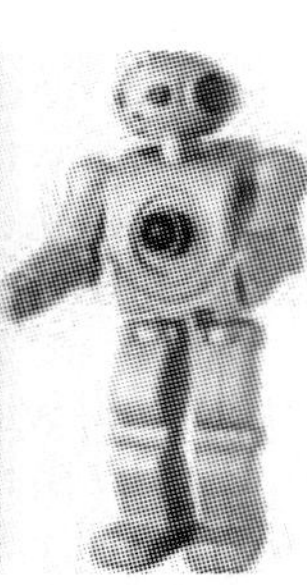
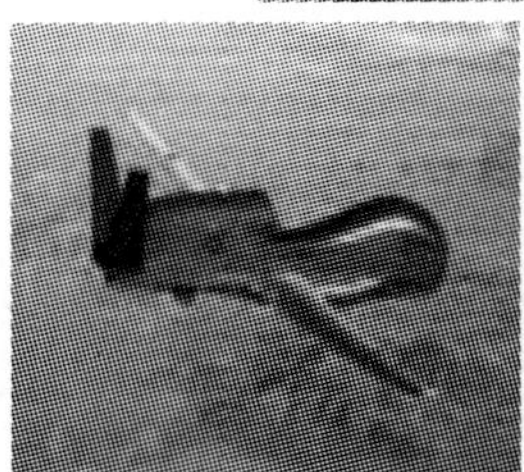
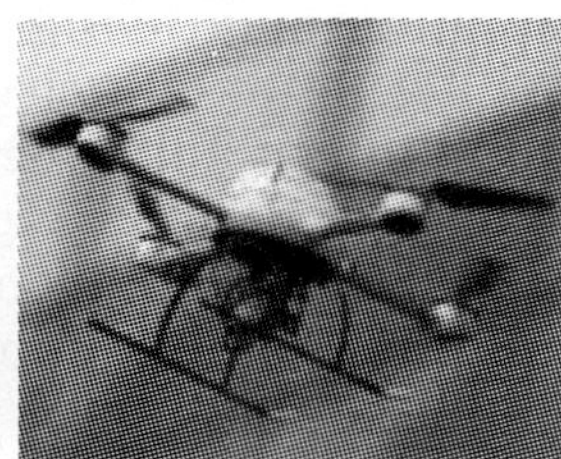

Fig. 68.1

ROBOTS IN DISASTERS

In modern day disasters, the recovery mission is considered a top priority and smart autonomous robots are playing a significant role in such missions like search for life under earth quake hit rubbles, tsunami hit islands, de-mining in war affected areas and many other situations.

Robotics Can Contribute Toward

1. Assisting search and rescue operations that are impossible or difficult to perform by humans.
2. Reducing risk of secondary damage.
3. Improving speed of operations and improve survival rates of victims in extreme conditions where first responders may not be able to access them.
4. Establishing communication network at disaster sites.

Rescue Robotics is a newly emerging field dealing with systems that support first response units in disaster missions. Especially mobile robots can be highly valuable tools in urban rescue missions after catastrophes like earthquakes, bomb- or gas-explosions or daily incidents like fires and road accidents involving hazardous materials. The robots can be used to inspect collapsed structures, to assess the situation and to search and locate victims. Rescue robots not only have to be designed for the harsh environmental conditions of disasters, but they also need advanced capabilities like intelligent behaviors to free them from constant supervision by operators.

Some of the robots available for such activities are elaborated.

Rugbots

Named for being rugged robots. Their designs range from basic mechatronics to the high-level behavior software and hardware components for fast robot prototyping and their operation can be tested in a simulated disaster scenarios. The weigh just 35 kg and have a small footprint (approximately 50 cm × 50 cm) that is highly beneficial in indoor scenarios and also renders them very agile and fast on open terrain. An active flipper mechanism allows Rugbots to negotiate stairs and rubble piles. They have significant on-board computation power and can be equipped with a large variety of sensors. The standard payload includes a laser-scanner, ultrasound sensors, four cameras, one thermo camera, and rate gyros that enables Rugbots to cooperate in multi-robot-teams. The onboard software is capable of mapping, detection of humans using special sensors like CO_2 detectors, infrared cameras and thermal imaging. They have fully autonomous control and teleoperation in varying degrees and the on-board batteries allow for 2.5 to 3 hours of continuous operation. For operation in rough environments they are fitted with tracks to negotiate large obstacles and loose soil.

Safety Security and Rescue Robots (SSRR)

Lead Zeppelin and Survivor Buddy are autonomous underwater vehicles (AUV) programmed to move through an environment and to avoid obstacles, to recognize targets by computer vision, and to operate at specific desired depths with option to use an antenna-buoy to maintain wireless communication. Hull design is like ROVs. Its nose section contains a pressure sensor for depth measurement, a heading sensor with an integrated 3D compass, an embedded processor capable of calculating the roll, pitch and yaw in real time, a scanning sonar which enables it to scan the surrounding for obstacles and their distance by emitting sound signals of 550 kHz and measuring the time it takes until the sounds echo comes back. The sonar covers up to 360 degrees since it is being turned by a motor in steps of one degree or bigger, and it has a resolution of 1.5 degree. The range of the sonar is selectable to up to 80 meters. The sensor can also scan vertically with a coverage of ± 20 degrees. The horizontal scan rate is about 60degree per second at distances of up to 10 m. The nose has a forward looking camera. The middle section contains echo sounder vertical thruster embedded PC DC/DC converters, a down looking camera and four battery tubes each containing propulsion motor propeller with guards power amplifier for the motor battery. The submarine is trimmed slightly positively buoyant, i.e. it comes up to the surface in case of some error. Thus the middle thruster has to be used to force the vehicle under water. The maximum power of the four propulsion motors is 350 W of which up to 280 W are usable. The 3-blade propellers are protected by guards for safety. The robot has an operational depth of 300 meters. The echo sounder has a beam width is ± 3degrees, the accuracy ± 5 cm and the depth range 0.5 to 9.8 meters. The on board cameras support a resolution of up to 640 × 480 pixel, and have a wide-angle lens which enables a field of view of 78 degrees. The camera at the bottom of the submarine can locate targets and guide the submarine directly over them and both cameras are inserted in a waterproof protective lid of transparent plastic.

"Aqua Box" series are handy, small underwater robots which can be operated by a few researchers.

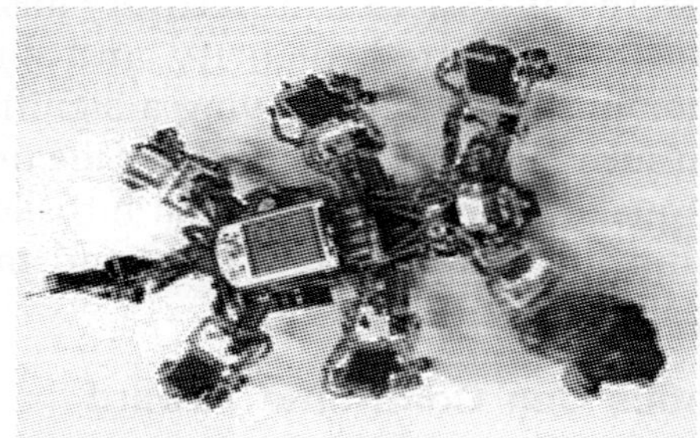

Fig. 68.2

Hexapod Robots

These can play significant role in disaster recovery missions as they can reach a hazardous field quite easily while wheeled robots have limited mobility in such missions. Given sufficient intelligence these robots can negotiate any kind of terrain as the hexapod provides additional degrees-of-freedom. The TITAN VIII four-legged walking robot, was developed as a general-purpose walking robot at the Tokyo Institute of Technology, Japan while COMET-I was the first six-legged robot developed at Chiba University, Japan, for rescue missions. This robot weighed nearly 120 kg and too heavy for real search and rescue missions COMET-IV weighed about one ton and ARIEL was developed for mine-recovery operations. The Defense Advanced Research Projects Agency (DARPA) and the US Office of Naval Research (ONR) are exploring methods for using this robot for underwater missions. The RIMHO-2 walking robot is being used for detecting and locating unexploded ordnance. Since a robot can be statically secure on three or more legs, a hexapod robot has a great deal of suppleness in how it can move. If legs become disabled, the robot may still be able to walk. Furthermore, not all of the robot's legs are needed for stability; other legs are free to reach new foot placements or manipulate a payload. A hexapod, can achieve higher speed than a quadruped, and it is well known that a hexapod achieves its highest speed when using a statically stable gait. A hexapod configuration using alternating tripods can increase its speed, albeit at the cost of slightly jeopardizing stability. To navigate in the hazardous field, it will rotate in any direction; heavy legs with powerful servo motors are chosen over other types as they can withstand heavy loads. Spider-like leg configurations are the most efficient leg configuration from the energy point of view because it requires lower torques. However, it is not very efficient in terms of stability. Insect-like legs seem to be more efficient stability-wise, but power consumption increases extraordinarily in an insect-like configuration. By reducing servo motors size, motion can be allowed in two joints simultaneously and this robot is able to navigate all kind of terrain in the hazard field, and move faster on even terrain, and more leisurely on uneven terrain. Bump sensors helps it to detect any obstacle like hill or ditch which it may encounter in the hazardous field. The Tripod Gait is the best-known hexapod gait. A tripod consists of the front-back legs on one side and the middle leg on the opposite side. For each tripod, the legs are lifted, lowered, and moved forwards and backwards in unison. During walking, a hexapod uses its 2 tripods not unlike a biped stepping from one foot to the other—the weight is simply shifted alternately from one tripod to the other. Since 3 legs are on the ground at all times, this gait is both "statically" and "dynamically" stable. With the Wave Gait, all legs on one side are moved forward in succession, starting with the rear most leg. This is then repeated on the other side. Since only one leg is ever lifted at a time, with the other five being down, the robot is always in a highly-stable posture. Hence this is often chosen because it provides the maximum stability margin for uneven terrain navigation.

Quadcopters

Germany's Ilmenau University of Technology have developed flying quadcopter robots that can be used to form a self-assembling ad-hoc wireless network in the event of a disaster. Built with off-the-shelf parts (including VIA's Pico-ITX hardware and a GPS unit) the robots are designed to provide both mobile phone and WiFi access — and they can do it far more quickly than a technician on the ground might be able to.

Robot operated vehicles to clear landslides: Once disasters such as landslides occur, emergency response should be rapid in order to minimize loss of human life and prevent secondary disasters. To ensure safety of emergency workers, construction vehicles used to remove the collapsed soil and rock should be remotely operated and purpose-built. Fujita Corporation has developed a remotely controlled portable robot that can be installed in construction vehicles viz. backhoes and crawler dump trucks for simultaneously carried out excavation/loading and transportation of earth using a wireless local area network (WLAN).

Search and Rescue Robots

In a life-threatening environment after a natural disaster, heat, dust and collapsed buildings can make a rescue mission using humans or animals too dangerous. A remote controlled flight robot can help by reconnoitering the situation and sending information like location of victims, put together maps of disaster scene by video signals to the rescue services on the ground.

The TALON robot is relatively light (man-transportable), but stable and maneuverable in varying ground conditions. It can be configured into different sizes and functions, including stealthy reconnaissance, intruder attack, underwater surveillance and remote sensor/monitoring. The basic platform is designed to be physically compatible with related hardware, weapons and sensor systems. More than 80 different payloads have been developed or adapted and mounted on the TALON robot platform including the following lethal and non-lethal payloads:

- Gripper manipulator.
- Smoke dropping module.
- Grenade dropping module.
- Breaching tool.

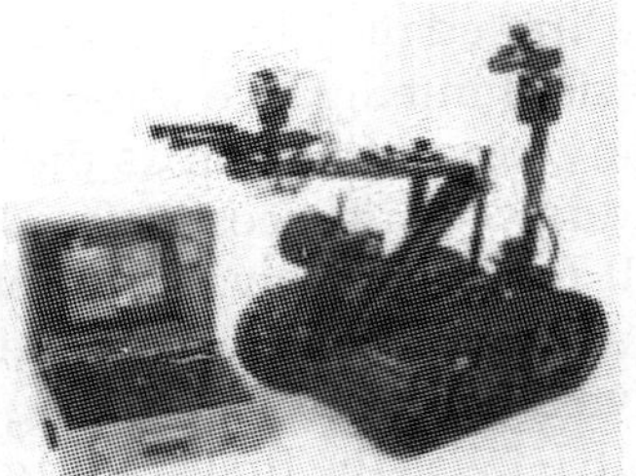

Fig. 68.3

- Night vision camera. NBC sensors.
- UXO/countermine systems/sensors.
- Anti-Tank (AT4) launcher.
- Light Anti-Tank Weapon (LAW) launcher.
- 40-mm grenade launcher (M203 barrel).
- 12-gauge shotgun.
- Mounts for remotely controlled weapons including: M240; M249: M16; M82A1 (50-cal).

TALON robots have been used in Special Operations missions including EOD and reconnaissance operations in Bosnia, Afghanistan and Iraq. They were the only American robots durable enough to be used in search and recovery missions at the World Trade Center after the September 11 attack, surviving 48 days of twice daily decontamination procedures. The robots are designed as rugged, all-weather platforms capable of operating reliably in desert or beach sand, snow, water, grassy or wooded terrain, and inside buildings. TALON robots are untethered and remotely operated, able to climb stairs, sustain falls and right themselves, and can be lowered into a landing zone from a helicopter, dropped from moving vehicles and thrown overboard offshore. The TALON robot is the only mobile platform currently certified by the Department of Defense for remotely controlled live firing of lethal weapons.

69 Nanotechnology in Disasters

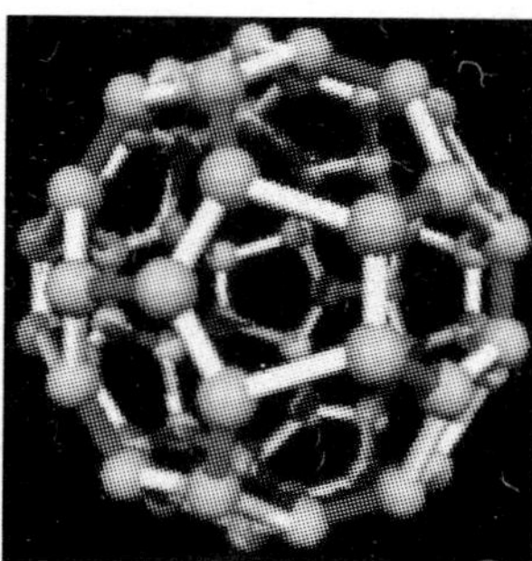

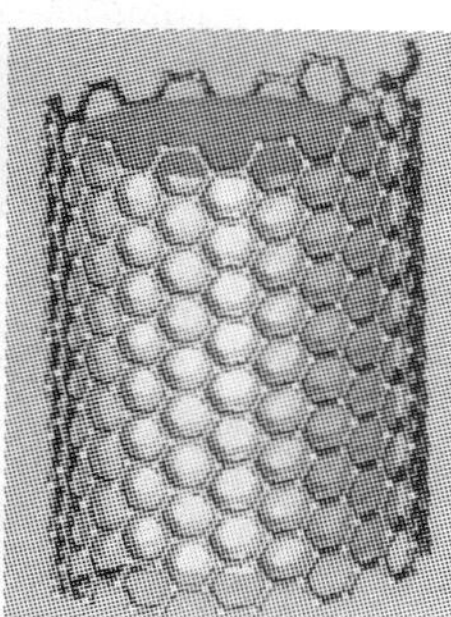

Fig. 69.1

Nanotechnology is being heralded as a new technological revolution, one so profound that it will touch all aspects of human society. Some believe that these influences will be overwhelmingly positive.

The "nano" prefix derives from the Greek noun nanos, meaning dwarf. A nanometre (nm) is one billionth (1 x 10-9) of a metre: the length of about ten atoms placed side-by-side, or 1/80,000th of the thickness of a human hair. Nanotechnology is commonly understood as a technology involving the manipulation and application of matter, based on its properties at the atomic scale. The term covers a family of technologies, including nanosciences and nanotechnologies.

Nanoscience is the study of phenomena and manipulation of materials at atomic, molecular and macromolecular scales, where properties differ significantly from those at a larger scale. Nanotechnologies are the design, characterisation, production and application of structures, devices and systems by controlling shape and size at nanometre scale. potential for nanotechnology to provide solutions to some of the global challenges we face (e.g., increasing energy efficiency to combat climate change, improving nutrition and protecting human health.

Food technology is regarded as one of the industry sectors where nanotechnology will play an important role in the future. It is commonly distinguished between two forms of nanofood applications: food additives (nano inside) and food packaging (nano outside). Nanoscale food additives may for example be used to influence product shelf life, texture, flavour, nutrient composition or even detect food pathogens and provide functions as food quality indicators. In the context of food packaging, nanotechnologies are mainly considered to be of use to increase product shelf life, indicate spoilt ingredients or generally increase product quality, e.g. by preventing gas flow across product packaging. Promising applications combining nanotechnologies and food are also expected to result from new encapsulation technologies. Such nano encapsulation systems can be used to add additional nutrients without changing a product's flavour or quality. This might enable producers to integrate nutrients which are not naturally occurring, or which could so far not be integrated due to reasons of chemistry. The advantages of such encapsulation systems also encompass extended shelf life, protection of the encapsulated ingredients from the surrounding media and undesired interaction during food processing, as well as delivery of certain contents to a specific target site within the body. makes use of silver's antibacterial properties by implementing silver nanoparticles into food containers.

The potential impact areas for nanotechnology in water applications is for treatment and remediation, sensing and detection and pollution prevention. Advanced filtration materials like nanostructured filters either carbon nanotubes or nanocapillary arrays together with nanoreactive membranes coupled with dendritic polymers will enable greater water reuse, recycling and desalination. Biological and chemical contaminants can be detected at very low concentration levels. Remediation is the process of removing, reducing or neutralizing contaminants. This can be achieved by novel nanomaterials like zeolites, carbon nanotubes, self-assembled monolayer on mesoporous supports (SAMMS), bipolymers, single enzyme nanoparticles, zero valent iron/bimetallic iron nanoparticles and nanoscale semiconductor photocatalysts with high affinity capacity and selectivity. Silver and titanium oxide catalysts have photocatalytic disinfection properties. Their enhanced reactivity, surface area and sequestration characteristics can be used to clarify inductrial effluents, surface and drinking water.

As far as nanotechnology's role in responding to climate change is concerned, the report correctly states that nanotechnologies are a platform technology and as such, by itself, nanotechnology will not have a dramatic impact on climate change–but its incorporation into larger systems, such as the hydrogen based economy, solar power technology or next generation batteries, potentially could have a profound impact on energy consumption and hence greenhouse gas emissions. The report highlights the role of nanotechnology in innovation in three broad categories, namely the development of efficient hydrogen powered vehicles, enhanced and cheaper photovoltaics or solar power technology, and the development of a new generation of batteries and supercapacitors.

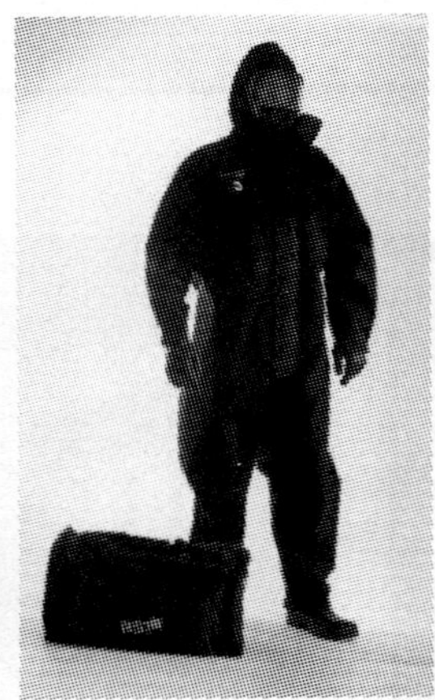

Fig. 69.2

Demron, which also has many other U.S. and international patents, consists of an advanced radiopaque nanopolymeric compound fused between layers of fabric and manufactured into lightweight nuclear-radiation blocking garments including full-body suits, vests, blankets and medical X-ray vests and aprons.

Demron's nanotechnology surpasses current NBC suits, which provide limited radioactive protection. Its patent describes and protects the use of nanopolymeric compounds that enable the latest version of Demron, called "Demron-W," to provide enhanced chemical, biological, radiation and flame protection. Demron-W is the world's first and only NFPA 1994-2007 Certified Fabric for Protective Ensembles for First Responders to CBRN Terrorism Incidents.

Demron is a lead-free, toxin-free and PVC-free material that allows heat dissipation and resists chemical penetration and cracks. Made of liquid metal, Demron nuclear protection fabrics feel cool and, unlike traditional nuclear suits, they're lightweight, flexible and foldable. Demron has proved to block gamma rays, X-rays and other nuclear emissions Scientists have selected it for thermo-mechanical suits for future space travel.

Nanotechnology will remain prohibitively expensive, limiting access to those who could benefit the most. Given the precedent of unequal access to recent technological development, e.g., advances in information technology, it is unlikely that access to nanotechnologies will be different without considerable intervention and guidance. There is concern that the development of this technology could just widen the divide between the industrialised and the developing world.

A Futuristic Concept

The river floods. The village is destroyed. Five thousand farming families are suddenly homeless, without even clean water to drink. The roads are washed out, and supplies must be delivered by helicopter. In 2004, this would have been a humanitarian disaster in the making. Today, however, a few flights can deliver all the necessary supplies. How is this possible?

Thousands of technological advances have made relief supplies more compact and effective. But the major advance is the portable nanofactory. Using local materials, it can build a wide range of humanitarian supplies. Let's watch as the first helicopter is unloaded.

The first crate is the water system. For only 25,000 people, this can be pre-supplied. The pipes are folded plastic; they look too flimsy to hold pressure, but they do the job. A few intakes are thrown into the still-muddy river, a block of fuel is loaded into the small generator, and the filter goes to work. Within minutes, clean water is inflating the pipes into a grid with 500 spigots; these outline the plan of the temporary refugee camp, supplying 100,000 gallons per day of purified water.

The second crate has already been unpacked. This is the heart of the system — the portable factory. Packed with nanotechnology and robotics, weighing 200 pounds and standing half as tall as a person, it can produce two tons per day of products. Control is simple: A touch screen selects the type and number of products to produce. After rapidly surveying the situation, the decision is made: the air is warm, but night is falling, so tents are needed first. Five thousand family-sized tents, each weighing two ounces, will take three hours to produce. A two-ton tank of oil is dropped from the belly of the helicopter, and connected to the factory. Within the factory, the oil is turned into nanotubes and sheets, which are rapidly stitched together. The finished product can inflate itself, though it must be staked or weighed down with rocks. By 10:00 pm, all the refugees are housed.

Other helicopters have brought food, but the expense of transporting many tons per day by helicopter would tax the local budget. Besides, the people should not have to continue living in tents. This is not a problem. The morning of the second day, 250 people receive training in running the factory, and 5,000 more are sent out to gather organic matter. The factory has been working overnight-making more factories. In one hour, it can duplicate itself. In the second hour, each of those duplicates makes another. Eight hours later, there are 256 factories ready to use, and the oil tank is half empty. The factories now use the rest of the oil to make an equal number of compact chemical plants, each one capable of distilling almost any organic matter into oil. The camp is divided into 250 units of 100 people each. Each unit receives one factory and one chemical plant. The people will be able to request a variety of common supplies, including clothing, building materials, and small prefab houses or greenhouses. The factory can also supply a bland food; vitamin and mineral supplements must be added, but transportation costs for these are negligible. The factory can produce 40 pounds of supplies per person per day-adequate to house the entire camp the first day, and build greenhouses on the second day. Human waste is dumped, and later piped, into the chemical plants.

The living environment is comfortable, but strange. As the flooded land dries, the village is slowly rebuilt. Vacant houses are deflated and burned (fed back to the chemical plants). Most of the factories are also burned, but the village keeps a few. Some of the farmers now prefer growing crops in greenhouses—and the next time the river floods, no outside aid will be required.

That's one scenario. Some of the details may change, but in broad terms, this shows the remarkable humanitarian potential of responsible nanotechnology.

70 Nuclear, Biological Chemical (NBC) Warfare

> "War is a series of disasters which result in a winner."
>
> —*George Clemenceau*

NBC operations represent the fourth dimension of warfare and have added financial and operational costs of establishing an effective medical support system to counter the threat. The separation of chemical and biological agents is considered to be an unnecessary add on, as the latters chemical component, the effect of toxins, is susceptible to conventional antidotes and treatments.

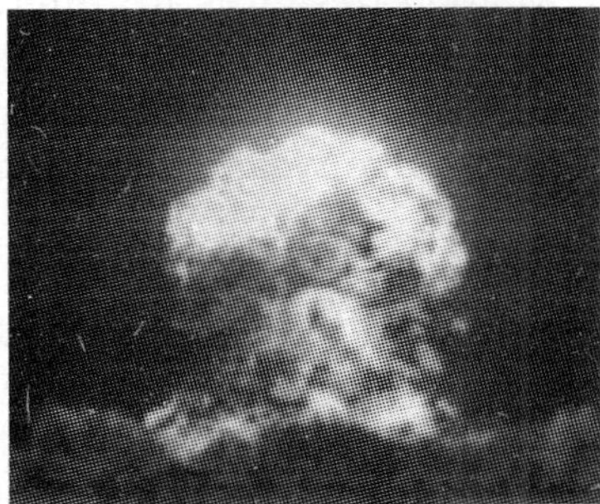

Fig. 70.1

THE ATOMIC WEAPON SPECTRUM

There are two basic types of nuclear weapon. The first type produces its explosive energy through nuclear fission reactions alone. Such fission weapons are commonly referred to as atomic bombs or atom bombs (abbreviated as A-bombs), though their energy comes specifically from the nucleus of the atom.

In fission weapons, a mass of fissile material (enriched uranium or plutonium) is assembled into a supercritical mass—the amount of material needed to start an exponentially growing nuclear chain reaction—either by shooting one piece of sub-critical material into another (the "gun" method), or by compressing a sub-critical sphere of material using chemical explosives to many times its original density (the "implosion" method). The latter approach is considered more sophisticated than the former, and only the latter approach can be used if plutonium is the fissile material.

A major challenge in all nuclear weapon designs is to ensure that a significant fraction of the fuel is consumed before the weapon destroys itself. The amount of energy released by fission bombs can range between the equivalent of less than a ton of TNT upwards to around 500,000 tons (500 kilotons) of TNT.

The second basic type of nuclear weapon produces a large amount of its energy through nuclear fusion reactions. Such fusion weapons are generally referred to as thermonuclear weapons or more colloquially as hydrogen bombs (abbreviated as H-bombs), as they rely on fusion reactions between isotopes of hydrogen (deuterium and tritium). However, all such weapons derive a significant portion – and sometimes a majority – of their energy from fission (including fission induced by neutrons from fusion reactions). Unlike fission weapons, there are no inherent limits on the energy released by thermonuclear weapons. Only six countries—United States, Russia, United Kingdom, People's Republic of China, France and India—have conducted thermonuclear weapon tests.

Thermonuclear bombs work by using the energy of a fission bomb in order to compress and heat fusion fuel. In the Teller-Ulam design, which accounts for all multi-megaton yield hydrogen bombs, this is accomplished by placing a fission bomb and fusion fuel (tritium, deuterium, or lithium deuteride) in proximity within a special, radiation-reflecting container. When the fission bomb is detonated, gamma and X-rays emitted first compress the fusion fuel, then heat it to thermonuclear temperatures. The ensuing fusion reaction creates enormous numbers of high-speed neutrons, which then can induce fission in materials which normally are not prone to it, such as depleted uranium. Each of these components is known as a "stage", with the fission bomb as the "primary" and the fusion capsule as the "secondary", In large hydrogen bombs, about half of the yield, and much of the resulting nuclear fallout, comes from the final fissioning of depleted uranium. By chaining together numerous stages with increasing amounts of fusion fuel, thermonuclear weapons can be made to an almost arbitrary yield; the largest ever detonated (the Tsar Bomba of the USSR) released an energy equivalent to over 50 million tons (50 megatons) of TNT. Most thermonuclear weapons are considerably smaller than this, due for instance to practical constraints in fitting them into the space and weight requirements of missile warheads.

There are other types of nuclear weapons as well. For example, a boosted fission weapon is a fission bomb which increases its explosive yield through a small amount of fusion reactions, but it is not a fusion bomb. In the boosted bomb, the neutrons produced by the fusion reactions serve primarily to increase the efficiency of the fission bomb. Some weapons are designed for special purposes; a neutron bomb is a thermonuclear weapon that yields a relatively small explosion but a relatively large amount of neutron radiation; such a device could theoretically be used to cause massive casualties while leaving infrastructure mostly intact and creating a minimal amount of fallout. The detonation of a nuclear weapon is accompanied by a blast of neutron radiation. Surrounding a nuclear weapon with suitable materials (such as cobalt or gold) creates a weapon known as a salted bomb. This device can produce exceptionally large quantities of radioactive contamination. Most variety in nuclear weapon design is in different yields of nuclear weapons for different types of purposes, and in manipulating design elements to attempt to make weapons extremely small.

Other Uses

Apart from their use as weapons, nuclear explosives have been tested and used for various non-military uses, and proposed, but not used for large scale earth moving. When long term health and clean-up costs were included, there was no economic advantage over conventional explosives.

Synthetic elements, such as einsteinium and fermium, created by neutron bombardment of uranium and plutonium during thermonuclear explosions, were discovered in the aftermath of the first thermonuclear bomb test. In 2008 the worldwide presence of new isotopes from atmospheric testing beginning in the 1950s was developed into a reliable way of detecting art forgeries, as all paintings created after that period contain traces of Cesium-137 and Strontium-90, isotopes that did not exist in nature before 1945.

Nuclear explosives have also been seriously studied as potential propulsion mechanisms for space travel (Project Orion).

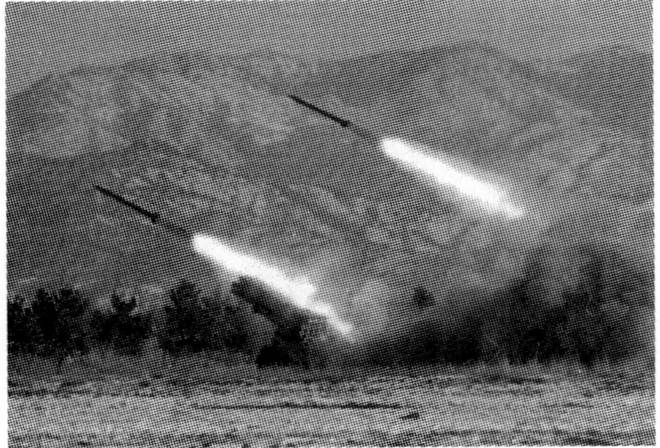

Fig. 70.2

NUCLEAR WEAPONS DELIVERY

The first nuclear weapons were gravity bombs, such as the "Fat Man" weapon dropped on Nagasaki, Japan. These weapons were very large and could only be delivered by heavy bomber aircraft.

Nuclear weapons delivery: The technology and systems used to bring a nuclear weapon to its target—is an important aspect of nuclear weapons relating both to nuclear weapon design and nuclear strategy. Additionally, developing and maintaining delivery options is among the most resource-intensive aspects of nuclear weapons: according to one estimate, deployment of nuclear weapons accounted for 57% of the total financial resources spent by the United States in relation to nuclear weapons since 1940.

Historically the first method of delivery, and the method used in the two nuclear weapons actually used in warfare, is as a gravity bomb, dropped from bomber aircraft. This method is usually the first developed by countries as it does not place many restrictions on the size of the weapon, and weapon miniaturization is something which requires considerable weapons design knowledge. It does, however, limit the range of attack, the response time to an impending attack, and the number of weapons which can be fielded at any given time. Additionally, specialized delivery systems are usually not necessary; especially with the advent of miniaturization, nuclear bombs can be delivered by both strategic bombers and tactical fighter-bombers, allowing an air force to use its current fleet with little or no modification. This method may still be considered the primary means of nuclear weapons delivery; the majority of U.S. nuclear warheads, for example, are represented in free-fall gravity bombs, namely the B 61.

More preferable from a strategic point of view are nuclear weapons mounted onto a missile, which can use a ballistic trajectory to deliver a warhead over the horizon. While even short range missiles allow for a faster and less vulnerable attack, the development of intercontinental ballistic missiles (ICBMs) and submarine-launched ballistic missiles (SLBMs) has allowed some nations to plausibly deliver missiles anywhere on the globe with a high likelihood of success. More advanced systems, such as multiple independently targetable reentry vehicles (MIRVs) allow multiple warheads to be launched at several targets from any one missile, reducing the chance of any successful missile defense. Today, missiles are most common among systems designed for delivery of nuclear weapons. Making a warhead small enough to fit onto a missile, though, can be a difficult task.

Tactical weapons (see above) have involved the most variety of delivery types, including not only gravity bombs and missiles but also artillery shells, land mines, and nuclear depth charges and torpedoes for anti-submarine warfare. An atomic mortar was also tested at one time by the United States. Small, two-man portable tactical weapons (somewhat misleadingly referred to as suitcase bombs), such as the Special Atomic Demolition Munition, have been developed, although the difficulty to combine sufficient yield with portability limits their military utility.

Nuclear Warfare

The great destructive possibilities of the atomic bomb and other thermonuclear weapons has added another dimension to man made disasters. The scale of deaths and injuries would number hundreds of thousands and an enormous effort would be required to care for even a modest number of seriously injured victims. A great majority of casualties would occur as a result of the blast and heat effects of the explosion and only about 15 to 20% of the fatalities would be from effects of radiation. A thermonuclear device can be exploded in three ways. A high air-burst similar to that used in Hiroshima and Nagasaki causes a maximum degree of destruction by blast effect, thermal radiation, secondary fires and radiation. This can kill by acute exposure as well as persistent effects due to the slow decay of fission products and unfissioned bomb material. In a surface burst near ground level, the overall blast damage and destruction by heat and secondary fires would be considerably less. Because of the smaller radius of effectiveness of the explosion, the results of acute and delayed radiation would also be moderate in comparison to an air burst. Near the centre of the explosion, there would be an area of intense destruction and persistent radiation. In an underwater burst similar to the one at Bikini, the effect of blast and fires would be minimum but the spread of radioactive contamination would be significantly greater. Gamma radiation and neutron beams would be rapidly absorbed by the water, but a radioactive rain of gamma radiation from fission products would contaminate a wide area. Alpha radiation from unfissioned bomb material will persist and remain unchanged until removal by decontamination methods. Alpha emission is not dangerous unless absorbed into the body by ingestion, inhalation or through open wounds.

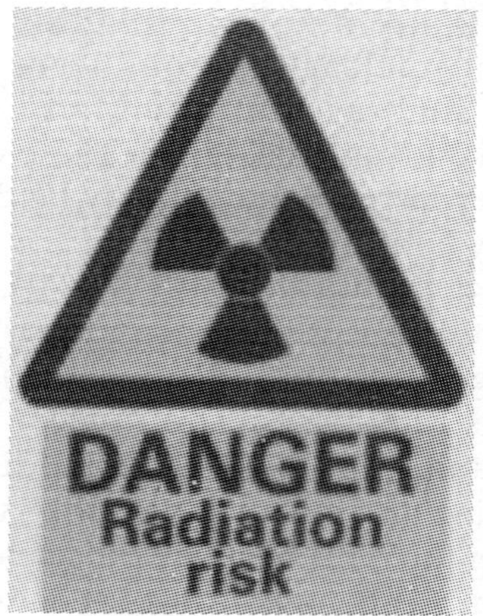

Fig. 70.3

THE INFLUENCE OF RADIATION ON TRIAGE

The triage procedure has to be modified for patients exposed to a source of ionizing radiation, the main aim being to contain contamination. Movements of such patients and the attending staff must be restricted by isolation. All clothing, soiled dressings, washings and body fluids must be collected separately for disposal by a specialist agency. The examiner must wear gloves and apron at all times and the time of onset of CNS, gastrointestinal and hemopoetic abnormalities after exposure are useful guidelines towards prognosis. Triage must be completed speedily as the patient will never be fitter to withstand surgical intervention than on the first day of exposure. In general, an atomic blast affects personnel by radiation fallout upto 10000km (2.6 to 3.2 km) from site of explosion, by shock wave upto 4.13 km, by thermal injury upto 9.1 km and by intense light causing visual injury upto 100 km. The four major types of ionizing radiation include alpha particles, beta particles, neutron radiation and gamma rays. Alpha particles are a low energy source of radiation and do little damage since they are easily absorbed by a layer of clothing, a few inches of air, paper or by the outer layer of the skin. Beta particles are higher in energy level but can be stopped by heavy clothing. Both alpha and beta particles are dangerous when inhaled, when they contaminate open wounds or are ingested when consuming irradiated foodstuff. Once inside the body, they produce cell damage until they are removed or until their decay. The more serious effects of radiation effects are mostly due to gamma rays and neutron radiation as they carry high levels of energy and can penetrate thick shielding and inflict extensive cell damage. Their activity persists from time of blast to 48 hours afterwards. Since ionizing radiation cannot be seen or felt, their presence is measured by a Geiger counter. The rate of radiation exposure is measured in roentgens per hour (r/hr) or milliroentgens per hour (mr/hr, 1000 mr=1r). Depending on the dosage of the exposure, ionizing radiation causes changes in cell division, cell structure and cellular chemical activities. Radiation can cause leukaemias and cancers and certain death above certain levels. How much radiation a person receives depends upon the source of radiation, the duration of exposure, the distance from the source and the shielding between the person and the source. Acute radiation sickness occurs after an exposure of 600 rads and above and is fatal within 48 hours. Exposure to below 100r/h is well tolerated. Above 200r/h exposure will cause moderate illness while above 300r/h is considered a serious exposure.

RADIATION EXPOSURE

- 1 Gray=100 rad=1 joule/kg.
- >10 rad – testis spermatogenesis depression.
- >500 rad – permanent sterility.
- >500 rad – skin burns.
- 75-240 rad – prodromal syndrome.
- 50-1000 rad – haemopoetic syndrome-lymphopenia <300-poor prognosis >1200 good prognosis.
- 400-5000 rad – GI syndrome-ulcerations and hemorrhage.
- >5000 rad – cerebral syndrome-vasculitis, meningoencephalitis, edema.
- >600 rads – over few hours is fatal.

Note: >100 rad exposures can cause fetal anomalies.

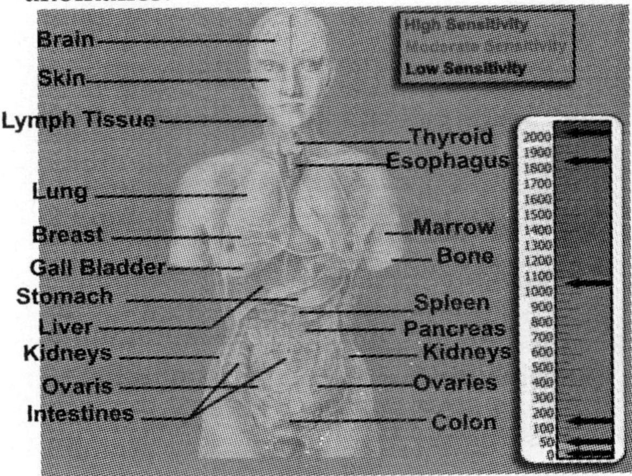

Fig. 70.4

While all personnel within the citadel would be safe, others will have to be decontaminated, after dossimetric assessment, by removal of all clothing, water hosing of the body and isolation. Ambulances must be parked upwind, as far behind the scene of contamination as possible, behind a shielding of thick concrete. Personnel must wear thick protective clothing and use breathing equipment with NBC filters. The rule for EMTs is 'get in and out quickly', with three EMTs taking turns to minimise exposure. All contaminated clothing and accessories must be placed in a metal container with a tight fitting lid. All vomitus and body wastes must also be sealed and labeled in metal containers. Surface decontamination is effected by showering with copious quantities of water, careful scrubbing of the entire body with particular attention to the hair, orifices and parts of the body that usually stay in contact like medial arm and lateral chest etc. The shower must be allowed to run after completing the wash to flush contaminants into the sanitary system. The victim is draped in a thick blanket with his/her head draped in a towel, leaving only the face exposed during transportation. Follow-up check by radiation experts and a physician must be ensured (Table 70.1).

Potassium Iodide tablets in an adult daily dose, taken for 120 days after exposure.

Table 70.1: Types of atomic burst

Effect	*Air burst*	*Ground surface*	*Under water*	*Under-ground*[1]
Anti-personnel effects				
Blast (50-60% of fatalities)	+ + + +	+ + +	+	+ +
Heat (20-30% of fatalities)				
"Flash", infra-red and				
ultraviolet..	+ + + +	+ + +	0	+
Secondary (foes)	+ + + +	+ + +	+	++
Radiation (15-20% of fatalities)				
Prompt				
gamma...............	+ + + +	+ + +	0	++
neutron.	+ + + +	+ + +	0	++
Delayed				
gamma..	+	++	++++	+++
beta[2].................	+	++	++++	+++
alpha..	0		+	++++
neutron	0	+	0	+
Persistent				
gamma.............	+	++	++++	+++
beta[2]..............	+	++	++++	+++
alpha......... ...	0	+	++++	++
Induced	+	++	0	+
Fall out (dust or rain)				
near.................	+	+	++++	++
distant	++	++	+	+
Structural damage				
Buildings destroyed	++++	++	+	++
Fires...........	++++	++	0	++
Transportation.	++++	++	+	++
Communication	++++	++	+	++

Small coated tablets overcome typical KI bitterness when dosing children 3+ years old with single whole tablet. Bottles containing 60 tablets of 85 mg each are double safety sealed, with childproof cap and contain desiccant for extended storage life. Also, this dose is sized for adults although it can be broken in half and quarters to dose for children. Potassium Iodate, KIO3 will shield (or block) the thyroid gland and prevent it from absorbing Radioactive Iodine during a nuclear emergency-War, Terrorism, Spills, Reactor Leaks, Melt-downs, or during Uranium enrichment.

Bibliography

Medical aspects of an atomic disaster plan King ER. US naval Medical Bulletin, Mar-Apr ,1948).

NUCLEAR DISARMAMENT

Beginning with the 1963 Partial Test Ban Treaty and continuing through the 1996 Comprehensive Test Ban Treaty, there have been many treaties to limit or reduce nuclear weapons testing and stockpiles. The 1968 Nuclear Non-Proliferation Treaty has as one of its explicit conditions that all signatories must "pursue negotiations in good faith" towards the long-term goal of "complete disarmament". However, no nuclear state has treated that aspect of the agreement as having binding force. The ongoing 3S (safeguards, safety and security)dialogue between USA, Australia and Japan under the auspices of the International Atomic Energy Agency aims at a world of decreased nuclear risk.

Only one country—South Africa—has ever fully renounced nuclear weapons they had independently developed. A number of former Soviet republics—Belarus, Kazakhstan, and Ukraine—returned Soviet nuclear arms stationed in their countries to Russia after the collapse of the USSR.

MANAGEMENT OF RADIATION EXPOSURE

Introduction

Emergency personnel are rarely familiar with the topics of radiation exposure and/or radioactive contamination, and few emergency physicians have experience in managing a case of acute radiation syndrome or local radiation injury. Although many emergency personnel have had training regarding procedures for handling the patient contaminated with radioactive materials, most training has focused on the more likely situation of handling only one or two accident patients. Sadly, today's international environment is such that the real possibility exists that emergency department personnel might have to deal with not just one or two victims of a radiation accident, but overwhelming numbers injured in a malevolent act. The types of catastrophes involving radiological or nuclear materials. Triage and distribution of patients to distant hospitals would be a necessity should such a malevolent act occur. Victims could be irradiated, contaminated with radioactive materials and injured by the heat and force of explosions. On-scene triage, should be based on the severity of conventional injuries, while triage during the first 24 hours of hospitalization should include considera-tion of exposure to penetrating radiation. Although irradiation does not cause early, life-threatening symptoms, it can, in time, cause serious or life-threatening illness if the radiation dose is high. If irradiation is combined with trauma, recovery is threatened. Triage and subsequent early treatment decisions are based on the signs and symptoms evident in the first 24 to 48 hours and on the results of laboratory tests completed during that time.

Types of Radiation Injury

Irradiation: Irradiation (sometimes called "exposure") occurs when a person is exposed to penetrating radiation (gamma rays, neutrons, X-rays) from a source external to the body. The total body or a large portion of it can be irradiated in an incident, or a small, localized area can be affected. Time, distance, and shielding can reduce exposure from a source. Once the source of penetrating radiation is removed, or the victim is moved away from the source, no further exposure will occur. Irradiation of the whole body or a significant part of it can result in acute radiation syndrome. Acute radiation syndrome begins with a prodrome that starts after exposure and lasts 24 to 48 hours. During this prodrome, the kind and severity of symptoms and their timing is dependent on the total amount of energy deposited in the body (i.e., the dose), the dose rate, and the volume and location of involved tissue. The prodromal period is followed by a symptom-free latent period lasting a few hours when exposures are high, or as long as two or three weeks or more for lower levels of exposure. A period of manifest illness follows, with the type of symptoms and their severity dependent on radiation dose. Dose is measured in "rads", (or, in SI units, in Grays. One hundred rads = 1 Gray). The LD 50/60, without treatment, is estimated to be 350 rads, or 3.5 Grays. In general, loss of stem cells and rapidly dividing cells from hematopoietic, gastrointestinal, and other tissues can lead to bleeding, infection, diarrhea, mucositis, skin lesions and other problems, followed by recovery or death. The symptoms occurring in the first 24 hours after a total or partial body exposure are seldom life-threatening. Examples of these are nausea, vomiting, fatigue, headache, diarrhea, parotitis, erythema, and fever. However, loss of fluids and electrolytes can be problematic in infants, children, and the elderly; in addition, some *lethal* exposures have resulted in severe hypotension.

Early symptoms of a localized skin injury from contact with a small but highly radioactive source of penetrating radiation include itching, tingling, erythema, and edema. Lesions do not appear for days to weeks. Unless symptomatic, emergency care is not needed urgently. However, these lesions can be debilitating and life threatening, and a significant amount of medical care could be forthcoming. If resources are sufficient, a baseline CBC and differential should be completed and repeated in 24 hours.

Medical follow-up is essential, and victims should be cautioned to avoid trauma to involved areas.

Contamination: External contamination occurs when radioactive materials are deposited on the external surface of the body. Internal contamination occurs when radioactive materials are ingested, inhaled, or absorbed through skin or wounds, or when neutron irradiation occurs. If radioactive atoms enter cells, they are said to be "incorporated". As long as radioactive materials are on or in a person, the person is being irradiated. Contamination does not cause symptoms, unless the contaminants are corrosive, toxic, or thermally hot. However, note that fission product fallout (i.e., from a nuclear weapon or nuclear reactor core damage) should be brushed off the skin and clothing as soon as possible, since it can be highly radioactive. Caregivers should use strict isolation precautions (including wearing cap, mask, gown, shoe covers, and double gloves) when handling contaminated victims, and gloves should be changed frequently to avoid cross contamination. In most cases, external contamination can be readily detected with survey instruments and readily removed.

Decontamination (removal of contaminants) can be accomplished by removal of the victim's clothing and thorough, careful washing with warm water and soap, followed by a radiation survey to determine if the washing procedure was sufficiently effective. Except for victims of serious trauma, decontamination can be accomplished prior to admission to hospital emergency care. Uninjured individuals do not require hospitalization unless they are vomiting, have diarrhea, or have conventional reasons for seeking emergency care. Detection of internal contamination is accomplished by whole body counting and/or with excreta analysis. Internal contamination does not cause early signs or symptoms. During the first 24 hours, those who are not injured (but are suspected of being internally contaminated) should be advised to seek assistance from public health authorities. Public health authorities may recommend excreta collection and/or lung or whole body counts.

If the radioactive contaminants have been identified, appropriate treatment will be instituted. For example, in the event of releases of radioactive iodines, public health officials would recommend administration of potassium iodide, especially to children and pregnant women.

Total body, partial body, or localized radiation injury can occur with external or internal contamination. Any of these radiation injuries can be complicated by the coincidental presence of trauma, chemical or thermal injury, as well as by serious pre-existing conditions (such as infections, uncontrolled diabetes, immune deficiencies, etc.).

Combined Injury: Combined injury is present when trauma, thermal, or chemical injury occurs along with a radiation exposure sufficient to cause immunosuppression, delayed healing, pancytopenia, and other problems. Combined injury is not likely with use of an explosive device such as a "dirty bomb", unless victims are trapped near sources of penetrating radiation. An overwhelming number of combined injury victims (and deaths) would be likely with a nuclear weapon detonation. Morbidity and mortality from thermal injury combined with the radiation injury would likely be high. Victims with serious trauma, thermal or chemical injury require prompt assessment, stabilization, and subsequent treatment to conserve life and limb. Radiation exposure increases the probability of mortality when combined with other injuries or pre-existing conditions that result in immunosuppression, blood loss, and danger of infectious complications. Early management of trauma and early recognition and assessment of radiation injury are essential if lives are to be saved.

Guidelines

The following guidelines are for dealing with an influx of victims of a nuclear or radiological catastrophe. They provide a fast, logical, and useful mechanism for gathering information and determining appropriate disposition of these patients. The guidelines are not intended to serve as a hospital's disaster plan. Ideally, such a plan should include a designated, rearranged triage area, and arrangements for the walking wounded, the worried well, concerned family members, etc. The guidelines could be useful for any hospital, clinic, or emergency care center receiving victims in the first 24 hours following a nuclear event. The hospital staff should not hesitate to admit victims because of fear of radiation or because of concern about contamination. Contaminants can be readily located with radiation detection devices, and facility decontamination can be accomplished once an emergency is over. It is important to note that the health physicists, medical physicists, radiation technicians, and others who are skilled in radiation detection, measurement must be involved in contamination control, and decontamination of personnel and facilities.

Initial Actions

(Hospital authority, emergency department supervisor, and/or emergency physician, according to existing hospital disaster plan.) Assign a non-medical person the responsibility of gathering incident information and keeping track of updates. Request that a written log be kept of this information, including who provided the information, where they are, and how they can be contacted. Have this person contact fire, police, and EMS to remind them to remove victims' clothes and leave them at the scene, if possible. Prepare for reception of victims. Initiate hospital disaster plan. Mobilize hospital radiation experts (i.e., radiation safety officer, nuclear medicine and radiation oncology specialists and all nuclear medicine and radiation oncology staff, as well as any radiologists not needed for trauma diagnostic studies). Request radiation monitoring and survey instruments. Request dosimeters for staff.

Request extra security for the emergency department. *Be aware that a terrorist could be among the victims.* Request police assistance for traffic and crowd control, assistance with gathering evidence, etc.Identify areas on the hospital grounds for incoming (1) "walking wounded" victims and (2) "worried well" individuals. Assign security and appropriate staff to areas.

Prepare the ED: Identify the area where contamination will be tolerated. Use ropes, tape, signs or other means to designate "clean" or "dirty" areas. Establish control lines. Request MANY large plastic bags and extra containers for waste, MANY boxes of plastic gloves, and necessary medical supplies. Prepare the staff. Staff should wear a scrub suit covered with a water resistant gown, or a Tyvek suit or other clothing to keep contaminants off skin. They should also wear a cap, face mask, boots or shoe covers. Two pairs of plastic gloves should be worn at all times. The first pair of gloves should be taped to the gown or Tyvek suit. The second pair of gloves should be changed after handling contaminated items and between patients. Dosimeters, if available, should be worn at the collar, but under protective clothing.

Guide for First 24 Hours in a Mass Casualty Situation

Possibly irradiated victims: No trauma:

- Focused history of exposure.
- Ask and record:
  - Where were you when the incident happened? (Specific address/location)
  - Were you inside a building/ house?
  - About how long were you outside?
  - Have you vomited or had diarrhea? About what time did it start?
  - How much do you weigh?
- Document if the person was decontaminated prior to admission.
- Document if a brief period of unconsciousness was reported.

RATIONALE

- Information about shielding and proximity of the victim to the source aids in determining the likelihood of radiation exposure. Subsequently, the information will be useful in dosimetry. Vomiting and diarrhea are symptoms of radiation injury. The time to onset of vomiting is roughly correlated to dose.
- Note that periodic measurements of patient's weight can guide fluid replacement for individuals with vomiting and diarrhea, since an overwhelmed professional staff will be unable to keep careful track of output.

- This is especially important for infants, children, the elderly and pregnant females.
- Patients who are incapacitated because of vomiting, diarrhea or shock might be contaminated on arrival at the hospital.
- Removal of clothing and decontamination should be accomplished at the earliest opportunity.
- Focused physical exam.
- Take vital signs, including temperature. Repeat every 2 hours for symptomatic patients.
- Note especially the occurrence of vomiting and diarrhea.
- Document the severity and timing.
- Note and record erythema of skin and/or mucosa, nausea, parotitis, headache, unusual fatigue, abdominal cramps.
- Note and record a history and/or evidence of altered CNS function. Rule out trauma as a cause.
- *Laboratory tests:* Obtain baseline CBC with differential and absolute lymphocyte count (i.e. total white count times the percent of lymphocytes on the differential).

RATIONALE

- Baseline measurements are important, since elevated temperature is related to dose, and development of hypotension is possible with high levels of exposure. (Rule out other causes).
- Less than 10% of persons vomit if the radiation dose is less than 1 Gray, whereas most vomit if the dose is more than 2 Gray. The time of vomiting is roughly correlated to dose.
- The acute onset of diarrhea is associated with doses greater than 9 Gray. Abdominal cramps and strong bowel contractions could also be present. Some symptoms of the acute radiation syndrome (such as fatigue, weakness, anorexia, headache) could be due to the physical and emotional stress of the situation or other causes. Vomiting and diarrhea can also be due to stress, but if present, radiation injury must be assumed until proven otherwise.
- If there is a history of loss of consciousness or evidence of cerebral edema or other CNS abnormality not due to physical trauma or stress, with a history of early vomiting (within minutes) and diarrhea, the victim's dose is likely greater than 15 Gray. Long term survival is unlikely, since multiorgan failure will ensue.
- Radiation exposure will cause early changes in blood cell counts.
- *Note:* If the initial lymphocyte count is below 1000/microliter, suspect significant radiation exposure.
- If vomiting and diarrhea occurred in the first 2 to 3 hours, consider the need for blood typing, HLA-sub-typing, and cytogenetic dosimetry. Obtain samples of blood before the lymphocyte count falls. Draw blood in heparinized tubes. If necessary, save for later analysis. Refrigerate but do not freeze. If history indicates that inhalation of radioactive materials was possible, ask patient (or parent of child) to collect a 24 hour urine specimen. (Any sealed container, properly labeled, is adequate. Refrigeration of the urine is not necessary).
- Collection of stools might be necessary in some cases, but public health or radiation experts will advise regarding this.
- Request serum amylase (if situation allows it and depending on laboratory capabilities).

Initial Treatment

- Anti-emetics, as needed. Ondansetron, granisetron, or other 5HT3 receptor antagonist.

- *Anti-diarrheals:* Loperamide hydrochloride, (diphenoxylate/atropine).
- Replace fluids and electrolytes as necessary.
- *Follow-up labs:* Repeat CBC with differential and absolute count at 6, 12 and 24 hours.

RATIONALE

- Bone marrow, cord blood or peripheral blood stem cells might be needed in treatment of patients at risk for pancytopenia.
- Cytogenetic dosimetry provides the most reliable whole body dose measurement.
- Excreta analysis is useful in determining if radioactive materials have been inhaled or ingested.
- Some elements are poorly absorbed in the GI tract and are excreted in the feces.
- Others "recycle" through the GI tract and their presence in the body can be detected through measurements of the elements in the feces.
- Initial results provide a baseline.
- Greater than 0.5 Gray (50 rads) to the total body or parotid glands causes a significant rise in serum amylase. (*Note:* Repeat measurement in approximately 24 hours.)
- Review hematology lab results: Absolute lymphocyte count, Neutrophil count, at 24 hours repeat serum amylase and review results in relation to baseline measurement. Request serum electrolytes as necessary.
- Follow-up physical exam at 6 and 12 hours
- Did the body temperature change in the first 5 to 6 hours after the incident?

RATIONALE

Lymphocytes are extremely sensitive to ionizing radiation. A drop in the absolute lymphocyte count indicates radiation exposure. procedures for estimating dose like Andrew's normogram for general severity estimates. A temporary rise in neutrophils with a decreased absolute lymphocyte count occurs with serious radiation exposures. Greater than 0.5 Gray (50 rads) to the whole body or parotid gland areas cause a significant rise in serum amylase. The rise reaches a maximum between 4 and 10 Gray, but the level is not well correlated with dose. Elevated temperature up to 5 hours after a radiation exposure is related to a dose greater than 2.5 Gray. The sooner the temperature rises, the higher the radiation dose

Note and record location of any erythema of skin and/or mucosa. Ask, observe, and record continuing or developing symptoms of the acute radiation syndrome: unusual fatigue, anorexia, nausea, vomiting and diarrhea (record frequency, timing, and severity), headache, muscle weakness, altered reflexes, abdominal cramps, parotitis, hypoxemia, hypotension. Observe for evidence of dehydration.

RATIONALE

Note that erythema can disappear from one area and reappear in another area. Early (occurring in less than 6 hours after exposure), widespread erythema could be a sign of a whole body dose of greater than 4 Gray and a skin dose much higher. Persons with extensive erythema will require care in a burn center or in a specialized facility. Documentation of areas of erythema will aid in determining the uniformity of the exposure, the general direction of gamma radiation and areas with highest levels of beta exposure. Erythema of mucosa portends development of radiation mucositis.

Considerations for Patient Disposition

Note: Disposition of patients might take place before laboratory test results are available.

If a patient is transferred to another facility, the receiving hospital should complete the test sequence and, as soon as feasible, contact the original hospital for transfer of initial test results. Test results will provide valuable information that will be useful in determining the subsequent medical treatment.

SIGNS AND SYMPTOMS

Vomiting a few minutes after exposure, diarrhea in less than an hour, fever in less than an hour, severe headache, possible history of a period of unconsciousness or altered consciousness, possible hypotension, abdominal cramps, erythema, parotid pain. Onset of vomiting less than 30 minutes after exposure incident, early fever, severe headache, possible diarrhea within 2 hours, parotid pain, possible erythema. Prodromal symptoms are severe.

DECISION AND FOLLOW-UP

Supportive/palliative care is needed. Draw blood for CBC and differential and cytogenetic dosimetry. Evaluate daily CBC and re-evaluate as more information is available. (*Note:* If resources are NOT scarce, treat as following group.) Prolonged survival is possible with intensive medical care, but prognosis is poor. Intensive care needed beginning day 1. If transfer is necessary because of the number of patients or because other expertise is needed, transfer on day 1 or as soon as feasible. The latent period of the acute radiation syndrome (ARS) might be short or absent with higher doses, with the prodromal period followed by a continuing severe illness. Cytogenetic dosimetry is recommended. Blood and tissue typing are needed. Hematopoietic growth factor therapy should begin early. Viral prophylaxis recommended. CBC daily. Consult with hematologist. Consider cord blood transplant for children and peripheral blood stem cell transplant for adults.

SIGNS AND SYMPTOMS

Onset of vomiting in less than 1 hour of incident, fever in 1 to 2 hours, diarrhea in 3 to 8 hours in less than 10% of victims. Parotid pain and erythema possible in some patients. Nausea, vomiting with onset 1 to 2 hours after exposure.

DECISION AND FOLLOW-UP

Hospitalization necessary. Prodrome lasts approximately 48 hours. Latent period follows, lasting 1 to 3 weeks. Intensive care might be needed during period of severe illness. Patient can be transferred to another hospital for intensive care if necessary. CBCs with differentials daily. Cytogenetic dosimetry needed. Blood and tissue typing recommended. Viral prophylaxis recommended. Hematopoietic growth factory therapy needed. Consult with hematologist or radiation oncologist regarding use. Consider consult with pediatric hematologist regarding cord blood transplant for children. Peripheral blood stem cell transplant might be indicated for some victims.

Hospitalization or careful medical observation recommended. If hospital beds are scarce, hospitalization can be delayed unless patient is symptomatic. Patients can be transferred to other facilities if hospitalization is needed because of age, pre-existing medical condition, or other problem.

Prodrome lasts approximately 48 hours. A latent period follows, lasting 1 to 3 weeks. CBCs with differentials should be scheduled every 3 days or as necessary. Expect neutrophil and platelet count to reach nadir in 2 to 3 weeks. Cytogenetic dosimetry is recommended but not urgent. Some patients might need growth factors.

SIGNS AND SYMPTOMS

Anorexia, nausea, no vomiting more than 2 hours after irradiation.

DISCUSSION AND FOLLOW-UP

Provide instructions if hospitalization is delayed: Make every attempt to avoid infections or injury; take temperature every day and notify physician of elevation; report for CBCs as requested; notify physician and report for hospitalization if fever, infection, bleeding from body orifice or injury occurs.

Collect blood for CBC and differential. Discharge with instructions to return for CBC and differential in 1 week or earlier if problems arise. Out-patient follow-up is recommended.

GUIDELINES: FIRST 24 HOURS IN A MASS CASUALTY SITUATION; INJURED VICTIMS, POSSIBLY IRRADIATED

1. Attend to ABCs and standard trauma resuscitation.
2. Determine YES/NO if contaminated with radioactive material. (If personnel and survey instruments are not available, assume contamination).
3. Remove clothing if not accomplished previously.
4. Delay further decontamination until patient is stable. However, if visible pieces of metal are embedded in tissue, assume they are radioactive and promptly use long forceps to remove the metal particles. Store them in a labeled container in a shielded area away from people.
5. Obtain abbreviated medical and exposure history (from rescuer or patient).
6. Mechanism of injury, allergies, medications in use, etc. Focused history of exposure. Where was patient located at time of event (address, inside or outside, proximity to source if known, approximate time trapped in radiation area).
7. Note report of or evidence of vomiting or diarrhea.

RATIONALE

Radiation does not cause immediate life-threatening problems. Serious injury takes priority over concerns about contamination. Note that most contamination is removed with clothing. Quick action will reduce exposure to staff and patient. Distance and shielding will reduce exposure to staff and patient. Routine. Information about shielding and proximity of the victim to the source of radiation aids in estimating the likelihood of radiation exposure. Subsequently the information will be useful in dosimetry estimates. Vomiting and diarrhea are symptoms of acute radiation injury. The time of onset of GI symptoms is roughly correlated to dose.

If patient is able to respond, ask weight. Physical exam: routine, plus: Note and document vital signs and temperature every 2 hours or as necessary. Note and document erythema (noting areas and distinguishing between flame/flash burns and erythema due to radiation).

Record frequency and timing of vomiting and diarrhea.

Record presence of parotitis or parotid edema.

Evaluate CNS symptoms. Rule out trauma as case of symptoms.

Labs: Obtain CBC, differential and absolute lymphocyte count. Request serum amylase. Type and cross-match prn. *If blood transfusion is needed, use irradiated blood if available.* Routine labs (as necessary for patient's condition).

RATIONALE

Hypoxemia and hypotension have occurred in victims after very high radiation doses. Elevated temperature in the first 5 to 6 hours occurs with a radiation dose greater than 2.5

Gray. Flame and flash burns are painful and there is loss of hair in the involved area along with tissue loss (depending on the depth of the burns). The primary erythema caused by radiation is not accompanied by obvious loss of tissue and there is no hair loss. (Epilation does not occur for 2 to 3 weeks after an exposure). Although the irradiated tissue might be somewhat edematous and feel "stretched" or "itchy", it is not painful. Cells of the parotid are sensitive to radiation exposure. The presence of parotitis is an indication of radiation exposure. Irradiation of blood prevents the transfusion of live WBC and reduces the chance of subsequent graft versus host disease.

If patient has signs and symptoms of the ARS, consider the need for tissue typing and cytogenetic dosimetry. (Obtain samples early, before the lymphocyte count falls). Begin 24 hour urine collection. Treat serious injuries according to usual protocols. Open wounds are considered to be contaminated, even if there is no visible material in the wound. Clean the area around the wound and drape. Flush wounds copiously using standard wound management. Debride as necessary. Close open wounds, or use biological wound dressings. If surgery is needed and there are indications of acute radiation syndrome, *necessary surgery should be completed* as soon as possible – *within the first 48 to 72 hours of the radiation injury.*

Plan to avoid additional surgery until hematopoiesis is restored. Follow procedure for ARS. Note that lymphocyte dosimetry *may* beless reliable because of the physiologic response to trauma and thermal injury, as well as hemoconcentration or hemodilution associated with injury or therapy, use of transfusions, etc.

RATIONALE

Peripheral blood stem cell transplants (or cord blood for children), platelet, or RBC transfusions might be needed. Excreta analysis is useful in determining if radioactive materials have been inhaled or ingested. Wounds that are closed are less likely to allow entrance of infectious agents. These patients will become leukopenic, thrombocytopenic, immunosuppressed, and anemic. Expect nadir at approximately 2 to 3 weeks, although it could occur sooner if significant blood loss occurred. (Note that the severity is dependent on the radiation dose.) These patients are at risk for prolon-ged healing times, delayed callous formation in fractures, and other complications.

Serious trauma or other stress can cause an initial lymphocytosis which is followed in a short time (hours) by lymphopenia. Other signs and symptoms indicating exposure (vomiting, diarrhea, erythema, and elevated temperature) might still be present, although vomiting is less reliable as an indicator of ARS if a patient is in pain, shock, or reacting to medication. Serum amylase (parotid) should not be affected by trauma unless parotids are involved.

Considerations for patient disposition:

- Decisions to transfer for surgery, burn care or supportive care are based on the patient's injuries, clinical condition, age, the number of patients, etc.
- *Transfers should be carried out during the first 72 hours when possible.*
- *Necessary surgery should be completed within 72 hours.*

Trauma or burn victims in serious or critical condition after initial stabilization, who have also been determined to be significantly irradiated (based on accident history, history of early vomiting, diarrhea, early elevated temperature, erythema, elevated serum amylase in first 24 hours) should be given palliative/compassionate care. Patients with radiation injury and trauma or thermal injury (greater than 10% BSA) should be *hospitalized or under watchful medical surveillance* because of the risk of immunosuppression and pancytopenia. Reverse isolation is recommended. If neutrophil or platelet counts are low, if infection, pre-existing illness, or other complicating factors are present, hospital care is recommended. Victims with simple fractures, after stabilization and decontamination, should be triaged according to ARS guide. Expect delayed callous formation. Victims with minor injuries will most likely have to wait for treatment. They should be showered and have clean clothing prior to hospital admission, if possible. Superficial skin wounds should be thoroughly washed while showering. After the wound is treated and covered, the patient should be triaged according to the ARS guide.

Information or experience regarding combined injury in infants, young children, or the elderly is not available. Summary: With few exceptions, radiation accidents over the past 60 years have generated small numbers of patients requiring emergency or intensive care. Notable exceptions are the Chernobyl accident (1986) and the Cs-137 accident in Goiania, Brazil (1987). However, with the real threat of nuclear/ radiological terrorism, an emergency department staff may be overwhelmed by individuals requiring or seeking medical attention after a malevolent act. Leadership, command and control, security and communication capability will be essential. Emergency department personnel would find it challenging to triage, evaluate, and treat large numbers of irradiated/contaminated victims. Specific guidance and the associated rationale are presented and provide a stepwise approach to patient care.

Life threatening trauma should be dealt with promptly and injured managed according to usual accepted practice with some exceptions regarding timing of surgical intervention and wound closure. It is important to stress that good clinical medicine should be practised in spite of the distractions of the situation and personal concerns about contamination and radiation exposure.

Types of Nuclear/Radiological Catastrophes

1. *Detonation of a "dirty bomb"*, (an explosive device used to disperse radioactive material) or detonation of the high explosives in a nuclear weapon without a nuclear yield:

   Problems:
   - Explosive dispersal of radioactive material in the environment.
   - Blast injuries, burns, and trauma, with possible entrapment of some victims.
   - Possible localized radiation injuries due to radioactive material blown onto skin or embedded in wounds.
   - Internal contamination of victims if material is vaporized or dispersed in ultra-fine particles.
   - Acute radiation syndrome not likely unless victims are trapped near high activity sources emitting penetrating gamma radiation (such as Ir-192, Cs-137, Co-60).
   - Widespread psychological trauma.
   - Vaporization/aerosolization of radioactive materials and subsequent dispersal by wind and weather could cause contamination of the environment and economic disruption.
2. *Explosive destruction of a nuclear reactor:*

   Problems:
   - Blast injury to those in vicinity.
   - Radiation exposure and contamination to those onsite and in surrounding areas.
   - Widespread psychological trauma.
   - Airborne dispersal of radioactive materials which would cause contamination of the environment and economic depression.

- Release of radioactive iodine would necessitate administration of thyroid blocking potassium iodide (KI) to children, pregnant women and others.

Note that implementation of existing and well rehearsed emergency response plans would substantially minimize the number of injuries caused by radiation.

3. *Detonation of a nuclear weapon:*
   Problems:
   - Massive widespread destruction with catastrophic consequences from blast, heat, and radiation.
   - Hundreds to thousands of immediate deaths.
   - Hundreds to hundreds of thousands of victims with burns, blast injuries and trauma, radiation exposure, contamination, flash blindness, etc.
   - Destruction of medical facilities, fire, EMS services, and emergency management capabilities in the involved area, with loss of personnel.
   - Widespread contamination of environment.
   - Nationwide psychological trauma.
   - Computer, electrical equipment, phone system, etc., malfunction due to an electromagnetic pulse that can occur with a nuclear detonation.

Ways to Reduce Exposure from a Source of Radiation

- Reduce time near a radiation source to lower exposures. Work quickly and efficiently.
- Increase distance from a radiation source to lower exposure. When not involved in care of a contaminated patient, remain a few feet away from the patient. Use long handled forceps to remove contaminated particles, dressings, etc.
- Shielding (such as from buildings, walls or debris) lowers exposure. Put contaminated metal or glass in lead containers. Place bags of contaminated waste in secure concrete walled areas away from the immediate work area.

Types of Radiation Injury

Radiation injury can occur in any of the following ways:

Total or partial body irradiation (exposure) can be present with or without any of the following:

- Internal and/or external contamination.
- Trauma.
- Local radiation injury.

Local radiation injury can be present with or without:

- Internal and/or external contamination.
- Trauma.

External contamination can be present with or without:

- Internal contamination.
- Trauma.

Estimation of Dose Related to Onset of Vomiting

For *single, acute exposure,* note time of onset of vomiting and estimated dose range. The timeframe for onset of symptoms varies if dose rate was low (i.e., total exposure was spread over time).

Onset time of vomiting	*Estimated dose*
After exposure	
Less than 10 minutes	>8 Gy
10-30 minutes	6-8 Gy
Less than 1 hour	4-6 Gy
1-2 hours	2-4 Gy
More than 2 hours after	< 2 Gy

Procedure for Determining Approximate Dose Based on Lymphocyte Count

Determine initial lymphocyte count and subsequent counts at 6 or 12 hours. Divide initial count (L1) by (L2). Take natural log of quotient. Divide result by the time change in 24 hours (number of hours between counts divided by 24) to determine K. Refer to table below for estimated dose:

(K=)	*Estimated dose in Gy*
0.1	1.24
0.2	2.27
0.4	3.90
0.6	5.11
0.8	6.06
1.0	6.82
1.5	8.18
2.0	9.09
2.5	9.73
3.0	10.22

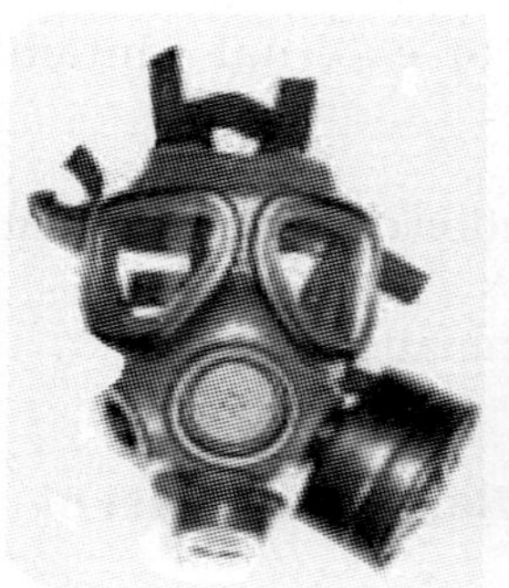

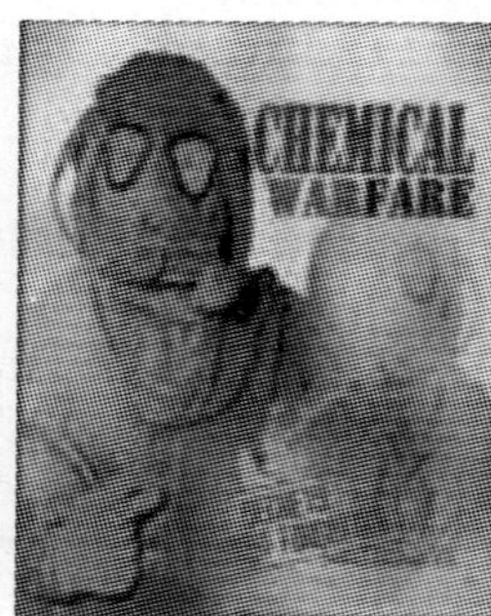

Fig. 70.5

Chemical Warfare

The horror of chemical death has an undermining effect on the psychology of the troops and poses a difficulty in diagnosis for the physician. Many of the symptoms of poisoning mimic those of battle stress. Fast pulse rate, stomach cramps, narrowed vision, headaches, vomiting and involuntary defecation and shock state can occur in both settings. At times, it would be difficult to differentiate between a shell-shocked soldier from a gassed one, and unnecessary use of antidotes may compound the problem further. It becomes important, therefore, that the field medic is in the know of how his colleagues react to stress. Chemical agents have been called "the poor man's atomic bomb" because of their ease of acquisition, production and potential use.

Definition

Chemical warfare agents, as defined by the United National Chemical Weapons Convention, are "any chemical which, through its chemical effect on living processes, may cause death, temporary loss of performance, or permanent injury to people and animals.

HISTORICAL ASPECTS OF CHEMICAL WARFARE

Some instances where Chemical Weapons have been used:

42 BC: Spartans ignite pitch and sulphur to create toxic fumes in the Peloponnesian War.

424 BC: Toxic fumes used in siege of Delium during the Peloponnesian War.

1456: City of Belgrade defeats invading Turks by igniting rags dipped in poison to create a toxic cloud.

April 24, 1863: The US War Department issues General Order 100, proclaiming the use of poison in any manner, be it to poison wells, or foods, or arms, is wholly excluded from modern warfare.

World war I: The use of chemical agents in WWI caused an estimated 1,300,000 casualties, including 90,000 deaths.

1914: French begin using tear gas in grenades and Germans retaliate with tear gas in artillery shells. This was the first significant use of chemical warfare in WW I.

April 22, 1915: Germans attack the French with chlorine gas at Ypres, France. This was the first significant use of chemical warfare in WWI.

September 25, 1915: First British chemical weapons attack; chlorine gas is used against

Germans at the Battle of Loos

February 26, 1918: Germans launch the first projectile attack against US troops with phosgene and chloropicrin shells. The first major use of gas against American forces.

June 1918: Fist US use of gas in warfare.

June 28, 1918: The US begins its formal chemical weapons program with the establishment of the Chemical Warfare Service.

1911: British use Adamsite against the Bolsheviks during the Russian Civil War.

1922–1927: The Spanish use chemical weapons against the Rif rebels in Spanish Morocco.

1936: Italy uses mustard gas against Ethiopians during its invasion of Abyssinia.

1942: Nazis begin using Zyklon B (hydrocyanic acid) in gas chambers for the mass murder of concentration camp prisoners.

Dec 1943: A US ship loaded with mustard bombs s attacked by Germans in the port of Bari, Italy; 83 US troops die in poisoned waters.

April 1945: Germans manufacture and stockpile large amounts of tabun and sarin nerve gases but do not use them.

1962–197: US uses treat gas and four types of defoliant, including Agent Orange, in Vietnam.

1963-1967: Egypt uses chemical weapons (phosgene, mustard) against Yemen.

1975-1983: Alleged use of Yellow Rain (trichothecene mycotoxins) by Soviet-backed forces in Laos and Kampuchea. There is evidence to suggest use of T-2 toxin, but an alternative hypothesis suggests that the yellow spots labelled Yellow Rain were caused by swarms of defecating bees.

1979: The US government alleges Soviets use of chemical weapons in Afghanistan, including Yellow Rain.

August, 1983: Iraq begins using chemical weapons (mustard gas), Iran-Iraq War.

1984: First ever use of nerve agent tabun on the battlefield, by Iraq during Iran-Iraq War.

1987-1988: Iraq uses chemical weapons (hydrogen cyanide, mustard gas) in its Anfal Campaign against the Kurds, most notably in the Halabja Massacre of 1988.

March 20, 1995: The Tokyo Subway sarin gas attack killed nearly a dozen people and incapacitating or injuring approximately 5,00 others. Thousands did not die from the Tokyo attack due to impurity of the agent. A tiny drop of sarin, which was originally developed in Germany in the 1930s, can kill within minutes after skin contact or inhalation of its vapour. Like all other nerve agents, sarin blocks the action of acetylcholinesterase, an enzyme necessary for the transmission of nerve impulses.

SPECTRUM OF CHEMICALS FOR WARFARE

About 700 different chemicals have been used or stockpiled as Chemical Weapons (CW) agents during the 20th century. These chemicals are in liquid, gas or solid form and blister, choke and affect the nerves or blood. Chemical warfare agents are generally classified according to their effect on the organism and can be roughly grouped as Nerve Agents, Mustard Agents, Hydrogen Cyanide, Tear Gases, Arsines, Psychotomimetic Agents, Toxins and Potential CW Agents.

Under the Chemical Weapons Convention (CWC) chemicals are divided into three groups, defining their purpose and treatment:-

- Schedule One are those typically used in weapons such as sarin and mustard gas and tabun.

- Schedule Two include those that can be used in weapons such as amiton and BZ.
- Schedule Three chemicals include the least toxic substances that can be used for research and the production of medicine, dyes, textiles, etc.

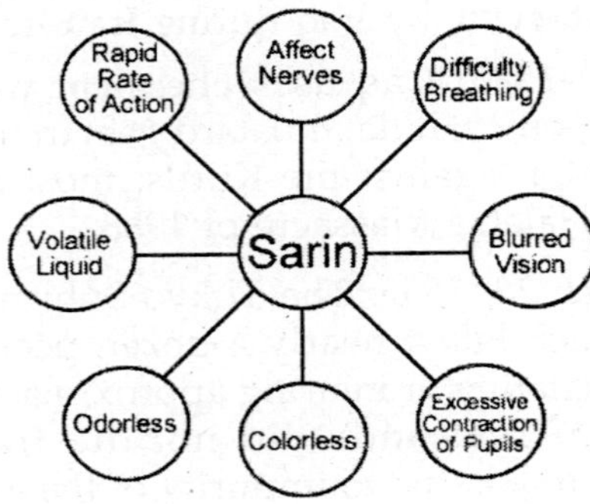

Fig. 70.6

CW agents mainly used against people are divided into lethal and incapacitating categories. A substance is classified as incapacitating if less than 1/10 of the lethal dose causes incapacitation, e.g., through nausea or visual problems. The limit between lethal and incapacitating substances is not absolute but refers to a statistical average.

Classification of CW agents

- Chemicals that blister, e.g., sulphur mustard, lewisite, nitrogen mustard, mustard-lewisite, phosgene-oxime.
- Chemicals that affect the nerves, e.g., VX, Sarin, Soman, tabun, novichole agents.
- Chemicals that cause choking, e.g., chlorine, phosgene, diphosgene, chloropicrin.
- Chemicals that affect the blood, e.g., herygem, cynanide, cyanogen chlorine.
- Chemicals for riot control, e.g., tear agent 2 (SN gas), tear agent (CS gas), psychedelic agent 3 (BZ).

Incendiary agents such as napalm and phosphorus are not considered to be CW agents since they achieve their effect mainly through thermal energy. Certain types of smoke ammunition are not classed as a chemical weapon since the poisonous effect is not the reason for their use.

The most dreaded chemical is cyanide. It inhibits mitochondrial ferricytochrome oxidase enzymes and blocks electron transport. This results in decreased oxidative metabolism and utilization prompting anaerobic metabolism and lactic acidosis.

Protection Against Chemical Warfare

The principles of protection in the event of a chemical warfare attack are:

Avoidance by reconnaissance, detection, identification, location, quantification, warning/alarm and by reporting. All these must be in real time.

Verification and Identification

In order to reach decisions on the level of protection required, it is necessary to know the type of agent present in the area and whether the concentration exceeds the threshold level. If alarms are sounded on the basis of vague detection reports (direct observations), the suspicions should be confirmed by verification. In order to reach tactical decisions, more detailed information on CW agents is necessary.

Detection (enzyme) tickets and detection tubes are sufficient to demonstrate nerve agents and mustard agent under field conditions. A manual suction pump is used to draw air through the detection tube or against the ticket. Subsequently, the material is developed in order to see whether CW agents have affected the tube or ticket. A small device called the BUTTON that fits inside a gas mask is an efficient chemical detector containing its own liquid to moisturise reagents contained within and indicate to the soldier on the field if the atmosphere is free of nerve gas.

In order to reach tactical decisions, more detailed information on CW agents is necessary. This identification can be done to some extent by means of a combination of manual vapor detection (tickets and tubes) and detection paper. Information on an even higher reliability level will require analysis in a laboratory. Samples can then be taken in the field for subsequent analysis.

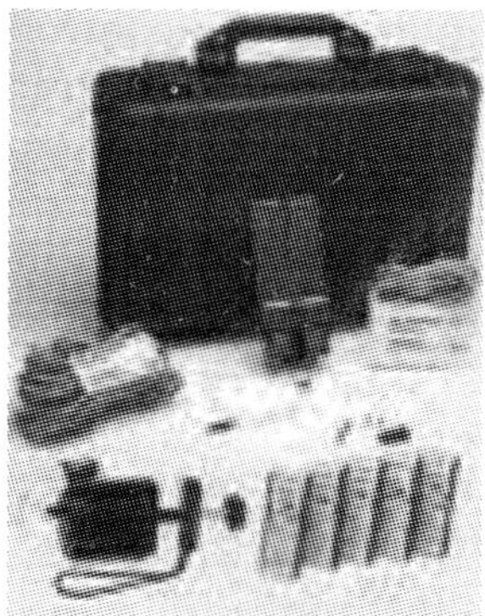

Fig. 70.7

MANUAL DETECTION METHODS

They must be sensitive, selective, have a low probability of false positives or negatives and give results in real time (less than 60 seconds), inexpensive, heavy duty, easy to operate, work over a wide range of temperatures and have agent specific alarm modes. The various techniques available are as follows:

Detection Paper

Chemical detection paper can detect and identify airborne chemical warfare agents. The paper is attached as patches to the chemical-defense overgarment using either an adhesive backing or Velcro like bonding material. The paper is impregnated with dyes sensitive to different types of chemical warfare agent, and will indicate which type of agent is present by its corresponding pigment signal. Detection paper is based on certain dyes being soluble in CW agents. Normally, two dyes and one pH indicator are used, which are mixed with cellulose fibers in a paper without special coloring (unbleached). When a drop of CW agent is absorbed by the paper, it dissolves one of the pigments. Mustard agent dissolves a red dye and nerve agent a yellow. In addition, VX causes the indicator to turn to blue which, together with the yellow, will become green/green-black. Detection paper can thus be used to distinguish between three different types of CW agents. A disadvantage with the papers is that many other substances can also dissolve the pigments. Consequently, they should not be located in places where drops of, e.g., solvent, fat, oil or fuel can fall on them. Drops of water give no reaction. On the basis of spot diameter and density on the detection paper, it is possible to obtain an opinion on the original size of the droplets and the degree of contamination. A droplet of 0.5 mm diameter gives a spot sized about 3 mm on the paper. A droplet/cm^2 of this kind corresponds to a ground contamination of about 0.5 g/m^2. The lower detection limit in favorable cases is 0.005 g/m^2.

Detection Tubes

The detection tube for mustard agent is a glass tube containing silica gel impregnated with a substrate (DB-3). Detection air is sucked through the tube using a special pump. The reaction between the mustard agent and substrate (see below) is speeded up by heating the tube with, e.g., a cigarette lighter. A developer is then added, and the result can be read-off. If the silica gel in the tube turns blue, then the vapor in the sample contains mustard agent.

Detection Tickets

Detection tickets for nerve agents are used in a similar way. The ticket consists of two parts, one with enzyme-impregnated paper and the other with substrate-impregnated paper. When the package is broken and the enzyme paper wetted, the substrate part of the ticket is exposed to the test vapor by means of a pump. Subsequently, the two parts are put together for two minutes. If the enzyme part of the ticket has turned a weak blue color, nerve agent is not present in the air. The detection limit is 0.02-0-05 mg/m^3 depending on the number of strokes of the pump. The ticket can also be used without a pump (by waving it in the air) but this gives a slightly poorer sensitivity. An example of the enzyme substrate reaction used in detection tickets for nerve agents can be seen below. Note that the blue change of color requires an active enzyme – some form of cholinesterase. In the presence of nerve agents, the enzyme is inhibited and no change of color occurs. Detection tickets of this kind cannot distinguish between the different nerve agents.

1. ONE-DIMENSIONAL SENSORS (SELECTIVE DETECTORS)

The simplest approach for chemical detection is to target the specific compound of interest and selectively detect it in the presence of other background compounds and interferences.

Surface Acoustic Wave (SAW) Sensors

One of the most popular approaches for selective sensing of CW agents is the SAW sensor. First reported by Wohltjen and Dessy in 1979 and based on the GC piezoelectric response demonstrated by King in 1964 this sensor detects adsorption of an analyte on the surface of a piezoelectric crystal. When a time-varying electric field is applied to one side of a piezoelectric material, it sets up an acoustic wave that is propagated along the surface of the piezoelectric material and detected by electrodes located at the other end of the material. Changes in amplitude or phase of this wave occur when an analyte adsorbs onto the surface of the piezoelectric material. When the surface is coated with a thin film, which adsorbs chemicals selectively, a selective sensor is produced. Early work on the application of SAW instruments to CW agent detection reported the development of a temperature-controlled array of SAW devices with automated sample preconcentration and pattern recognition. Detection limits as low as 0.01 mg/m for organophosphorus analytes and 0.5 mg/m for organosulfur analytes were obtained within 2 min. Besides the difficulty of developing selective coatings for SAW sensors, polymer films can dewet the surface and produce isolated droplets The major advantage of SAW detectors is that they can be made small and portable. A small sensor based on SAW technology called the joint chemical agent detector (JCAD) unit has a threshold detection level of 1 mg/m^3 for both V- and G-type nerve agents. Threshold detection levels for vesicant blister agents such as lewisite were found to be slightly higher at 50 mg/m. However, in 1 min, typical blood agents like AC or CK can be detected at 22 mg/m and 20 mg/m respectively. The JCAD unit is portable weighing under a kilo and can operate over a wide range of environmental temperatures. The SAWRHINO is based on the SAW system and has been developed for vehicular mounted field applications. It is an automated chemical agent detector, providing reversible responses for G-nerve and H-mustard agents. The SAWRHINO is reported to provide 7 orders of magnitude from a detection limit of 200 parts per trillion.

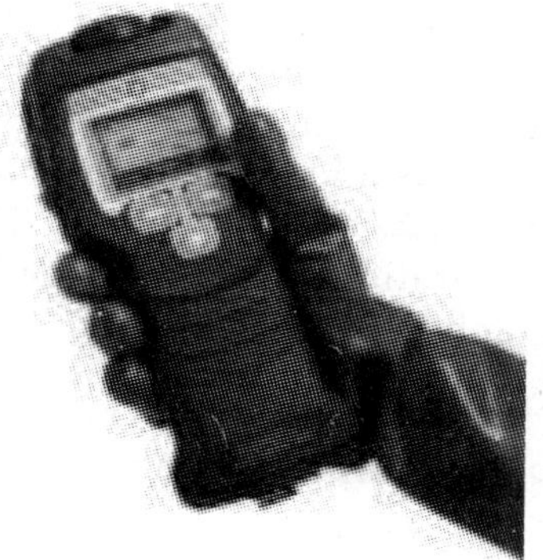

Fig. 70.8

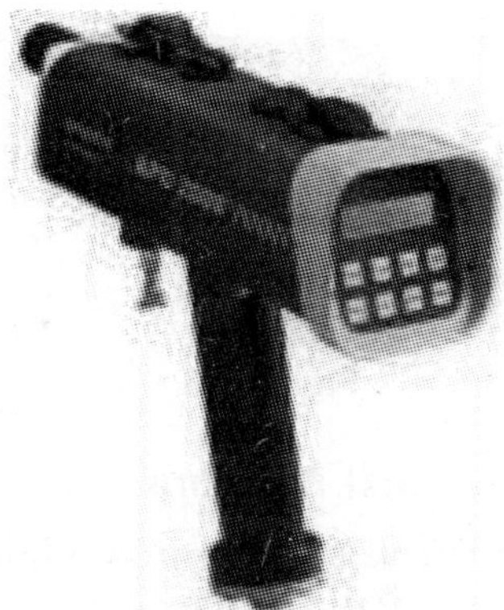

Fig. 70.9

Electrochemical Sensors

Direct determination of organophosphate nerve agents can also be accomplished using the amperometric response of an enzyme biosensor. In this approach, the biosensor incorporated the enzyme organophosphorus hydrolase by covalently immobilizing it on glass beads. The enzyme hydrolyzes organophosphate to an electroactive species, which can be determined amperometrically. Best results were achieved with organophosphates containing a nitrophenyl group. This approach has been incorporated into a single-channel microchip for the rapid screening of organophosphate nerve agents. Chemiresistive vapor detectors for nerve agent simulants have also been reported. They use a conducting polymer composite that changes electrical resistance when an agent adsorbs onto the surface. The detection limit for this sensor is in the range of 47–240 μg/m of dimethyl methyl phosphonate (DMMP) in air.

Spectrophotometric Sensors

The least expensive approach to chemical agent detection is the use of the color spot test. Chemical agent detector kits are available that can identify field concentrations of nerve agents (GB, GA, GC, GF, and VX), vesicant agents (mustard, phosgene oxime, mustard-lewisite, and lewisite), and blood agents (hydrogen cyanide and cyanogen chloride) in about 15–20 min. Chemical agents are adsorbed onto a pretreated test spot, and when a "developer" reagent is added, specific color changes indicate the presence or absence of chemical agents. The problem with the spot test approach is that it is too slow and insensitive for early warning detection and not sufficiently selective to provide reliable verification. Nevertheless, for CW veri-fication, the spot test approach is a convenient method for initial screening. More sophisti-cated color detection relies on the use of spectrophotometers. Techniques of molecular imprinting have been combined with sensitized lanthanide luminescence to create a selective sensor for nerve agents. When hydrolysis products of a chemical warfare nerve agent such as sarin or soman adsorb to the imprinted polymer, a narrow luminescence band in the 610 nm region of the Euspectrum appears due to a shift in the ligand field. The limit of detection for this method is on the order of 7 ppt in solution with a linear range up to 10 ppm. Immobilized whole-cell photosynthetic microorganisms have been used for stand-off detection of airborne chemical warfare agents and simulants using well-known principles of fluorescence induction. The fluorescence signal from the sensors is stable for up to 40 days.

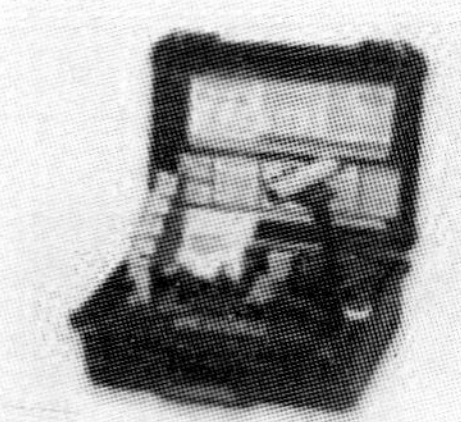

Fig. 70.10

Immunochemical Sensors

Immunochemical sensors potentially offer a more specific alternative to the relatively nonspecific color reactions involved with spot tests. In this approach, a protein antibody is developed that binds specifically to the chemical agent and elicits some type of analytical response. Fluorescence and electrochemical responses have been used. However, enzyme-linked immunoabsorbent assays (ELISA) have proven most useful for the detection of a variety of nerve agents. For example, soman, even in the presence of its major hydrolysis product, can be detected down to levels of 180 ng/ml (180 ppb). A major problem with immunochemical sensors is that they are slow, taking up to 2 h in some cases. While this is a problem for early warning of a chemical attack, specific ELISA sensors could be used for verification. In general, immunochemical assays are expensive to develop, but can be inexpensive for large numbers of assays. Another problem for field analysis is the stability of the antibody in a variety of environmental conditions and for long periods of time. For these reasons, immunochemical assays have not reached their potential as a simple, sensitive, and selective assay for chemical warfare agents.

2. TWO-DIMENSIONAL SENSORS

Due to the complex nature of the agents and their matrices, nonseparation-based analytical methods often experience interferences, which result in false positive or negative responses. Thus, some type of separation method is often coupled to an analytical detector to provide more specificity of response and a broader range of application. The most common separation devices are GC, liquid chromatography (LC), capillary electrophoresis (CE), IMS, and mass spectro-metry (MS).

Gas Chromatography (GC)

For vapor-phase chemical warfare agents, GC is usually the analytical separation method of choice. In general, a high-resolution gas chromatographic separation can require up to 30 min for complete separation and detection of a complex mixture. However, when selective detectors are used in combination with GC, the separation time can be reduced significantly. For example, using a pulsed-flame photometric detector, which is highly selective for phosphorus and sulfur-containing compounds, detection of 20 ng/m of organophosphorus compounds and 200 ng/m for organosulfur compounds can be accomplished within 30s. Collection and concentration in tubes packed with selected adsorbents followed by thermal desorption of the agent and gas chromatographic separation proved to be useful for both high- and low-volatility analytes. Collection and concentration are also convenient for GC using solid-phase microextraction (SPME) methods. Selective SPME prior to sample introduction into a GC increases the select-ivity of the analysis for sarin. Sulfur mustard has also been detected by SPME in soil samples.

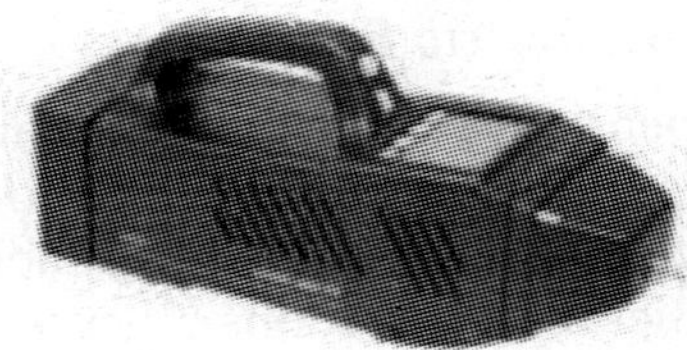

Fig. 70.11

Liquid Chromatography (LC)

For compounds that are not volatile or thermally labile, LC rather than GC is often the method of choice for separation prior to detection. However, high pressures and small particle sizes limit column length and, therefore, the ultimate resolving power possible by LC. In addition, low diffusion rates in liquids make LC a relatively slow analytical method for the detection of CW agents. Nevertheless, a number of applications have been reported. For example, hydrolysis products of sulfur mustards can be determined at the ppm level in about 20 min per sample by reversed-phase liquid chromatography (RPLC) coupled with a sulfur flame photometric detector. Simi-larly, aqueous samples of alkylphosphonic acids can be analyzed at the ppt level in about 20 min/sample by reversed-phase LC coupled with phosphorous selective flame photometric detection.

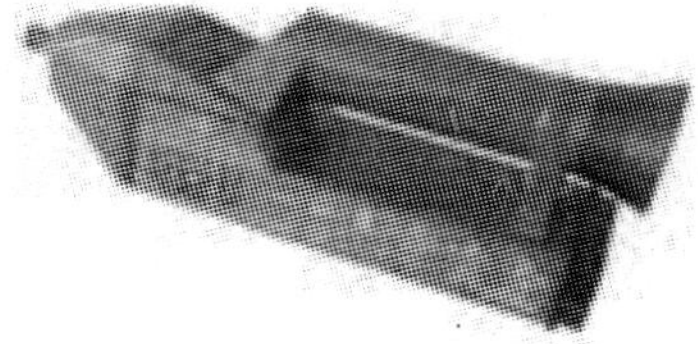

Fig. 70.12

Capillary Electrophoresis (CE)

For higher resolving power than is possible with RPLC (or faster analysis times with similar resolving power), CE is the separation method of choice for ionic and ionizable compounds. Coupled with selective detectors such as the flame photometric detector, CE can detect alkylphosphonic acids in water at the 0.1–0.5 μg/ml level in less than 10 min Indirect UV absorbance detection has also been reported for the detection of these compounds after CE The use of electrokinetic injection improved detection limits for a number of degradation products. For example, methylphosphonic acid (MPA), ethylmethylphosphonic acid (EMPA), isopropylmethylphosphonic acid (IMPA), and pinacolyl-methylphosphonic acid (PMPA) were detected at the ppb level in 3 min from water samples. A miniaturized analytical system has been reported for the separation and detection of nerve agents using CE microchips with mperometric detection

Ion Mobility Spectrometry (IMS)

IMS is a separation method in which gas-phase ions, created by the vapor-phase ionization of neutral molecules using photon-corona or radioactive ionization processes (or by the liquid-phase ionization of both neutral, ionic, and ionizable molecules using electrospray or coronospray ionization processes), are separated according to their differences in velocities through a gas in an electric field. In IMS, ions separate according to their size-to-charge ratio. Ion mobility instruments that have been used for the field detection of CW agents are the chemical agent monitor (CAM) and the improved chemical agent monitor (ICAM). Using a radioactive ionization source, they require only 1 min of exposure time to detect vapors of H-type vesicant agents as well as G- and V-type nerve agents. In addition to the CAM and ICAM, the automatic chemical agent detection alarm (ACADA) is also based on IMS technology. Used as a man-portable and point-sampling alarm system, the ACADA provides concurrent nerve and vesicant agent detection at improved sensitivity. To date, all ion mobility measurements made for CW agents have been direct mobility measurements made under low electric field conditions in which the ion mobility is directly proportional to the electric field strength. However, a new and promising method for using ion mobility for monitoring gas phase ions takes advantage of the nonlinear behavior of ion mobilities under high electric field strength conditions Unfortunately, the resolving power of this novel approach is currently too low to provide adequate selectivity for CW agent detection, but the absence of an ion gate promises improved sensitivity over traditional IMS instruments.A third type of IMS that is used for the detection of CW agents is called aspiration IMS. In this system, the ions travel through an orthogonal electric field in which the ions are deflected to multichannels located on the collecting electrode. Ions with higher mobilities are deflected to electrodes faster than ions with lower mobilities. Although these types of detectors also suffer from low resolving power, they also have the advantage of not requiring an ion gate. They have been applied to the detection of soman and VX degradation products.

Mass spectrometry (MS)

Unlike IMS, MS is an ion separation method in which gas-phase ions separate according to their mass to charge ratio as they move through a vacuum. Due to the lack of ion–molecule interactions and the rapid analysis time (on the order of μs), typical mass spectrometers have resolving powers 1 to 2 orders of magnitude better than IMS and chromatographic instruments. However, the complexity of requiring a vacuum limits the practical application of MS as a field analytical technique. An ion trap mass spectrometer with a high-pressure negative ion source and selected reactant negative ions has been used to insure unambiguous detection of phosphorus- and nitrogen-containing chemical warfare agents Ion traps can also be used for the direct determination of VX- and nitrogen-containing vesicant agents on the surface of soils at the ppm level using secondary ionization MS Matrix-assisted laser desorption ionization with time-of-flight mass spectrometry (MALDI-TOFMS) has been used for the determination of sulfur mustard exposure. When hemoglobin and metallothioneine are exposed to sulfur mustard, alkylation and cross-linking occurs. Over the years, there have been a number of attempts to miniaturize the mass spectrometer. Recent approaches have been reported for the miniaturization of a time-of-flight mass spectrometers; one with an electron impact ionization source and another with a photoionization ion source for the detection of phosphonates at the 10–100 ppb level. Miniaturization of ion traps using a cylindrical design produced a detection limit for methyl salicylate of 1 pg with a resolution of 100. Ion trap MS has also been reported for the detection and identification of both chemical and biological agents in the field. With this design, detection was based on respirable particle collection followed by liberation of derived biomarkers into the mass spectrometer. MS, however, usually requires an additional separation step prior to the introduction of the sample into the spectrometry. This additional separation step serves to both kept the MS clean and to reduce the number of interferences in the ionization process or in the mass separational.

3. THREE-DIMENSIONAL SENSORS

Even with high-resolution, two-dimensional sensors, mistakes can be made with respect to identification of unknown analytes. Thus, for absolute identification, data obtained using three-dimensional sensors are normally recommended. Because of the complexity of these instruments, they are difficult to operate in the field without the support of a full mobile laboratory.

Gas Chromatography/Mass Spectrometry (GC/MS)

GC/MS is the only analytical method of analysis that has been approved for chemical warfare verification, but due to the complex nature of this instrument, it has not been employed for field verification of chemical agents. However, GC/MS can provide some of the most reliable analytical information.

Liquid Chromatography/Mass Spectrometry (LC/MS)

In addition to GC/MS, LC is often employed to identify an unknown sample of chemical warfare agents. Degradation products of CW agents are particularly difficult to determine due their lack of volatility for gas chromatographic separation and lack of chromophores for detection. Several ionization methods after liquid chromatographic separation have been found to be useful for the determination of CW degradation products. These ionization methods include particle beam ionization (PBI), electrospray ionization (ESI), and atmospheric pressure chemical ionization (APCI) Each ionization method was found to provide complementary information. But it has been the introduction of ESI that has enabled the most successful applications of LC methods coupled with MS. Thus, the determination of sarin, soman, and their hydrolysis products is now possible at the 10 μg/g level with liquid chromatographic separation followed by mass separation and detection.

Ion Mobility/Mass Spectrometry (IM/MS)

As with MS, the development of ESI has enabled the introduction of nonvolatile compounds into the IMS. Using the IMS as a preseparation device, IMS serves as a rapid replacement for LC prior to the introduction into a mass spectrometer. CW degradation products have been separated and detected from water samples by using an IMS coupled to a quadruple mass spectrometer (QMS) Not only do IMS separations have a greater resolving power than LC separations, they are also faster. Complete ion mobility spectra can be obtained within 20 ms. Even when several spectra are averaged to improve signal-to-noise ratio, separations occur in less than 10 s compared with 10–30 min for LC. With IMS/QMS separation and detection, the IMS is scanned continuously while the QMS is scanned slowly to produce the mobility-mass spectrum in about 10 min. Recently, however, IMS has been interfaced to a time-of-flight mass spectrometer, and complete mobility-mass spectra can be obtained in a few seconds. In both IM/MS instruments, the detection limit for the CW degradation products is similar at about 100 ppb. The primary advantage of adding an IMS to the front of a mass spectrometer is to keep the mass spectrometer clean and to reduce the noise from that electrospray process in the mass spectrum. IM/MS data can also be collected for volatile CW simulants using a Ni ionization source or a secondary ESI source.

Other Three-Dimensional Sensors

Other three-dimensional analytical devices have been reported, although not specifically applied to CW agents. CE/MS can be interfaced similarly as LC, except that the high voltage at the end of the capillary column requires special approaches to isolate the voltage and assure proper potential on the electrospray needle. Thus, CE/MS has not found widespread use due to the complexity of its interface design. GC/GC utilizes a rapid switching technique to collect and inject a GC peak from a first high-resolution separation into a second fast chromatograph with a stationary phase of a different polarity from that of the first column. This approach supplies added information that can be used for qualitative analysis. LC/GC is also possible but has limited use due to the fact that compounds separated by LC are normally not amenable to gas chromatographic separation.

4. FOUR - AND MORE - DIMENSIONAL SENSORS

Given that chromatographic separations occur on the order of minutes, ion mobility separations on the order of milliseconds, and mass separations on the order of microseconds, four-dimensional sensors are possible when these separation techniques are coupled in series. Moreover, with some mass spectrometers it is possible to obtain MS/MS spectra or even MS spectra. Thus, it might be possible to have more than four-dimensional sensors such as GC/IMS/MS/MS/MS. Increasing the dimensional space in which a compound identification is determined decreases the possibility of false responses, although it does increase the complexity of the sensor.

Biosensors

The three different optical biosensing mechanisms that can be implemented in a multibiosensor technology platform: surface are plasmon resonance, magnetooptical surface plasmon resonance and optoelectronic biosensing (evanescent wave detection) using integrated Mach-Zehnder interferometer devices. In the last case, the use of standard silicon microelectronics technology opens the possibility for integration of optical, fluidics based and electrical functions within a single optical sensing circuit leading to a complete lab-on-a-chip design solution. All three mechanisms can be efficiently used as an early warning system for biological and/or chemical warfare. A biointegrated detection system (BIDS) has been developed iconfigured to provide real time analysis of samples from air, liquid, solids, and soil for chemical warfare agents. The military has used the instruments to screen, detect, identify, quantify, and confirm agents in weapons defense, monitoring, and demilitarization. The system has proven to be effective in the detection and confirmation of many nerve agents such as sarin gas and VX as well as for blister agents such as mustard gas.

Developmental Trends

Development of detection methods today is mainly concentrated on instruments. New manual methods, e.g., for toxins, may be developed but the development mainly concerns instruments for detection and monitoring. In some cases, instruments capable of both tasks are being constructed. Several lines of development are presently being followed as regards detection principles. The most common line of development is some form of ion mobility detector IMS (Ion Mobility Spectroscopy). The Chemical Agent Monitor (CAM) also belongs to this group, as well as detectors for warning such as the Finnish M86 and the more recent M90. Another principle used is flame photometry FPD (Flame Photometric Detector). A flame of hydrogen is allowed to burn the sample of air after which the color of the flame is investigated by a photometer. In this way, the presence of phosphorus and sulfur can be demonstrated. Examples of instruments using this principle are the French monitor AP2C and Israeli combined detector and monitor CHASE. A third principle is to use enzymes, as in the manual methods for nerve agent detection. Detectors operating on this principle have been developed in the United Kingdom, in the Netherlands and the former Soviet Union, among others. Methods for long-range monitoring using optical methods (IR) are being developed in France and the U.S.A.

A research sector attracting great interest is the use of biologically active molecules as sensors. These biosensors are believed to have extremely great potential and research is ongoing in several countries. The advan-tage of biosensors is that, at least in theory, they can be given the sensitivity and specificity desired. This is possible since the biosensor uses the same mechanisms that influence the human body when exposed to poisoning. A simple type of biosensor is the enzyme ticket.

A more general type of biosensor may also be useful in the early detection of potential threats. Instead of studying toxic substances, investigations can be made of which receptors in the body may be sensitive to, e.g., a toxin. These receptors could then be used in a biosensor.

Alarm

The simplest form of alarm is based on direct observations like a visible cloud drifting in or when someone in the unit shows symptoms of poisoning, masses of dead animals/birds etc. Earlier and more reliable alarms require continuous and automatic monitoring of the gas concentration. For this purpose, specialized instrumentation is necessary. An alarm detector must be capable of operating continuously for long periods. It should require no particular attention except for changing batteries, etc., and might be operated by personnel with short training periods. At a predetermined concentration of the relevant substance, the instrument must emit both visual and acoustic alarms. An added refinement would be if the device can emit different types of sound or different signal colors for different agents.

It must always be considered that other substances than chemical warfare (CW) agents may trigger the alarm. It is important not only that these are as few as possible but also that they are known so that situations with false alarms can be avoided. Detection paper placed onsite in advance is a simple manual method. It can be used as a warning for CW agents in the form of liquid fallout. In such cases, it is necessary to have continuous monitoring with specially trained personnel.

All-Clear

Wearing a protective mask and protective clothing implies a major physical and mental strain for personnel. Consequently, it is of major importance to sound the all-clear as soon as possible after a CW attack. Protective measures can be terminated when the concentration of CW agents in the air has fallen below the threshold limit. A continuously operating all-clear system is preferable. The need to sound the alarm may soon arise again if the conditions change. As regards the all-clear, an instrument which can be directly read-off is of great value. Such instruments like the British CAM (Chemical Agent Monitor) illustration) show the air concentration for different types of substances. Changes can then be observed and a temporary fall in concentration can be utilized to decrease the level of protection, e.g., in order to eat. Correct utilization of an instrument with direct-reading facilities requires an operator and also someone with sufficient knowledge to reach correct decisions. Provided there is access to other information, e.g., mapping of the ground contamination has been completed, manual methods using detection tubes or detection tickets may be sufficiently accurate when reaching decisions on sounding the all-clear.

Protection: Individual and Collective

The immediate action to a chemical attack is by closing all openings to outside air, running breathing air through filters, and starting a system that continually washes down the exterior surfaces. On ships the area that has these features is called the Citadel.

Personal Protection by Individual Protective Equipment (IPE)

History and development of the gas mask

A primitive respirator to be used by miners was introduced by Alexander von Humboldt already in 1799, when he worked as a mining engineer in Prussia.

The gas mask was patented on June 12, 1849, by American Lewis Haslett in Louisville, Kentucky. It was an "Inhaler or Lung Protector", issued for an air purifying respirator. Haslett's device filtered dust from the air.

Early versions were constructed by the Scottish chemist John Stenhouse in 1854 and the physicist John Tyndall in the 1870s.

One such design began as a "Safety Hood and Smoke Protector" invented by African American inventor, Garrett A. Morgan in 1912, and patented in 1914. It was a simple device, consisting of a cotton hood with two hoses which hung down to the floor, allowing the wearer to breathe the safer air found there. In addition, moist sponges were inserted at the end of the hoses in order to better filter the air. Morgan won acclaim for his device when in 1916 he, his brother, and two other volunteers used his device to rescue numerous men from the gas and smoke-filled tunnels beneath Lake Erie in the Cleveland Waterworks.

The first use of poison gas on the Western Front was on 22 April 1915, by the Germans at Ypres, against Canadian and French colonial troops. The initial response was to equip troops with cotton mouth pads for protection. Soon afterwards the British added a long cloth which was used to tie chemical-soaked mouth pads into place, and which was called the Black Veil Respirator. Dr. Cluny MacPherson of The Royal Newfoundland Regiment brought the idea of a mask made of chemical absorbing fabric and which fitted over the entire head to England, and this was developed into the British Hypo Helmet of June 1915. This primitive type of mask went through several stages of development before being superseded in 1916 by the canister gas mask of 1916. This had a mask connected to a tin can containing the absorbent materials by a hose.

In 1915, American chemist and inventor credited with the invention of the gas mask James Bert Garner read a newspaper article describing a gas attack on British forces which he hypothesized had employed chlorine gas. Remembering experiments he had performed while teaching at the University of Chicago, he set about creating the first gas mask which he tested on two of his associates in a gas filled chamber. Following the successful completion of the test, he provided the results to the British government. Garner's mask was the first to be used on the Western front during World War I. Also in World War I, since dogs were frequently used on the front lines, a special type of gas mask was developed that dogs were trained to wear.

The British Royal Society of Chemistry claims that British scientist Edward Harrison developed the first practical gas mask for mass production, a claim supported by a thank-you note written by Winston Churchill.

In America thousands of gas masks were produced for American as well as Allied troops. Mine Safety Appliances was a chief producer. This mask was later used widely in industry.

Gas masks development since has mirrored the development of chemical agents in warfare, filling the need to protect against ever more deadly threats, biological weapons, and radioactive dust in the nuclear era. However, where agents that cause harm through contact or penetration of the skin occurs, such as blister agent or nerve agent, a gas mask alone is not sufficient protection, and full protective clothing must be worn in addition, to protect from contact with the atmosphere. For reasons of civil defense and personal protection, individuals often purchase gas masks in the belief that they protect against the harmful effects of an attack with nuclear, biological, or chemical (NBC) agents; which is only partially true, as gas masks protect only against respiratory absorption. Whilst most military gas masks are designed to be capable of protection against spectrum of NBC agents, they can be coupled with filter canisters that are proof against those agents (heavier) or just against riot control agents and smoke (lighter, and often used for training purposes); likewise there are lightweight masks solely for use in riot control agents and not for NBC situations.

Although thorough training and the availability of gas masks and other protective equipment can render the casualty-causing effects of an attack by chemical agents nullified, troops who are forced to operate in full protective gear are less efficient in completing their given tasks, tire easily, and may be affected psychologically by the threat of attack by these weapons. During the Cold War era, it was seen as inevitable that there would be a constant NBC threat on the battlefield, and thus troops needed protection in which they could remain fully functional; thus protective gear, and especially gas masks have evolved to incorporate innovations in terms of increasing user-comfort, and in compatibility with other equipment (from drinking devices to artificial respiration tubes, to communications systems etc). The gas mask has thus now arrived at a 'fourth generation' of development.

History of Absorbents and Neutralizers

Activated charcoal is a common component of gas masks. It is a carbon with an extremely high surface area and which attracts all manner of pollutants from air and water. Pollutants do not react with the carbon but are bonded to it in a process called adsorption. Over time the activated carbon becomes thoroughly coated and it ceases to remove pollutants. However, the charcoal can be reactivated and restored to its original state by baking the charcoal with high heat, which either evaporates or burns off the pollutants.

In the first gas masks of World War I, it was initially found that wood charcoal was a good adsorbent of poison gases. In about 1918 it was found that charcoals made from the shells and seeds of various fruits and nuts such as coconuts, chestnuts, horse-chestnuts, and peach stones performed much better than wood charcoal. These waste materials were collected from the public in recycling programs to assist the war effort. Two filter canisters are issued for the S10, as with the S6; a light pressed metal type for riot control situations or training (marked with a painted red stripe or red tape), and a heavier plastic encased type for protection against NBC agents. The latter have a maximum shelf-life of 10 years, and the mask itself (the facepiece) of 20 years. World War II gas masks contained blue asbestos in their filters, and this material continued to be used until at least 1956. Breathing blue asbestos in the factories resulted in death from mesothelioma of 10% of workers, and between 2.5 and 3.2 times the normal incidence of lung or respiratory cancers.

Variants include the SF10, intended for security and special forces use, the AR10 for police forces, and the N10, a commercial version. S10s issued to British nationals in Saudi Arabia during the 1991 Gulf War were marked by a blue coloured PSM fitting or a blue painted spot on the forehead; although meant to be returned to the authorities after the Iraqi threat (from Scud missile attacks, potentially carrying chemical warheads) had expired, large numbers were unaccounted for in the wake of the conflict. The S10 is widely available on the army surplus market and is usually reasonably priced. The S6 NBC Respirator was the protective gas mask issued to the British armed forces from the 1960's (not from 1966) up until the introduction of the current-issue S10 in 1986, after which it was withdrawn from service.

The S6 was developed by the Defence Science and Technology Laboratory, Porton Down from the 1950s and manufactured by the Birmingham and Leyland Rubber Company. Although made obsolete by the S10, production of the S6 continued in Turkey after the adoption of the new mask by the British forces.

The S6 features an innovative air seal around the inside of the facepiece to improve fit and comfort of the mask; the pressure inside the seal can be adjusted by means of a tap inside the nosecup.

During the widely documented Iranian Embassy Siege of 1980, the S6 is the mask seen being worn by SAS troops.

Ex-British army S6 masks are easily found on the army surplus market, but can no longer be relied upon to provide any degree of protection as the effective shelf-lives of even the most recently-produced example will have expired.

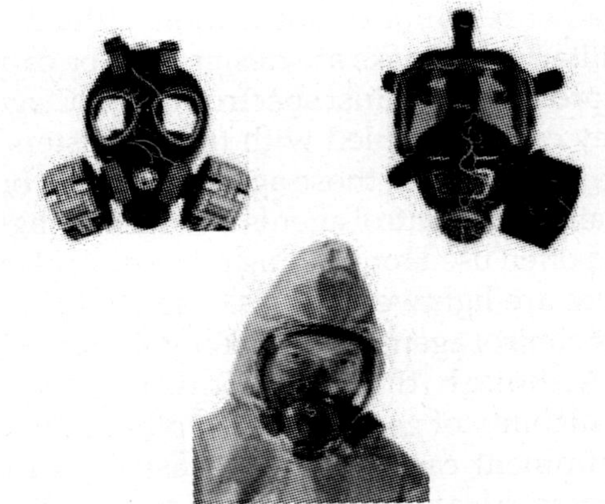

Fig. 70.13

Modern Day Gas Masks

The S1NBC Respirator is the protective gas mask currently in service with all branches of the British armed forces, and is generally accepted, along with its derivative, the FM12, as one of the best protective masks in the world today. The Advantage 320CBA-RCA (Chemical Biological Agent-Riot Control Agent) Respirator features a soft, pliable silicone facepiece with a test proven Advantage respirator seal that instantly conforms to the wearer's facial contours. It has a very low breathing resistance and a standard nosecup to help eliminate lens fogging besides being exceptionally comfortable, lightweight and stable and providing protection against all known biological, chemical and nuclear contamination. The Millennium MSA gas mask has a flexible, 1-piece polyurethane lens with wide field of vision bonded to a durable Hycar rubber facepiece. A drinking tube portal provides connection for fluid ingestion in contaminated atmospheres. A fully elastic, 6-point harness promotes easy on-off, easy adjustment without hair pulling. An internal nosecup with 2 check valves deflects air from the lens, reduces fogging. A standard mechanical speaking diaphragm is included. The Kareta M Mask manufactured by Draeger provides full protection against warfare gases and its dual eyepiece provides excellent vision and also a standard thread connection accepting NATO NBC (Nuclear, Biological, Chemical) cartridges and all Drager NIOSH-approved cartridges. A drinking device connection is included. The Panorama Standard (Draeger) Mask provides the wearer with full protection against gases, vapors and particles with full face protection. Panorama's unique double sealing frame forms a double seal around the user's face allowing the face piece to fit firmly and comfortably without exerting pressure. Air supply is cleansed by mechanical filtration through a highly efficient filter media or by absorption of contaminants by activated charcoal The Bardas Child Protective Wrap can be used by children between 3 and 8 years and is a

NBC (Nuclear, Biological, Chemical) rated youth protective wrap that allows for a non-intrusive seal on a young child. It also provides positive pressure to the youngster and allows for hydration with a drink device. Bardas has a blower that is powered by LiSo2 batteries which provides positive pressure and cooling airflow to the child. It is extremely lightweight and provides greater mobility and wear time. Bardas also offers wide, clear and comfortable viewing. The M 40 and M42 have replaced the M17 and M25 masks while the A/P23P-14(V) N respiratory assembly gives total protection. A small device called the BUTTON that fits inside a gas mask is an efficient chemical detector containing its own liquid to moisturise reagents contained within and indicate to the soldier on the field if the atmosphere is free of nerve gas.

NBC SUITS

In military operations, NBC suits are intended to be quickly donned over a soldiers uniform and can continuously protect the user for up to several days. Most of the older varieties are made of impermeable material such as rubber coated canvas, but some incorporate a filter, allowing air, sweat and condensation to slowly pass through. The CBRN (Chemical, Biological, Radiological, Nuclear) suit of the British Armed Forces also known as the Noddy suit because if its pointed hood, is made of reinforced nylon with charcoal impregnated felt. It is more comfortable because of the breathability but has a shorter useful life, and must be replaced often. The Soviet style suit, also nicknamed Womble, protects the wearer at higher concentrations than the British suit but is less comfortable due to the build-up of moisture within it. In Canadian terminology, an NBC suit or any kind of similar protective over-

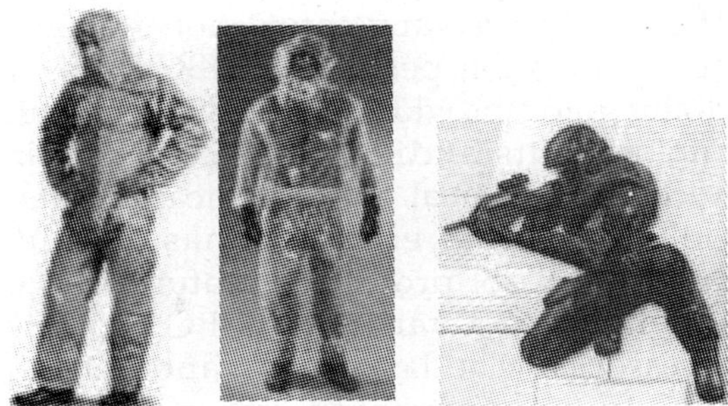

Fig. 70.14

suit is also known as a Bunny suit. Protective NBC Clothing such as Tyvek and Hagor NBC suits protect body skin against most harmful biological agents and chemical agents, but do not offer protection against radiation. Gloves, booties and duct tape are recommended to ensure a full body seal. Demron is the only non-lead radiation suit offering protection against X-ray and low energy Gamma emissions. Nomex Suits provide primary flash fire protection for the wearer. Tyvek F has been tested and certified to meet the standards NATO tests for chemical warfare protection but this suit does not offer protection against radiation. Chemical protective undergarment (CPU), self contained toxic environment protective outfits (STEPO) and improved toxicological agent protectives (ITAP) with a 'second skin' design for better protection, fit, comfort and ease of filter change are available. Some even incorporate personal ice cooling systems (PICS) for desert conditions. Demron radiation shielding garments are effective against various forms of ionizing radiation like X-rays, low energy gamma emissions, as well as high and low energy alpha and beta particles. It is also highly resistant to chemical vapors. The Demron coverall is constructed with an integrated hood, heat sealed seams, and seam seal tape for total protection. The Karcher Safeguard 3002-A1 consists of several textile layers including an activated carbon layer.

This highly innovative protection system is a new generation permeable NBC protective clothing and provides better wearer comfort and an outstanding protection against nuclear, biological and chemical threats as well as thermal effects. It has an added unique aerosol protection feature. DuPont also markets a variety of NBC protective accessories. The latest generation Demron NBC suit has advanced radiopaque nano-polymeric compound fused between layers of fabric having lightweight nuclear-radiation blocking properties.It's nanotechnology surpasses all other NBC suits by providing total radioactive protection. Demron-W provides enhanced chemical, biological, radiation and flame protection, and is the world's first and only NFPA 1994-2007. Certified fabric for First Responders in CBRN Terrorism Incidents. It is lead and PVC free, and allows heat dissipation besides resisting chemical penetration and cracks. Made of liquid metal, Demron nuclear protection fabrics feel cool and, are lightweight, flexible and foldable and completely block gamma rays, X-rays and other nuclear emissions

MOPP (Mission Oriented Protective Posture Gear) Criteria

MOPP Level 0: In MOPP Level 0, the mask is worn in a carrier on the military member's hip. Chemical-protective gear is issued, prepared, and located so the member can retrieve it within 5 minutes. MOPP Level 0 is used during periods of increased alert when the enemy has chemical/biological employment capability, but there is no indication of use in the immediate future.

MOPP Level 1: In this level, the chemical overgarment (pants and jacket) are worn, and the rest of the equipment is carried. MOPP Level 1 is used when it is determined that chemical/biological attack within the theater of operations is possible.

MOPP Level 2: In MOPP Level 2, the overgarment is worn, and the overboots are worn. The mask, hood and gloves are carried in the mask-carrier, strapped to the hip. MOPP Level 2 is initiated when chemical/biological attack is probable.

MOPP Level 3: In this MOPP level, the overgarment, mask/hood, and overboots are worn, but the protective gloves may be carried. MOPP Level 3 is used after chemicals have been used by the enemy, but in areas with negligible hazard.

MOPP Level 4: Everything is worn. This condition is used during/after an attack when chemical weapons have been used or are suspected.

MOPP Level Alpha: The mask, hood, and gloves are worn, but the protective overgarment is not. MOPP Level Alpha is called only during certain circumstances, such as when upwind from a negligible vapor hazard agent, or when inside buildings or aircraft.

Collective protection methods are also now available and known as Integrated Environmental Control (IEC). These deploy chemical and biological protective shelters (CBPS) and advanced integrated collective protective systems (AICPS) with their own power, NBC filtration and environmental control that allows continued functioning of groups of people during operations. These shelters can be fixed, mobile, or improvised. With ordinary buildings, this may be as basic as plastic sheeting and tape, although if the protection needs to be continued for any appreciable length of time, there will be requirement of NBC enabled air supply.

Passive and active chemical and biological laminates for inflatable tents, framed tents, and other temporary structures for chem-bio defense uses a passive barrier system in the form of an impermeable, chemical and biological resistant material that is durable, lightweight, and flexible. An active chemistry system takes the protection features of the passive barrier and incorporates active decontamination properties into the material. In this way, the chem-bio threat is prevented from entering the structure and also neutralized over time, which is critical when live chemical and biological warfare agents are present. In addition, active chemical agent barriers are rechargeable (i.e., allow repeat decontamination).

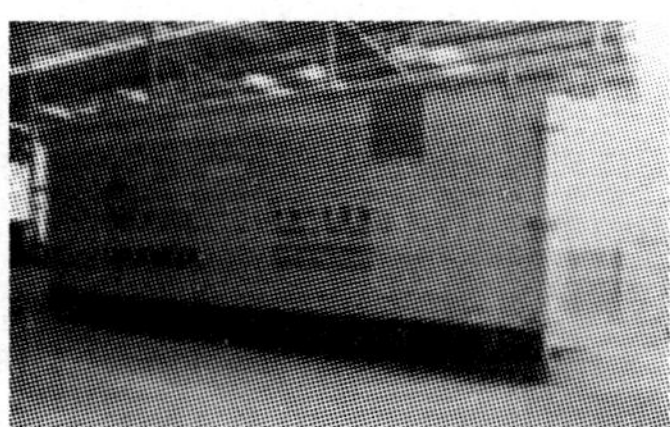

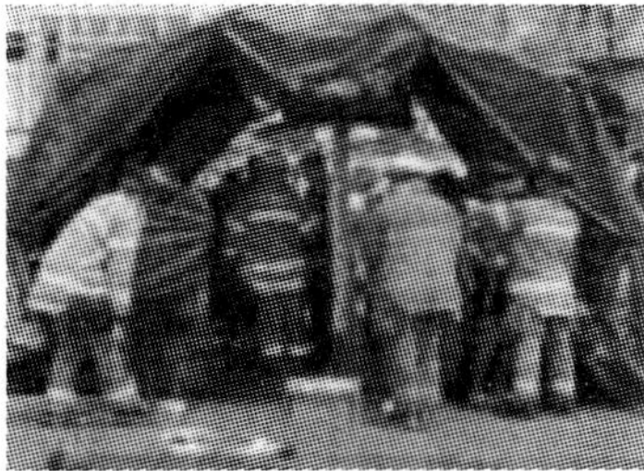

Fig. 70.15

Self-Decontaminating Emergency and Military Shelters

Active chemical barriers for defense designed to be more robust and lower in weight, when compared to previously fielded tent offerings. Temporary military shelter materials designed with rechargeable, active chemistry laminates that reliably destroy chem-bio agents. These self-decontaminating chemical warfare shelters provide protection against fugitive chemical and biological agents. Chemical warfare tent laminates are designed to perform with a variety of base structural models, including low-pressure and high-pressure inflatable systems, as well as metal, composite, and folding frames. These patented laminates integrate chem-bio barrier protection while delivering the necessary protective structure properties of low weight, flame resistance, weather resistance, durability, packing volume, structural heat seal, and thermal management to meet challenging chemical defense goals set by DTRA (Defense Threat Reduction Agency), JECP (Joint Expeditionary Collective Protection), and CBPS (Chemical and Biological Protective Shelters).

Decontamination Individual and Ground

Decontamination varies with the particular chemical agent used. For non-persistent pulmonary agents, like chlorine, phosgene and the nerve gas GB, their dissipation can be ensured by employing powerful exhaust fans to clear out buildings where they have accumulated. Whatever the chemical agent used, it is vital that decontamination efforts are instituted promptly. Casualties must be evacuated to safe zones with controlled air flow systems and given a thorough shower with soap and water. All contaminated clothing and equipment are destroyed. Wounds are washed with an alkaline solution. Whole body decontamination is an expensive process. Mass decontamination is a less common requirement for people than for equipment, since soldiers are immediately symptomatic and specific treatment is the action required. However, decontamination is indicated when people have been contaminated with blistering agents, VX and others made persistent with a thickener. Treatment and decontamination may need to be simultaneous, with the medical personnel protecting themselves with IPE so they can continue to function. A decontamination-emulsion spray suction system (Mediclean) is available from Karcher of Germany that dislodges particles, and cleans the body surface within a decontamination room fitted with controlled air flow to create a safe zone. The military issues special personnel decontamination kits, called M291 and M295 individual decontamination kits. They are the most effective method of removing chemical agents from the skin. In the absence of a personal decontamination kit, military personnel can use a 5 percent chlorine bleach solution to remove the chemical agent from equipment and a 0.5 percent solution to remove agents from the skin. The eyes are very vulnerable when exposed to nerve and blister agents. If one of these agents gets in the eyes, military personnel are trained to irrigate them with water.

Decontamination powder is intended by the military for decontaminating soldiers skin and personal equipment from liquid NBC agents. The powder is usually finely ground to give it a larger surface area, making it an extremely effective adsorbent. Generally the main ingredients are chloride of lime and magnesium oxide which provide both absorption and neutralisation properties.

MAPPING OF GROUND CONTAMINATION

In some cases, it is necessary to map which parts of an area are and which are not contaminated with CW agents in liquid form. This is essential if, for example, a convoy of vehicles has to pass through an area where CW agents have been used. Several methods are available. Traditionally, detection paper has been used. Detection papers prepared before an attack could give the information required. In such cases, this must have been made over the entire area in question and at several different places in the area. However, such information is probably not available or deficient. Detection paper can be used in post factum detection. However, this method is not entirely reliable, particularly if a long period has passed between the contamination and detection occasions. Considerable quantities of CW agents may have been absorbed into the soil layer and still imply danger without giving any response on detection paper. Consequently, soil detection with paper should be complemented with some kind of vapor detection.

Another problem is that traditional methods of soil detection take a long time. The speed of a convoy of vehicles will decrease to a few km/h if detection must be conducted at the same time as the convoy makes progress. In this way, an aggressor achieves a considerable tactical advantage already with a low or moderate CW attack. By vapor detection with detectors or monitors, the speed of vehicles could be increased to about 30 km/h, provided that the instruments react sufficiently rapidly and are sufficiently sensitive.

Vapor detection is not a fully reliable method, and particularly not for CW agents with low volatility or at low temperatures. There is a risk that vehicles, ordnance, etc., may be contaminated after transport without this being detected using the actual transport. Military personnel are trained to avoid kneeling, sitting, or walking in contaminated areas if possible, and not to touch anything unless it is absolutely necessary.

MAPPING OF DECONTAMINATION REQUIREMENT

Mapping of the decontamination requirement involves approximately the same problems as mapping ground contamination although generally on a smaller scale. Detection with paper generally works well but is not sufficient in all situations. CW monitors are important in controlling the need for decontamination. Persons suspected or known to be contaminated must be decontaminated immediately without previous time-consuming controls. This should also apply to personal equipment if it is reasonably easy to decontaminate. Checks of the decontamination requirement should be concentrated to heavier and more difficulty decontaminated equipment.

Water Safety

A compact water-purifier the size of two packets of cigarettes is available to process contaminated water and render it safe with absolute reliability. A process of super-chlorination, adsorption by activated charcoal, coagulation, flocculation and filtration purifies 750 ml of suspected water in 15 minutes time. Water testing kits are also available to detect chemical warfare agents. These can detect a wide spectrum of chemical agents even if low in strength. The agents screened are:

- Sarin 0.02 mg/l.
- Soman 0.20 mg/l.
- Tabun 0.04 mg/ml.
- VX 0.02 mg/ml.
- Mustard gas 2.0 mg/l.
- Aresenic 1-2 mg/l.
- Cyanide 8 mg/l.
- CLCN 5 mg/l.
- CL2 5 mg/l.
- Phosgene 6.5-9.0 mg/l.

Chemical Warfare Treatment Options

A. Pre-emptive Treatment

Organophosphorus nerve gases are organic esters of substituted phosphoric acids. such as tabun, sarin, soman and VX. These compounds are highly volatile and easily disseminated in vapor form. They are readily absorbed through the lungs and eyes, and also the skin and intestinal tract without producing any irritation or other sensation. They are sufficiently potent that even brief exposure may be fatal. Depending on the concentration of the poison, death may occur in as little as one minute, or it may be delayed for 1-2 hours. Chemically related insecticides include parathion, methyl parathion and malathion, and these exhibit similar toxicity, although they are generally less potent. They act mainly by inhibiting cholinesterase at cholinergic synapses. Hence they are termed as anticholinesterase agents affecting both main types of cholinergic receptor—muscarinic and nicotinic. The nerve agents act in a 3 step fashion:

Step 1 Formation of AChE-nerve agent complex.

Step 2 Phosphorylation and inactivation of the enzyme.

Step 3 Aging reaction, in which a leaving group separates, providing a monophosphoric acid residue bound to the enzyme. Following the aging process, the nerve agent can no longer be pulled off the AChE molecule by pralidoxime. Sarin's half time to aging (time at which aging has occurred in half the sarin-AChE complexes) is several hours giving ample time following exposure to administer an oxime before aging of the nerve agent-AChE complex occurs. The aging half-time is even longer for tabun, cyclosarin and VX. However, the half-time of aging for soman is approximately two minutes, inadequate for even highly trained personnel to administer atropine and oxime.

Skeletal muscle effects are among the so-called nicotinic effects. Early skeletal muscle symptoms include twitching and cramps and coincide with axonal backfiring in which a signal travels up the axon, the nerve process that relays signals, in the reverse direction to that by which signaling ordinarily occurs.

Twitching is first seen in eyelids, and it spreads to face and calves and then becomes generalized. This reaction occurs in the first 24 hours and may be followed by weakness or paralysis, depending on the severity of the intoxication. Paralysis involves all skeletal muscles, including the breathing muscles, and results in labored, shallow, and rapid breathing. Respiratory failure and cyanosis (turning blue) may ensue in some cases. Weakness of the tongue and pharyngeal muscles (muscles in the pharynx, or back of the throat) further enhances respiratory failure by promoting airway obstruction. Muscarinic receptors are found in the smooth muscle of viscera(internal organs), heart muscle, secretory glands, and in the endothelial cells lining blood vessels—as well as in the brain. Muscarinic effects from action of ACh at smooth muscles, glands, and the heart include spasm of smooth muscles, increased glandular secretions, and slowing of the heart rate. Specific examples of smooth muscle spasm and increased secretions include increased abdominal motility and intestinal secretions, with possible consequent abdominal cramping, nausea, vomiting, and diarrhea; excessive salivation (with drooling); lacrimation (increased secretions from tear ducts); rhinorrhea (runny nose); bronchorrhea (increased bronchial, or airway, secretions); bronchospasm (constriction of the airways); laryngospasm (constriction of the larynx area); diaphoresis (sweating); ureteral spasm with frequent urination or bladder incontinence; and sphincter relaxation, which may promote bowel incontinence. Miosis, or pupillary constriction, is almost always present. In addition, there may be reddening of the eyes and slowing of the heart. Nicotinic and muscarinic effects on the heart rate are opposed, so theoretically either an increased or reduced heart rate may occur, but bradycardia (slowed heart rate) is more common. ACh influences autonomic ganglia through both muscarinic and nicotinic mechanisms. Effects also include release of catecholamines such as adrenaline (nicotinic). Consequences of these effects may include pallor and transitory elevation of blood pressure followed by low blood pressure.

So-called central effects result from accumulation of ACh at central synapses. Central receptors are themselves characterized as muscarinic or nicotinic, but because it is often not well known which receptors are responsible for which effects, effects are commonly referred to simply as central. Early signs include anxiety, restlessness, emotional lability, insomnia, and excessive dreaming. Larger doses may lead to headaches, tremor, drowsiness, memory impairment, apathy, fatigue, and depression. Severe intoxication results in confusion, ataxia, dysarthria and absent muscle-stretch (myotatic) reflexes and progresses to coma, Cheyne-Stokes respirations (an abnormal breathing pattern), generalized grand mal-like seizures, and central respiratory depression (breathing problems produced by abnormal action of the breathing center in the brain).

Delayed or chronic CNS effects may include giddiness, tension, anxiety, jitteriness, restlessness, emotional lability, excessive dreaming, insomnia, nightmares, headaches, tremor, withdrawal and depression, bursts of slow waves of elevated voltage in EEG (especially on hyperventilation), drowsiness, difficulty concentrating, slowness of recall, confusion, slurred speech, and ataxia (incoordination with walking).

Treatment of nerve agent poisoning at present relies on two approaches. In the first, an oxime is given to detach the agent from cholinesterase, thus reactivating the enzyme

This mitigates both nicotinic and muscarinic effects, for those nerve agents against which oximes are effective (which do not include soman). In the second, the muscarinic antagonist atropine is used to quell the effects of excessive acetylcholine action. Atropine is of special value when the nerve agent is oxime-resistant or when symptoms are already severe. However, atropine targets only excessive muscarinic activity and not the nicotinic effects. Nicotine is a convulsant poison, and nerve agents enhance nicotinic depolarizations and modulate nicotinic receptor ion channels directly by an allosteric effect—as does pyridostigmine, which is used as a protective measure against nerve gases. Organophosphate exposure causes persistent changes in both muscarinic and nicotinic function. With repeated low-level exposure chronic changes have been reported in muscarinic (M1 and M3) receptors. But, in addition, persistent downregulation of nicotinic receptor expression has been demonstrated when exposed to a cholinesterase inhibitor causing impaired function on cognitive tests, and the nicotinic character of the impairments was confirmed by reversal with nicotine. Thus it would seem appropriate to examine nicotinic antagonists as well as muscarinic ones, as possible therapeutic agents for anticholinesterase nerve gas toxicity.

Upon suspicion, it is advisable for soldiers to take a 30 mg dose of the anticholine esterase pyridostigmine bromide three times a day as prophylaxis In some cases, it might be necessary to decontaminate them chemically, as with ammonia for hydrogen cyanide or chlorine. Riot control agents such as CS will dissipate in an open area, but articles contaminated with CS powder needs to be aired or spray washed by people wearing protective gear.

Artificial respiration: Mouth to mouth ventilation is contraindicated in suspected chemical warfare victims, instead the MARK III F type of Ambu manual resuscitator that has a butyl outer cover with gas filter adaptors can be safely used in a chemical gas warfare setting.

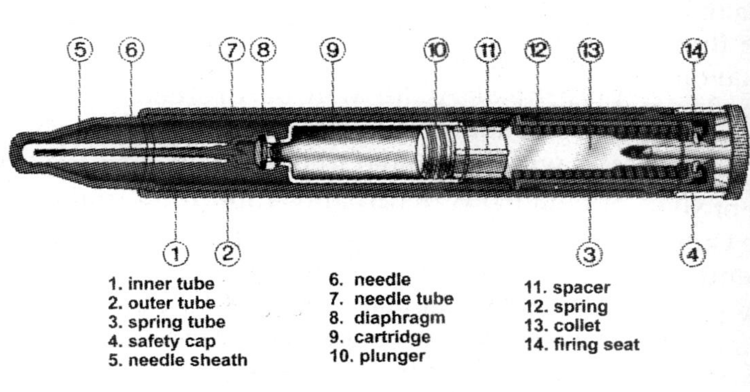

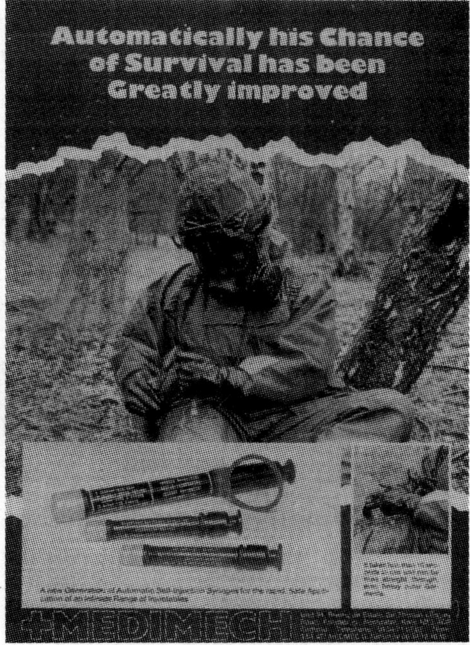

Fig. 70.16

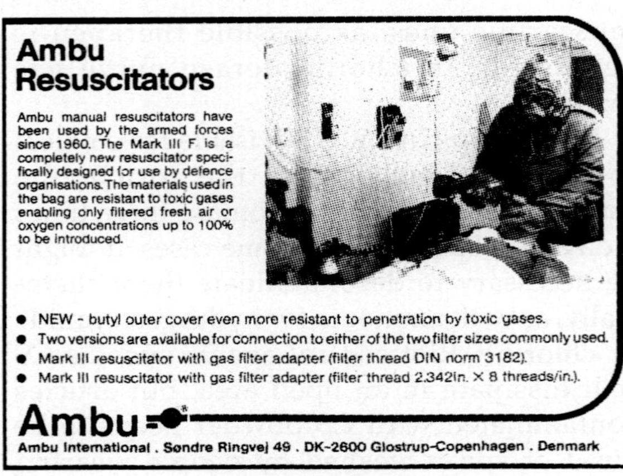

Fig. 70.17

B. Specific Treatment:

Samples for analysis: Quantity of sample: 12 ml total, either 4 ml × 3 vacutainers or 3 ml × 4 vacutainers. The glass/plastic containers must be inverted 6-8 times and bottle tops are purple or green topped by convention. Urine samples will be needed in chemical poisoning cases. Biological samples must be passed through a particle analyzer and samples are preferably collected from the "fluffy cloud" and unexposed to uv rays or direct sunlight.

History

Physostigmine (also known as eserine from éséré, West African name for the Calabar bean) is a parasympathomimetic, specifically, a reversible cholinesterase inhibitor alkaloid. The chemical was synthesized for the first time in 1935 by the chemists Percy Lavon Julian and Josef Pikl. Pyridostigmine bromide (PB) has been in use since 1955 to treat myasthenia gravis. It was given to 250000 to 300000 American troops in a daily dose of 90 mg for a maximum of seven days in the Gulf war, as a "pretreatment" against potential Iraqi attacks with the nerve gas soman.

Treatment Rationale

It has been estimated that, for adequate protection against nerve agents in combat conditions, a protective ratio of at least 5 is desired. That is, the treatments we give must allow exposure to five times the usual lethal dose. The protective ratio (PR) is the LD50 with treatment (the dose that is lethal in 5 percent of subjects, if treatment is given) divided by the LD50 without treatment (the dose that is lethal in 50 percent if treatment is not given. In the absence of PB, the PR of atropine and oxime against the nerve agent soman does not reach this goal but is around 1.6. However, adding PB brings the ratio to in excess of 50 in primates, providing more than adequate protection against death from soman. PB enhances the protection of oxime and atropine against a nerve agent, perhaps by reversibly binding to the AChE site at which the nerve agent or other cholinesterase inhibitors (like the OP DFP) would normally bind, preventing the nerve agent from binding. In particular, soman cannot bind to a PB-bound AChE molecule. This prevents aging of soman-AChE from taking place. (Without PB, this would lead to irreversible inhibition of the soman-bound AChE molecules, and recovery of AChE activity would require several weeks for full regeneration of AChE.) The stated goal of PB pretreatment is to bind (and thereby inhibit) approximately 30 percent of AChE; carbamylation of about 30 percent of circulating (RBC, or erythrocyte) AChE corresponds to a great increase in the effectiveness of the antidotes. This 30 percent of AChE will be protected from binding and irreversible inhibition by soman and will be restored to normal function once spontaneous decarbamylation (dissociation of PB from the AChE molecule) occurs. (Meanwhile, there is enough time for oxime to be given, so that PB decarbamylates, and any residual nerve agent that binds the now-functional AChE can be pulled off).

Because PB and nerve agents both inhibit AChE, it might be supposed that the toxicity would be additive—that a smaller amount of a nerve agent would be needed to produce toxicity if PB were given in advance. For reasons not well understood (which may relate to the ability of PB to desensitize the ACh receptor, as noted above), an additive effect on performance and on lethality evidently does not occur.

Other mechanisms have been proposed that may contribute to protection by PB pretreatment, including desensitization of the neuromuscular endplate and ACh receptor; decreased quantal release of ACh; and decreased frequency of miniature endplate potentials (small voltage changes in the cell receiving a signal).

PB is preferred over other carbamates, particularly physostigmine, because it has fewer side effects, longer duration of action, and a greater margin of safety. Physostigmine has been viewed as a candidate for pretreatment, but it has several disadvantages for field use it has quite a short half-life in vivo, protecting dosing levels produce side effects, and it penetrates the CNS. CNS penetration leads to concerns that use of physostigmine could result in adverse effects on troops' performance.

PB does not cross the blood-brain barrier under ordinary circumstances, because of its positive charge. Thus CNS side effects from PB are not thought to be an issue with normal use. While PB does not protect AChE in the CNS from nerve agents, it also presumably does not itself induce CNS symptoms and potentially deleterious performance changes (by inhibiting brain AChE. (Protection of the CNS is done post exposure, using atropine, oximes, and diazepam). PB's ability to confer protection in doses without substantial side effects has made it the preferred pretreatment over physostigmine.

It should be noted, however, that if PB is given after nerve agent rather than before, additive effects might be expected.

Pre Treatment

Prophylactic pretreatment for nerve gas and pesticide poisons which can be administered orally at 12 hourly intervals for 5 days comprising of the following agents, in combination:

a. Pyridostigmine bromide 30–60 mg or physostigmine 0.5–2.0 mg. The pyridostigmine and physostigmine doses are selected with a view to lowering serum cholinesterase activity to 70-80% of the initial value over a period of 10-12 hours. PB is used as a pretreatment or, more precisely, as a pretreatment adjunct for poisoning by nerve agents. It confers no protection on its own but enhances the protection conferred by postexposure treatment in the form of atropine and pralidoxime (2-PAM). AChE inhibition of 20 to 40 percent should be maintained to provide adequate protection against death from soman poisoning; generally, 30mg each eight hours orally has been found to provide that range of inhibition in people, although the inhibition may fall below 20 percent six hours after dosing. Dosing every eight hours has been estimated to leave five hours a day in which AChE inhibition falls below 20 percent. Nonetheless, the recommended dosing schedule for nerve agent pretreatment is 30mg orally every eight hours.
b. Diazepam 3.0-5.0 mg or clonazepam 0.5-2.0 mg.
c. 3-8 mg G3063, 5-15 mg Arpenal, 2-10 mg Sycotrol (pipetabanate hydrochloride), 5-15 mg caramiphen (caramiphene hydrochloride) or 3-20 mg benactyzine (benactyzine hydrochloride.

Caramiphen is an anticonvulsant, anticholinergic drug with anti-glutamatergic properties, and seen to dramatically attenuate the process of cell death as assessed by the binding of [3H]RoS-4864 to peripheral benzodiazepine receptors (omega 3 sites) on microglia and astrocytes. In addition, caramiphen but not scopolamine, blocks the soman-evoked down-regulation of [3H] AMPA binding to forebrain membrane preparations and capable of abolishing the effects of soman intoxication on learning. The beneficial use of drugs exhibiting both anticholinergic and anti-glutamatergic properties for the protection against changes in cognitive parameters caused by nerve agent poisoning is proven. The effects of pipethanate (sycotrol) and two newly synthetized cholinolytics, DPX-8 and ANC-51 has shown that the anticholinergic activity of pipethanate, DPX-8, and ANC-51 was weaker than that of atropine. However, the therapeutic effect of pipethanate was higher than that of atropine in organophosphate poisoning whereas DPX-8 and ANC-51 afforded a better antidotal effect than atropine only in DDVP-poisoning.

Benactyzine is an anticholinergic drug. It is a glycolic acid ester, related to other drugs such as the piperidinyl benzilates and 3-Quinuclidinyl benzilate but with much less potent anticholinergic effects. Benactyzine has also been used as an antidepressant Certain muscarinic antagonists like atropine, aprophen, and benactyzine aprophen and benactyzine are effective non-competitive inhibitors of the AChR.

Mark I™, Nerve Agent Antidote Kit (NAAK) (atropine and pralidoxime chloride injection).

Contains: AtroPen® 2 mg Auto-Injector (atropine injection) Pralidoxime Chloride 600 mg Auto-Injector (pralidoxime chloride injection).

The Mark I NAAK, or MARK I Kit, is a "Nerve Agent Antidote Kit". It is a dual-chamber autoinjector: Two anti-nerve agent drugs—atropine sulfate and pralidoxime chloride—each in injectable form, constitute the kit. The kits are only effective against the nerve agents Tabun (GA), Sarin (GB), Soman (GD) and VX.

Typically, soldiers are issued three MARK I Kits when operating in circumstances where chemical weapons are considered a potential hazard. Along with the three kits are issued one CANA (Convulsive Antidote, Nerve Agent) for simultaneous use. (CANA is the drug diazepam or *Valium*, an anticonvulsant.) Both of these kits are intended for use in "buddy aid" or "self aid" administration of the drugs prior to decontamination and delivery of the patient to definitive medical care. Dose may be repeated every 5 minutes until the mucous membranes dry.

A newer model, the ATNAA (Antidote Treatment Nerve Agent Auto-Injector), has both the atropine and the pralidoxime in one syringe, allowing for simplified administration.

The use of a Mark 1 or ATNAA kit inhibits the nerve agents' purpose, thereby reducing the number of fatal casualties in the advent of chemical warfare. The kits should only be administered if nerve agents have been absorbed or inhaled and symptomatic.

Mild symptoms: Rhinorrhea (runny nose) and Miosis (pinpoint pupils).

Moderate symptoms: D–diarrhea, U–urination, M–miosis, B–bronchospasms, E–emesis, L – lacrimation, S–salivation (Mnemonic DUMBELS).

Severe symptoms: Loss of consciousness, seizures and apnea.

Contraindications: None known.

Physostigmine salicylate injection is available in 2 mL ampuls, each mL containing 1 mg of Physostigmine Salicylate in a vehicle composed of sodium metabisulfite 0.1% benzyl alcohol 2.0% as a preservative in Water for Injection.

Newer generation of automatic self-injection syringes are now available from Medimech (UK) and DUPHAR (Netherlands) like AtroPen etc, ComboPen and MultiPen which are preloaded with atropine and oximes. An optional third antidote in desired concentration can be rapidly and safely injected by the soldier himself straight through even heavy outer protective garments. Pre-filled syringes containing 4-DMAP (4-dimethylaminophenol hydrochloride 250mg/5 ml is also available from Dr Franz Kohler Chemie GmbH, Alsbach, Federal Republic of Germany. This is effective against hydrocyanic acid, cyanide, nitrite and hydrogen sulphide poisoning. Dose required is 3-4 mg/kg body weight for poisoning cases and 1-2 mg/mg following smoke inhalation intravenously. For cyanide poisoning, this can be supplemented with continuous inhalation of oxygen and intermittent inhalation of amyl nitrite ampoules over a one minute period. Intravenous sodium nitrite 2.5 to 5.0 ml over one minute and repeated till a maximum of 10-15 ml (300 to 450 mg). For children 0.33 ml/kg or 10 mg/kg. This is followed by 50-100 ml/kg of sodium thiosulphate intravenously over 1 to 2 minute period for adults {For children dose is 1.65 ml/kg or 0.5mg/kg}. Half this dose can be repeated if blood cyanide levels are in excess of more than 0.1 mg/dl. These drugs convert hemoglobin to methemoglobin as the latter has greater affinity for cyanide. Once symptoms like flushing and tachycardia are controlled and the victim is fully awake and alert, 2-4 mg/kg of methylene blue can be administered I/V to tackle methemoglobinemia. Dexamethasone aerosol spray is indicated where pulmonary irritant inhalation has occured to minimise pulmonary edema and interstitial fibrosis. Prior to evacuation to a hospital, a Grasebys chemical agent monitor must be used to establish safety.

Prior to surgery, a solution of alkaline sodium hypochlorite solution can be used to wash the wound to neutralize most chemical agents. Over-pressure systems offer protection, but generate heat in the process and vitiate the air conditioning. Use of NBC gloves, gas masks, protective suits and specific antidotes based on chemical identification would be required to counter a chemical offensive.

Accidental Chlorine gas leakage can occur from water treatment plants, swimming pools, paper, plastic and fabric manufacturing units and cylinder bursts. Inhalation produces severe respiratory and ocular irritation, cough, choking, vomiting, pulmonary edema and cyanosis. Exposure to 3-5 ppm chlorine gas can produce symptoms and exposure to concentrations above 25 ppm can be fatal .Oxygen inhalation, irrigation of skin and eyes with saline/water, parenteral and inhaled corticosteroids, bronchodilators, antibiotic prophylaxis and ventilator therapy will be indicated, depending on the severity of the symptoms.

In Lewisite poisoning, the oil based British Anti Lewisite (BAL) is the specific antidote given in a dose of 0.5 ml/1kg body weight deep intramuscularly. Maximum dose permitted is 4 ml. Dose has to be repeated 4 hourly, at 4 h, 8 h and 12 h after the first dose. The interval may be reduced to 2 hrly in very symptomatic patients. In nerve poisoning cases, Inj. Atropine 6 mg I/M (paed=0.05 mg/kg) and Inj Pralidoxime 1.g slow I/V (Paed = 15 mg/kg) may be life saving.

CONCLUSIONS

The detection of targeted compounds does seem to be possible with relatively simple instrumentation, however, broad-spectrum analysis is more difficult. Lab-on-a-chip technology and the resolving power/instrument size ratio is increasing each year. The suggested approach to the problem of verifying the presence or absence of chemical weapons in the field is:

The first, and least expensive, is to use the one- and two-dimensional approaches outlined above to screen compounds in the field.

For example, field-portable gas chromatographs are readily available and relatively easy (much easier than the approved GC/MS instrument) to operate under field conditions. IMSs are also relatively reliable these days (they are now used for explosive detection in most airports). Thus, it should be possible to use a variety of simple analytical instruments to obtain on-site supporting data on the presence or absence of chemical weapons.

The second and more expensive approach would be to convert an airplane into a verification laboratory with full capabilities of a trace analysis laboratory for the identification and quantification of CW agents and their degradation products in all types of samples. This mobile laboratory could be flown anywhere in the world and located near the site under evaluation. Samples could then be taken and analyzed on (or near) site within a few hours. Whatever the final solution, it does seem possible, even with conventional analytical methods, to provide confirmatory analytical data for verification activities mandated through the CWC of 1993.

THE CHEMICAL WEAPONS CONVENTION (CWC)

The experience of large-scale chemical warfare was so horrifying that it led to the 1925 Geneva Protocol, which forbids the use of chemical and bacteriological agents in war. Images of victims gasping, frothing and choking to death had a profound impact. The text of the protocol reflects the global sense of abhorrence. It affirmed that these weapons had been justly condemned by the general opinion of the civilized world.

The Chemical Weapons Convention (CWC) reinforces aspects of the Geneva Conventions that also dealt with these agents and was negotiated over a period of 24 years. In 1992, after a decade of long and painstaking negotiations, the Conference on Disarmament in Geneva agreed to the text of the (CWC), which was adopted by the General Assembly on 03 November 1992, in its resolution entitled Convention on the Prohibition of the Development, Production, Stockpiling and Use of Chemical Weapons and on Their Destruction (A/RES/47/39). More than 17countries have signed the CWC, and 130 have ratified it. The treaty entered into force on April 29, 1997, 18 days after Hungary, the 65th country, ratified. Countries that ratify must destroy all chemical weapons over a ten year period with the treaty providing a leveling out principle that ensures possessors destroy their stockpiles at roughly the same time.

Five years after entry into force, destruction of 20% of the stockpile is to be completed. After seven years, 45% of the destruction should be complete. Under the treaty countries must to stop any development, produc-tion, acquisition, stockpiling and retention of chemical weapons. The CWC requires States Parties to report the location of chemical weapons storage sites, the location and characteristics of chemical weapons produc-tion and research facilities and also prohibits trade in certain chemicals with countries not party to the treaty.

The verification provisions of the CWC not only affect the military sector but also the civilian chemical industry, world-wide, through certain restrictions and obligations regarding the production, processing and consumption of chemicals that are considered relevant to the objectives of the Convention. The Convention also contains provisions on assistance in case a State Party is attacked or threatened with attack by chemical weapons and on promoting the trade in chemicals and related equipment among State Parties.

Chemical Warfare Threat

At least 23 nations are reported to have stockpiles of nerve agents, though these are prohibited for use in war by the 1925 Geneva Convention and the 1987 Paris Convention on Chemical Weapons (which not all nations have signed). As of 2009, 188 states are a party to the CWC.The nations reported to have chemical weapons include not only Iraq and Iran, but Egypt, Syria, Libya, Israel, Ethiopia, Burma, Thailand, North Korea, South Korea, Cuba, Vietnam, Taiwan, China, and South Africa. In addition, the Iraqis not only have CW capability, but have militarized nerve agents and used them against Iranians and against the Kurds. Use of nerve agent was confirmed by chemical examination of casualties. Typically, Iranian casualties were exposed after the explosion of artillery shells or bombs between 4 and 20 meters away. After 1984, chemical warfare intensified and became more frequent, despite numerous UN missions to investigate use of CW in the Iran-Iraq conflict, and repeated appeals by the UN. Iraq used chemical weapons more extensively and more frequently than Iran. Therefore, CW was justifiably understood to represent a valid Iraqi threat in the PGW. This threat was subsequently confirmed by the discovery of nerve agent munitions, including those containing sarin and cyclosarin, in the Khamisiyah ammunitions storage facility in Iraq. Although no direct intelligence indicated that soman stockpiles were present in Iraq, it was known that the former Soviet Union had stockpiled soman. With the dissolution of the Soviet Union and the consequent political and economic destabilization and fragmentation, the military was concerned that arms of many sorts were for sale to the highest bidder, possibly including Iraq. Schedule 1 (mustard and nerve gases) production is in excess of 100 grams/year has to be declared and any country can possess a maximum of 1 tonne of these materials. Schedule 2 chemicals like thiodiglycol manufacture has to be declared and its export is restricted. Schedule 3 chemicals (phosgene,triethanolamine etc) production in excess of 200 tonnes/year or 30 tonnes if it contains phosphorus, sulfur or fluorine, must be declared and these plants can be inspected.

Further Reading

1. IUPAC Workshop: Impact of Scientific Developments on the Chemical Weapons Convention,Bergen, Norway, 1–3 July 2002.
2. *Chemical and Biological Defense Program*, U.S. Department of Defense (2002).
3. H. Wohltjen and R. Dessy. "Surface acoustic wave probe for chemical analysis. I. Introduction and instrument description", *Anal. Chem. 51*, 1458–1464 (1979).
4. W. H. King, Jr. "Piezoelectric sorption detector", *Anal. Chem. 36*, 1735–1739 (1964).
5. D. J. Ballantine, Jr., S. J. Martin, A. J. Ricco, G. C. Frye, E. T. Zellers, R. M. White, H. Wohltjen. *Acoustic Wave Sensors: Theory, Design and Physico-Chemical Applications*, Academic Press, San Diego (1996).
6. J. W. Grate, S. L. Rose-Pehrsson, D. L. Venezky, M. Klusty, H. Wohltjen. "Smart sensor system for trace organophosphorus and organosulfur vapor detection employing a temperature-controlled array of surface acoustic wave sensors, automated sample preconcentration, and pattern recognition", *Anal. Chem.65*, 1868–1881 (1993).
7. J. W. Grate and R. A. McGill. "Dewetting effects on polymer-coated surface acoustic wave vapor sensors", *Anal. Chem. 67*, 4015–4019 (1995).
8. *Department of Defense Chemical and Biological Defense Program, Vol. 1: Annual Report toCongress*, U.S. Department of Defense (2002).
9. R.A. McGill, VK. Nguyen, R. Chung, RE. Shaffer, *et al.* "The 'NRLSAWRHINO': A nose for toxic gases", *Sens. ActuatorsB 65*, 10–13 (2000).
10. A. Mulchandani, P. Mulchandani, W. Chen, J. Wang, L. Chen. "Amperometric thick-film stripelectrodes for monitoring organophosphate nerve agents based on immobilized organo-phosphorus hydrolase", *Anal. Chem.71*, 2246–2249 (1999).
11. P. Mulchandani, W. Chen, A. Mulchandani. "Flow injection amperometric enzyme biosensor for direct determination of organophosphate

nerve agents", *Environ. Sci. Technol. 35*, 2562–2565 (2001).

12. J. Wang, M. Pumera, M. P. Chatrathi, A. Escarpa, M. Musameh, G. Collins, A. Mulchandani, Y. Lin, K. Olsen. "Single-channel microchip for fast screening and detailed identification of nitroaromatic explosives or organophosphate nerve agents", *Anal. Chem. 74*, 1187–1191 (2002).
13. H. HILL, JR. AND S. J. MARTIN © 2002 IUPAC, *Pure and Applied Chemistry* 74, 2281–22912288.
14. A. R. Hopkins and N. S. Lewis. "Detection and classification characteristics of arrays of carbon black/organic polymer composite chemiresistive vapor detectors for the nerve agent simulants dimethylmethylphosphonate and diisopropylmethylphosponate", *Anal. Chem.*73, 884–892 (2001).
15. A. L. Jenkins, O. M. Uy, G. M. Murray. "Polymer-based lanthanide luminescent sensor for detection of the hydrolysis product of the nerve agent Soman in water", *Anal. Chem.* 71, 373–378(1999).
16. C.A. Sanders, M. Rodriguez, Jr., E. Greenbaum. "Stand-off tissue-based biosensors for the detection of chemical warfare agents using photosynthetic fluorescence induction", *Biosens.Bioelectron. 16*, 439–446 (2001).
17. D. E. Lenz, A. A. Brimfield, L. A. Cook. "Development of immunoassays for detection of chemical warfare agents", in *Immunochemical Technology for Environmental Applications*, D. A. Agaand E. M. Thurman (Eds.), pp. 77–86, ACS Symposium Series 657, American Chemical Society, Washington, DC (1997).
18. G. Frishman and A. Amirav. "Fast GC–PFPD system for field analysis of chemical warfare agents", *Field Anal. Chem. Technol. 4*, 170–194 (2000).
19. W.A. Carrick, D. B. Cooper, B. Muir. "Retrospective identification of chemical warfare agents by high-temperature automatic thermal desorption-gas chromatography–mass spectrometry", *J.Chromatogr. A 925*, 241–249 (2001).
20. S.D. Harvey, D. A. Nelson, B. W. Wright, J. W. Grate. Selective stationary phase for solid-phase microextraction analysis of sarin (GB). *J. Chromatogr. A954*, 217–225 (2002).
21. G.L. Kimm, G. L. Hook, P. A. Smith. "Application of headspace solid-phase microextraction and gas chromatography–mass spectrometry for detection of the chemical warfare agent bis(2-chloroethyl) sulfide in soil", *J. Chromatogr. A 971*, 185–191 (2002).
22. E. W. J. Hooijschuur, C. E. Kientz, A. G. Hulst, U. A. Th. Brinkman. "Determination of hydrolysis products of sulfur mustards by reversed-phase microcolumn liquid chromatography coupled on-line with sulfur flame photometric detection and electrospray ionization mass spectrometry using large-volume injections and peak compression", *Anal. Chem. 72*, 1199–1206 (2000).
23. E.W.J. Hooijschuur, CE Kientz, UA. Th. Brinkman. "Determination of alkylphosphonic acids by microcolumn liquid chromatography with gradient elution coupled on-line with flame photometric detection", *J. Chromatogr. A907*, 165–172 (2001).
24. C.E. Kientz, E. W. J. Hooijschuur, UA. Th. Brinkman. "Capillary electrophoresis coupled online with flame photometric detection: Determination of alkylphosphonic acids", *J. Micro. Sep 9*, 253–259 (1997).
25. J. E. Melanson, B. L.-Y. Wong, C. A. Boulet, C. A. Lucy. "High-sensitivity determination of thedegradation products of chemical warfare agents by capillary electrophoresis-indirect UV absorbance detection", *J. Chromatogr. A* 920, 359–365 (2001).
26. A-E.F. Nassar, S. V. Lucas, L. D. Hoffland. "Determination of chemical warfare agent degradation products at low-part-per-billion levels in aqueous samples and sub-part-per-million levels in soils using capillary electrophoresis", *Anal. Chem.* 71, 1285–1292 (1999).
27. J. Wang, M. P. Chatrathi, A. Mulchandani, W. Chen. "Capillary electrophoresis microchips for separation and detection of organophosphate nerve agents", *Anal. Chem.* 73, 1804–1808 ,2001).
28. R.A. Miller, E. G. Nazarov, G. A. Eiceman, A. T. King. "A MEMS radiofrequency ion mobilityspectrometer for chemical vapor detection", *Sens. Actuators A* 91, 301–312 (2001).
29. K. Tuovinen, H. Paakkanen, O. Hanninen. "Determination of soman and VX degradation products by an aspiration ion mobility spectrometry", *Anal. Chim. Acta* 440, 151–159 (2001).
30. T. Faye, J. C. Mathurin, A. Brunot, J. C. Tabet, G. Wells, C. Fuche. "High-pressure ion source combined with an in-axis ion trap mass

spectrometer. Application of selective low-pressure negative ion chemical ionization", *Anal. Chem.* 72, 5063–5069.

31. A. J. Bell, J. Murrell, C. M. Timperley, P. Watts. "Fragmentation and reactions of two isomericO-alkyl S-(2-dialkylamino)ethyl methylphosphonothiolates studied by electrospray ionization/ion trap mass spectrometry", *J. Am. Soc. Mass Spectrom.* 12, 902–910 (2001).
32. G.S. Groenewold, A. D. Appelhans, GL. Gresham, J.E. Olson, M. Jeffery, JB. Wright." Analysis of VX on soil particles using ion trap secondary ion mass spectrometry", *Anal. Chem.*71, 2318–2323 (1999).
33. G.L. Gresham, G.S. Groenewold, J.E. Olson. "Identification of the nitrogen-based blister agents bis(2-chloroethyl)methylamine (HN-2) and tris(2-chloroethyl)amine (HN-3) and their hydrolysis products on soil using ion trap secondary ion mass spectrometry", *J. Mass Spectrom.* 35,1460–1469 (2000).
34. E.O. Price, J. R. Smith, C. R. Clark, J. J. Schlager, M. L. Shih. "MALDIToF/MS as a diagnostic tool for the confirmation of sulfur mustard exposure", *J. Appl. Toxicol.* 20, S193–S197 (2000).
35. VD Berkout, RJ Cotter, DP Segers. "Miniaturized EI/Q/oa TOF mass spectrometer", *J. Am.Soc. Mass Spectrom. 12*, 641–647 (2001).
36. J.A. Syage, M.A. Hanning-Lee, K.A. Hanold. "A man-portable, photoionization time-of-flightmass spectrometer", *Field Anal. Chem. Technol.4*, 204–215 (2000).
37. G.E. Patterson, A.J. Guymon, L.S. Riter, M. Everly, J. Griep-Raming, B. C. Laughlin, Z.Ouyang, R. G. Cooks. "Miniature cylindrical ion trap mass spectrometer", *Anal. Chem.* 74,6145–6153 (2002).
38. L.S. Riter, Y. Peng, R. J. Noll, G. E. Patterson, T. Aggerholm, R. G. Cooks. "Analytical performance of a miniature cylindrical ion trap mass spectrometer", *Anal. Chem. 74*, 6154–6162(2002).
39. W.H. Griest, M.B. Wise, K.J. Hart, S.A. Lammert, C. V. Thompson. "Biological agent detection and indentification by the Block II Chemical Biological Mass Spectrometer", *Field Anal.Chem. Technol.5*, 177–184 (2001).
40. Ch. E. Kientz. "Chromatography and mass spectrometry of chemical warfare agents, toxins and related compounds: state of the art and future prospects", *J. Chromatogr. A 814*:1–23 (1998).
41. J.R. Smith, M.L. Shih, E. O. Price, G. E. Platoff, J. J. Schlager. "Army medical laboratory telemedicine: Role of mass spectrometry in telediagnosis for chemical and biological defense", *J.Appl. Toxicol. 21*, S35–S41 (2001).
42. BA Eckenrode. Environmental and forensic applications of field-portable GCMS: An overview", *J. Am. Soc. Mass. Spectrom.12*, 683–693 (2001).
43. J.A. Syage, B. J. Nies, M. D. Evans, K. A. Hanold. "Field-portable, high-speed GC/TOFMS", *J.Am. Soc. Mass Spectrom. 12*, 648–655 (2001).
44. M.D. Brickhouse, W. R. Creasy, B.R. Williams, K. M. Morrissey, R. J. O'Connor, H. D. Durst."Multiple-technique analytical characterization of a mixture containing chemical-weapons simulant from a munition", *J. Chromatogr. A883*, 185–198 (2000).
45. J.R. Smith and M. L. Shih. "Analysis of the degradation compounds of chemical warfare agents using liquid chromatography/mass spectrometry", *J. Appl. Toxicol. 21*, S27–S34 (2001).
46 P.A. D'Agostino, J. R. Hancock, L. R. Provost. "Determination of sarin, soman and their hydrolysis products in soil by packed capillary liquid chromatography–electrospray mass spectrometry", *J. Chromatogr. A912*, 291–299 (2001).
47. G.R. Asbury, C. Wu, W. F. Siems, H. H. Hill, Jr. "Separation and identification of some chemical warfare degradation products using electrospray high resolution ion mobility spectrometrywith mass selected detection", *Anal. Chim. Acta 404*, 273–283 (2000).
48. H.HILL, JR. AND S. J. MARTIN© 2002 IUPAC, *Pure and Applied Chemistry* 74, 2281–2291 48. W. E. Steiner, B. H. Clowers, L. M. Matz, W. F. Siems, H. H. Hill, Jr. "Rapid of aqueous chemcal warfare agent degradation products: Ambient pressure ion mobility mass spectrometry", *Anal.Chem. 74*, 4343–4352 (2002).
49. C.M. Harris. "GC to go", *Anal. Chem.74*, 585A–589A (2002).
50. E.W.J. Hooijschuur, A.G. Hulst, A.L. deJong, L. P. de Reuver, S. H. van Krimpen, B. L. M.van Baar, E.R.J. Wils, C.E. Kientz, U.A. Th. Brinkman. "Identification of chemicals related to the chemical weapons convention during an interlaboratory proficiency test", *Trends Anal. Chem.*

> *"The one that scares me to death, perhaps even more so than tactical nuclear weapons, and the one we have the least capability against is biological weapons."*
>
> *—General Colin Powell, 1993*

BIOLOGICAL WARFARE

Introduction

The natural outbreak of dangerous diseases like plague, anthrax, cholera, Ebola fever, lassa fever and small pox led to the deployment of such pathogenic micro organisms and/or their toxins to deliberately cause epidemics among the enemy. This new dimension to modern day warfare is unique in that they are self-propagating and require no additional effort from the hostile quarter to enhance damage whereas, explosives and chemical weapons have to be used repeatedly to succeed in annihilation. The clandestine nature of biological warfare has the advantage over other forms as it is difficult to prove or disprove the intentional nature of an outbreak of disease, especially if it is endemic to the region. Biological agents do not destroy installations and properties and also, the troops employing such agents can be protected by vaccinating them in advance. Biological warfare is best suited for high density population living in temperate regions.

Historical Perspective

- The use of biological agents is not a new concept, and history is filled with examples of their use.
- Attempts to use biological warfare agents date back to antiquity.
- Scythian archers infected their arrows by dipping them in decomposing bodies or in blood mixed with manure as far back as 40 BC.
- Persian, Greek and Roman literature from 30 BC quotes examples of dead animals used to contaminate wells and other sources of water.

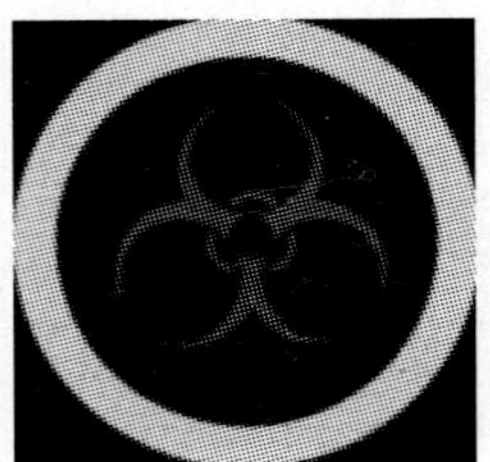

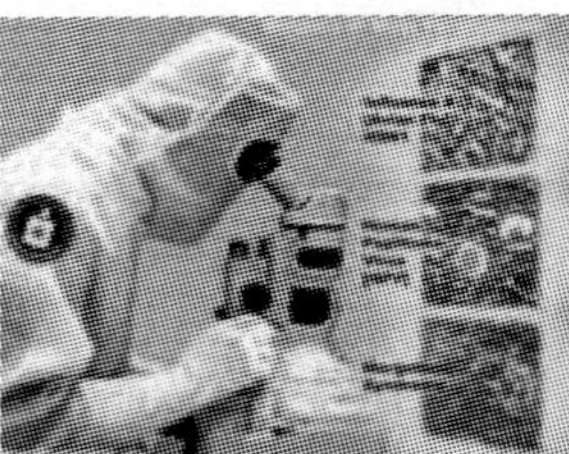

Fig. 70.18

- In the Battle of Eurymedon in 19 BC, Hannibal won a naval victory over King Eumenes II of Pergamon by firing earthen vessels full of venomous snakes into the enemy ships. During the battle of Tortona.

In the 12th century AD, Barbarossa used the bodies of dead and decomposing soldiers to poison wells. An early BW attack took place in the Black Sea port of Kaffa (now Feodossia, Ukraine) in 1346. Rats and their fleas carried the disease to attacking Tatar soldiers. The Tatars catapulted the bodies of victims at the defending Genoese who contracted plague and left Kaffa. The same rats afflicting the Tatars brought disease to the Genoese.

This was repeated in 1710, when the Russians besieging Swedish forces at Reval in Estonia catapulted bodies of people who had died from plague.

During the French and Indian War, British forces under the direction of Sir Jeffrey Amherst attempted use of biological warfare between 1754 and 1767 by passing smallpox-infested blankets to unsuspecting American Indians. Smallpox decimated the Indians, but it is unclear if the contaminated blankets or endemic disease brought by the Europeans caused these epidemics.

Allegations were made during the American Civil War by both sides, but especially against the Confederate Army, of the attempted use of smallpox to cause disease among enemy forces.

Biological warfare reached sophistication during the 1900s when, during World War I, the German Army developed anthrax, glanders, cholera, and a wheat fungus specifically for use as biological weapons. They allegedly spread plague in St. Petersburg, Russia, infected mules with glanders in Mesopotamia, and attempted to do the same with the horses of the French Cavalry.

The Geneva Protocol of 1925 was signed by 108 nations. This was the first multilateral agreement that extended prohibition of chemical and biological agents. Unfortunately, no method for verification of compliance was addressed.

In 1932 during the course of World War II, Japanese forces operated a secret biological warfare research facility (Unit 731) outside Harbin, Manchuria that carried out human experiments on prisoners. 11 Chinese cities were attacked with the agents of anthrax, cholera, shigellosis, salmonella, and plague, and at least 10,000 died during their gruesome experiments. They also exposed more than 3000 prisoners to plague, anthrax, and syphilis in an attempt to develop and observe the disease. Some victims were executed or died from their infections. Autopsies were also performed for greater understanding of the effects on the human body.

In 1942, the United States formed the War Research Service. Anthrax and botulinum toxin initially were investigated for use as weapons. Sufficient quantities of botulinum toxin and anthrax were stockpiled by June 1944 to allow unlimited retaliation if the German forces first used biological agents. The British also tested anthrax bombs on Gruinard Island off the northwest coast of Scotland in 1942 and 1943 and then prepared and stockpiled anthrax-laced cattle cakes for the same reason. The United States started an offensive biological warfare program at Camp Detrick (today Fort Detrick) in Frederick, Maryland in 1943. Ten years later, the defensive program began when, from 1951-1954, harmless organisms were released off both coasts of the United States to demonstrate the vulnerability of American cities to biological attacks. This weakness was tested again in 1966 when a test substance was released in the New York City subway system.

By 1969, the U.S. had weaponized the agents causing anthrax, botulism, tularemia, brucellosis, Venezuelan equine encephalitis, and Q fever.

During the Vietnam War, Viet Cong guerrillas used needle-sharp punji sticks dipped in feces to cause severe infections among US GIs who fell into traps and impaled on these devices.

In 1979, an accidental release of anthrax from a weapons facility in Sverdlovsk, USSR, killed at least 66 people. The Russian government claimed these deaths were due to infected meat, and maintained this position until 1992, when Russian President Boris Yeltsin finally admitted to the accident.

In September and October of 1984, 751 people were intentionally infected with Salmonella typhimurium, an agent that causes food poisoning, when followers of the Bhagwan Shree Rajneesh contaminated restaurant salad bars in Oregon.

In 1985, Iraq began an offensive biological weapons program producing anthrax, botulinum toxin, and aflatoxin. During Operation Desert Storm, the coalition of allied forces faced the threat of chemical and biological agents. Following the Persian Gulf War, Iraq disclosed that it had bombs, Scud missiles, 122 mm rockets, and artillery shells armed with botulinum toxin, anthrax, and aflatoxin. They also had spray tanks fitted to aircraft that could disseminate biological agents over a specific target.

In 1994, a Japanese sect of the Aum Shinrikyo cult attempted an aerosolized (sprayed into the air) release of anthrax from the tops of buildings in Tokyo.

In 1995, 2 members of a Minnesota militia group were convicted of possession of ricin, which they had produced themselves for use in retaliation against local government officials.

In 1996, an Ohio man attempted to obtain bubonic plague cultures through the mail. In 2001, anthrax was delivered by mail to US media and government offices. There were 4 deaths.

In December 2002, 6 terrorist suspects were arrested in Manchester, England; their apartment was serving as a ricin laboratory.- Among them was a 27-year-old chemist who was producing the toxin. Later, on January 5, 2003, British police raided-2 residences around London and found-traces of ricin, that led to an investigation of a possible Chechen separatist plan to attack the Russian embassy with the toxin.

On February 3, 2004, 3 US Senate office buildings were closed after the toxin ricin was found in mailroom that serves Senate Majority Leader Bill Frist's office.

Definition

Biological Warfare (BW) is defined as the employment of biological agents to produce casualties in man or animals or damage to plants.

Characteristics of an Ideal Biological Warfare Agent

The properties of an ideal biological warfare agent are as follows:

- Must be inexpensive.
- Easy to produce.
- Easily disseminated and dispersible with aerosolizable potential (1 to 10 μm diameter).
- Survive sunlight, drying, and heat and cold.
- Cause lethal or disabling disease.
- Result in person-to-person transmission.
- Have no effective therapy or prophylaxis.
- Have a short incubation period.

Anthrax comes closest to being the ideal biological warfare agent.

Disadvantages of BW

The disadvantages of using BW agents as weapons include hazards to the user, their dependence on optimal weather conditions to result in effective dispersal, and their possible inactivation by solar irradiation and other climatic conditions.

Opportune Time for Biowarfare

BW attacks would most likely occur late at night or early in the morning when agents would be less likely to undergo inactivation by ultraviolet radiation. At these times, atmospheric temperature inversions would allow an agent cloud to travel at low altitude to cover its target.

Epidemiologic Clues of a Biowarfare Attack

- Large epidemic with similar disease in a discrete population.
- Many cases of unexplained disease.
- More severe disease than expected.
- Disease unusual for the population.
- Disease normally transmitted by a vector uncommon in the affected area.
- Uncommon disease.
- Unusual strains of pathogens.

BIOWARFARE AGENTS

Category A

Definition

High-priority agents include organisms that pose a risk to national security because they:

- Can be easily disseminated or transmitted from person to person.

- Result in high mortality rates and have the potential for major public health impact.
- Might cause public panic and social disruption and
- Require special action for public health preparedness.

Agents/Diseases

- Anthrax (*Bacillus anthracis*).
- Botulism (*Clostridium botulinum* toxin).
- Plague (*Yersinia pestis*).
- Smallpox (Variola major).
- Tularemia (*Francisella tularensis*).
- Viral hemorrhagic fevers (filo viruses [e.g., Ebola, Marburg] and arena viruses [e.g., Lassa, Machupo]).

Category B

Definition

Second highest priority agents include those that

- Are moderately easy to disseminate.
- Result in moderate morbidity rates and low mortality rates and
- Require specific enhancements of CDC's diagnostic capacity and enhanced disease surveillance.

Agents/Diseases

- Brucellosis (*Brucella* species).
- Epsilon toxin of *Clostridium perfringens*.
- Food safety threats (e.g. *Salmonella* species, *Escherichia coli* O157:H7, *Shigella*).
- Glanders (*Burkholderia mallei*).
- Melioidosis (*Burkholderia pseudomallei*).
- Psittacosis (*Chlamydia psittaci*).
- Q fever (*Coxiella burnetii*).
- Ricin toxin from *Ricinus communis* (castor beans).
- Staphylococcal enterotoxin B.
- Typhus fever (*Rickettsia prowazekii*).
- Viral encephalitis (alpha viruses [e.g., Venezuelan equine encephalitis, eastern equine encephalitis, western equine encephalitis]).
- Water safety threats (e.g., *Vibrio cholerae*, *Cryptosporidium parvum*).

Category C

Definition

Third highest priority agents include emerging pathogens that could be engineered for mass dissemination in the future because of

- Availability.
- Ease of production and dissemination and
- Potential for high morbidity and mortality rates and major health impact.

Agents

- Emerging infectious diseases such as Nipah virus and hantavirus.

Dissemination of BW Agents

1. Through the air by aerosol sprays: To be an effective biological weapon, airborne germs must be dispersed as fine particles. To be infected, a person must breathe a sufficient quantity of particles into the lungs to cause illness.
2. Used in explosives (artillery, missiles, detonated bombs): The use of an explosive device to deliver and spread biological agents is not as effective as the delivery by aerosol. This is because agents tend to be destroyed by the blast, typically leaving less than 5% of the agent capable of causing disease.
3. Put into food or water: Contamination of a city's water supplies requires an unrealistically large amount of an agent as well as introduction into the water after it passes through a regional treatment facility.
4. Absorbed through or injected into the skin: This method might be ideal for

assassination, but is not likely to be used to cause mass casualties.

Countering Biowarfare

During a biological attack one has to:
a. First detect the agent; and
b. Then initiate protection efforts.

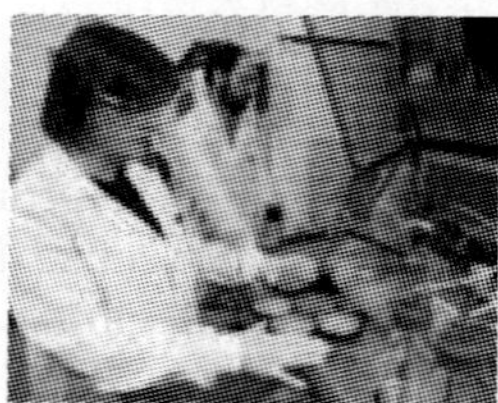

Fig. 70.19

a. *Detection:*

This is easier said than done, as detection of small quantities of a pathogenic microorganism from a large volume of the environment is difficult. Also the environment may have harmless microorganisms similar to that of the agent injected. Detection and identification poses a great challenge and the need for speedy detection conflicts with sensitivity and specificity of the tests. Classically, microorganisms have been identified by bacteriological means. Typically, this would involve plating of the specimen on suitable growth media, incubation at least overnight to allow growth, streak purification of individual suspect colonies followed by another overnight incubation and inoculation of specific biochemical reactions that are useful for differentiation of the organism from other genera or species possibly followed by a third overnight incubation. Thus, the "gold standard" for the identification of bacteria that might be used to identify an organism included in a bioweapon is cultivation followed by differential testing to specifically identify the agent. In the best case, the amount of time needed to identify these organisms could be reduced if specific antiserum was available that could be used after the initial specimen has been plated and incubated to obtain individual bacterial colonies. Thus, a presumptive identification using antibody-based methods would be available after approx 24 h. Besides being time consuming, this process produces a large burden in terms of logistics to get the reagents and equipment to the site of testing. The above scenario is for a bacterial agent and the logistical burden is even heavier for viral agents given the specialized reagents and equipment needed for their identification.

This is simply not acceptable because therapy for infections caused by these agents generally must begin within the first few hours after exposure if the patient is to survive. With rapid identification of a threat, one can be armed with information to fight bioterrorism, and, the quicker one can identify an agent, the quicker a physician can make an accurate diagnosis and commanders can start taking action.

Sampling is advised at night between 6:30 PM and 6:30 AM, the period when biological warfare agents would be most effective. During the day, higher temperatures and relative humidity, faster wind speed, and more ultraviolet light accelerate biological warfare agents' decay—these factors are less severe during darkness. Even anthrax spores, which strongly resist environmental degradation, degrade when exposed to bright sunlight. Inversion conditions are more likely to exist between dusk and dawn, restricting the distributed agent cloud between the ground and the inversion layer, thereby making the agent more effective and less likely to dissipate.The joint biological agent identification and diagnostic system (JBAIDS) is a 40-pound device small enough to slip into a rucksack, and designed to vastly increase the speed and accuracy of biological warfare agent detection. The device looks deceptively simple, just a laptop connected to an analyzer. Lab technicians load suspect samples into a carousel within the analyzer. Real-time DNA analysis requires many copies of a DNA sample, which are made by the polymerase chain reaction. PCR requires repeated cycles of an aqueous sample being heated close to the boiling point and then cooled(they're "cooked and cooled" repeatedly so strands of DNA break apart and reform to make copies of themselves. Each time heating and cooling occur, more DNA copies are formed, which takes something from undetectable to identifiable). To detect DNA in a sample, a synthesized DNA probe or primer tagged with a fluorescent dye is introduced into the sample before it is inserted into the heater chamber. Each probe or primer is designed to attach to a specific organism-anthrax, plague, etc. If that organism is present in the sample, the probe attaches to its DNA. By measuring the sample's fluorescence, the instrument reports the presence (or absence) of the targeted organism. The thermal cycling process takes place in a micromachined, silicon heater chamber that has integrated heaters, cooling surfaces, and windows through which detection takes place. The PCR reaction and DNA analysis take place in a disposable polypropylene reaction tube inserted into the heater chamber. Because of the low thermal mass and integrated nature of the silicon heater chambers, they require very low power and can be heated and cooled much faster than conventional units. So the unit is not only portable but also much faster and more energy-efficient than bench-top models. A multiple-chamber unit that allows the examination of many samples at the same time has been field tested and the device can simultaneously identify up to 10 different biological warfare agents in a given sample, including smallpox, anthrax, plague and encephalitis. The unit can accurately identify the presence of a biological warfare agent on the spot in 40 minutes.

Flow cytometers have been used in laboratories to analyze cells and their features, perform blood typing, test for diseases and viruses, and separate out particular cells or chromosomes. The Biowarfare miniFlo system is small, portable and sensitive. Its novel system eases alignment and increases the accuracy of flow cytometry. In a flow cytometer, the cells flow in single file in solution while the experimenter directs one or more beams of laser light at them and observes the scattered light, which is caused by variations in the cells or DNA. Instead of using a microscope lens or an externally positioned optical fiber as a detector, this method uses the flow stream itself as a waveguide for the laser light, capturing the light and transmitting it to an optical detector. This approach not only eliminates the alignment problems that plague traditional flow cytometers but also collects ten times more light than a microscope lens does. Simpler alignment and more light mean better, faster analysis. Bacteria are large enough for individual detection but viruses and proteins are not. So beads large enough to be detected are coated with an antibody and added to the sample. The virus or protein attaches itself to the bead and can then be detected. When different beads are coated with different antibodies, simultaneous detection of several biological agents is possible. Recombinant antibodies to biological warfare threat agents including F. tularensis, Y. pestis, Brucella spp., V. cholerae O1 and O139, ricin, staphylococcal enterotoxins B and C, botulinum toxins A, B, and E and cholera toxin have been developed through the use of phage display technology. Both recombinant scFvs and Fabs have been produced. Substitutions of currently available monoclonal antibodies with these recombinant antibodies in immunological based detection systems have been successful. The recombinant antibodies exhibited equal sensitivity and equal or lower background across a number of platforms including ELISA assays, ECL based platforms and hand-held immunochromatographic assays. In addition, incorporation of the recombinant antibodies into current detection systems provides a stable genetic source for maintaining critical immunological reagents. The use of recombinant antibodies has allowed for improved detection and identification of biological warfare agents.

One can now continuously monitor the air to detect and identify specific biological warfare agents in near real-time using handheld, fully field portable PCR identifier to detect bacterial and viral pathogens in just 40 minutes. The unique lab-on-a-chip technology system provides robust, reliable analysis of countless harmful microorganisms.

Rapid Diagnostic Tests Biological Agents

Enzyme-linked immunosorbent assay (ELISA)

Direct fluorescent antibody (DFA) testing.

- Rapid immunochromatographic flow assay (RFA) for the detection of immunoglobulin M (IgM) and IgG antibodies.
- Indirect fluorescence assay (IFA).
- Branch-chained DNA assays (molecular markers).
- Hybrid antigen capture particle agglutination immunoassay.
- Nucleic acid–based sequence amplification.
- Polymerase chain reaction (PCR).
- Multiplex PCR.
- Real time PCR.
- Multiplex reverse transcription PCR.
- Real time fluorescence PCR assay.
- Reverse transcription–polymerase chain reaction.
- Quantitative competitive polymerase chain reaction.
- Polymerase chain reaction–based sequencing assay.
- DNA microarray.
- Mass spectrometry.
- NMRI immunoassay.

b. *Protective measures:*

Protective measures can be taken against biological warfare agents. These should be started early (if enough warning is received) but definitely once it is suspected that a biological agent has been used. *Masks:* Currently, available masks such as the military gas mask or high-efficiency particulate air (HEPA) filter masks filter out most biological warfare particles delivered through the air. However, the face seals on ill-fitting masks often leak. For a mask to fit properly, it must be custom fitted to a person's face. *Clothing:* Most biological agents in the air do not penetrate unbroken skin, and few organisms stick to skin or clothing. After an aerosol attack, the simple removal of clothing eliminates a great majority of surface contamination. Thorough showering with soap and water removes 99.99% of the few organisms that may be left on the victim's skin. *Medical protection:* Health care providers treating victims of biological warfare may not need special suits but should use latex gloves and take other precautions such as wearing gowns and masks with protective eye shields. Victims would be isolated in private rooms while receiving treatment. *Drugs:* Victims of biological warfare might be given antibiotics orally (pills) or through an IV, even before the specific agent is identified. Ribavirin is a nonimmunosuppressive nucleoside analogue with broad antiviral properties, and is of proven value for some of the VHF agents. Ribavirin reduces mortality from Lassa fever in high-risk patients, and presumably decreases morbidity in all patients with Lassa fever, for whom current recommendations are to treat initially with ribavirin 30 mg/kg, administered intravenously, followed by 15 mg/kg every 6 hours for 4 days, and then 7.5 mg/kg every 8 hours for an additional 6 days. Treatment is most effective if begun within 7 days of onset; lower intravenous doses or oral administration of 2 g followed by 1 g/d for 10 days also may be useful. The only significant side effects have been anemia and hyperbilirubinemia related to a mild hemolysis and reversible block of erythropoiesis.

The anemia did not require transfusions or cessation of therapy. Ribavirin is contraindicated in pregnant women, but, in the case of definite Lassa fever, the predictability of fetal death and the need to evacuate the uterus justify its use. Safety of ribavirin in infants and children has not been established.

A similar dose of ribavirin begun within 4 days of disease is efficacious in patients with HFRS. Ribavirin has been shown to reduce virological parameters of Junin virus infection (i.e., Argentine hemorrhagic fever), and is now used routinely as an adjunct to immune plasma. However, ribavirin does not penetrate the brain and is expected to protect only against the visceral, not the neurological phase of Junin infection.

Small studies investigating the use of ribavirin in the treatment of Bolivian hemorrhagic fever and Crimean-Congo hemorrhagic fever have been promising, as have preclinical studies for Rift Valley fever. Ribavirin will be ineffective against both the filoviruses and the flaviviruses.

No other antiviral compounds are currently available for the VHF agents.

Interferon alpha has no role in therapy, with the possible exception of Rift Valley fever, where fatal hemorrhagic fever has been associated with low interferon responses in experimental animals. However, as an adjunct to ribavirin, exogenous interferon gamma holds promise in treatment of arenaviral infections.

Passive Immunization

Antibody therapy (i.e., passive immunization) also has a place in the treatment of some VHFs. Argentine hemorrhagic fever res-ponds to therapy with two or more units of convalescent plasma that contain adequate amounts of neutralizing antibody (or an equivalent quantity of immune globulin), provided that treatment is initiated within 8 days of onset. Antibody therapy is also beneficial in the treatment of Bolivian hemorrhagic fever. Efficacy of immune plasma in treatment of Lassa fever and Crimean-Congo hemorrhagic fever is limited by low neutralizing antibody titers and the consequent need for careful donor selection.

In the future, engineered human monoclonal antibodies may be available for specific, passive immunization against the VHF agents. In HFRS, a passive immunization approach is contraindicated for treatment, since an active immune response is usually already evolving in most patients when they are first recognized, although plasma containing neutralizing antibodies has been used empirically in prophylaxis of high-risk exposures.

Active Immunization

The only established and licensed virus-specific vaccine available against any of the hemorrhagic fever viruses is yellow fever vaccine, which is mandatory for travelers to endemic areas of Africa and South America. For prophylaxis against Argentine hemorrhagic fever (AHF) virus, a live attenuated Junin vaccine strain (Candid #1) was developed at USAMRMC and is available as an Investigational New Drug (IND). Candid

#1 was proven to be effective in Phase III studies in Argentina, and plans are proceeding to obtain a New Drug license. This vaccine also provides some cross-protection against Bolivian hemorrhagic fever in experimentally infected primates. Two IND vaccines were developed at USAMRMC against Rift Valley fever; an inactivated vaccine that requires three boosters, which has been in use for 20 years; and a live-attenuated RVF virus strain (MP-12), which is presently in Phase II clinical trials.

For Hantaa virus, a formalin-inactivated rodent brain vaccine is available in Korea, but is not generally considered acceptable by U.S. standards. Another USAMRMC product, a genetically engineered vaccinia construct, expressing hantaviral structural proteins, is in Phase II safety testing in U.S. volunteers. For dengue, a number of live attenuated strains for all four serotypes are entering Phase II efficacy testing. However, none of these vaccines in Phase I or II IND status will be available as licensed products in the near term. For the remaining VHF agents, availability of effective vaccines is more distant.

Currently, protective vaccines (given as shots) are available for anthrax, botulinum toxin, tularemia, plague, Q fever, and smallpox. The widespread immunization of non-military personnel has not been recommended by any governmental agency so far. Immune protection against ricin and staphylococcal toxins may also be possible in the near future.

Protective shelters: Self contained collective protection system that provides a contamination free, environmentally controlled working area for medical, combat services, and combat service support personnel to work freely without continuously wearing chemical-biological protective clothing. Unique systems that combine sensors and technologies, integrating multiple levels of chemical-biological security in order to protect troops.

Differential diagnosis of chemical nerve agent, botulinum toxin and seb intoxication following inhalation exposure

	Chemical nerve agent	*Botulinum toxin*	*SEB*
Time to symptoms	Minutes	Hours (12-48)	Hours (1-6)
Nervous	Convulsions, muscle twitching	Progressive paralysis	Headache, Muscle aches
Cardiovascular	Slow heart rate	Normal rate	Normal or rapid heart rate
Respiratory	Difficult breathing, airway constriction	Normal, then progressive paralysis	Nonproductive cough; Severe cases; chest pain/difficult breathing
Gastrointestinal	Increased motility, pain, diarrhea	Decreased motility	Nausea, vomiting and/or diarrhea
Ocular	Small pupils	Droopy eyelids, Large pupils	May see "red eyes" (conjuntival infection)
Salivary	Profuse, watery saliva	Normal; difficulty swallowing	May be slightly increased quantities of saliva
Death	Minutes	2-3 days	Unlikely
Response to Atropine/ 2PAM-CL	Yes	No	Atropine may reduce gastrointestinal symptoms

Comparative lethality of selected toxins and chemical agents in laboratory mice

Agent	*LD_{50} (mg/kg)*	*Molecular weight*	*Source*
Botulinum toxin	0.001	150,000	Bacterium
Shiga toxin	0.002	55,000	Bacterium
Tetanus toxin	0.002	150,000	Bacterium
Abrin	0.04	65,000	Plant (Rosary Pea)
Diphtheria toxin	0.10	62,000	Bacterium
Maitotoxin	0.10	3,400	Marine Dinoflagellate
Palytoxin	0.15	2,700	Marine Soft Coral
Ciguatoxin	0.40	1,000	Marine Dinoflagellate
Textilotoxin	0.60	80,000	Elapid Snake
C. perfringens toxins	0.1 – 5.0	35-40,000	Bacterium
Batrachotoxin	2.0	539	Arrow-Poison Frog
Ricin	3.0	64,000	Plant (Castor Bean)
Alpha-Conotoxin	5.0	1,500	Cone Snail
Taipoxin	5.0	46,000	Elapid Snake
Tetrodotoxin	8.0	319	Puffer Fish
Alpha-Tityustoxin	9.0	8,000	Scorpion
Saxitoxin	10.0 (Inhal 2.0)	299	Marine Dinoflagellate
VX	15.0	267	Chemical Agent
SEB (Rhesus/Aerosol)	27.0 (ED_{50}~pg)	28,494	Bacterium
Anatoxin-A(s)	50.0	500	Blue-Green Algae
Microcystin	50.0	994	Blue-Green Algae
Soman (GD)	64.0	182	Chemical Agent
Sarin (GB)	100.0	140	Chemical Agent
Aconitine	100.0	647	Plant (Monkshood)
T-2 Toxin	1,210.0	466	Fungal Myotoxin

Lab Identification of biological warfare agents

Immunoassays						
Agent	*Gold standard*	*Antigen detection*	*IgG*	*IgM*	*PCR*	*Animals*
Aflatoxins	Mass spectrometry					
Arboviruses (incl. alphaviruses	Virus isolation/ FA, neutralization	X	X	X	X	X
Bacillus anthracis	FA/Std. Microbiology	X (PA)	X	X	X	X
Bacillus globigii	Std. Microbiology				X	
Bacillus thuringiensis	Std. Microbiology				X	
Bot Toxins (A-G)/ *C. botulinum*	Mouse neutralization/ standard microbiology	X (A,B,E Toxin)			X	X
Brucella sp.	FA/Std. Microbiology	X	X	X	X	X
C. burnetii	FA/eggs or cell Cx/serology	X	X	X	X	X
C. perfringens/ Toxins	Std. Micro./ELISA (alpha and enterotoxin	X	X		X	
F. tularensis	FA/Std. Microbiology	X	X	X	X	X
Filoviruses	Virus isolation/ neutralization	X	X	X	X	X
Hantaviruses	Virus isolation/ FA/neutralization	X	X	X	X	X
Orthopox Viruses	Virus isolation/ FA/neutralization	X	X		X	X
Ricin Toxin	ELISA	X	X	X	X	X
Saxitoxin	Bioassay		(neutralizing antibodies)			X
SEA Toxin	ELISA	X	X		*	
SEB Toxin	ELISA	X	X		*	X
Shigella sp.	Std. Microbiology	X			X	
TetrodoToxins	Bioassay	X	(neutralizing antibodies)			X
Vibrio cholerae	Std. Microbiology/ serology	X(toxin)	X	X	X	
Yersinia pestis	FA/Std. Microbiology	X (F1)	X	X	X	X

*Toxin gene detected.

ELISA - enzyme-linked immunosorbent assays.

FA - indirect or direct immunofluorescence assays.

Std. Micro./serology - standard microbiological techniques available, including electron microscopy.

Biological warfare agent characteristics

Disease	*Transmit man to Man*	*Infective dose (Aerosol)*	*Incubation period*	*Duration of illness*	*Lethality (approx. case fatality rates)*	*Persistence of organism*	*Vaccine efficacy (aerosol exposure)*
Inhalation anthrax	No	8,000–50,000 spores	1-6 days	3-5 days (usually fatal if untreated)	High	Very stable-spores remain viable for > 40 years in soil	2 dose efficacy against up to 1,000 LD_{50} in monkeys
Brucellosis	No	10 -100 organisms	5-60 days (usually	Weeks to months 1-2 months)	<5% untreated	Very stable	No vaccine
Cholera	Rare	10-500 organisms	4 hours-5 d (usually 2-3 days)	≥ 1 week	Low with treatment, high without	Unstable in aerosols and fresh water; stable in salt water	No data on aerosol
Glanders	Low	Assumed low	10-14 days via aerosol	Death in 7-10 days in septicemic form	> 50%	Very stable	No vaccine
Pneumonic plague	High	100-500 organisms	2-3 days	1-6 days (usually fatal)	High unless treated within 12-24 hours	For up to 1 year in soil; 270 days in live tissue	3 doses not protective against 118 LD_{50} in monkeys
Tularemia	No	10-50 organisms	2-10 days (average 3-5)	≥ 2 weeks	Moderate if untreated	For months in moist soil or other media	80% protection against 1-10 LD_{50}
Q Fever	Rare	1-10 organisms	10-40 days	2-14 days	Very low	For months on wood and sand	94% protection against 3,500 LD_{50} in guinea pigs
Smallpox	High	Assumed low (10-100 organisms)	7-17 days (average 12)	4 weeks	High to moderate	Very stable	Vaccine protects against slarge doses in primates
Venezuelan equine encephalitis	Low	10-100 organisms	2-6 days	Days to weeks	Low	Relatively unstable	TC 83 protects against 30-500 LD_{50} in hamsters
Viral hemo-rrhagic fevers	Moderate	1-10 organisms	4-21 days	Death between 7-16 days	High for Zaire strain, moderate with sudan	Relatively unstable - depends on agent	No vaccine
Botulims	No	0.001μmg/ kg is LD_{50} for type A	1-5 days	Death in 24-72 hours; lasts months if not lethal	High without respiratory support	For weeks in nonmoving water and food	3 dose efficacy 100% against 25-250 LD_{50} in primates
Staph Ent-erotoxin B	No	0.03mmg/ person incapaci-tation	3-12 hours after inhalation	Hours	< 1%	Resistant to freezing	No vaccine
Ricin	No	3-5 μmg/ kg is LD_{50} in mice	18-20 hours	Days-death within 10-12 days for ingestion	High	Stable	No vaccine
T-2 Mycotoxins	No	Moderate	2-4 hours	Days to months	Moderate	For years at room temperature	No vaccine

Specimens for laboratory diagnosis during biological warfare

Agent	*Face or nasal swab*[1]	*Blood culture*	*Smear*	*Acute& convales-cent sera*	*Stool*	*Urine*	*Other*
Anthrax	+	+	Pleural and CS fluids mediastinal lymph node spleen	+		-	Cut. lesion aspirates
Brucellosis	+	+	-	+	-	-	Bone marrow and spinal fluid cultures; tissues, exudates
Cholera	-	-	-	+	+	-	
Plague	+	+	Sputum	+	-	-	Bubo aspirate, CSF, sputum, lesion scraping, LN aspirate
Tularemia	+	+	+[2]	+	-	-	
Q-fever	+	[4]	Lesions	+			Lung, spleen, lymph nodes, bone marrow
Congo-Crimean hemorrhagic Fever	+	[3]	-	+	-	-	Liver
VEE	+	[3]	-	+	-	-	CSF
Clostridial toxins	+	-	Wound tissues	+	+	-	
SEB Toxin	+	-	-	+	+	+	Lung, kidney
Ricin Toxin	+	-	-	+	+	+	Spleen, lung, kidney

[1] Within 18-24 hours.
[2] Fluorescent antibody test on infected lymph node smears. Gram stain has little value.
[3] Virus isolation from blood or throat swabs in appropriate containment.
[4] *C. burnetii* can persist for days in blood and resists desiccation. EDTA anticoagulated blood preferred. Culturing should not be done except in BL3 containment.

NBC LEGISLATIONS

At the first regional symposium on chemical emergency preparedness held in Metepec, Mexico in July 1984, the following observations were made by professionals from public and private sector from 16 nations:

Major differences exist between countries regarding the amount of information available on the geographical distribution of chemical manufacturing plants.

Regulations on the routes for the transport of hazardous chemicals are inadequate.

Information on the nature and quantity of chemicals manufactured is inadequate, as is the system to register chemicals that are imported, transported, distributed and stored.

Reporting systems for chemical accidents are not centrally coordinated, nor is there usually a long term follow up of their consequences.

There are, as yet, no comprehensive contingency plans in operation in most participating countries and, at the most, only partial plans for specific emergencies are in force.

The committee has advised high priority be given to risk assessment especially in areas where there is a high concentration of both industry and population and also a free exchange of information on the points mentioned above. Labeling systems for hazardous chemicals has to be standardized and adopted and better preparedness has to be evolved to handle chemical and toxic waste emergencies. The experiences at Bhopal and Mexico, have amply reflected the fact that there is little time to lose and urgent steps have to be taken to meet the spectrum of emergencies likely to be caused by technological hazards.

The Biological Weapons Convention of 1975 and the 5th Review Conference held at Geneva have attempted to put forward a legally binding draft protocol to outlaw activities related to biological warfare, control access to dangerous pathogens, and preclude high risk experiments including genetic engineering. Extradition and punishment of individuals implicated in biological weapons offences was also sought. International investigation by United Nations inspectors of suspicious disease outbreaks and alleged biological weapons incidents was encompassed in the draft. The draft is however, yet to be ratified and does not have the force of international law to make it legally binding on all constituent 65 countries and remains a political effort in the right direction.

NBC ORGANIZATIONAL ELEMENTS

A. NBC Reconnaissance Teams

Mission: NBC reconnaissance operations include search, survey, surveillance, and sampling missions.

1. Search Reconnaissance undertaken to obtain significant information about the NBC condition of routes, areas, and zones. This information confirms or denies the presence of NBC hazards with detection and identification equipment. Visual observation or the collection of samples in the specified location or region can also provide this information.
2. Surveys missions conducted to collect detailed information of NBC contamination hazards. The survey determines the type of contamination, the degree (extent/intensity), and the boundaries.
3. *Surveillance:* The systematic observation of an area to provide early warning.
4. *Sampling:* Provides physical evidence of NBC attacks and technical intelligence concerning NBC weapons systems.

Units employed: Each team must train a platoon-sized element to perform reconnaissance operations.

Employment: These elements should be prepared to deploy to an incident site after an incident to assist the incident commander to confirm or deny contaminated areas and also confirm the area is clear of contamination.

B. NBC Patient Decontamination Element

Mission: Provide patient decontamination support to the local Incident Commander and prepare to:

- Perform casualty decontamination near the incident site, prior to evacuation, or establish decontamination/detection stations at community hospitals.
- Decontamination of non-ambulatory casualties is normally performed prior to evacuation. However, in a terrorist incident, many ambulatory casualties will self evacuate, arriving at the hospital still contaminated. Hospitals must have the capability to detect contamination, and decontaminate when necessary.

- Casualty decontamination is done by trained non-medical personnel under the supervision of the medical personnel. Each decontamination team will consist of twenty non-medical personnel and capable of decontaminating 12 casualties per hour. Three teams are required per decontamination site to run 24-hour operations (4 hours on and 8 hours off shifts). This team requires three to five medical personnel from either the supported hospital/EMS or a medical unit to supervise the process and perform triage and immediate treatment of casualties.

C. NBC Medical Response Element

The medical response plan requires coordination with both the private and public sector and provides medical advice to incident commander and local authorities on protection of first responders and health care personnel in an NBC environment. They also provide advice on casualty decontamination procedures, first aid and initial medical treatment, medical threat information and assess the health risks to civilian and military populations and provide initial medical advice to include signs, symptoms, and first aid. NBC Medical elements consist of 6 medical personnel and is capable of providing medical advice to include signs, symptoms, and first aid of NBC agents and the teams consist of 1 Preventive Medicine Officer, 1 Acute Care Physician, 1 Nurse, 1 Nuclear Medical Science Officer, and 1 Nuclear Medicine Specialist/ Health Physics Specialist. After the initial assessment the NBC medical elements will provide periodic updates to the incident commander and local authorities on protection of first responders and health care personnel in an NBC environment. Elements may elect to use telemedicine reach back capabilities to provide medical advice to local hospitals on appropriate management of care issues. These elements are deployed at an incident site between 8-72 hours after an incident.

D. Triage Medical Response Element

They provide triage support to the Incident Commander including the sorting and assignment of treatment priorities to various categories of wounded, and providing immediate emergency care.

Units Each triage team will be trained to perform triage using the Simple Triage and Rapid Treatment (START) system and deploy to an incident site within 72 hours to assist the Incident Commander with a Mass Casualty Incident (MCI). Each triage team will consist of 26 personnel and is capable of treating 10 patients per hour.

E. Trauma Medical Response Element

They provide expertise in triage, resuscitation, and damage control medicine near the incident site or at a definitive care location. Specific tasks are:

- Perform damage control surgery for up to four patients.
- Augment community hospital systems overwhelmed by NBC casualties.
- Augment hospital after 24 hours to conduct sustainment operations.
- Provide support to local hospitals, triage and immediate treatment of casualties.
- Provides Analgesia and anesthesia for patients under their care.
- Each trauma team will be trained in the treatment of chemical, biological and radiological casualties and associated effects from blasts and crush injuries. Teams consist of 2 General Surgeons, 1 Anesthesiologist, 1 Emergency Medical Physician/Orthopedic Surgeon, 1 Maxillofacial surgeon, 1 Critical Care Nurse, 1 ER Nurse and deployed at an incident site between 8-72 hours after an incident to assist the Incident Commander.

F. Preventive Medicine Element

They provide initial disease and environmental health threat assessments during early or continuing assistance stages of a disaster. Specific tasks are:

- Provide medical threat information and characterize the health risks to civilian and military populations.
- Prepare preventive medicine estimates; conduct rapid hazard sampling, monitoring and analysis.
- Sampling including endemic and epidemic disease indicators.
- Provide initial disease and environmental health threat assessments prior to or in the initial stages of a disaster.
- Each preventive medicine team will be trained in initial disease and environmental health threat assessments. Teams may require information from the Center for Disease Control and other agencies with endemic disease and environmental effect information to prepare their database for the area. Teams consist of 1 Preventive Medicine Officer, 1 Industrial Hygienist/ Health Physicist, 1 Environmental Science/ Engineering specialist, 1 Community Health Nurse, 1 Entomologist, 1 Biologist, 1 Preventive Medicine NCO. This team should attend to public health aspects of natural disasters and civil emergencies and deployed at an incident site between 8-72 hours after an incident to assist the Incident Commander. Personnel are alerted using pagers.

G. Stress Management Element

They provide initial stress management for military and civilian responder and incident survivors and composed of personnel highly trained in stress management and neuropsychiatry. They are capable of providing limited neuropsychiatric triage and stabilization of clinical cases in order to reduce the disabling effects associated with post traumatic stress disorder. Each element will consist of 6 medical personnel consisting of 1 Psychiatrist , 1 Clinical Psychologist, 1 Social Work Officer, 1 Psychiatric Nurse, 2 Mental Health NCOs, 1 Priest, 1 Occupational Therapy Officer, 1 Occupational Therapy NCO capable of handling victim assistance, psychological trauma, post traumatic stress disorder, mental health risks associated with relief workers (burn out syndrome) and deployed at an incident site between 18 and 48 hours after an incident to assist the Incident Commander.

H. Security/Law Enforcement Element

The team selected must provide support to the state and local emergency response plans to assist in maintaining order, ensuring public safety and providing assistance to the law enforcement officials. Specific tasks and capabilities include:

Access control: The potential for mass panic following a weapon of mass destruction (WMD) incident will overwhelm the ability of hospitals to function effectively without additional personnel to control access to the facilities. Troops could be called upon to augment law enforcement and hospital security personnel to maintain efficient access control in the hospitals. Because arriving victims may be contaminated, the personnel assigned this function require both awareness level knowledge and training in performing security operations in personal protective equipment (PPE). The units assigned this responsibility need ready access to PPE that allows for rapid mobilization from a local armoury to an incident site. Once the limits of the contaminated area are established, a cordon will need to be established to prevent people from entering the area. Because this mission will be performed outside the hot zone and

Guard units regularly perform this type of mission in other disaster situations, no additional training beyond basic awareness will be required. The potential for lawlessness and disorder will exist following any WMD incident. Units designated with on-street civil disturbance missions need to be aware of the aspects of crowd control. The Guard could be called on to assist in the implementation of a quarantine, if public health officials determine that a biological attack using a communicable disease agent occurs.

Evacuation Guard units will be required to assist in any evacuation ordered by the local officials. Military Police and other types of units may be called upon to assist in managing the flow of traffic during an evacuation.

I. Mass Care Elements

They provide support to the incident commander in providing shelter, feeding, emergency first aid, and bulk distribution of emergency relief supplies. Specific tasks and capabilities include:

The provision of emergency shelter for disaster victims includes the use of pre-identified shelter sites in existing structures. Creation of temporary facilities such as tent cities, or the temporary construction of shelters.

Use of similar facilities outside the disaster-affected area, should evacuation be necessary. Military installations and facilities such as the armories and reserve centers can be used. The military can also be tasked to provide tentage, cots, etc. in the event of an incident.

The provision for feeding disaster victims and emergency workers through a combination of fixed sites, mobile feeding units, and bulk food distribution. Such operations will be based on sound nutritional standards and will include provisions for meeting dietary requirements of disaster victims with special dietary needs. Mobile kitchens may be requested from the military to support mass feeding operations.

Emergency first aid services will be provided to disaster victims and workers at mass care facilities and at designated sites within the disaster area. This emergency first aid service will be supplemental to emergency health and medical services established to meet the needs of disaster victims.

Bulk Distribution of Emergency Relief Items: Sites will be established within the affected area for distribution of emergency relief items. The bulk distribution of these relief items will be determined by the requirement to meet urgent needs of disaster victims for essential items. Military units can be tasked to man these operations.

J. Mortuary Affairs Element

They provide mortuary support to include identification, processing, storage, and disposition of remains following a mass casualty incident. Specific tasks and capabilities include:

Assist in providing victim identification and mortuary services, temporary morgue facilities; victim identification utilizing latent fingerprint, forensic dental, and/or forensic pathology/anthropology methods; and processing, preparation, and disposition of remains.

K. Communications Element

This element provides telecommunications support to the response forces following an emergency. They will coordinate the establishment of required temporary telecommunications in link with Government-furnished telecommunications, commercially leased communications and telecommunications. Tactical Army, Navy, and Air Force communications units may provide communications elements to link key command and control and deployed assets. Each NBC command element will consist of an information specialist deployed at an incident site between 8-72 hours after an incident to assist the incident commander. Personnel are alerted using pagers and mobilized to incident site. They form the core group for planning and use of military telecommunications assets and resources in a WMD emergency.

L. Engineering Element

They provide technical advice and evaluations, engineering services, construction management and inspection, emergency contracting, emergency repair of wastewater and solid waste facilities, and real estate support in and around the incident site for:

- Emergency clearance of debris for reconnaissance of the damage areas.
- Ensure safe passage of emergency personnel and equipment for lifesaving, life protecting, health and safety purposes during the initial response phase.
- Temporary construction of emergency access routes which include damaged streets, roads, bridges, ports, waterways, airfields, and any other facilities necessary for passage of rescue personnel.
- Emergency restoration of critical public services and facilities including supply of adequate amounts of potable water, temporary restoration of water supply systems, and the provision of water for fire fighting.
- Emergency demolition or stabilization of damaged structures and facilities designated by State or local government as immediate hazards to the public health and safety, or as necessary to facilitate the accomplishment of life saving operations (undertake temporary protective measures to abate immediate hazards to the public for health and safety reasons until demolition is accomplished).
- Technical assistance and damage assessment, including structural inspection of structures.
- Military Engineer units and Civil Engineering units could be tasked.

M. Transportation Elements

They provide transportation at assigned WMD response missions and consist of Air Force personnel tasked:

- To transport both civil and military response assets and elements to the site of an incident.
- To provide transport of patients (post-decontamination) to medical facilities around the nation.

Rotary wing assets will be critical to the operations of the other military response elements and in support of the local Incident Commander. Potential missions include:

- *Air Ambulance:* The potential for mass casualties in an incident will quickly overwhelm the hospital capacity in a local community. The use of aeromedical ambulance companies to transport patients to more distant treatment facilities can help to alleviate this problem. This transport capability is post decontamination and outside the hot zone. (Helicopters should not be used within a chemically contaminated area because their rotors tend to spread agents/contamination.)
- *Survey/Reconnaissance:* Helicopters may be used to conduct an aerial reconnaissance of a radiologically contaminated area to determine the spread/level of contamination. Pilots need to receive training in the conduct of this type of operation. Ground/ Military vehicles, trucks, etc. can be operated in support if not otherwise required to carry out the units emergency mission.
- *Manpower movements:* Dropping assigned drivers of vehicles operating within the hot zone (such as ambulances) wearing protective clothing, decontamination personnel, medical personnel etc.

71 Terrorism

> "Out of clutter, find Simplicity. From discord, find Harmony. In the middle of difficulty lies opportunity."
> — *Albert Einstein*

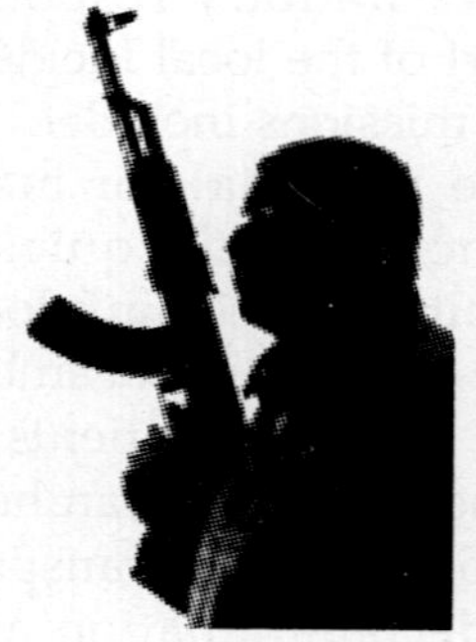

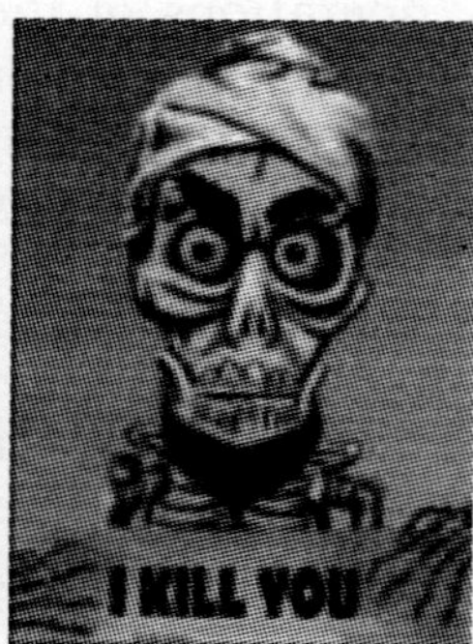

Fig. 71.1

The world is witnessing an upsurge in terrorist attacks. They are often sensational, senseless, devastating and leave one feeling very insecure indeed. Terrorist attacks are the unlawful use of force and violence against persons or property in order to intimidate or coerce the government or population targeted to further political and social objectives. They are perpetrated by small fundamentalistic and often suicidal groups, designed to call attention to a cause, spread fear and influence the public and decision makers. The primary objectives of most terrorist groups are to:

1. Gain publicity.
2. Stimulate loss of confidence in the government.
3. Attract recruits.
4. Get public support.
5. Gain support from financial institutions, and ultimately.
6. Weaken and overthrow the government.

Techniques used to gain an audience for their platform include hostage-taking, product-tampering, criminal extortion, arson, sabotage, threats against individual family members, assassinations, kidnapping, explosive bombings, and armed attacks. The most likely targets of these forms of terrorism are political leaders, key military personnel, foreign missions, military facilities, corporate executives and facilities, and celebrities. Terrorist attacks can take a wide variety of forms:

A. *Biological weapons:* These weapons use infectious microbes or toxins to produce illness or death in people, animals, or plants. Potential biological weapons include anthrax, botulism, smallpox, viral hemorrhagic fevers, water safety threats (e.g. cholera), and food safety threats (e.g. salmonella). Biological weapons are relatively difficult to cultivate and disseminate.

B. *Chemical weapons:* Chemical weapons cause severe health reactions designed to incapacitate or cause death. There is a wide array of potential chemical agents that could be used as weapons. These agents vary in how their effects on the body, required dose, exposure mechanism, length of exposure, toxicity, origination, and form (e.g. liquid, gas). Examples of chemical agents include sarin, mustard agent, VX and cyanide.

C. *Radiological and nuclear weapons:* Although there has been much speculation by media and various governmental agencies regarding the potential for a terrorist to obtain fissionable material or a nuclear bomb, there are no known unclassified cases of any such organization or group actually obtaining weapons grade material. Constructing a nuclear bomb would be relatively difficult and require special resources, training, and materials.

D. *Cyberterrorism:* Attacks computers and networks, and the information contained within them. A cyber attack could potentially disrupt communications, banking systems, power systems, and emergency networks.

Terrorist attacks typically occur without prior warning. There may, in some cases, be a heightened sense of hazard or alert, but there is rarely sufficient information available prior to an incident to allow for predicting the specific nature and time of an attack. The effects of terrorism can vary significantly from property damage and disruption of services (power, water, transportation, and communication), to injury and/or loss of life. An incident could directly impact a relatively small area (e.g. a single building) or a large area (multiple buildings or disrupted services throughout a city). Even a small terrorist incident could have multiple impacts spreading throughout a community, such as disruption of services, interruptions to businesses, banking and communications systems, false alarms and long term trauma to responders, witnesses, caregivers and others.

Terrorism is often categorized as domestic or international. This distinction refers not to where the terrorist act takes place but rather to the origin of the individuals or groups responsible for it. For the purposes of consequence management, the origin of the perpetrator(s) is of less importance than the impacts of the attack on life and property; thus, the distinction between domestic and international terrorism is less relevant for the purposes of mitigation, preparedness, response, and recovery than understanding the capabilities of terrorist groups and how to respond to the impacts they can generate.

Both the public and law enforcers as well as intelligence agencies have to be alert at all times to terrorist machinations and preempt their schemes. It is always difficult to predict how, why and when terrorists may attack and these threats have to be identified, defined and quantified and then detected, deterred, denied and devalued. Areas that may suffer collateral damage will also have to be identified.

The following mitigating efforts are suggested to combat terrorist attacks:

1. Identify all attractive targets i.e. assets at greater risk of attack like iconic commercial properties, symbolic governmental buildings, others with significant emotional and economic value. Signboards, etc. identifying such establishments may be toned down or removed altogether. It must have layers of defence to delay and thwart attacks. Deception methods can be used to make the protected critical areas look less attractive or non critical areas made to look more appealing to misdirect the attackers. Avoid clustered designs of concentrating people, property and operations in any one wing of a building. Some form of dispersal is advisable.
2. Adopt regulatory and legislative measures to earmark those responsible to protect the community and its assets. Draw up new designs, construction codes and zoning in cities to improve safety in the event of terrorist attacks

to prevent building collapse and flying debris.

3. Heighten alertness of intelligence agencies and screen arrivals at airports, railway stations etc especially with regard to red corner notices issued by agencies like Interpol, CIA , RAW etc
4. Attractive targets must have a standoff distance for vehicles and a buffer zone between them and other public utilities. Perimeter walls must be 7 feet high minimum and topped with barbed wires, triple standard concertina wire or tangle foot wire. Straight line and perpendicular approach to such buildings must be avoided as high speed vehicles can ram through barriers and crash/penetrate targeted buildings. Sufficient barriers and obstacle course with speed breakers, rumble strips, bollards and high curbs etc must be created. Single, well illuminated entry and egress points are preferred. Dense vegetation and hiding places in the immediate perimeter must disallowed. Thorny plants can be planted to create natural barriers. Fuelling points and trash receptacles must be located a minimum 10 feet away from the main building. There must be no parking of vehicles allowed within or below the building and there must be no access to the roof by unauthorized personnel. External plumbing, electrical wiring and utility lines are best avoided. Manhole covers greater than 10" must be secured. Large sized drains must have secured barred iron grilles. The building must have emergency back up power generation with auto mains failure panel for immediate switch over to UPS. Electronic security systems like fence sensors, buried line sensor probes, microwave intrusion detection systems, video motion sensors, passive ultrasonic sensors, glass break sensors, structural vibration sensors, CCTV (one camera for 100 feet level ground and 30 feet undulating ground) and internal PA system may be installed in high threat areas. Water sprinklers and sophisticated automatic fire protection systems, blast resistant doors, hardened reinforced concrete walls are advisable. Background check on new employees must be made and biometric identification systems installed. Employees must wear distinctive identification badges at all times and be conversant with emergency drills and procedures, evacuation plans and emergency shelters. Drinking water supply must be tested periodically and airconditioning must incorporate NBC filters and detection systems. Universal fit escape hoods must be available for key personnel. Activated carbon sorbents and impregnated carbon sorbents (ASZM-TEDA), in-duct ultraviolet germicidal irradiation, Ion mobility spectrometry/Surface acoustic wave/ mass spectrometry chemical detection systems will help combat chemical and biological contamination. Windows in high vulnerable areas must be minimized and fitted with tempered, reinforced, laminated or thermoplastic glass panes as they are 4 to 5 times stronger than annealed glass. Intake ports of air handling units must be located at least 12 feet above ground level and capable of external and internal filtration and air purging.

General Safety Guidelines During Terrorist Situation

- Be aware of your surroundings.
- Move or leave if you feel uncomfortable or if something does not seem right.
- Take precautions when traveling. Be aware of conspicuous or unusual behavior.

Do not accept packages from strangers. Do not leave luggage unattended. You should promptly report unusual behavior, suspicious or unattended packages, and strange devices to the police or security personnel.

- Learn where emergency exits are located in buildings you frequent. Plan how to get out in the event of an emergency.
- Be prepared to do without services you normally depend on electricity, telephone, natural gas, gasoline pumps, cash registers, ATMs, and Internet transactions.
- Work with building owners to ensure the following items are located on each floor of the building:
  - Portable, battery-operated radio and extra batteries.
  - Several flashlights and extra batteries.
  - First aid kit and manual.
  - Hard hats and dust masks.
  - Fluorescent tape to rope off dangerous areas.

Bomb Threat

- If you receive a telephoned bomb threat, you should do the following:
  - Get as much information from the caller as possible. Try to ask the following questions:
  - When is the bomb going to explode?
  - Where is it right now?
  - What does it look like?
  - What kind of bomb is it?
  - What will cause it to explode?
  - Did you place the bomb?
  - Why?
  - What is your address?
  - What is your name?
  - Keep the caller on the line and record everything that is said.
  - Notify the police and building management.

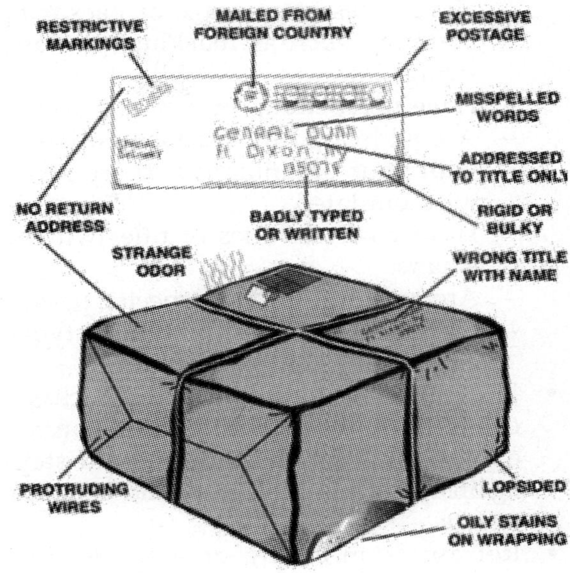

Fig. 71.3

Suspicious Packages and Letters

- Bewar of suspicious packages and letters. They can contain explosives, chemical or biological agents. Be parti-cularly cautious at your place of employ-ment.
- Some typical characteristics postal inspectors have detected over the years, which ought to trigger suspicion, include parcels that:
  - Are unexpected or from someone unfamiliar to you.
  - Have no return address, or have on that cant be verified as legitimate.
  - Have protruding wires or aluminum foil, strange odors, or stains.
  - Show a city or state in the postmark that doesn't match the return address.
  - Are of unusual weight given their size, or are lopsided or oddly shaped.
  - Are marked with threatening language.
  - Have inappropriate or unusual labeling.

  - Have excessive postage or packaging material, such as masking tape and string.
  - Have misspellings of common words.
  - Are addressed to someone no longer with your organization or are otherwise outdated.
  - Have incorrect titles or titles without a name.
  - Are not addressed to a specific person.
  - Have hand-written or poorly typed addresses.
- With suspicious envelopes and packages other than those that might contain explosives, take these additional steps against possible biological and chemical agents.
- Refrain from eating or drinking in a designated mail handling area.
- Place suspicious envelopes or packages in a plastic bag or some other type of container to prevent leakage of contents. Never sniff or smell suspect mail.
- If you do not have a container, then cover the envelope or package with anything available (e.g., clothing, paper, trash can, etc.) and do not remove the cover.
- Leave the room and close the door, or section off the area to prevent others from entering.
- Wash your hands with soap and water to prevent spreading any powder to your face.
- If you are at work, report the incident to your building security official or an available supervisor, who should notify police and other authorities without delay.
- List all people who were in the room or area when this suspicious letter or package was recognized. Give a copy of this list to both the local public health authorities and law enforcement officials for follow-up investigations and advice.
- If you are at home, report the incident to local police.

During an Explosion

If there is an explosion, you should:

- Get under a sturdy table or desk if things are falling around you. When they stop falling, leave quickly, watching for obviously weakened floors and stairways. As you exit from the building, be especially watchful of falling debris.
- Leave the building as quickly as possible. Do not stop to retrieve personal possessions or make phone calls.
- Do not use elevators.
- Once you are out:
  - Do not stand in front of windows, glass doors, or other potentially hazardous areas.
  - Move away from sidewalks or streets to be used by emergency officials or others still exiting the building.
- If you are trapped in debris:
  - If possible, use a flashlight to signal your location to rescuers.
  - Avoid unnecessary movement so you don't kick up dust.
  - Cover your nose and mouth with anything you have on hand. (Dense-weave cotton material can act as a good filter. Try to breathe through the material).
  - Tap on a pipe or wall so rescuers can hear where you are.
  - If possible, use a whistle to signal rescuers.
  - Shout only as a last resort. Shouting can cause a person to inhale dangerous amounts of dust.

Bibliography

FEMA Reference manual to mitigate potential terrorist attacks against building and people, Dec 2003.

72 Characteristics of Pyridostigmine Bromide (PB)

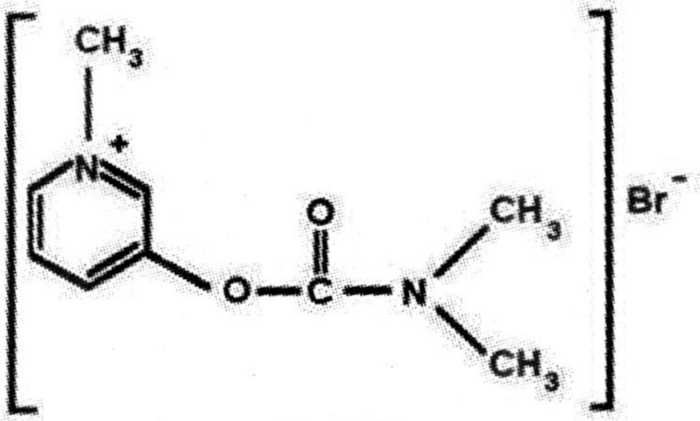

Fig. 72.1

PB is a positively charged quaternary ammonium carbamate compound, which binds to (carbamylates) two sites on acetylcholinesterase (AChE), a negatively charged site and an esteratic site, preventing acetylcholine (ACh) from binding to these same sites and being broken down by the enzyme. This inhibition leads to buildup of ACh, which is not being hydrolyzed, resulting in increased action of ACh on its receptor.

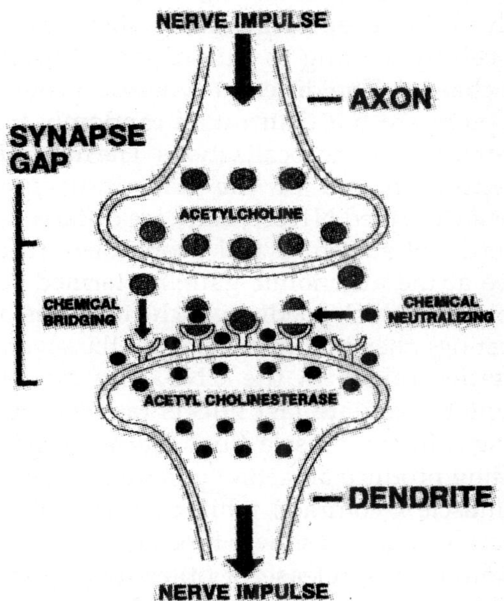

Fig. 72.2

ACETYLCHOLINE RECEPTORS

Not all ACh receptors are alike. Receptors belong to one of two groups, nicotinic and muscarinic, so termed because of specific chemicals—nicotine and muscarine—initially shown to bind to these receptors. Both types of receptors occur both in the CNS (central nervous system, including the brain and spinal cord) and peripherally (as part of the PNS or peripheral nervous system, which includes nerve cells and their connections located in the rest of the body).

NICOTINIC RECEPTORS

Nicotinic receptors exist in skeletal muscle (the neuromuscular junction), autonomic ganglia, the adrenal medulla, and the central nervous system. Nicotinic receptors consist of five protein subunits—classically, two alpha subunits, a beta, a gamma, and a delta. These produce nicotinic receptors with different structures (though all share the property of having five subunits) and functional characteristics. They also have different affinity for binding to different acetylcholine agonists (substances that bind to acetylcholine receptors and activate them) and show different predilections for desensitization. These characteristics are of importance in considering possible effects of PB on the acetylcholine system. Of note, receptors with the alpha subunit are actually stimulated by both nicotine and muscarine and have atypical nicotinic/muscarinic pharmacology. In each case the subunits are believed to form an ion channel. Binding of ACh to the receptor produces signaling in the cell by leading to flux of ions through this channel. The different types of nicotinic receptors are not distributed randomly but have characteristic localizations. The nicotinic receptors found at the neuromuscular junction (termed N1receptors) are different—in terms of structure and properties—from those at the autonomic ganglia (termed N2 receptors, which mediate such functions as sweating); they in turn differ from the several varieties found in the CNS. The muscle receptors mediate fast effects (as electrical changes in the muscle fiber following ACh binding produce an action potential, causing the muscle to contract), while central nicotinic effects may have a slower time-course, acting by influencing release of other neurotransmitters, such as dopamine, GABA (gamma amino butyric acid), and glutamate. Although the nicotinic acetylcholine receptor is the best characterized neurotransmitter receptor because of the differences in properties of different nicotinic receptors—and new nicotinic receptors have continued to be characterized—quite a lot remains unknown.

MUSCARINIC RECEPTORS

Muscarinic receptors are found in the smooth muscle of viscera (internal organs), heart muscle, secretory glands, and in the endothelial cells lining blood vessels—as well as in the brain. Muscarinic receptors do not make up ion channels, as nicotinic receptors do. Rather, muscarinic effects are produced more indirectly, through chemicals termed second messengers. There are at least five distinct muscarinic receptor types (at least five genes have been cloned and sequenced), which differ in their ability to couple to different second messenger GTP binding proteins,or G-proteins. These in turn exert other chemical effects, which lead ultimately to muscarinic actions. (The effects of G-proteins are fairly technical and include inhibition of cyclic AMP formation, stimulation of phospholipase C and regulation of ion channels—but in this case regulation is not direct, as with nicotinic receptors, but mediated by G-proteins).

FUNCTIONAL LOCALIZATION OF ACH RECEPTORS

As mentioned previously, nicotinic and muscarinic receptors predominate in different places in the body – for example, nicotinic receptors occur in skeletal muscle while muscarinic receptors are found in the smooth muscle of viscera. Moreover, different nicotinic receptors (and different muscarinic receptors) themselves are characteristically found in different parts of the rest of the body—such as N1 nicotinic receptors at the neuromuscular junction, and N2 receptors at the autonomic ganglia. Analogously, different receptors dominate in different functions and different parts of the brain. For instance, some areas of the brain (such as the optic tectum) rely primarily on nicotinic receptors. Some areas—such as the hippocampus (which is critically involved in memory function) and the cerebral cortex—have predominantly muscarinic receptors of the type that bind with high affinity to the chemical pirenzapine (which antagonizes the action of ACh and serves as a major factor in distinguishing different types of muscarinic receptors), while the cerebellum and brainstem have predominantly muscarinic receptors that bind this chemical more sluggishly. As scientists begin to understand more clearly what the effects are of AChE inhibition with such agents as PB on each different receptor type—and begin to understand more clearly which brain effects rely on which receptors—a more satisfactory resolution to the possible contribution of PB to symptoms in POST GULF WAR veterans may be obtained. This knowledge is still fairly rudimentary.

TERMINOLOGY ISSUES

Inhibition of AChE is produced by PB, by other carbamates (compounds which, like PB, reversibly carbamylate and inactivate the AChE), or by organophosphates (OPs), such as nerve agents or pesticides, which irreversibly phosphorylate and inactivate the AChE. A major difference is that since little PB normally crosses the blood-brain barrier into the brain, central effects from PB are normally minimal. In contrast, the related carbamate physostigmine does cross into the brain, as do many OPs.

MUSCARINIC, NICOTINIC AND CENTRAL EFFECTS OF ACHE INHIBITORS

AChE inhibitors, including both PB and nerve agents, exert their effects by blocking AChE at ACh receptor sites, increasing ACh and ACh activity, causing first hyperactivity of smooth and of skeletal muscles and then paralysis (with high enough doses). If the agent penetrates the CNS, then CNS effects also occur. Nerve agents penetrate the CNS; however, PB does not, or at least not much, when taken under normal conditions. Limited evidence suggests that PB does penetrate the CNS when it is taken under stressful conditions.

Enzymes Regulate ACh Activity. ACh activity is regulated in large part by the enzyme acetylcholinesterase (also called red blood cell cholinesterase or RBC cholinesterase or true cholinesterase and abbreviated AChE), which binds to and breaks down ACh that has accumulated in the synapse, preventing inappropriate excessive signaling. Butyrylcholinesterase (also called plasma cholinesterase or pseudocholinesterase and abbreviated BChE) plays a less critical role. It is made in the liver and circulates in the plasma. But it is thought that very little ACh will diffuse far from the synapse, so this enzyme plays a small direct role.

PHARMACOKINETICS AND PHARMACODYNAMICS OF PB

PB is a positively charged compound that exerts its primary action by inhibiting the enzyme AChE. (It has other actions, including direct binding to, and stimulation of, the ACh receptor). Because of its charge, PB has difficulty passing through biological membranes, which are relatively impermeable to charged molecules. Perhaps in part for this reason, PB is poorly and erratically absorbed from the gastrointestinal tract into the bloodstream. It has also been suggested that the low oral bioavailability of PB may result from first pass metabolism by the gut or liver. Recommended oral doses are 3 times those of intravenous doses to achieve similar levels of activity in the body, as only 4 percent of PB is absorbed following oral administration.

PB makes its way to many sites throughout the body and is detected in most tissues except the brain, intestinal wall, fat, and thymus. It crosses the placenta and decreases fetal plasma cholinesterase activity after large oral doses.

Most of the orally administered dose is eliminated in the feces. Most of the absorbed dose is eliminated through the kidneys unchanged or as the major metabolite, 3-hydroxy-N-methyl pyridium (3HMP); other metabolites, including 3-hydroxyphenyl-trimethylammonium (3HP) are present to a lesser degree. Liver enzymes are involved and 9 percent of the absorbed dose is metabolized by the liver on first pass; 75 to 90 percent is excreted in the urine and a third of the amount excreted may be the 3HMP metabolite. The 3HMP product is an acetylcholine antagonist and also inhibits AChE. Even after intravenous administration, in which there is no time burden getting the drug into the bloodstream, some PB activity can be detected in the urine 72 hours later . The half-time of elimination (estimates for the half-life with oral dosage are on the order of two to four hours) is not stable but lengthens as PB is excreted; this could relate to the putative sequestering of PB in sites such as cartilage. Because PB enhances the propulsive movement of the intestines, it may reduce its own absorption with continued use by encouraging its own elimination before the GI tract has had adequate time to absorb the PB. Patients with severe myasthenia gravis seem to metabolize and excrete PB faster than patients with milder disease, which has been offered as an explanation for the resistance to anticholinesterase medication that occurs with some severely ill patients. Dosage requirements in myasthenia vary widely due to individual differences in absorption, metabolism, and excretion of PB so that dosage is usually determined individually for each patient. Many of the same individual variations are probably present in normal subjects; PB reportedly has a variable duration of action in patients with myasthenia gravis, supposedly depending on the physical and emotional stress suffered by the patient and the severity of the disease, though other biological factors may be important. Moreover, individual muscle groups in the same patient may respond differently to the same dose of PB, producing weakness in one muscle group while increasing strength in another. The muscles of the neck and of chewing and swallowing are usually the first to be weakened by overdose, followed by the muscles of the shoulder and upper extremities, and finally the pelvic girdle, the muscles that control eye movement, and leg muscles.

ACCUMULATION OF PB IN THE BODY

PB may bind specifically to cartilage chondroitin sulfate.

OTHER ACTIONS ON THE CHOLINERGIC SYSTEM

Partial Agonist

PB is considered an AChE inhibitor but PB also reacts directly with the ACh receptor as a partial agonist; it produces some of the same effects that ACh itself would produce acting at the same receptor.

ACh Receptor Desensitization

PB either alone or in combination with ACh induces an altered, desensitized species of the nicotinic receptor-ion channel complex. That is to say, PB use produces ACh receptors (binding sites) that are less sensitive to the action of ACh. (This has been proposed as one of the methods of conferring protection against nerve agent.) Normally, when ACh binds, certain ion channels open and produce an electrochemical signal. The frequency of these channel openings is decreased when PB is given, and ACh ion channel currents are modified. Other carbamates (chemicals in the same family as PB) produce similar but not identical effects. This desensitization could have a role in cholinergic down regulation.

Autoregulation

Most ACh receptors considered clinically are those that exist at the postsynaptic membrane—the membrane of a signal-receiving cell. ACh released from a signaling or presynaptic cell (a nerve cell or neuron) binds to these receptors on the postsynaptic cell (typically either a nerve or muscle cell), allowing the presynaptic cell to communicate with the receiving cell. However, ACh receptors also exist at the presynaptic membrane—the membrane of the signaling cell—where they play an important role in autoregulation of ACh release from the terminal axon (the extension of the signaling cell that grows out and forms connections with the receiving cell). When ACh binds to and activates these presynaptic receptors, the effect is to inhibit further release of ACh from the presynaptic membrane (that is, from the signaling cell). (However, nicotinic action presynaptically increases release in the brain of other neurotransmitters, including both glutamate and GABA). The factors that regulate the degree to which this inhibition occurs are not understood. Thus, inhibition of ACh breakdown by PB will lead to increased binding by ACh on these presynaptic sites, potentially reducing continued release of ACh.

ACh Receptor Heterogeneity

Neuronal ACh receptors exhibit considerable heterogeneity with respect to their distribution, pharmacological sensitivity and functional role. Many receptor types have been identified in the CNS since these have different characteristics, they are presumably differently affected by such carbamates as PB, in the event that PB reaches the CNS.

Nonsynaptic Cholinergic Effects

It has been noted that the presence of acetylcholine and its receptors at locations not related to synaptic activity raises the possibility that acetylcholine may have receptor-mediated cellular functions other than transmission of nerve signals, i.e., that acetylcholine may act as a local hormone modulating cellular functions. For example, both nicotinic and muscarinic ACh receptors, similar to those seen in the brain and autonomic ganglia, evidently regulate migration and cell stickiness of skin cells (epidermal keratinocytes). Immune and blood cells also have cholinergic mechanisms, as do sperm and ovaries.

Effects on Other Transmitter Systems

ACh (nicotinic) stimulation can cause release of neurotransmitters including GABA, dopamine, and glutamate.Moreover, there appears to be a relation to serotonin action. It has been speculated that in addition to the actions of ACh in the usual signaling-cell/receiving-cell interactions (the wiring transmission mode), ACh may also be released in a paracrineor volume transmission fashion—acting more or less like a local hormone, drifting to modulate release of other neurotransmitters (not necessarily just at a site at which the ACh-releasing cell synapses). Evidence in favor of this is that the cell bodiesof the neurons that release ACh are restricted to a few nuclei located mainly in parts of the brain termed the basal telencephalon and dorsal pons, but the ends of the nerve cell processes from these cells are spread throughout the brain in a somewhat diffuse way, and no consistent match exists between the known distribution of the nicotinic ACh receptors in the brain and that of the acetylcholinergic terminals (release sites from the signaling cell). Further complicating matters, muscarinic receptors are known to regulate synaptic transmission in some instances with actions opposite to nicotinic receptors, so that the effects depend on the relative distribution of these types of receptors. This distribution, however, has not yet been established. The information provided below should be considered with these provisos in mind.

ACh may also stimulate release of catecholamines—epinephrine particularly, and also norepinephrine—and hormones, including cortisol, prolactin, growth hormone, beta-endorphin, and others.

Glutamate

The glutamatergic (i.e., glutamate-related) transmitter system shares elements with the acetylcholinergic system, including its ability to be influenced by carbamates (such as PB). In the mammalian central nervous systems, the NMDA (N-methyl-D-aspartate) type of glutamatergic receptor as well as the ACh receptor are involved in a number of processes. These range from control of transmitter release (described above), to postsynaptic membrane depolarization (changes occurring in the membrane of the signal-receiving cell) with mobilization of intracellular second messengers. Second messengers, such as calcium, in turn participate in mechanisms of protein synthesis, learning (through a process termed long-term potentiation), outgrowth of nerve processes to allow connections to other cells, cell death, and other functions. Glutamate receptor overactivation can induce delayed neuronal cell death (toxic effects by overactivation are termed excitotoxicity). Such effects may be mediated by breaking of DNA strands.

Indeed, it has been shown that low (nanomolar) concentrations of nicotine enhance both glutamatergic and acetylcholinergic synaptic transmission by activating presynaptic nicotinic ACh receptors that increase presynaptic calcium concentrations.

Studies have demonstrated that carbamates and OPs (including the OP agents diisopropylfluorophosphate (DFP) and the nerve agent VX) affect properties of the glutamate system, including such presynaptic properties (properties of the signal-sending side) as increasing transmitter release and such postsynaptic properties (properties of the signal-receiving side) as reducing the peak size of the current induced by binding of glutamate to its receptor. Moreover, carbamates may cause unstimulated endplate synaptic potentials, or voltage changes in the receiving cell side, large enough to provoke action potentials(full self-propagating signals down a nerve process that are normally produced in response to input from one or more signaling cells). This response could disrupt the specificity of signaling, since action potentials are more typically driven by specific inputs to the neuron. These data derive from work on insects' neuromuscular junctions, however, and insects employ glutamate rather than ACh at their neuromuscular junctions. The degree to which PB per se affects glutamate neurons in the mammalian CNS remains to be evaluated but would likely depend in part on the degree to which PB has access to the brain. (It has been observed that ACh receptors and NMDA-sensitive receptors on central neurons share much functional homology with ACh receptors in muscle fibers,suggesting that similar effects may apply if PB were to reach the CNS).

GABA

Carbamates may also affect signaling through another neurotransmitter system, the GABA (gamma amino butyric acid) system. GABA is the chief inhibitory neurotransmitter in the mammalian nervous system. ACh acts presynaptically to modulate GABA release. Preterminal nicotinic receptors on GABAergic axons have been identified in rats, e.g., the interpeduncular nucleus, and ACh has been shown to modulate the release of GABA.

Dopamine

By a similar mechanism, ACh acts via presynaptic nicotinic receptors to modulate the release of dopamine. Indeed, in some parts of the brain (but not others), the release of GABA by nicotine is mediated by dopamine release. Nicotine evokes dopamine release (from the rat corpus striatum as well as frontal cortex) in vivo and in vitro. Chronic treatment with nicotine has been shown to increase the density of nicotine-binding sites (that is, nicotinic receptors) in the frontal cortex but to produce no increase in striatal preparations. A reduction in dopamine release is evoked by the same amount of nicotine in the frontal cortex but not in the striatum. There are also antidopamine muscarinic effects -and perhaps wholly or partly because of different distribution of muscarinic and nicotinic receptors, ACh stimulation regulation of dopamine activity may be opposite in different brain regions. (For instance, it is opposite in the nigraland striatal regions of the brain. The clinical relevance of an effect of ACh on dopamine is suggested by reports of development and of exacerbation of parkinsonism (a condition of reduced motor movement combined with tremor that results from problems in the dopamine-rich nigrostriatal system in the brain, following PB and Ops or unspecified pesticides. Also, the beta 2-containing neuronal nicotinic ACh receptor is believed to assist in mediating the reinforcing properties of nicotine (and other substances of abuse), by contributing to release of dopamine in the mesolimbic system of the brain.

Substance P

The cholinergic system, specifically AChE—and by extension PB—affects breakdown of substance P, a neurotransmitter involved in pain signaling.

Serotonin

Serotonin is known to be involved in important functions including regulation of mood, pain, impulsivity, and sleep. Several lines of evidence suggest important interactions between the ACh system and the serotonergic system.

Briefly, PB binds to the same site on the ACh receptor that serotonin is believed to bind to, a relatively new finding. (This site has also been called the galanthamine binding site). Although many identified classes of nicotinic receptors are in the brain that differ by which of a set of subunits make up their five parts, this binding site is highly conserved across different types of nicotinic receptors—that is, while other properties of the receptor change, this property remains constant. Carbamate and OP AChE inhibitors, including nerve agents and PB, have been shown to reduce platelet serotonin uptake, increase serotonin turnover, and reduce nighttime enhancement of serotonin in the pineal gland, and nighttime rise of melatonin measured in blood. Some serotonergic drugs have been found to augment the AChE-inhibiting effects of PB and slow the time-course of recovery. Others have been shown to have similar effects to PB in some circumstances, such as enhancing release of growth hormone from the pituitary gland in response to growth hormone releasing hormone from the hypothalamus. Finally, there has been an unsubstantiated (non-peer reviewed) report of benefit from combined serotonergic/dopaminergic treatment of ill PGW veterans. This treatment used the drug combination fenfluramine and phentermine. (Fenfluramine is no longer available, after reports of heart valve abnormalities with this drug or with the fenfluramine-phentermine drug combination).

Opioids

The opioid codeine has, like serotonin, been shown to bind to the galanthamine binding site on nicotinic ACh receptors, acting as a modulation of central nicotinic function. It is known that the opioid system, the serotonin system, and the acetylcholinergic system are all involved in regulation of pain. High levels of opioids and serotonin are related to increased tolerance to pain.

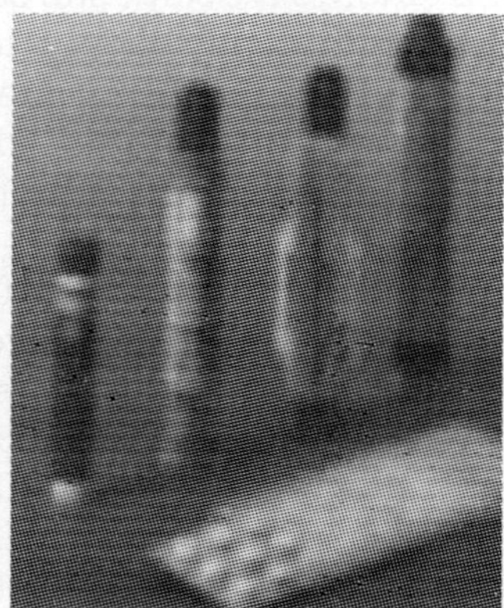

Fig. 72.3

Shelf Life

PB can be maintained for long periods without refrigeration Because of the desire for long storage, the military policy is to maintain PB under refrigeration and dispose of PB that has remained unrefrigerated for a period exceeding six months. Refrigeration off PB is desired because prolonged storage without refrigeration may affect its potency. PB does not break down into toxic products.

Breakdown Products

As noted above, the chief metabolite of PB is 3-hydroxy-N-methylpyridium. Although it has traditionally not been thought to contribute to the action of PB, it may have some AChE inhibiting activity.

Side Effects

In two decades of PB testing in the military, the incidence of side effects with PB administration was reputedly under 1 percent. Most side effects were mild, principally involving the GI tract (increased flatus, loose stool). The drug is usually tolerated well. The most common side effects reported are gastrointestinal (abdominal cramps, nausea, and diarrhea), with other effects including weakness, light-headedness, exacerbation of asthmatic symptoms, fatigue, sleep disturbances, and reduced mental concentration. Urinary urgency or frequency is also seen. Less than 5 percent incidence of runny nose, sweating, and tingling of the extremities is reported. However, these symptoms do not noticeably interfere with performance of the full range of demanding physical and mental tasks required. The effects may continue as long as PB was taken or it may abate after one to two days of use.

73 Humanitarian Sites

Dmoz Open Directory:
http://dmoz.org/Society/Organizations/Humanitarian/European forum on International cooperation: http://www.euforic.org/framed
Development resource centre:
http://www.drc.org.nz/links/
European Community Humanitarian Office (ECHO):
http://europa.eu.int/en/comm/echo/
UK humanitarian relief:
http://bubl.ac.uk/link/H/humanitarianrelief.html
Institute of development studies:
http://ids.ac.uk/eldis/aid/rdb lorg.html
Reuters Foundation (AlertNet):
http://www.foundation.reuters.com/aid/main/alertnet.html/
Oxfam International:
http://www.caa.org.au/world/emergencies/
Voluntary Organizations in Cooperation in Emergency (VOICE):
http://www.oneworld.org/voice/
International Federation of Red Cross and Red Crescent Societies:
http://www.ifrc.org
International Labor Organization:
http://www.ilo.org
United Nations Children's Fund:
http://www.unicef.org
United Nations Economic and Social Development Council:
http://www.un.org/esa
United Nations High Commission for Human Rights (OHCHR):
http://www.unhcr.ch/
World Bank:
http://www.wbg.org
World Health Organization:
http://www.who.int
World Trade Organization:
http://www.wto.org
FAO:
www.fao.org
CARE :
www.care.org
Food:
www.fh.org (food for the hungry)
Relief:
www.amurt.org (Ananda Marga)
Relief:
www.worldrelief.org
Relief:
www.disasterrelief.org
Relief:
www.charity.org
Relief:
www.helpindisaster.org
Relief:
www.duo.org
Relief:
www.salvationarmy.org
US Agency for International Development:
http://www.info.usaid.gov/
Amnesty International:
http://www.amnesty.org
Care International:
http://www.careinternational.org
Doctors of the World:
http://www.doctorsoftheworld.org
Doctors without Borders:
http://www.dwb.org
Medicins Sans Frontiers:
http://msf.org
Oxfam International:
http://www.oxfam.org
Save the Children:
http://www.savethechildren.org
Red R:
http://www.redr.org/resources/links/hr.htm

Medicines:
http://www.who.int/medicines/edl.html & http://www.masta.org
Medical equipment:
http://www.999supplies.com,
http://www.pltsu.com,
http://www.equipped.com/drperskit.html, http://www.echohealth.org.uk
Vaccines:
http://www.cdc.govt/travel/ and
http://www.org/about/index.html

Food:
www.friendsofthewfp.org
Medicines:
www.AmeriCares.org
Disaster assistance:
www.fema.gov
Disaster assistance:
www.new.paho.org
Relief, Search and Rescue:
www.wwdr.org

Index